Miriam Offer

WHITE COATS IN THE GHETTO

Jewish Medicine in Poland during the Holocaust

This publication has been supported by a grant from
The Conference on Jewish Material Claims Against Germany

Claims Conference ועידת התביעות
The Conference on Jewish Material Claims Against Germany

This book was published under the auspices of the
Center for Research on the Holocaust in Poland,
generously supported by the Aaron Gutwirth Fund and the
Danek Gertner Yad Vashem Scholarship.

Miriam Offer

WHITE COATS IN THE GHETTO

Jewish Medicine in Poland during the Holocaust

Translated from the Hebrew by Naftali Greenwood

יד ושם
YAD VASHEM
THE WORLD HOLOCAUST REMEMBRANCE CENTER
THE INTERNATIONAL INSTITUTE FOR HOLOCAUST RESEARCH
The Center for Research on the Holocaust in Poland

Miriam Offer
Haluk Lavan Bageto
Mabat Al Korot Harefu'a Hayehudit BePolin Bitkufat Hashoah

Language and Production Editor: Dania Valdez

P.O.B. 3477, Jerusalem 9103401, Israel
publications.marketing@yadvashem.org.il
First published in Hebrew by Yad Vashem, 2016.

ISBN 978-965-308-602-9

Typesetting: Hava Salzman

Printed in Israel by Offset Natan Shlomo Press, Jerusalem

This book is lovingly dedicated to my parents, Shimon and Martha Gerstenfeld, and to my father-in-law and mother-in-law, Chaim and Shulamit Offer, who survived the Holocaust and who, together with the remaining refugees, were granted the privilege of participating in building the State of Israel, establishing their homes, and raising their children, grandchildren, and great-grandchildren.

And to the memory of my grandparents, aunts, and uncles, who were murdered in the Holocaust: Yona and Tova Gerstenfeld, and their daughters, Primat and Mela, who were murdered in Bełżec; Avraham Yehoshua and Bracha Retek, and their children, Yehuda Yechiel, Alexander Isaac, Bryna, Feige, Saul, Ze'ev, and Sheva Rachel, who were murdered in Auschwitz.

Table of Contents

Part Two
The Jewish Medical System in Warsaw in the Face of Unprecedented Conditions
Its Organization and Challenges

Part Three
The Challenges to the Medical Profession
Living Conditions, Diseases, and Ethical Dilemmas

Preface

A last few words to honor you, the Jewish doctors. What can I tell you, my beloved colleagues and companions in misery? You are a part of all of us. Slavery, hunger, deportation, those death figures in our ghetto were also your legacy. And you by your work could give the henchman the answer Non omnis moriar, *I shall not wholly die.*[1]

Dr. Israel Milejkowski, Director, Judenrat Health Department in the Warsaw Ghetto, October 1942

The history of the more than 400,000 Jews of the Warsaw ghetto has been the subject of extensive research. In 2020, seventy-seven years after the Germans burned to the ground the vestiges of the largest ghetto, the heroic Jewish armed uprising—the first urban rebellion in the Nazi-occupied lands—remains the dominant event in the collective historical memory of what occurred there. In contrast, little attention has been paid to the daily challenges that the leaders and inhabitants of the ghetto faced, foremost the war on the diseases and the epidemics that swept the ghetto and the efforts to preserve the lives of its inhabitants.

The conditions in the Warsaw ghetto induced morbidity seen only in other cases of mass atrocities, ethnic cleansing, and genocide. In blood-drenched confrontations such as these, what is usually most striking is the total collapse of the persecuted group's

1 Myron Winick, ed., *Hunger Disease: Studies by the Jewish Physicians in the Warsaw Ghetto* (New York: Wiley, 1979), p. 5.

medical systems, leaving medical aid for the casualties mainly in the hands of outside elements. However, the readers of this book will find that this was not the case in the Warsaw ghetto and in other Jewish ghettos. Amid the grim ghetto conditions, the Jews, that is, the persecuted society, established a professional and modern health care and medical system on their own, despite the many restrictions—a phenomenon unparalleled in history.

The historical portrait of the medical system in the ghetto that is revealed in this book invites readers to reconsider the patterns of the Jewish response in the Nazi-era ghettos as those of a modern oppressed society; to set them in a broad historical context; and to examine them from various perspectives—research on genocide, the modern centralized nation-state, East European Jewry, the Holocaust, and medical ethics under conditions of extreme stress. This study affords readers an opportunity to listen to the voices of the doctors and nurses who came forward to provide medical services under impossible conditions and faced tragic dilemmas that health care staff do not confront in ordinary times. Through the media of diaries and other contemporary sources produced by the medical teams in the ghetto, this book discusses fundamental issues that affected the lives of the ghettoized Jews.

There is no doubt that alongside my intellectual curiosity and the desire to investigate the events of World War II and the Holocaust, the memories of my parents—Holocaust survivors—and the absence of their parents, my grandparents, who perished in the Holocaust along with most of my uncles and aunts, prodded me to embark on treks of research into Jewish history, in general, and Holocaust history, in particular. When I met my in-laws, Shulamit and Chaim Offer, survivors of the ghetto in Shavli (Šiauliai), Lithuania, I was awed to discover that they were part of the group of child survivors of the ghetto and was honored to learn about their astounding history firsthand. These survivors had stayed in touch over the years and we, the second and third generation, had the privilege of basking in the fraternity and camaraderie that prevailed among them. In 1993, they and their friends alerted me to the diary of Dr. Aaron Pik, and I thereupon began to probe the history of Jewish medicine in the Holocaust.

Dr. Israel Milejkowski, head of the Judenrat Health Department in the Warsaw ghetto, wrote that although the documentation and research endeavors of the doctors in the Holocaust had been cut short by the deportation and murder of the doctor–researchers themselves, the "work was stopped but not liquidated." If discussed in historical terms, it is truly "an unfinished symphony" written by Jewish doctors in 1942.[2] This book invites you to listen to this unfinished symphony—its characteristics, uniqueness, historical context, and universal implications.

2 Ibid., p. 3.

Acknowledgments

This book, published in Hebrew in 2015 by Yad Vashem,[1] stirred much interest in Israel, both among scholars and among the public at large. Since its publication, the book has been updated to the extent possible. However, in order to publish an English version of reasonable length, it was necessary to omit the appendices in the Hebrew edition, which included selected contemporary archive sources that were translated from various languages. I hope that a book devoted to the subject of documentation on medicine and the Holocaust will appear one day.

This study owes its inception to my PhD dissertation, presented to Bar-Ilan University. I am indebted to Prof. Dan Michman, my advisor, for cultivating my abilities in research and scholarship, orienting me in historiography and research methods, and developing my sensitivity to comprehensive perspectives and the quest for historical insights. While guiding me as I proceeded, he firmly protected my authority as a researcher and raised the bar at every stage of my work, which entailed the challenging demand that I adopt a comprehensive comparative view of the Warsaw ghetto medical system and its functioning. Without Prof. Michman, this study would not have been published, and I thank him from the bottom of my heart.

1 Miriam Offer, *Haluk Lavan Bageto: Mabat Al Korot Harefu'a Hayehudit BePolin Bitkufat Hashoah* (*White Coats in the Ghetto: Jewish Medicine in Poland during the Holocaust*) (Hebrew) (Jerusalem: Yad Vashem, 2015).

I am also deeply indebted to the late Prof. Israel Gutman, a survivor of the Warsaw ghetto who participated in the uprising and a world-renowned expert on Holocaust research and especially on the history of the Warsaw ghetto. I was privileged to have him read my studies thoroughly and we were both moved to tears during the professional discussion that followed. He shared his personal history with me and described the fate of his family in the ghetto from a medical perspective, while emphasizing its consistency with the historical picture presented in this book.

I wish to thank the Yad Vashem International Institute for Holocaust Research for encouraging and supporting me in publishing this book, and the entire staff of Yad Vashem Publications, particularly Dr. Ella Florsheim, the editor-in-chief; Idit Zaken, the director; and Yasmine Garval, who labored and accompanied me from the first steps I took to the publication of the book. Their professional recommendations left an imprint on the final version. I am extremely grateful to Naftali Greenwood for his masterfully crafted translation. I note with abundant appreciation the contribution of the language and production editor, Dania Valdez, whose painstaking attention and professionalism were worth more than their weight in gold. It is by dint of her dogged, consistent, professional devotion that the job was completed. Thank you to Sarah Veeder, who accompanied me in all the challenges involved in publishing the English edition of this comprehensive work.

The English edition of my book was made possible foremost by a grant from the Israel Office of the Conference on Jewish Material Claims against Germany, Inc., for which I am profoundly grateful. I also thank all the institutions and foundations that granted me stipends and prizes, which allowed me to advance and complete my research: the Mozes S. Schupf Fellowship, Bar-Ilan University; a donation in the name of the late Yitzchak Shavit, chair of the Jewish Federations of North America; the Jewish Agency for Israel; the United Israel Appeal; the Karev Program for Educational Involvement, its former director general, Nissim Matalon, and its director, Dr. Janet Aviad; the Yad Penina and Shimon Yehuda Association for Love of the Torah, the Jewish

People, and *Eretz Israel*, headed by Ezra Hartman; the annual Yehiel Ozer, Yona (Tova) Hinde, and Moshe Yehezkel, Klar Family Memorial Prize, bestowed through the Faculty of Jewish Studies and the Arnold and Leona Finkler Institute for Holocaust Studies at Bar-Ilan University; the Norbert and Lisa Schechter Memorial Foundation Prize, conferred by the International Institute for Holocaust Studies at Yad Vashem; the Chaya and Yitzhak Urbach Foundation Prize, awarded under the auspices of the Arnold and Leona Finkler Institute for Holocaust Studies at Bar-Ilan University; the Jacob and Clara Egit Foundation Award for Holocaust and Jewish Resistance Literature; and the Memorial Foundation for Jewish Culture in New York.

It was also my privilege to take part in an international seminar, "The Holocaust in Poland: Antecedents, Execution, Aftermath," held in July 2005 at New York University, The Center for Advanced Holocaust Studies, and the United States Holocaust Memorial Museum, Washington, D.C. I express special gratitude to the staff of the Hadassah–Brandeis Institute and, in particular, to the director, Prof. Lisa Fishbayn Joffe, and the assistant director, Debby Olins, who in 2017 gave me a scholar-in-residence stipend that allowed me to spend two months at Brandeis University. During this period, I enjoyed exceptional hospitality and was able to advance my research for the updates to this book on the contribution of women doctors and nurses to the establishment of the Warsaw ghetto medical system.

As I wrote the study and as the English version was being produced, many professionals contributed their expertise and encouragement in ways that I found immensely helpful. First, I extend my heartfelt gratitude to, among others, Dr. Daniel Nadav of Tel Aviv University, Prof. Dalia Ofer of the Avraham Harman Institute of Contemporary Jewry at the Hebrew University in Jerusalem, Prof. Gershon Bacon of Bar-Ilan University, Prof. Shifra Shvarts of the Moshe Prywes Center for Medical Education at Ben-Gurion University of the Negev, Prof. Daniel Statman of the University of Haifa, Prof. Yair Auron, and Dr. Natalia Aleksiun. In regard to the medical aspect, I thank several senior physicians, whose generous help throughout was invaluable in the presentation of my research findings: Prof. Bill Seidelman, Prof. Shaul Shasha, Prof. Avi Ohry, and Dr. Dan Reich. I also thank Dr. Yoram Keness, Dr. Danny Meron, Prof. Arnon Afek, Prof. Nachman Ash, Prof. Yoram Epstein, and Prof. Shmuel Reiss, with whom it was my privilege to organize the Second International Conference on Medicine in the Holocaust and Beyond, held in the Western Galilee in Israel in 2017. This event spawned a series of projects and publications, some of which have enriched my research.

For the past ten years, it has been an honor to participate in research symposia and discussions on medicine in the Holocaust with dozens of associates and colleagues from all over the world, who have devoted their lives to studying the history of medicine during and after the Holocaust. By meeting, communicating with, and learning from my peers, I acquired knowledge, support, strength, and inspiration to sustain the demanding research effort, which impacted the publishing of this book. Unable to list them all, I will mention only the most prominent among them: Prof. Michael Grodin, Prof. Sabine Hildebrandt, and Prof. Paul Weindling; as well as my colleagues, who direct international academic symposia, Prof. Sheldon Rubenfeld, Dr. Esther Cuerda, Dr. Matthis Krischel, Dr. Herwig Czech, and Dr. Maria Ciesielska, among others.

My heartfelt thanks to the Holocaust survivors and to the offspring of medical personnel who worked in the ghettos, who translated documents from various languages for me and entrusted me with valuable personal documentation: Chava Sachs, the late Shulamit Tzeder, Aviva Blum-Vaks, Ruti Ben Shahar, the late Sarah Urbach, the late Edith Rosenberg and her daughter, Dina Inbar, Miriam Shmuel, Miriam Harel, the late Haim Piotrkowski, the late Prof. Yaacov Lensky and his wife, Dr. Miri Lensky, the late Benjamin Anolik, Rami Nowodworski, and Chaya Pik. Without their assistance, I could not have researched this topic.

I wish to thank the staff of the Yad Vashem Archives, who always responded to my every request courteously and devotedly. A huge thank you to my friend Elisheva Shaul, whose expertise in the recesses of the Yad Vashem Archives and in the many languages necessary for this research were a tremendous help in updating this edition. I thank the archives of the Ghetto Fighters' House Museum for the cooperation I received from the former director of the archives, Mr. Yossi Shavit, and for the devoted assistance of the current director, Anat Bratman-Elhalel, her staff, and the director of the library, Dafna Itzkovich; the staff of the Alfred Goldschmidt Medical Sciences Library at the Technion for their professional and courteous service, especially Margie Serling and Hedva Razieli; the YIVO Archives in New York for their library and archive services and, in particular, for sharing material from a medical symposium that took place in 1996; the American Jewish Joint Distribution Committee Archives in New York, with special gratitude to Misha Mitsel for his loyal service during my stay there; the United States Holocaust Memorial Museum Library and Archives in Washington, D.C., for their professional and devoted service; the Emanuel Ringelblum Archive at the Archiwum Żydowski Instytut Historyczny (Archives of the Jewish Historical Institute), AŻIH, in Warsaw for allowing me to photocopy—efficiently, rapidly, and in unlimited quantities—rich, original material written in the Warsaw ghetto; the Wiener Archive and Library for the Study of the Nazi Era and the Holocaust at Tel Aviv University; and the devoted librarians at the National Library of Israel. I also wish to thank my friends on the staff of the Western Galilee College Library for their professional assistance, and their willingness to help me answer any question and to satisfy my every request.

Finally, I thank the president of Western Galilee College, Prof. Nissim Ben-David, and the administration for giving me a warm academic home and much support throughout the publication of this book. Gratitude is also due to my professional colleagues: Dr. Haim Sperber, head of the multidisciplinary program; Dr. Boaz Cohen, who heads the college's Holocaust Studies Program; and Dr. Yaron Pasher, my colleague on the teaching faculty. Our collaborative work to advance Holocaust teaching and research was a source of encouragement and support as I worked on this book.

I would like to note that I first took an interest in Holocaust research during my term as director of the Hedva Eibschitz Holocaust Studies Program in Haifa in 1988–1993. My years of work at this institute and with its founder, the late Holocaust survivor Yehoshua Eibschitz, definitely helped to solidify my views on how the Holocaust should be studied, taught, and commemorated.

I am especially appreciative of the contribution of my neighbors, members of the community of Hoshaya. Many of them assisted me in diverse ways, but several were particularly and immeasurably helpful, including Yona and Yehuda Zusman, Binny and Miriam Shalev, Rivka and Danny Statman, Ronit and Yedidya Lotan, and Yael and Itamar Kehati, and their children—my research assistants—Nitzan, Amit, and Tamar.

Last, but not least, I am profoundly grateful to the members of my core and expanded family, particularly my husband, Shmulik, and my beloved children, sons-in-law, and daughter-in-law: Irit and Yoel, Einav and Matan, Yishai and Tal, and Yaara and Efi. Their understanding, appreciation, and willingness to share the burden of my research and work allowed me to conclude the book. My dear grandchildren give me an added dimension of mental fortitude and I am keenly hopeful that they and their generation will continue to study, investigate, and teach the history and meaning of the Holocaust.

The dozens of people to whom I am thankful constitute, in effect, a quasi-virtual multidisciplinary research team that made it possible to write this book. *White Coats in the Ghetto* also stands on the shoulders of numerous studies that preceded mine. Therefore, I thank all the researchers who paved the way for me in this field, most notably, the late Prof. Mark Meir Dworzecki, a physician, Holocaust survivor, and pioneer of the study of medicine during the Holocaust; and the late Prof. Charles Roland, who made a comprehensive and outstanding contribution to research on medicine in the Warsaw ghetto. Above all, I thank those who pioneered the documentation and research of Jewish medical activity in the Holocaust—the Jewish physicians in the ghettos, who were murdered in the camps together with the rest of their fellow Jews.

Miriam Offer
Hoshaya, April 20, 2020
Holocaust Martyrs' and Heroes' Remembrance Day 2020

Introduction

Among the masses of martyrs who fell victim to the Nazi slaughter, the Jewish people will remember the doctors who risked their lives in a dual struggle—against the murderers' sword and against epidemics and disease.

Jewish physicians in exile have performed an exalted public mission since time immemorial. Many served in the courts of kings and ministers; many—towering personalities in Torah and science—served as exilarchs, leaders, and teachers of Jewish law for the dispersed. Their deeds transcended the bounds of professional medicine and extended to all areas of life, particularly social assistance and public hygiene.

Amid the assault on the body and soul of the European Diaspora, doctors took up a special place, knowing how to preserve the human image amid the agonies of the ghetto and to instill hope and comfort in hearts until the last moment....

May these pages be a modest memorial from doctors who were graced by fortune with the ability to take part in building new lives in the homeland to those fated to fall on the sword of the exile in the struggle for the rescue of Jewish souls.[1]

Dr. Mark Meir Dworzecki, 1946

1 Mark Meir Dworzecki, ed., "Hama'vak Al Hakiyum Vehabriyut Bageta'ot Biymei Hakibush Hanatzi" (The Struggle for Existence and Health in the Ghettos during the Nazi Occupation), *Dapim Refu'iyim* (Hebrew), 6 (1946), p. 2.

These lines from "Yizkor for the Doctors" were penned in 1946 by Dr. Mark Meir Dworzecki, a physician who survived the Vilna ghetto and subsequently became a historian as well. Dworzecki described Jewish doctors as fighters who "risked their lives in a dual struggle" against both the Nazis, on one hand, and epidemics and morbidity, on the other. He wrote that the doctors' place in the history of the Holocaust was unique—in their efforts to comfort and encourage the masses, they were exemplars and paragons in maintaining the image and values of humankind. As he saw it, the Jewish doctors died a hero's death. Did the Jewish medical tradition, alluded to in "Yizkor for the Doctors," contribute to the doctors' actions during the Holocaust? Were these physicians exemplars and paragons of the preservation of the human image? This study shows that the reality was complex. The doctors, like others in the ghettos who held official posts, faced impossible moral trials. Some failed; others endured admirably.

In this book, I describe the working conditions of the doctors under Nazi rule and the medical resources available to them. I inquire into the German policy on illness and health among the Jewish population in Warsaw, the way the Jews perceived this policy, and the insights that may be gained from the discipline of medicine about the everyday lives of Jews under Nazi rule, among other matters. I also investigate the precipitants of morbidity and mortality in the ghetto, the specific diseases that occurred there, and their treatment. Did the doctors have a special status in the ghetto and did they influence the complexion of the ghetto leadership? What was the nature of their collaboration with the Judenrat (Jewish Council)? What moral dilemmas did members of the medical staff confront? These questions have served as a point of departure for past research on Jewish medicine during the Holocaust. Some of these studies concern the reconstruction of history, others the evaluation of history, and yet others moral and national reckoning. In this book, I wish to place these matters in a broader context and argue that the patterns of the Jewish response and the establishment of the Jewish medical system in the Warsaw ghetto were largely characteristic of Jewish society in Poland in the modern era in general and particularly in the interwar years.[2]

The idea of researching this topic came up in 1992, when I had the privilege of disclosing the diary of the physician Dr. Aaron Pik from the Šiauliai ghetto in Lithuania. My first exposure to the diary and the discovery of the medical aspects that it describes prompted me to investigate the history of Jewish medicine in that ghetto.[3] This research sparked my interest in studying the history of medicine in the ghettos, and I outlined a comparative interdisciplinary study on a range of aspects of medicine in selected ghettos in Poland and Lithuania. However, after discovering the plethora of archive documentation and additional sources that describe the medical system in the Warsaw ghetto, I came to the conclusion that the variegated medical activity in the Warsaw ghetto—the largest ghetto in Europe—and the copious documentation that exists about it warrant deeper research that would relate to this ghetto.

Thus, this work aims to present a comprehensive and systematic portrait of the medical and health care system in the Jewish community of the Warsaw ghetto, the epitome of a "coerced community" under Nazi rule. Its main topic is an examination of the elements that affected the patterns that the Jewish community, as a modern and rather well-developed society,[4] adopted to cope

2 Miriam Offer, "Coping with the Impossible: The Developmental Roots of the Jewish Medical System in the Ghettos," in Marcin Moskalewicz, Ute Caumanns, and Fritz Dross, eds., *Jewish Medicine Health Care in Central Eastern Europe: Shared Identities, Entangled Histories*, vol. 3, (Cham: Springer International Publishing, 2019), pp. 261–277.

3 Miriam Offer, "Refu'a Verof'im Begeto Shavli Be'ikvot Hasifat Yomano Shel Harofe Aaron Pik, Reshimot Migai Hahariga: Zihronot Ktuvim Bageto Hashavla'i (Lita), 1942, 1943, 1944" (Medicine and Doctors in the Shavli [Šiauliai] Ghetto Following the Discovery of the Diary of Dr. Aaron Pik, Notes from the Valley of Death: Written Notes from the Shavli Ghetto in Lithuania from the Years 1942, 1943, 1944) (Hebrew) (Master's thesis, University of Haifa, 1993); Miriam Offer, "Medicine in the Shavli Ghetto: In Light of the Diary of Dr. Aaron Pik," in M. Grodin, ed., *Jewish Medical Resistance in the Holocaust* (New York and Oxford: Berghahn, 2014), pp. 164–172.

4 On Jewish society in Poland in general and specifically in Warsaw, see Israel Bartal and Israel Gutman, eds., *Kiyum Veshever: Yehudei Polin Ledoroteihem* (The Broken Chain: Polish Jewry through the Ages) (Hebrew), 2 vols., (Jerusalem: Zalman Shazar Center, 1997 and 2001).

with the medical catastrophe that the Germans' decrees brought upon it. This study also seeks to set the functioning of the Warsaw ghetto medical system in the context of the development of public health values in modern countries and their internalization in Jewish society. The book describes how, despite the grim conditions in the Warsaw ghetto, and in other ghettos, the Jews themselves, i.e., the persecuted society, managed to establish a hierarchical and rather strongly disciplined health care and medical system. This mechanism undertook to meet the public health challenges inside the ghetto in accordance with modern standards, such as sanitation, inoculation, quarantine of infected persons, inspection of food and water quality, and so on. It even set up a system of study, in-service activities, and research. In this book, I will show that it is truly unique among cases of genocide, and will attempt to shed light on its origins and to explain it as thoroughly as possible.

The definition of "Jewish medicine" in this book relates not to a specific medical discipline but to the attitude of Jewish society and tradition toward issues of health, morbidity, and medicine. This study traces the actions taken by the Jews in Warsaw to maintain health and prevent, diagnose, and treat diseases from the organizational, scientific, and ethical standpoints. This book, which spans the period from 1918 to 1943, notes the characteristics of Jewish medicine in the interwar era as the background for the infrastructure of Jewish medicine and the operation of the Jewish medical system in Nazi-era Poland until the liquidation of the Warsaw ghetto in 1943.

A study of the history of medicine and health calls for a method involving the "research of everyday life." Within a few years after the Holocaust, diaries, chronicles, and excerpts from Holocaust memoirs that documented diurnal life during that time were being published. Among the survivor–historians who began to engage in Holocaust research, some called attention to these questions.[5] Only since the 1980s has the description of quotidian life become an accepted and systematic current in historical

5 On this matter, see Boaz Cohen, *Israeli Holocaust Research: Birth and Evolution* (London: Routledge, 2013).

research. This shift of approach originates in social perceptions that sociologists and historians, mainly in Germany and the United States, have embraced with growing celerity since the 1970s. These views place the individual in the middle of the processes that drive history and promote marginal groups in society to the forefront of the historical debate.[6]

Given the topics that converged under the umbrella of research of everyday life, it is necessary to gather a wide variety of sources from different fields and invoke interdisciplinary research methods as a methodological basis.[7] Although my study is historical, it concerns itself with medicine and its place in a given society. Accordingly, my research integrates sources and literature from additional disciplines: medicine, sociology, and ethics. To achieve this integration, I consulted medical journals,

6 Daniel Blatman, "Idiologiya Vehayei Yom-Yom Be'itonut Hamahteret Begeto Varsha" (Ideology and Daily Life in the Warsaw Ghetto Underground Press), in Israel Gutman, ed., *Migniza Letziyunei Dereh Historiyim: Hartza'ot Mitoh Hakinus: Ringelblum Ve'arhiyon Oneg Shabbat, Arhiyonim Yehudiyim Mitkufat Hamilhama Vehashoah* (Hidden Treasures to Historical Landmarks: Lectures from the Conference on Ringelblum and the Oneg Shabbat Archive, Jewish Archives from the World War II and the Holocaust Period) (Hebrew) (Jerusalem: Yad Vashem, 1997), pp. 90–91. On research on everyday life during the Holocaust, see Yehoyakim Kochavi and Asher Cohen, eds., "Hayei Yom-Yom Bitkufat Hashoah" (Everyday Life during the Holocaust), *Dapim Leheker Tkufat Hashoah* (DAPIM) (The Journal of Holocaust Research, formerly known as Studies on the Holocaust) (Hebrew), 10 (1993). On research on daily life in Nazi Germany, see, for example, Detlev Peukert, *Inside Nazi Germany: Conformity, Opposition, and Racism in Everyday Life* (New Haven: Yale University Press, 1987). On research on everyday life in Poland, see Jan Tomasz Gross, *Polish Society under German Occupation: The Generalgouvernement 1939–1944* (Princeton: Princeton University Press, 1979).

7 Much has been written about the methodological aspects of research on everyday life. The historian Yehuda Bauer believes that integrative historiography, manifested in the everyday-life research method, makes an important contribution to our understanding of the history of the Holocaust. He mentions Saul Friedländer's *Nazi Germany and the Jews: The Years of Persecution, 1933–1939* (New York: HarperCollins, 1997), as a model of integrative writing that deserves emulation. See Yehuda Bauer, *Rethinking the Holocaust* (New Haven: Yale University Press, 2002), pp. 116–117. See also Dalia Ofer, "Heker Hayei Yom-Yom Tahat Hakibush Hanatzi" (The Study of Daily Life under the Nazi Occupation: Methodological Problems), *Dapim Leheker Tkufat Hashoah* (Hebrew), 10 (1993), pp. 7–39.

materials from organizational and policy research, and literature on medical ethics and emergency medicine.

I gathered my source material from various archives, mainly: Yad Vashem, the Ghetto Fighters' House Museum, the Wiener Archive at Tel Aviv University, the YIVO and the JDC Archives in New York, and the Archiwum Żydowski Instytut Historyczny in Warsaw. These diverse sources, some Jewish and others not, present a spectrum of aspects of medicine from various perspectives: those of the officials in the ghetto medical system, of the Jewish entities and organizations in the ghetto and elsewhere, of the Red Cross, and of the German authorities.

Development of Research on Jewish Medical Activity during the Holocaust

Writing about Jewish medicine in the Holocaust began in the very midst of World War II and continues to this day. Five stages in its development, in general, and in the specific context of Warsaw may be identified.[8]

Stage 1: Medical Research in Ghettos and Camps, 1940–1945

The pioneers in this research were the doctors in the ghettos and camps. They focused on describing the physiological aspects of morbidity and medicine, studied the diseases that afflicted the ghetto and camp populations, and secretly documented specific medical phenomena in order to relieve those who suffered from them and to document their occurrence as testimony to the free world. There were attempts in the field of research to develop vaccinations and medicines as well.

8 Miriam Offer, "The Study of Jewish Medicine during the Holocaust: Its Creation and Preliminary Steps," *Korot*, 22 (2013–2014), pp. 129–154; Miriam Offer, "The Study of Jewish Medicine during the Holocaust: Trends and Characteristics of Development," *Korot*, 23 (2015–2016).

Doctors in many ghettos engaged in research. The most famous studies were conducted in the Warsaw ghetto, where doctors investigated the physiology, pathology, and clinical manifestations of hunger in 1942. The report on the study, headed by Dr. Israel Milejkowski, the director of the Judenrat Health Department in the Warsaw ghetto, was smuggled to the "Aryan" side and first published in 1946.[9] Similarly, a large study on typhus was carried out in the Warsaw ghetto. The chief researcher in this project, Dr. Jakub Penson, head of the typhus department at Czyste Hospital in the ghetto, survived and published the findings in a Polish journal in 1946.[10] Some Jewish doctors kept diaries during the Holocaust, which provide an overview of the actions taken in various disciplines of health care and medicine from the vantage point of the eyewitnesses and the participants.[11]

9 Emil Apfelbaum, ed., *Choroba Głodowa: Badania kliniczne nad głodem wykonane w getcie warszawskim z roku 1942* (Warsaw: American Jewish Joint Distribution Committee, 1946); Emil Apfelbaum, ed., *Maladie de Famine: Recherches Cliniques sur La Famine Exécutée dans La Ghetto de Varsovie en 1942* (Warsaw: American Jewish Joint Distribution Committee, 1946). For a Yiddish translation by Ludvig Korn of part of this study, see "Hunger-krankhayt kolektive arbet fun yidishe doktoyrim in varshever geto" (Hunger Disease, Collective Work by Jewish Physicians in the Warsaw Ghetto), YIVO Archives, Poland Collection, RG–116–3.1. In 1948, Martin Gumpert, physician and researcher, wrote that he had seen the study in Yiddish on official German Army letterhead two years earlier. One may adduce from this that the work was written originally in Yiddish. See Martin Gumpert, "The Physicians of Warsaw," *The American Scholar*, 18 (1948), pp. 285–290. This article is also available in the American Jewish Joint Distribution Committee Archives (JDC), AR 33–44, file 840.

10 Jakub Penson, "Cechy kliniczne epidemii duru plamistego w latach 1940 i 1940/1941 w Warszawie. Badania nad przemiana azotowa ze szczegolnym uwzgl´dnieniem nerek. Metoda wczesnego rozpoznawania," *Polski Tygodnik Lekarski*, 46–52 (1946), pp. 1399–1404, 1478–1487, 1538–1542, 1553–1569; Boleslaw Rutkowski, "Jakub Penson and His Studies on Acute Renal Failure during Typhus Epidemics in Warsaw Ghetto," *Journal of Nephrology*, 17 (2004), pp. 175–179. See also M. Małecka, *Prof. dr med. Jakub Penson (1899–1971): życie, działalność i dokonania* (Gdansk: Akademia Medyczna w Gdansku Zakład Historii Filozofii Nauk Medycznych, 2008).

11 Among the published diaries, see, for example, Regina Brodinger, *Yomana Shel Ahot Bamilhama Neged Hanatzim, 1941–1945* (Diary of a Nurse in the War against the Nazis, 1941-1945) (Hebrew) (Tel Aviv: Afikim, 1982); Baruch Milch, *Can Heaven Be Void* (Jerusalem: Yad Vashem, 2003); Aaron Pik, "*Reshimot Migai Hahariga*": *Zihronot Ktuvim Bageto HaShavla'i (Lita) Bishnot*

Stage 2: Documentation and Investigation by Doctors Who Survived the Holocaust, 1946–1960s

The first two postwar decades were characterized by extensive documentary and research writing by doctors who survived the Holocaust. The writings of Dr. Mark Meir Dworzecki, a physician who survived the Holocaust and became one of the few researchers in Israel or elsewhere to discuss diverse aspects of the topic of Jewish medicine during the Holocaust from both a scientific medical perspective and a historical one, are particularly noteworthy among the studies that appeared at this time. Dworzecki also helped to lay the foundations of research on the history of Nazi medicine.[12]

1942, 1943, 1944 (Notes from the Valley of Death: Written Notes from the Shalvi Ghetto in Lithuania from the Years 1942, 1943, 1944) (Hebrew) (Tel Aviv: Igud Yotzei Lita, 1998); Valeria Stark, *Ahat Mini Elef: Yomana Shel Rofa BeBergen-Belsen* (One Out of a Thousand: The Diary of a Doctor in Bergen-Belsen) (Hebrew) (Tel Aviv: Neografica, 1951). On physicians' diaries that were written in Warsaw during the Nazi occupation, see, for example, two diary notebooks by Dr. Chaim Einhorn, Yad Vashem Archives (YVA), O.3/1836; two diary notebooks by Dr. Adolf Polisiuk, Ghetto Fighters' House Archives (GFH), no. 3182.

12 Dworzecki's writings and his contribution to research on medicine in the Holocaust deserve a separate comprehensive study. The scale of his research on Jewish medicine is extensive and unprecedented. See, for example, Dworzecki, "Hama'vak Al Hakiyum Vehabriyut Bageta'ot Biymei Hakibush Hanatzi"; Dworzecki, "Heker Mahalot Tkufat Hashoah" (Research on Diseases during the Holocaust), *Niv Harofe* (Hebrew), 3–4 (1955), pp. 5–9; Dworzecki, "Hapatalogiya Shel Tkufat Hashoah Vehasha'eret Hapatologiya Etzel Nitzolei Hashoah" (The Pathology of the Holocaust Era and Its Persistence among Holocaust Survivors), *Dapim Refu'iyim* (Hebrew), 15 (1956), pp. 3–11; Dworzecki, "Hamada Harefu'i Vehamatzpun Harefu'i" (Medical Science and the Medical Conscience), *Dapim Refu'iyim* (Hebrew), 12 (1953), pp. 3–13; Dworzecki, "Hasterilizatziya Vehakastratziya Haplilit Bekarnei Harentgen" (Sterilization and Criminal Castration Using X-Rays), *Dapim Refu'iyim* (Hebrew), 13 (1954), pp. 3–20; Dworzecki, "Prof. Klauberg, Miyozmei Hasterilizatziya Hahamonit" (Prof. Klauberg, an Instigator of Mass Sterilization), *Niv Harofe* (Hebrew), 1–2 (1956), pp. 3–20; Dworzecki, "Hameri Harefu'i Hayehudi Vaharefu'a Haposha'at Hanatzit Bitkufat Hashoah" (The Jewish Medical Uprising and Nazi Criminal Medicine during the Holocaust), *Niv Harofe* (Hebrew), 9–10 (1953), pp. 3–15; Dworzecki, ed., *Hama'avak Lakiyum Velabriyut Biymei Hashoah: Sidrat Hartza'ot Al Be'ayot Habriyut Bageta'ot, Bemahanot Harikuz Uvaye'arot* (The Struggle for Existence and Survival during the Holocaust: Lecture Series on Problems of Health in the Ghettos, the Concentration Camps, and the Forests) (Hebrew) (Jerusalem: World Jewish Congress and Physicians Association and

A descriptive style and the perception of Jewish medical activity as an act of heroism run like crimson threads throughout the doctors' writings during those years. Nonetheless, Dworzecki and his colleagues provide a systematic and painstaking account of medical activity in the ghettos.

Testimonies and the first flicker of research on the history of Jewish medicine in the Holocaust were published in Israel and elsewhere during the 1950s, when academic research about the Holocaust first began to appear.[13] However, since most articles by

Holocaust Survivors, 1958), p. 2; Dworzecki, "Tofa'ot Patologiyot Begeto Vilna Ubemahanot Harikuz: Ma Hayta Hadmut Hasanitarit Shel Geto Vilna Vehahayim Bo" (Pathological Phenomena in the Vilna Ghetto and the Concentration Camps: What Were the Sanitary Image and Living Conditions in the Vilna Ghetto?) in Dworzecki, *Hama'avak Lakiyum Velabriyut Biymei Hashoah*, pp. 33–36; Dworzecki, *Yerushalayim DeLita Bemeri Uvashoah* (Jerusalem of Lithuania in Rebellion and Holocaust) (Hebrew) (Tel Aviv: Mifleget Po'alei Eretz Israel, 1951), pp. 286–308; Dworzecki, "Adjustment of Detainees to Camp and Ghetto Life and Their Subsequent Readjustment to Normal Society," Yad Vashem Studies, 5 (1963), pp. 193–220; Dworzecki, "Be'yot Psiho-sotziologiyot Shel Yeladim Yehudim Shehuhbe'u Etzel Lo Yehudim Bitkufat Hashoah" (Psychosocial Problems of Jewish Children Who Hid with Non-Jews during the Holocaust), *Dapim Refu'iyim* (Hebrew), 1–6 (1966), pp. 244–250; Dworzecki, "The Day-to-Day Stand of the Jews" in Israel Gutman and Livia Rothkirchen, eds., *The Catastrophe of European Jewry: Antecedents, History, Reflections: Selected Papers* (Jerusalem: Yad Vashem, 1976), pp. 386–399; Dworzecki, *Mahanot Hayehudim Be'Estonia 1942–1944: Hatmurot Beshitat Hahovalot Uveshitat Hamahanot, Amidat Ha'asirim, Hamahteret, Habrihot Laye'arot* (The Jewish Camps in Estonia 1942–1944: Changes in the Transport Method and the Camps Method, Prisoners' Steadfastness, Resistance, and Escape to the Forests) (Hebrew) (Jerusalem: Yad Vashem, 1970), pp. 168–187, Dworzecki, "Asthenia Hronit Progresivit Vehizdaknut Mukdemet Etzel Nitzolei Shoah" (Progressive Chronic Asthenia and Premature Aging among Holocaust Survivors), *Rofe Hamishpaha* (Hebrew), 1 (1970), pp. 3–7.

13 Mordechai Lensky, "Beit Haholim Hayehudi Tzhista," (Czyste Jewish Hospital), *Dapim Leheker Hashoah Vehamered* (Hebrew), 1 (1951), pp. 102–107; Lensky, Mordechai, "Problems of Disease in the Warsaw Ghetto," *Yad Vashem Studies on the European Jewish Catastrophe and Resistance*, vol. 3, (Jerusalem: Jewish Agency, 1959), pp. 283–293. In 1955, Dworzecki's article about the Jewish medical uprising and Nazi criminal medicine during the Holocaust was published in the Ghetto Fighters' House newsletter, allowing Holocaust medical research to sustain a small-scale presence in the first journals that dealt with Holocaust research and not only in medical journals. Mark Meir Dworzecki, "Hameri Harefu'i Hayehudi Bitkufat Hashoah" (The Jewish Medical Uprising

doctors at that time appeared in medical journals—because they contained medical information and because academic research forums on the Holocaust had not yet developed—historians did not investigate them sufficiently. Most of the articles, like works in the memoir and testimony genres, lacked the genuine attributes of research.[14]

This period is noted for ramified documentary activity on medicine in the Holocaust. Most of the writers were doctors who had survived the inferno, and research on morbidity continued to dominate. Concurrently, however, initial indications of historical research appeared. In these writings, the question of the German policy on illness and health in the Warsaw ghetto, as observed from a Jewish point of view, was raised for the first time, and a pioneering attempt was made on the theoretical level to survey the history of Jewish medicine in Poland from its inception to the formation of the Jewish medical system under Nazi rule in Poland.

In 1953, Isaiah Trunk, a survivor and historian, published the first historical study on Jewish medicine in the Holocaust in his article, "Epidemics and Mortality in the Warsaw Ghetto, 1939–1942."[15] According to Trunk, ghettoization was a scheme that the Germans had planned in order to annihilate the Jews by means of bacteria. Although some took issue with this view, the research conception and the breadth of the documentation on which Trunk rested his case served researchers for decades after his study appeared.[16]

and Nazi Criminal Medicine during the Holocaust), *Yediyot Beit Lohamei Hageta'ot* (Ghetto Fighters' House Newsletter) (Hebrew), April 1955, pp. 20–22.

14 This kind of writings by doctors during those years is unique, because it is neither historical research nor medical research by academic standards, but it is also difficult to define as mere personal testimony or memoir. The material was pressed into the structure of systematic articles in which the authors mirrored the medical outlooks and hypotheses that were current among ghetto physicians in regard to the medical phenomena described in the articles. A few doctors conducted research on the topics of their writings, although the sources they could access were limited.

15 Isaiah Trunk, "Epidemics and Mortality in the Warsaw Ghetto, 1939–1942," *YIVO Annual of Jewish Social Sciences*, 8 (1953), pp. 82–122.

16 See, for example, Paul Julian Weindling, *Epidemics and Genocide in Eastern Europe, 1890–1945* (New York: Oxford University Press, 2000).

In 1963, the first comprehensive study on the martyrology of Jewish physicians in Poland was published in the United States.[17] The Medical Alliance–Association of Jewish Physicians from Poland in the United States initiated the research and the book that it yielded. Although their study does not focus on any particular ghetto and provides neither an overview nor a comparison of all the ghettos, it remains a basic text in research on the history of Jewish medicine in Poland, in general, and that of the Holocaust era, in particular.

This period also witnessed the publication of articles and documentary materials, and the organization of international and national conferences.[18] Prompted by the conviction that the doctors' activity in the Holocaust is part of the broader story of Jewish heroism and, as such, deserves commemoration, groups of doctors, such as the Union of Holocaust Survivor Physicians in Israel and the Medical Alliance–Association of Jewish Physicians from Poland in the United States, mobilized to commemorate the feats of doctors who had perished in the Holocaust and to promote research on the subject of Jewish medicine. During this period, Dr. Dworzecki also endeavored to establish an institute for research on Holocaust pathology.[19] Although his vision was not

17 Leon Wulman et al., *The Martyrdom of Jewish Physicians in Poland*, ed. by Louis Falstein (New York: Medical Alliance–Association of Jewish Physicians from Poland, by Exposition Express, 1963). Dr. Wulman, a coauthor of the book and one of the leaders of this research and commemoration project, served in the interwar years as general secretary of TOZ, the Jewish health care organization in Poland.

18 Congrès international de la pathologie des déportés, Paris, October 4–5, 1954; "Conference Médico-Social Internationale sur la Pathologie des Anciens Déportés et Internés," Copenhagen, June 5–7, 1954; "Internationale Medizinische Konferenz über die Therapeutik, Wiederherstellung und Umschulung der Kriegsinvaliden: Widerstandskämpfer und Deportierte, Moscow," June 25–28, 1957; "Medizinische Konferenz anlässlich der Internationalen Studientage über die Gesetzgebung und die Rechte der Widerstandskmpfer," Brussels, October 22, 1955. See also the conference lectures of the Internationalen Foderation der Widerstandskämpfer, Vienna, April 21, 1956; Dworzecki, *Hama'avak Lakiyum Velabriyut Biymei Hashoah*; Dworzecki, "Hacongres Habeinle'umi Leheker Mahalot Tkufat Hashoah, *Yedi'ot Yad Vashem* (Hebrew), 3 (December 1954), pp. 4–7.

19 Letter from Dr. Mark Meir Dworzecki to the Medical Association on the establishment of a Research Institute for Medicine and the Holocaust, YVA,

fulfilled, his efforts to realize it reflect his belief in the importance of the cause, the intensive work that was conducted in this field, and the furtherance of the research that the establishment of this entity was meant to assure.

Stage 3: Deceleration of Research and Documentary Activity, Mid-1960s to Mid-1980s

From the mid-1960s to the mid-1980s, research on Jewish medicine slackened perceptibly. Some survivor–doctors passed away. Dworzecki, the living spirit behind the study of Jewish medicine in the Holocaust, died of an illness in 1974, leaving a gaping void in this field of research.[20] Although Holocaust research was burgeoning in Israel, it focused on matters related to the Jewish leadership, the Judenräte (Jewish Councils), and the nexus between the *Yishuv* (pre-independence Israel), the Holocaust, and the Jewish armed resistance. While Jewish medicine did not totally vanish from the research scene, it and other topics were marginalized.[21]

P.10/38. In this file, I found a letter concerning the creation of such an institute, including an explanation of the proposed entity and its goals, and a list of doctors who were members of the founding committee. The author of the letter went on to say, "A large-scale public council with fifty-three members will soon be formed, composed of doctors, biologists, researchers, and scientists at higher institutions in Israel, heads of hospital departments, and representatives of various survivors' organizations."

20 Dworzecki's last study concerned the activities of the International Committee of the Red Cross during the Holocaust. See Mark Meir Dworzecki, "The International Red Cross and Its Attitude toward the Jews in the Nazi-Occupied Countries," in Israel Gutman and Efraim Zuroff, eds., *Rescue Attempts during the Holocaust: Proceedings of the Second Yad Vashem International Historical Conference* (Jerusalem: Yad Vashem, 1977), pp. 71–110.

21 Some of the few studies written at this time make direct reference to medical matters; others do so indirectly while focusing on other themes such as the Judenrat and the Warsaw Ghetto Uprising. See Leonard Tushnet, *The Uses of Adversity: Studies of Starvation in the Warsaw Ghetto* (New York and London: Thomas Yoseloyf, 1966); Ryszard Zabłotniak, "Epidemia duru plamistego wśród ludności żydowskiej w Warszawie w latach II wojny światowei," *Biuletyn Żydowskiego Instytutu Historycznego* (*BŻIH*), vol. 4 (1971), pp. 3–21; R. Zabłotniak, "Wydział lekarski w getcie warszawskim," *BŻIH*, vol. 74 (1970), pp. 81–85; Isaiah Trunk, *Judenrat: The Jewish Councils*

This period saw no meaningful development of the research trends that had surfaced in previous decades. However, doctors who had survived the Holocaust continued to publish memoirs and some of them did so in research forums. Doctors who had not gone through the Holocaust also took an interest in the topic, mainly in regard to the hunger studies that doctors in the Warsaw ghetto had performed. In 1979, Myron Winick, an expert on nutrition and pediatrics, published the first complete English translation of a manuscript on this hunger research.[22] The book presents the historical background of the instigation of the research, its performance, and a discussion from a scientific-research perspective of each area studied by the ghetto physicians, including an assessment of the scientific accomplishments of their probing work. Although this book was helpful in disseminating the studies of the Warsaw ghetto doctors, more than a decade passed until historians turned their attention to this research.

Alongside the doctors' studies, historical research appeared on a limited scale. Here Jewish medicine attracted the attention of historians as a medium through which the institution of the Jewish ghetto leadership could be better understood, or as background material for research on Jewish resistance to Nazi rule.

Stage 4: Rapid Development of Academic Research on Jewish Medicine among Historians and Doctors, Late 1980s Onward

Since the second half of the 1980s, there has been a tide of academic studies on Jewish medicine during the Holocaust. The reason may be traced to several concurrent social and political

in Eastern Europe under Nazi Occupation (New York: Macmillan, 1972), pp. 143–171; Israel Gutman, *The Jews of Warsaw 1939–1943: Ghetto, Underground, Revolt* (Bloomington: Indiana University Press, 1989), pp. 26–27, 29–30, 51–55, 62–63, 63–65, 83, 102–106, 107–110, 308–309.

22 Winick, *Hunger Disease*. In 2007, twenty-five years after publishing this book, Winick published a novella that he had written on the main theme of hunger research in the ghetto. See Myron Winick, *Final Stamp: The Jewish Doctors in the Warsaw Ghetto* (Bloomington: Author House, 2007).

processes, and the evolution of the discipline of history. With the crumbling of the Eastern Bloc and the end of the Cold War in the late 1980s, previously inaccessible archives were opened up, allowing research, in general, and medical research, in particular, to expand. An outpouring of studies on the Nazis' medical crimes, also published in the 1980s, expedited research on Jewish medicine at that time. The establishment of the United States Holocaust Memorial Museum and its archives in Washington in the early 1990s fostered the broadening of research.

The study of Jewish medicine in the Holocaust was also influenced by the development of research of everyday life, which acquired legitimacy in historical research at this time and widened the ambit of the discussion topics. This process liberated researchers from their intensive preoccupation with the Judenräte, the resistance, and the responses of the *Yishuv* leadership—issues that had commanded center stage in the two previous decades—and made room for a historical debate that expanded the ranks of participants from statespersons and leaders to individuals and other groups in society, such as physicians.

As the survivors of the Holocaust, including the doctors, grew older, a new dialogue ensued between them and second and third generation survivors. The dialogue was expedited by the March of the Living Project, which began in the late 1980s and has continued with trips to Poland by members of post-Holocaust generations from Israel and other countries. Feeling that time was running out, young people and researchers encouraged the last survivors to share hitherto suppressed documentation and thereby leave one last imprint in the corpus of testimony and commemoration. These developments, as well as Steven Spielberg's documentation project, triggered a reawakening among individual survivors and among landsmanshaften (associations of Holocaust survivors from the same city or region who provided mutual assistance and worked to commemorate their communities), which led to their cooperation in the collection of a new wave of testimonies. Finally, the discovery of new documentation impacted the field of Jewish medicine in the Holocaust, and the circle of researchers and geographic distribution expanded as more and more historians joined those from medical and nursing backgrounds who researched the topic.[23] The penchant for judging medical activity in heroic terms seems to have remained dominant. Nonetheless, a few studies began to pay attention to dilemmas related to medical activity, and this trend continues.[24]

In 1992, Prof. Charles Roland, a physician specializing in medical history in Canada, published his pathbreaking and

23 See, for example, Leah Koren, "Hasiyud Kehelek Misherutei Habriyut Begeta'ot Varsha, Vilna, Kovna, 1939–1944" (Nursing as Part of the Health Care Services in the Warsaw, Vilna, and Kovno Ghettos, 1939–1944) (Hebrew) (Master's thesis, Tel Aviv University, 1987). See also Barbara Engelking and Jacek Leociak, *Getto warszawskie: Przewodnik po nieistniejącym mieście* (Warsaw: Wydawnictwo IFiS PAN, 2001). The description of the ghetto health care services in this book is as extensive as the accounts of the Judenräte and armed warfare. For additional material on medical and health issues in the Warsaw ghetto, see Michal Grynberg, ed., *Words to Outlive Us: Eyewitness Accounts from the Warsaw Ghetto* (New York: Metropolitan Books, 2002); Ahuva Aricha, "Hasherut Hameditzini Bethum Briyut Hatzibur Bere'i Hahistoriya Haklalit Vehayehudit Ufo'alo Begeto Varsha, Kehelek Mipe'ilut Ma'arehet Habriyut Al Irguneha Umosdoteha Hashonim (Medical Service in the Field of Public Health through the Lens of General and Jewish History, and Its Operation in the Warsaw Ghetto as Part of the Activity of the Health Care System, Its Organizations, and Its Institutions) (Hebrew) (Master's thesis, The Hebrew University of Jerusalem, 2002).

24 See, for example, Miriam Offer, "Refua Verof'im Begeto Shavli"; Lea Prais, "Sugiyot Shel Refu'a, Etika Vemusar Begeta'ot Vilna, Kovna, VeShavli" (Issues of Medicine, Ethics, and Morals in the Ghettos of Vilna, Kovno, and Shavli), *Yalkut Moreshet* (Hebrew), 71 (2001), pp. 23–38; Yulian Rafes, *Doctors and Patients: Doomed to Destruction: Ethical, Human, and Professional Dimensions of Jewish Doctors in the Vilna Ghetto* (Danbury: Begell House, 2001); Miriam Offer, "Ethical Dilemmas in the Work of Doctors and Nurses in the Warsaw Ghetto," *Polin: Studies in Polish Jewry*, 25 (2012), pp. 467–449; Sari Siegel, "Treating Dr. Maximilian Samuel: A Case Study of an Auschwitz Prisoner Doctor," *Holocaust, and Genocide Studies* (2014); Offer, "Medicine in the Shavli Ghetto," pp. 164–172; Ross Halpin, *The Essence of Survival: How Jewish Doctors Survived Auschwitz* (Sydney: Sydney Jewish Museum, 2014); Miriam Offer, "Jewish Medical Ethics during the Holocaust: The Unwritten Ethical Code," *Wiener klinische Wochenschrift: The Central European Journal of Medicine*, 130 (2018), pp. 172–176; Sari Siegel, "Between Coercion and Resistance: Jewish Prisoner–Physicians in Nazi Camps, 1940–1945" (PhD diss., University of Southern California, 2018); Ross Halpin, *Jewish Doctors and the Holocaust: The Anatomy of Survival* (Berlin and Jerusalem: De Gruyter Publishing and Magnes Press, 2019).

probing book about starvation, disease, morbidity, and death in the Warsaw ghetto.[25] I refer to his findings extensively and rely strongly on his sources. Roland notes the nobility of spirit that the Warsaw ghetto doctors displayed in establishing their clandestine medical school and in engaging in research. His tendency to focus the reader's attention on hunger research and the study of medicine above all else parallels the earlier tendency to prioritize the ghetto uprising, as though this were the alpha and the omega of the ghetto era. In this sense, the emphasis on medical activities that were undertaken at mortal risk and in defiance of the Germans' decrees may be viewed as a "medical uprising" that contrasts with "medical survival." The "medical uprising," manifested in furtive research and underground medical studies, overshadows the account of the everyday medical struggle, and the dilemmas and crucial decisions that had to be faced under the circumstances of the dire reality. The tension between the Holocaust and heroism appears to have found expression in research on Jewish medicine, as well as elsewhere.

In 1996, a large conference that addressed research on Jewish medicine during the Holocaust, titled "Jewish Medical Resistance during the Holocaust," took place on the initiative of YIVO.[26] The first of its kind, the colloquium was the swan song of the doctor–survivors who had left their mark on the study of the history of Jewish medicine in the Holocaust.[27] In 2006, Dalia Ofer's article, "Another Glance through the Historian's Lens: Testimonies in the Study of Health and Medicine in the Ghetto,"[28]

25 Charles Roland, *Courage under Siege: Starvation, Disease, and Death in the Warsaw Ghetto* (New York: Oxford University Press, 1992).

26 The YIVO Institute for Jewish Research was established in 1925 as the yidisher visnshaftlekher institut (Yiddish Scientific Institute) in Vilna and had branches in Warsaw, Berlin, and New York City. Forced to relocate because of the war, it has been headquartered in New York City since 1940.

27 YIVO Institute for Jewish Research, New York, November 1996. I wish to thank the directors and staff of YIVO for graciously giving me a copy of the lectures delivered at the 64th International Conference of the YIVO Institute for Jewish Research entitled "Jewish Medical Resistance during the Holocaust," New York, 2005.

28 Dalia Ofer, "Another Glance through the Historian's Lens: Testimonies in the Study of Health and Medicine in the Ghetto," *Poetics Today*, 27:2 (2006), pp. 331–351. I wish to thank Prof. Dalia Ofer for discussing her research on the topic with me personally and for everything I learned from her lectures.

was one of the first to derive general insights from the medical realities of ghetto life. Daniel Nadav's *Medicine and Nazism*, the first single historical overview of both Nazi medicine and Jewish medicine published in Israel, appeared the same year.[29] Nadav is one of the few historians in Israel who specializes in researching both the history of medicine in the Nazi era and Jewish medical activity during the Holocaust. The primacy of this work is reflected in its dual historical perspective and its attempt to provide a comprehensive description of Jewish medicine in the ghettos and camps. His account of Nazi medicine points to the development, continuity and change, turning points, and decline of the German doctors' work from the late nineteenth century to the annihilation process of the Final Solution. Jewish medicine in the Holocaust, in contrast, is not described from a developmental point of view. Nadav concludes with several insights that construe the Nazi past as a warning and a demand for maximal caution in the treatment of contemporaneous bioethical issues.[30]

A collection of articles in Hebrew on medicine in the Holocaust, published in Israeli medical journals from the end of World War II to 2005, compiled by Dr. Julian Thomas (Tomi) Spenser, appeared in 2007 titled *Harefu'a Vehashoah: Ma'amarim Mitoh* Harefu'a *Ve* Mihtav Lehaver, (Medicine and the Holocaust: Articles from Harefu'a and Mihtav Lehaver, 1946–2005).[31] In addition to the importance of the collection for research—although it omits many articles that appeared in other forums during the relevant period—it reflects the keen interest in the history of medicine in the Holocaust that doctors in Israel had begun to show from the 1990s onward. Starting in the 2000s and continuing through the 2010s, important works devoted to Jewish medicine during the Holocaust were published by researchers from different countries around the world, for example, in 2014, a collection of

29 Daniel S. Nadav, *Medicine and Nazism* (Jerusalem: The Hebrew University Magnes Press, 2009).

30 Ibid., pp. 147–148.

31 Julian Thomas Spenser, ed., *Harefu'a Vehashoah: Ma'amarim Mitoh* Harefu'a *Ve* Mihtav Lehaver, *1946–2005* (Hebrew) (Ramat Gan: Israel Medical Association, 2007).

articles in the volume *Jewish Medical Resistance in the Holocaust*, edited by Michael Grodin. The book includes articles on Jewish activity in the ghettos, camps, and other areas during World War II.[32] Alongside this, during 2014 and 2015, another seven studies on Jewish medicine during the Holocaust were published by researchers from Germany, the Czech Republic, Australia, and Israel. In fact, the 2010s saw an enrichment of knowledge, with studies on the fate of Jewish physicians during the Holocaust in Holland,[33] Berlin,[34] Nuremburg,[35] Hamburg,[36] Warsaw,[37] Bohemia and Moravia,[38] Auschwitz,[39] and Theresienstadt,[40] etc.[41] Since

32 Grodin, *Jewish Medical Resistance.*

33 Hannah van den Ende, *Vergeet niet dat je arts bent, Joodse artsen in Nederland, 1940–1945* (Amsterdam: Boom, 2015).

34 Susanne Doetz and Christoph Kopke, "*Und dürfen das Krankenhaus nicht mehr betreten*": *Der Ausschluss jüdischer und politisch unerwünschter Ärzte und Ärztinnen aus dem Berliner städtischen Gesundheitswesen, 1933–1945* (Berlin: Hentrich & Hentrich, 2015); Rebecca Schwoch, ed., *Berliner Jüdische Kassenärzte und ihr Schicksal im Nationalsozialismus* (Berlin: Hentrich & Hentrich Teetz, 2009).

35 Bernd Höffken, *Schicksale jüdischer Ärzte aus Nürnberg nach 1933* (Berlin: Metropol, 2014).

36 Anna von Villiez, *Mit aller Kraft verdrängt: Entrechtung und Verfolgung "nicht arischer" Ärzte in Hamburg 1933 bis 1945* (Munich: Dölling u. Galitz, 2009).

37 Offer, *Haluk Lavan Bageto.*

38 Michal V. Šimůnek and Antonin Kostlán, eds., *Disappeared Science: Biographical Dictionary of Jewish Scholars from Bohemia and Moravia—Victims of Nazism, 1939–1945* (Červený Kostelec: Pavel Mervart, 2013).

39 Halpin, *The Essence of Survival.*

40 H. Jenss and P. Reinicke, *Der Arzt Hermann Strauß, 1868–1944: Autobiographische Notizen und Aufzeichnungen aus dem Ghetto Theresienstadt* (Berlin: Hentrich & Hentrich, 2014); Miriam Offer, "Review of *Der Arzt Hermann Strauß, 1868–1944: Autobiographische Notizen und Aufzeichnungen aus dem Ghetto Theresienstadt*, by H. Jenss and P. Reinicke," *Social History of Medicine*, 29:4 (2016), pp. 853–855: Anna Hájková, "Medicine in Theresienstadt," *Social History of Medicine*, hky066, August 30, 2018, https://academic.oup.com/shm/advance-article-abstract/doi/10.1093/shm/hky066/5087809 (accessed December 12, 2019).

41 Thomas Beddies, Susanne Doetz, and Christoph Kopke, eds., *Jüdische Ärztinnen und Ärzte im Nationalsozialismus: Entrechtung, Vertreibung, Ermordung* (Berlin: de Gruyter, 2014); Matthis Krischel, *Urologie und Nationalsozialismus: Eine Studie zu Medizin und Politik als Ressourcen füreinander* (Stuttgart: Franz Steiner Verlag, 2014); Kai Kranich, *Anpassung im Nationalsozialismus: die Universität Breslau und die Aberkennung von Doktortiteln* (Wrocław: Oficyna

2015, several important studies, specifically on the Warsaw ghetto, were published, including two comprehensive works. One is by the physician–historian Maria Ciesielska,[42] who researched and published inter alia the names of the 700 physicians who worked in the Warsaw ghetto, and the other is by Naomi Menuhin,[43] who wrote a biography of Dr. Israel Milejkowski, the head of the Judenrat Health Department in the Warsaw ghetto. In addition, shorter studies were published.[44] Since the mid-1990s, articles on Jewish medicine in the Holocaust have appeared in the Israeli print and electronic media as well. Almost every year since 2000, the print media has published these articles for Holocaust Martyrs' and Heroes' Remembrance Day, for example, thus admitting the topic

Wydawn, 2012); Robert Jütte, "Die Vertreibung jüdischer und staatsfeindlicher Ärztinnen und Ärzte," in Robert Jütte, ed., *Medizin und Nationalsozialismus: Bilanz und Perspektiven der Forschung* (Göttingen: Wallstein, 2011), pp. 83–93; Werner Kümmel, "Die Ausschaltung rassisch und politisch mißliebiger Ärzte," in Kudlien Fridolf, ed., *Ärzte im Nationalsozialismus* (Köln: Kiepenheuer & Witsch, 1985), pp. 56–81. Rachel Herzog, "Hitarutam Shel Rofim Nitzolei Shoah Bahevra Hayisra'elit Uvema'arehet Habriyut Beyisra'el, 1945–1957" (The Intermingling of Holocaust Doctors Survivors into Both the Israeli Society and the Israeli Health Care System in the Years, 1945–1957) (Hebrew) (PhD diss., Ben-Gurion University of the Negev, 2015).

42 Maria Ciesielska, *Lekarza Getta Warszawskiego* (Warsaw: Wydawnictwo Dwa Światy, 2017).

43 Naomi Menuhin, "Dr. Israel Milejkowski: Ha'intelektual Hayehudi BePolin Bein Shtei Milhamot Ha'olam: Doktor Izrael Milikovski Kemikreh Mivhan" (Dr. Israel Milejkowski: The World of a Jewish Intellectual in Poland between Two World Wars) (Hebrew) (PhD diss., Ben-Gurion University of the Negev, 2016).

44 Juliet D. Golden, "'Show that you are really alive,' Sara-Zofia Syrkin-Binsztejnowa's Emergency Medical Relief and Public Health Work in Early Interwar Poland and the Warsaw Ghetto," *Medizinhistorisches Journal*, 53:2 (2018), pp. 125–162; George M. Weisz, Andrzej Grzybowski, and William Randall Albury, "The Fate of the Warsaw Ghetto Medical Faculty," *IMAJ*, 14 (April 2012), pp. 209–213; Weisz, Grzybowski, and Albury, "Henryk, Thaddeus and Ludwik Stabholz: Three Outstanding Physicians from a Jewish Medical Family in Mid-20th Century Poland," *Korot*, 21 (2011–2012), pp. 363–372; Agnieszka Witkowska, "Anna Braude-Heller Seen from a Distance," *NASHIM: A Journal of Jewish Women's Studies & Gender Issues*, 36 (forthcoming, Spring 2020); Sean Martin, "Zofia Szymańska and Child Welfare in Twentieth Century Poland," *NASHIM: A Journal of Jewish Women's Studies & Gender Issues*, 36 (forthcoming, Spring 2020).

to the media discourse on remembrance.[45] The theme of Jewish medicine in the Holocaust has reverberated in the arts in different places in the world, including in painting, theater, and cinema, and there has been intense public interest in this field.[46]

45 Examples include Miriam Offer, "Rofim Yehudim Ne'eltzu Laharog Bageto Tinokot Yehudim" (Jewish Doctors Had to Kill Jewish Infants in the Ghetto), *Ma'ariv* (Hebrew), Weekend Supplement, Special Edition for Holocaust Martyrs' and Heroes' Remembrance Day, April 8, 1994, pp. 16–19; Chaim Braude, "Hihrihu Oti Lihyot Malah Hamavet" (They Forced Me to Be the Angel of Death), *Yediot Aharonot* (Hebrew), Special Issue for Holocaust Martyrs' and Heroes' Remembrance Day, May 2, 2000, p. 9; Iris Milner, "Shfanei Nisayon Shel Atsmam" (Their Own Guinea Pigs), *Ha'aretz* (Hebrew), April 28, 2000, p. 9; Ayelet Negev and Yehuda Koren, "Nisuyim Bivnei Adam" (Human Experiments), *Yediot Aharonot* (Hebrew), Weekend Supplement, April 25, 2003, Weekend Supplement, pp. 53–56. Daniel Nadav, "Limed Anatomiya Begeto Varsha, Nitzal Kshehithaze Lekatoli Nehe" (He Taught Anatomy in the Warsaw Ghetto, He Survived by Posing as a Disabled Catholic), *Ha'aretz* (Hebrew), April 16, 2004, p. 10; Meron Rappaport, "Hamahpehan MiNes Tziona" (The Revolutionary from Nes Tziona), *Ha'aretz* (Hebrew), Supplement, February 11, 2005, pp. 44–46; Tamara Traubman, "Im Kvar Anahnu Bageto, Lefahot Nahkor Et Hara'av" (If We're Already in the Ghetto, We Might As Well Do Research on Hunger), *Ha'aretz* (Hebrew), March 11, 2005, p. 10b; Guy Fishkin, "Ani Megiya Lamahlaka Vehagehenom Amiti" (I Reach the Ward and Real Hell), *Ma'ariv* (Hebrew) April 8, 2013, p. 5; Ronny Linder-Ganz and Rotem Starkman, "Yesh Mashehu She'anahnu Lo Yod'im Al Hashoah? Hamered Harefu'i Begeto Varsha" (Is There Anything We Don't Know about the Holocaust? The Medical Uprising in the Warsaw Ghetto), *TheMarker* (Hebrew), April 17, 2015, pp. 8–10; Arik Weiss, "Mered Intelektuali: Hamehkar Hamahtarti Shel Rofim Yehudim Begeto Varsha" (Intellectual Uprising: The Underground Research of Jewish Doctors in the Warsaw Ghetto) (Hebrew), Israeli Television, Channel 13, May 4, 2019, https://13news.co.il/item/news/abroad/europe/ghetto-research-235861/.

46 See, for example, Tim Blake Nelson, *The Gray Zone*, directed by Tim Blake Nelson (Santa Monica: Lionsgate, 2001), a film based on the book by Miklos Nyiszli, *Auschwitz: A Doctor's Eyewitness Account* (Herfortshire: Mayflower, 1973); Anne Meredith, *Out of the Ashes*, directed by Joseph Sargent (Buckinghamshire: Ardent Productions, 2003), based on Gisella Perl, *I Was a Doctor in Auschwitz*, http://www.tcm.turner. com/tcmdb/title/483355/Out-of-the-Ashes/; Ella Milch-Sheriff, *Baruch's Schweigen* (Baruch's Silence) (Braunschweig, 2010), https://www.ellamilchsheriff.com/baruchs-schweigen, an opera, and Avi Nesher, *Past Life*, directed by Avi Nesher (Tel Aviv: Metro Communications in co-production with Poland's Opus Film, 2016), the Israeli film, both based on the memoir of the physician Baruch Milch, *Can Heaven Be Void?* See also Anita Tarsi, ed., *Umanut Verefu'a Begeto Terezienstat (Terezin): Rishumim Mehashanim 1942–1944* (Art and Medicine in Ghetto

Stage 5: Public and Research Awakening among Doctors and Historians, Early 2000s

Stage 5 is marked by many innovative attempts to formalize the teaching of medical history in the Nazi era, including medical activity initiated by the victims, which is the subject of this book. An increase in international conferences and academic publications on the topic are part of this trend. Examples from the 2010s include, in Europe, in 2014, the international symposium titled "Medicine in Nazi Germany: Historical Perspectives and Ethical Reflections," organized by Esther Cuerda and Matthis Krischel, who initiated a series of biannual conferences in the field. In the United States, in 2015, the First International Scholars Workshop on Medicine after the Holocaust was held, on the initiative of Prof. Sheldon Rubenfeld, president of the Center for Medicine after the Holocaust in Houston, Texas. In Vienna, in 2017, an international conference titled "Medical Ethics 70 Years after the Nuremberg Code, 1947 to the Present" was led by Prof. Paul Weindling, Herwig Czech, and Christiane Drumi. In Israel, in the same year, another very large international conference on "Medicine in the Holocaust and Beyond" was held at Western Galilee College, led by Shmuel Reis and Miriam Offer. In Poland, in 2018, Maria Ciesielska initiated annual conferences under the title "Medical Review Auschwitz: Medicine behind the Barbed Wire," and Stacy Galin and Tessa Chelouche promote conferences on the Holocaust and bioethics within the framework of the Department of Bioethics and the Holocaust, UNESCO Chair of Bioethics (Haifa), and the Maimonides Institute for Medicine,

Theresienstadt [Terezín)]: Drawings from the Years 1942–1944) (Hebrew) (Haifa and Givat Hayim Ihud: The Technion, The Ruth and Bruce Rappaport Faculty of Medicine, and Beit Terezín, 2001); Dieter Kunz, ed., *Deadly Medicine: Creating the Master Race* (Washington, DC: United States Holocaust Memorial Museum, 2004); Yehoshua Sobol, *Geto* (Ghetto) (Hebrew) (Tel Aviv: Or Am, 1984); Sobol, *Bamartef* (In the Basement) (Hebrew) (Tel Aviv: Or Am, 1990); Michael Taub, "Joshua Sobol's Theater and the Shoah's Imperfect Heroes" (paper presented at the conference titled "Jewish Medical Resistance during the Holocaust," YIVO Institute for Jewish Research, New York, November 1996).

Ethics, and the Holocaust. All these conferences included discussions on the aspects of medical activities of both the victims and the perpetrators. The challenge, driven by researchers in the field, to make the study of the history of medicine during the Holocaust an inherent part of all health care professionals' training, was expressed through the Galilee Declaration, signed by the participants of the international conference on "Medicine in the Holocaust and Beyond" in 2017 at Western Galilee College. The declaration calls on all the medical faculties in the world to include in their curricula the study of the history of medicine during the Holocaust and its significance, which is deemed to be essential for all health care professionals worldwide to alert them to the potential of abusing the power of this noble profession.[47] This view was endorsed also by Richard Horton, editor-in-chief of *The Lancet*, in July 2019.[48]

Chronologically, this development originated in the mid-1990s but gained perceptible momentum in the 2000s. In 1992, at a conference of the World Medical Association, a delegation of physicians from Germany nominated a former SS doctor, Hans Joachim Sewering, who had been a member of the National Socialist Party and had been involved in the Nazi "euthanasia" measures, to serve as its chair. This reflected the large-scale integration of Nazi doctors into important positions in the postwar German medical system and the Germans' refusal to confront the medical research conducted during the Nazi era. The United States and Israel had the initiative struck from the agenda.[49]

47 See http://english.wgalil.ac.il/category/Declaration; http://www.medicineaftertheholocaust.org/galilee-declaration/; http://mededirect.org/mimeh/galilee.cfm; Shmuel P. Reis, Hedy S. Wald, and Paul J. Weindling, "The Holocaust, Medicine and Becoming a Physician: The Crucial Role of Education," *Israel Journal of Health Policy Research* (June 2019), https://doi.org/10.1186/s13584-019-0327-3.

48 Richard Horton, "Offline: Medicine and the Holocaust—it's time to teach," *The Lancet*, 394:10193 (July 13, 2019), https://www.thelancet.com/journals/lancet/article/ PIIS0140-6736(19)31608-3/fulltext.

49 See Volker Roelcke, Sascha Topp, and Etienne Lepicard, eds., *Silence, Scapegoats, Self-Reflection: The Shadow of Nazi Medical Crimes on Medicine and Bioethics* (Gottingen: V&R Unipress, 2014). On Sewering, see William E. Seidelman, "'Requiescat sine Pace': Recollections and Reflections on the World Medical

Under the influence of this event, the Israeli Association for Research on Medicine in the Nazi Era was established, and the Sackler Faculty of Medicine at Tel Aviv University has incorporated a regular program of studies on medicine and the Holocaust in its curriculum since the mid-1990s. The historian Daniel Nadav was among those who initiated the process and served as a main lecturer in the program. Additional doctors from the school researched the topic, including Prof. Avi (Avraham) Ohry, an expert on rehabilitative medicine and the nephew of one of the doctors who studied hunger in the Warsaw ghetto.

Since the turn of the twenty-first century, several additional medical institutions in various countries have begun to promote the teaching of medicine in the Holocaust. This process received expression in presentations at the aforementioned Western Galilee conference in 2017, during a one-day session devoted to "Learning Curricula and Teaching about Medicine in the Holocaust and Beyond," by physicians and historians from Europe, the United States, and Israel, who teach this field at universities.[50] At the same time, physicians and historians who

Association, the Case of Prof. Dr. Hans Joachim Sewering and the Murder of Babette Fröwis," in Roelcke, Topp, and Lepicard, *Silence, Scapegoats, Self-Reflection*, pp. 281–301; Gerrit Hohendorf, "The Sewering Affair," in Roelcke, Topp, and Lepicard, *Silence, Scapegoats, Self-Reflection*, pp. 131–147.

50 Lecturers who taught the subject of "Medicine and the Holocaust" to students of the health care professions included Therkel Straede, of the University of Southern Denmark; Sheldon Rubenfeld, of Baylor College of Medicine, Houston, Texas; Hedy S. Wald, of Warren Alpert Medical School of Brown University; Stacy Gallin, director of the Maimonides Institute for Medicine; Esteban González López, of Autonoma University of Madrid; Rosa Ríos, Spain; Kamila Uzarczyk, of the Medical University of Wrocław; Ashley K. Fernandes, of the Center for Bioethics and Medical Humanities, Ohio State University College of Medicine; and Elisabeth Rögler, of Hamburg, Germany. For academic publications on teaching "Medicine and the Holocaust" at faculties of medicine, see, for example, Ashley Fernandes, "Nazi Medicine and the Holocaust: Implications for Bioethics Education and Professionalism," in John J. Michalczyk, ed., *Nazi Law: From Nuremberg to Nuremberg* (London and New York: Bloomsbury Academic, 2018), pp. 139–153; Esteban González-López and Rosa Ríos-Cortés, "Medical Student's Opinions on Some Bioethical Issues before and after a Holocaust and Medicine Course," *IMAJ*, 18:5 (May 2016), pp. 257–260; Shmuel Reis and Hedy S. Wald, "Contemplating Medicine during the Third Reich: Scaffolding Professional

engage in this field encourage medical students and health care practitioners to visit memorial sites where the medical activity took place under the Nazi regime.[51]

This stage of the development of the study of medical activity in the Holocaust is especially conspicuous in Israel, "the land of the survivors." [52] The ascent of the medicine–Holocaust nexus to the daily agenda of doctors in Israel found edifying expression at the Eighteenth International Conference of the Israel Medical Association, held in April 2007. During the four-day colloquium, devoted to the topic of "Advanced Technologies and Medicine," a full day was reserved for discussions on medicine and the Holocaust. Twenty of the approximately 100 medical lectures delivered at the event centered on this theme.[53] All of the five faculties of medicine in Israel include courses on medicine during the Holocaust (still only optional rather than compulsory). One of the leading personalities in this activity in Israel is Prof. Shaul Shasha, who directed Western Galilee Hospital in Nahariya for

Identity Formation for Medical Students," *Academic Medicine: Journal of the Association of American Medical Colleges*, 90:6 (June 2015), doi: 10.1097/ACM.0000000000000716; Tessa Chelouche and Geoffrey Brahmer, *Casebook on Bioethics and the Holocaust* (Haifa: UNESCO Chair in Bioethics, Israel National Commission for UNESCO, and the Ministry of Education, 2013).

51 See, for example, Anthony S. Oberman, Tal Brosh-Nissimov, and Nachman Ash, "Medicine and the Holocaust: A Visit to the Nazi Death Camps as a Means of Teaching Medical Ethics in the Israel Defense Forces Medical Corps," *Journal of Medical Ethics*, 36:12 (December 2010), pp. 821–826. The Israel Medical Association's Witnesses in White Project offers its members medical tours for physicians to memorial sites in Poland and Germany; see https://www.ima.org.il/MainSiteNew/ViewCategory.aspx?CategoryId=8519.

52 Between 1946 and 1956, the young State of Israel handled the mass immigration of about 900,000 Jews, including approximately 380,000 Holocaust survivors. By 1956, the total population numbered 1,667,455. In other words, at that time, one in four Jews in Israel were survivors and the medical system in Israel had to cope with morbidity among many of them. This might be one reason for the heightened interest in this field among physicians in Israel. See Mark Meir Dworzecki, "Be'ayot Demografiyot Uviyologiyot Shel Aliyat Nitzolei Artzot Hashoah" (Demographic and Biological Problems of Immigrants from the Holocaust Countries), *Niv Harofe* (Hebrew), 3–4 (1957), pp. 3–14.

53 *Eighteenth Israel Medical Association World Fellowship International Conference: "Advanced Technologies and Medicine," Programs and Abstracts, 95th Year Anniversary, Jerusalem, April 11–15, 2007*, pp. 87–105.

eighteen years, and has been holding annual conferences on morbidity and medicine in the Holocaust era since 2001. He also encourages research on morbidity among Holocaust survivors. Many other physicians, who hold senior positions in various institutions, are part of this activity.[54]

What motivated the doctors at this specific point in time, sixty years after the fact, to engage in such intensive activity? Several factors appear to have converged. In his article on the mental state of the Holocaust survivors, Dr. Shmuel (Tommy) Steier finds that the attitudes of medical professionals toward the survivors reflect the changes that Israeli society underwent concerning this issue. As described in many studies, the host society in Israel's first three decades treated Holocaust survivors with empathy and a sense of obligation, but also stigmatized them as representatives of the "exile" who, in many cases, had "gone like lambs to the slaughter," or who were suspected of being "egotistic."[55] The survivors were denied due attention to their special needs. In addition, the medical caregivers found it difficult to cope with these patients' distress and to provide them with professional treatment to relieve their extreme traumas. However, since the late 1970s—after the public drew insights from the Eichmann trial in which the survivors had been allowed to speak

54 Another salient accomplishment was the establishment of a program of research on medicine and the Holocaust at the Faculty of Medicine of the Technion, the fruit of an initiative by Prof. Shmuel Reis and the late Dr. Tomi Spenser, a central actor in the field who had been saved by the Kindertransport in 1939. In 2008–2009, a research and teaching group on "Medicine and the Holocaust" began to operate at the Faculty of Health Sciences of Ben-Gurion University of the Negev, led by Prof. William Seidelman, a world-renowned researcher on Nazi medicine. Its participants include Prof. Alan Jotkowitz, head of the Lord Rabbi Immanuel Jakobovits Center for Jewish Medical Ethics, and Prof. Shifra Shvarts of the Moshe Prywes Center for Medical Education. The group operates in conjunction with the Project for Holocaust and Medicine at Boston University, headed by the psychiatrist Prof. Michael Grodin. This subject is taught also at the Faculty of Medicine of the Hebrew University of Jerusalem and the Azrieli Faculty of Medicine of Bar-Ilan University, located in Safed.

55 There is extensive literature on this subject; see, for example, Tom Segev, *The Seventh Million: The Israelis and the Holocaust* (New York: Farrar, Straus, and Giroux, 1993); Hanna Yablonka, *Survivors of the Holocaust: Israel after the War* (London: Macmillan, 1999).

out and after Israel had suffered a series of wars that threatened its very existence—this tendency in society has changed. Now the trend of thought took the form of identification and sympathy to the extent of idealization. This new propensity impacted medical research, yielding a perceptible upturn in studies by doctors on morbidity among the survivors. One may surmise that some of these doctors felt that it was necessary to correct the earlier distortion.[56]

Furthermore, the 1990s saw a profusion of studies about Nazi medicine in medical journals worldwide and one may presume that these works influenced the surge in the study of Jewish medical activity.[57] Historical studies on Jewish medicine, albeit few in number, also sparked their interest in the history of their colleagues during the Holocaust. The aging and death

56 Shmuel (Tommy) Steier, "Madua Hem Shatku Shuv? Al Matzavam Hanafshi Shel Nitzolei Hashoah Vehityahasut Hahevra Vehametaplim Eleihem"(Why Were They Silent Again? About the Psychological Condition of Holocaust Survivors and Attitudes of Society and Therapists), *Harefu'a* (Hebrew), 149:4 (April 2009), pp. 219–223. See also, for example, Steier, "Al Matzavam Habriyuti Shel Nitzolei Hashoah: Ha'im Kayemet Tahlua Organit Meuheret?" (On the Health Status of Holocaust Survivors: Is There Late Organic Morbidity?) *Israeli Journal of Family Practice* (Hebrew), 150 (October 2009); Anatol Livshitz, Avraham Ohry, and Shaul Shasha, "Tahlua Meuheret Bekerev Nitzolei Shoah" (Late Morbidity among Holocaust Survivors), *Harefu'a* (Hebrew), 148:4 (May 2009), pp. 224–228; Naama Fund, Avi Porath, Nachman Ash, et al., "Comorbidity Rates Between Holocaust Survivors and Individuals in the General Population in Israel." *JAMA Netw Open*, 2:1:e186643 (2019), doi: 10.1001/jamanetworkopen.2018.6643.

57 The fields of the academic study of Nazi medicine and of Jewish medicine developed later than other fields of Holocaust study—only from the 1980s onward, and for completely different reasons. The seeds of study on Jewish medicine, begun by survivor–physicians, were shunted aside in favor of other topics that troubled the historians who researched the "victims." As for the German physicians who had worked in the service of the Nazis and continued in senior positions after the war, they deliberately silenced the study of criminal German medicine during World War II. A description of the development of the study of Nazi medicine is beyond the scope of this book. However, for a comparison between the development of the study of Nazi medicine and of Jewish medicine, see Miriam Offer, "Ma'arach Harefu'a Begeto Varsha Bitkufat Hashoah: Irguno Ve'etgarav Hamiktzo'iyim Bithumei Harefu'a Veha'etika Beheksher Histori" (The Medical Services in the Warsaw Ghetto during the Holocaust: Its Organization and Its Medical and Ethical Challenges in Historical Context) (Hebrew) (PhD diss., Bar-Ilan University, 2010), pp. 25–32.

of the survivor–doctors fostered the conviction among many of their colleagues in this field that the testimonies and history of these Jewish physicians who had contended with medical issues under Nazi rule should be memorialized. Some doctors escorted groups on visits to Poland and returned with greater curiosity and motivation to investigate. Personal background as "second-generation Holocaust survivors," in the broad sense of the term, encouraged the developments described above. It is an exceptional phenomenon and, in all likelihood, unique to the medical profession.

Thus, the fifth stage is marked by the unique phenomenon of heightened public and academic interest in the study of medicine during the Holocaust among doctors, historians, ethicists, educators, and the general public. Toward the end of the 2000s, there was an awakening of the study of Jewish medicine. The present era sees growing cooperation among historians and doctors and in other disciplines in different countries. This cooperation breeds hope for the development of in-depth, comprehensive studies that will shed light on medical activity during the Holocaust—of which more is still hidden than known.

* * *

This overview of the evolution of research on medicine in the Holocaust shows that, given the public and research interest in the field, it is all the more necessary to present historical research that will yield the most comprehensive picture possible of the history of medicine in the Holocaust. The purpose of such research is to facilitate thorough discourse about the significance, conclusions, and undertakings that arises from this grim and trying period for the community of doctors and, no less, their patients.

The aim of this book is to impart an understanding of the uniqueness of the Holocaust—the Nazis' persecution and murder of the Jews—among genocides. I will describe, inter alia, how the scale, complexion, and relatively high level of the Jewish medical settings in Warsaw, and the speed with which they organized rested on an infrastructure of Jewish medicine that had been developed previously, with an emphasis on the interwar era. I will also show that nothing like this occurred in any other genocide.

Alongside the description of the impressive organizational work that this medical system entailed, this book describes the ghastly moral dilemmas that the medical staff in the ghetto had to confront—the kinds that doctors never face under ordinary circumstances—from having to select able-bodied men for dispatch to forced labor camps, knowing many would perish, and thus implicating themselves in sealing the fates of these men, to having to exercise unmediated, personal, and direct judgment, at the Germans' command, over who should live and who should die. The book reveals little-known and hair-raising testimonies and documents about the details of the selections that members of the medical staff carried out.

In the eyes of quite a few researchers and witnesses, nearly all the doctors, nurses, and other members of the medical staff were moral saints, who were willing to risk their lives and to toil unrelentingly on behalf of their ill and needy brethren. This study argues that such a description presents an embellished, one-dimensional picture. What really happened was much more complex. Heroic and courageous feats by doctors, worthy of awe and admiration, were accompanied by instances of deficient moral conduct. At the personal level, the behavior of doctors as individuals differed little from that of many other ghetto officials. All faced unparalleled moral tests that some failed and others passed valiantly. Collectively, however, the well-developed medical and health care system that operated in the Warsaw ghetto is a historical phenomenon that has no parallel. This book attempts to shed light on this unique phenomenon and to explain its origins as thoroughly as possible.

PART ONE

Jewish Medicine in Poland on the Eve of the Holocaust and the Onset of the Nazi Occupation

Chapter One

The Jewish Medical System in Interwar Warsaw and Its Collapse under Nazi Occupation

The situation of Jewish doctors worldwide worsens with each passing day. The global economic crisis, the economic shocks, are affecting their material conditions, burdening their lives, causing internal rivalry among them, and degrading their status morally and materially. Furthermore, in the Central and Eastern European countries, the new nation-states' politics of privation and annihilation seeks to destroy the Jewish doctor's livelihood, diminish his rights and his opportunities to develop, and enclose him in a ghetto of limited employment, with no possibility of unrestricted medical endeavor and scientific work. On top of everything, the Hitler government's destructive policy regarding the Jewish doctor and his profession aims not only to isolate him from the outside world behind a fortified wall, preventing any contact and trade, but also to subject the giants of Jewish medical science to indignities and humiliation, vigorously and contemptuously, thus slighting men of repute who have engraved their names into the medical profession in letters of gold. This toxin of atavistic hatred, flowing in the heart of Europe, poses an immense menace that strikes at the heart of the entire class of doctors worldwide, wherever they may be.[1]

1 David Aryeh Friedman, ed., *Sefer Hakongres Ha'olami Harishon Shel Rof'im Yehudim* (Book of the First World Congress of Jewish Physicians) (Hebrew) (Tel Aviv: Harefu'a, 1936), pp. 52–53. I thank Prof. Avi Ohry for calling my attention to this edition of the historically invaluable journal.

Dr. Leon (Lejb) Wulman, a Jewish physician from Poland, delivered these chilling words about the plight of the Jewish doctors in Europe at the First World Congress of Jewish Physicians, held at the Ohel Shem Hall in Tel Aviv in April 1936, three years after Hitler vaulted to the German chancellorship.

Approximately 1,200 people attended this inaugural conference, including 68 Jewish doctors from Poland,[2] who were among 213 physicians representing 14 Diaspora communities. Prominent among them were Dr. Wulman of Warsaw, then secretary general of the Jewish health care organization TOZ—Towarzystwo Ochrony Zdrowia Ludności Żydowskiej (Society for Safeguarding the Health of the Jewish Population)—and Dr. Israel Milejkowski, who four years later would bear the heavy and tragic burden of managing the Judenrat's Health Department in the Warsaw ghetto. The composition of the participants, the invitation to address the colloquium, and the contents discussed in the course of the event reflected the dire situation that Jewish doctors and Jewish communities faced across Europe and in Poland, which had a very large Jewish population at the time. No one at the conference imagined that World War II would erupt three years later, plunging the Jewish people into the Holocaust.

As they described the problems, the doctors at the congress reported on the development of the Jewish medical system in Poland and elsewhere in the Diaspora, despite the grim conditions. By studying the lectures that were delivered there, it is possible to acquire an additional and important level of appreciation of the primary factors that powered the development of Jewish medicine in the Diaspora, in general, and in Poland, in particular, in the interwar years—from the doctors' perspective.

In this part of the study, which describes the Jewish medical system in interwar Warsaw and the challenges presented to it by

2 For a partial list of doctors from Poland who participated in the Congress as committee members and as delegates, see Friedman, *Sefer Hakongres Ha'olami*, pp. 91–92.

the Nazi occupation, I refer to the research literature and archive documentation on the topic and integrate these doctors' voices into them. Within several years after returning from this congress to Poland, many of these physicians perished in the Holocaust.

Important Processes in Independent Poland and Their Impact on Jewish Life

Interwar Poland was Europe's sixth most populous country and about one-third of its population of 32,000,000 was composed of national minorities. The Jews were the second-largest of these minorities at around 3,500,000 persons, more than 20 percent of all Jews worldwide. Polish Jewry was Europe's largest Jewish center and the world's second-largest, surpassed only by the United States.[3] On the eve of World War I, there were approximately 337,000 Jews in Warsaw—more than 38 percent of its total population.[4]

At the end of the Great War, after approximately 150 years of enslavement by its neighbors to the west and the east, Poland was declared an independent state.[5] The process of assembling the new Poland was accompanied by political strains and suspicions of disloyalty on the part of the national minorities dwelling in the nascent country. In a section of the Versailles accord known as the Minorities Treaty, independent Poland undertook to honor the minorities' rights.[6] After the Poles were forced to sign this covenant,

3 Shlomo Netzer, "Polish Jewry between Two World Wars," in Nahman Tamir, ed., *Polish Jewry before the Holocaust, 1914–1939* (New York: Herzl Press Publication, 1986), pp. 212–216; Joseph Marcus, *Social and Political History of the Jews in Poland, 1919–1939* (London: Mouton, 1978), pp. 15–16; Raphael Mahler, *Yehudei Polin Bein Shtei Milhamot Ha'olam: Historia Kalkalit-Sotzialit Be'or Hastatistika* (Polish Jewry between the World Wars: A Socioeconomic History in the Light of Statistics) (Hebrew) (Tel Aviv: Dvir, 1969), p. 7.

4 Israel Gutman, "Warsaw: Jews during the Holocaust," in Gutman, ed., *Encyclopedia of the Holocaust*, vol. 4, (New York: Macmillan, 1990), p. 1,601; Shmuel Spector and Geoffrey Wigoder, eds., *Encyclopedia of Jewish Life before and during the Holocaust*, vol. 3, (New York: New York University Press, 2001), p. 1,428.

5 Mahler, *Yehudei Polin*, p. 9.

6 Shlomo Netzer, *Ma'avak Yehudei Polin Al Zehuyoteihem Ha'ezrahiyot*

which they considered prejudicial, a "Polish nation-state" mindset—"Poland for the Poles"—developed in the country.[7] The intent was to Polonize the ethnic minorities by assimilating them, except in the case of the Jews, who would be encouraged to emigrate.[8]

The years 1918–1920 saw a wave of anti-Jewish pogroms in Polish cities. In the late 1930s, the antisemitic predispositions of the Polish authorities and the public intensified. As unemployment rose, so did the hatred of minorities. The general xenophobia was amplified by a special dimension of hatred of Jews: political, economic, and religious antisemitism, which in Poland, as in other European countries, became interwar Jewry's greatest problem. The successors to Marshal Józef Klemens Piłsudski, the supreme leader of the Polish state until his death in 1935, introduced brutal anti-Jewish policies in order to promote Polish national unity and accommodated fascist nationalist elements that strove to oust the Jews from their occupations.[9] Antisemitism also gathered momentum in institutions of education, from high school up.[10]

Vehale'umiyot, 1918–1922 (Polish Jewry's Struggle for Its Civil and National Rights, 1918–1922) (Hebrew) (Tel Aviv: Tel Aviv University, 1980), pp. 146–160; Israel Gutman, ed., *Sugiyot Beheker Hashoah: Bikoret Vetruma* (Issues in Holocaust Scholarship: Research and Reassessment) (Hebrew) (Jerusalem: The Zalman Shazar Center, Yad Vashem, 2008), pp. 261–285.

7 Marcus, *Social and Political History*, pp. 10–11.

8 Ezra Mendelson, *Jews of East Central Europe between the World Wars* (Bloomington: Indiana University Press, 1983), pp. 32–43; Bartal and Gutman, *Kiyum Veshever*, vol. 2, pp. 11–12; Shlomo Netzer, "Hama'avak Haparlementari Hayehudi Beveit Hanivharim" (The Jewish Parliamentary Struggle in the Legislature), in Bartal and Gutman, *Kiyum Veshever*, vol. 2, pp. 550–551.

9 Marcus, *Social and Political History*, pp. 15–26; Bartal and Gutman, *Kiyum Veshever*, vol. 2, p. 12; Israel Gutman, "Yehudim–Polanim–Antishemiyut" (Jews–Poles–Antisemitism), in Bartal and Gutman, *Kiyum Veshever*, vol. 2, p. 630.

10 Emanuel Ringelblum, *Polish-Jewish Relations during the Second World War*, ed. by Joseph Kermish and Shmuel Krakowski (Jerusalem: Yad Vashem, 1974), pp. 10–22. This book is a translation into English of only part of the original work in Polish. When citing parts that were not translated, I refer to the Hebrew edition, Ringelblum, *Ktavim Aharonim: Yahasei Polanim–Yehudim, Yanuar 1943–April 1944* (Hebrew) (Jerusalem: Yad Vashem, 1994). See also Ezra Mendelson, *Zionism in Poland: The Formative Years, 1915–1926* (New Haven: Yale University Press, 1981), pp. 1–36.

In addition to the antisemitism that was aggravated by the political situation, the Jews were afflicted by the country's severe economic plight. About two-thirds of the Polish population derived its livelihood from agriculture. Nearly 2,500,000 peasants were unemployed and the resulting poverty sapped the purchasing power of the domestic market and slowed the country's industrial development. The country's rickety economic structure also impaired the Jews' livelihood and the unrest that gripped the Polish public was exploited for political struggles against the Jewish minority.[11]

The Polonization policy, compounded by antisemitic discrimination, barred Jews from employment in the country's principal industries.[12] With the Jews' job opportunities crimped in this manner, most Jews in Warsaw on the eve of the Holocaust were members of the hardscrabble lower-middle class.[13] A few belonged to the proletariat and there was a very thin stratum among the affluent bourgeoisie.[14] Polish Jewry, who accounted for about one-third of the Polish urban population, was mainly employed in manufacturing and trade.[15] The great global economic crisis of 1929–1933 did not overlook the Jews of Poland, including those in Warsaw. The Depression took a toll on the Jewish peddlers and merchants, toppling them into grave economic distress. Warsaw did experience an economic rebound in 1933–1939, but its Jewish townspeople remained in their economic doldrums due to the authorities' discriminatory policies.[16]

11 Marcus, *Social and Political History*, pp. 10–13; Mahler, *Yehudei Polin*, pp. 12–17; Gutman, "Yehudim–Polanim–Antishemiyut," in Bartal and Gutman, *Kiyum Veshever*, vol. 2, pp. 624–625.

12 Mahler, *Yehudei Polin*, pp. 144–151.

13 Ibid., p. 37.

14 Spector and Wigoder, *The Encyclopedia of Jewish Life*, p. 1,429; Tamir, *Polish Jewry before the Holocaust*, p. 240; Moshe Yosef Faigenbaum, ed., *Sefer Biała-Podlaska* (Book of Biała-Podlaska) (Yiddish and Hebrew) (Tel Aviv: Kupat Gmilut Hesed al szem Kehilat Biala-Podlaska, 1961), p. 42; for an English translation of this book, see https://www.jewishgen.org/yizkor/Biala_Podlaska/Biala_Podlaska.html (accessed July 2, 2019).

15 Mahler, *Yehudei Polin*, pp. 36–37.

16 Ibid., p. 189.

The relative preponderance of Warsaw's Jews in trade[17] gave right-wing circles a pretext for anti-Jewish propagandizing in the last five years of independent Poland. Jewish merchants were excoriated as parasites who exploited the Polish nation, leading to a demand to limit their participation in these vocations. As restrictions on trade multiplied, Jews turned increasingly to crafts. On the eve of World War II, about one-third of all Jewish breadwinners in Warsaw made their living in this manner. Jewish manufacturing was concentrated in very small factories that had grown out of workshops—home-based businesses in which extended families were co-opted into production.[18] Sometimes these breadwinners were worse off than the Polish proletarians, because they did not qualify for unemployment insurance, put in longer hours, and lacked health insurance.[19] As it became harder for Polish Jews to find positions in the state and municipal bureaucracies, Jewish academics increasingly returned to the liberal professions. Their proportion in the public services and the free trades exceeded their share in the population, but their presence in these fields centered on vocations and jobs in Jewish public institutions. In the civil service, they constituted a negligible 1 percent.[20]

17 Ibid., pp. 132–133; Raphael Mahler, *Toldot Hayehudim BePolin Ad Hame'a Ha-19: Kalkala, Hevra, Hamatzav Hamishpati* (History of Polish Jewry until the Nineteenth Century: Economy, Society, Legal Status) (Hebrew) (Merhavia: Hakibbutz Hameuchad, 1946), pp. 98–105.

18 Mahler, *Yehudei Polin*, pp. 84–85.

19 Gutman, "Warsaw: Jews during the Holocaust," in Gutman, *Encyclopedia of the Holocaust*, p. 1,601; Abraham Wein, ed., *Pinkas Hakehillot: Entziklopediya Shel Hayishuvim Hayehudiyim Lemin Hivasdam Ve'ad Le'ahar Shoat Milhemet Ha'olam Hashniya, Polin: VarshaVehagalil* (Pinkas Hakehillot: Encyclopedia of Jewish Communities from the Onset to the End of the Holocaust and World War II, Polin: Warsaw and the Environs) (Hebrew), vol. 4, (Jerusalem: Yad Vashem, 1989), p. 64.ed., Pinkas Hakehillot: Entziklopediya Shel Hayishuvim Hayehudiyim Lemin Hivasdam Ve'ad Le'ahar Shoat Milhemet Ha'olam Hashniya, Polin: VarshaVehagalil (Pinkas Hakehillot: Encyclopedia of Jewish Communities from the Onset to the End of the Holocaust and World War II, Polin: Warsaw and the Environs) (Hebrew), vol. 4, (Jerusalem: Yad Vashem, 1989), p. 64.

20 Mahler, *Yehudei Polin*, pp. 155–156, 160–163.

In the pre-World War II years, 50 percent of the Jewish population of Warsaw was impoverished and lacked a source of livelihood. In 1933, about half of the Jews in town were exempt from paying even symbolic community dues. On the brink of World War II, one-third of the Jews in Warsaw verged on starvation.[21] Even Polish Jews of means mobilized aid from Jewish organizations outside the country, such as ORT—Obchestvo Remeslenogo Truda (Association for the Promotion of Skilled Trades), ICA—Jewish Charitable Association, and AJJDC—American Jewish Joint Distribution Committee), commonly known as JDC.[22]

In the interwar period, with the Jewish centers cut off from Russia, Polish Jewry became the largest Jewish concentration in Europe, whose main struggle was recognition as a national minority with rights in the new Poland. The Jews of Poland demanded full equality of rights and freedom of political, cultural, and social expression as a separate national minority. These demands, however, did not square with the Polish state's political and social attitudes toward its national minorities. Although denied the recognition that they sought, the Jews took the initiative of organizing as an independent parliamentary group. They established an autonomous Jewish communal and partisan system that oversaw the formation of diverse, professional, Jewish educational and cultural services, and sustained the Jewish religious tradition to which many adhered. They also developed mutual-aid operations, and undertook supportive and protective actions for the Jewish population.[23]

The spiritual world of Polish Jewry was diverse, accommodating contrasts and disagreements. In the religious domain,

21 Michael Melamed, "Hevrot Legmilut Hasadim" (Free Loan Societies), in Itzhak Gruenbaum et al., *Entziklopediya Shel Galuyot*: *Varsha* (Encyclopedia of the Jewish Diaspora: Warsaw) (Hebrew), vol. 1, (Jerusalem and Tel Aviv: Encyclopedia of the Jewish Diaspora Co., 1953–1956), p. 599; Wein, *Pinkas Hakehillot*, pp. 64–65.

22 Melamed, "Hevrot Legmilut Hasadim," p. 225; Mahler, *Yehudei Polin*, p. 189.

23 Gutman, *The Jews of Warsaw*, p. 119; Netzer, "Polish Jewry between Two World Wars," pp. 206–212.

the Mitnaggedim and Hasidim maintained their differences vis-à-vis the rest of the Jewish world and even among themselves. In the second half of the nineteenth century, new and modern political and social organizations came into being, but the traditional schism persisted.[24] Ideological disparities were also vast, ranging from the Irgun Zvai Leumi to the Socialist–Yiddishist Bund. Nevertheless, Bartal and Gutman state, "The cultural mentality, the organizational patterns, and the modus operandi of all these groups belonged to one political culture. The similarities among the diverse groups and their cultural discourse indicate that they constitute a national collective, distinct from its surroundings and aware of its singularity."[25]

History of Jewish Medicine in Poland

Rabbi Moshe Avigdor Amiel, born in Porozów, a shtetl in Poland, was named chief rabbi of Tel Aviv in 1936. Inaugurating the World Congress of Jewish Physicians that year, he delivered greetings to the participants and stressed the importance that Judaism attributes to medicine and the preservation of health.

> In our Torah, safeguarding physical health has a primary place, because it is indeed a duty of life. "You must safeguard your souls"—this is the most important commandment of all. All [other] commandments in the Torah yield to it. There is no single commandment in the Torah that does not yield to the preservation of life. In relating to every commandment, we say, "[You shall] live by them [the commandments] and not die by them." The Hebrews, not the Romans, coined the

24 In this matter, see David Engel, "Hamegamot Hapolitiyot Vehatarbut Hapolitit Shel Yehudei Polin" (The Political Trends and Political Culture of Polish Jewry), in Bartal and Gutman, *Kiyum Veshever*, vol. 2, pp. 649–665.

25 Ibid., pp. 9–14. For a succinct summary of the characteristics of European Jewry on the eve of the Holocaust, see Saul Friedländer, *Nazi Germany and the Jews, 1939–1945: The Years of Extermination* (New York: Harper Perennial, 2007), pp. 4–10.

> adage "a healthy soul in a healthy body," which is fundamental in the Torah. Therefore, the Sages said, "The [Divine] presence resides only in the wise and the strong," because physical strength is as important in our eyes as psychological strength. And we add the prayer for "a life of the extrication of bones" to the prayer for "a life that has fear of heaven and fear of sin." These are the main fundamentals in our Torah. Therefore, we see the Deity at every sickbed, [as though] He Himself sits there, as it is stated, "May God nurse us on the deathbed." And it is no wonder that we find Jewish doctors to be the greatest experts, because to be an expert physician one needs not only a sharp mind but also a good heart, [a sense of] mercy that rues every person's anguish. Now, who is like the People of Israel, a people of mercy? Mercy is the Jews' foremost characteristic, it is typical that we even call God *Rahmana* [the Merciful One].[26]

Indeed, the Jews have developed great appreciation for the medical field throughout their history. Jewish medicine includes both preventive and therapeutic elements. The Torah lays down basic rules of sanitation, which many East European Jews strictly observed as they went about their lives. Many religious commandments address the prevention and control of morbidity throughout the life cycle. The Torah's stringencies pertaining to health originate in the Jewish perception of the body as a receptacle for the mind, the soul, and the heart—a gift

26 Friedman, *Sefer Hakongres Ha'olami*, p. 37. Rabbi Moshe Avigdor Amiel (1882–1946) was a rabbi, a rabbinical judge, a philosopher, and a leading personality in the religious Zionist movement. Ordained as a rabbi at the age of eighteen, he was named rabbi of the town of Święciany at twenty-three and served as a rabbi in Grajewo on the Russian–German border during World War I, rabbi of the community of Antwerp in 1920–1936, and chief rabbi of Tel Aviv from 1936. As for the attitude of the Halacha (rabbinical law) toward the medical profession, see, for example, Avraham Steinberg, ed., *Sefer Asiya: Ma'amarim, Tamtziyot Veskirot Be'inyanei Refu'a Vehalaha* (The Book of Health: Articles, Abstracts, and Overviews on Medicine and Halakha) (Hebrew) (Jerusalem: Reuven Mas, 1970–2009); Avraham Steinberg, *Entziklopediya Hilhatit Refu'it* (Encyclopedia of Jewish Medical Law) (Hebrew) (Jerusalem: Machon Shlezinger Leheker Harefu'a Al Pi Hatorah, 1988–2009).

from God that its recipient must protect.[27] This attitude toward health and illness was highly central in Jewish communities. An illness of a community member raised concern among those near and far, prompting the mobilization of nursing, healing, and moral support. The weak population received special attention.[28]

The Jewish community encouraged specialization within the medical profession and accomplished much within its own society in the modern era. Doctors in European Jewish society played a special role as providers of medical care and as leaders in all fields of intellectual, communal, and political endeavor. In the period preceding World War II, the Jewish medical world saw its greatest efflorescence in the history of Jewish medicine up to that time.[29] Jewish doctors from countries as diverse as Germany, Spain, and *Eretz Israel* had been practicing in Poland since the tenth century CE.[30]

27 Mark Zborowski and Elizabeth Herzog, *Life Is with People: The Jewish Little-Town in Eastern Europe* (New York: International University Press, 1953); F. H. Garrison, *An Introduction to the History of Medicine*, 4th Edition (Philadelphia and London: W. B. Saunders Company, 1929); Solomon R. Kagan, *Jewish Medicine* (Boston: Medico-Historical Press, 1952); Immanuel Jakobovits, *Jewish Medical Ethics—A Comparative and Historical Study of the Jewish Religious Attitude to Medicine and Its Practice* (New York: Bloch Publishing Company, 1975).

28 Jacob Jay Lindenthal, "Abi Gezunt: Health and the Eastern European Immigrant," *American Jewish History*, 70 (1981), pp. 420–441; Zborowski and Herzog, *Life Is with People*, p. 354.

29 Yulian Rafes, "The Ethical and Human Dimension of Jewish Medical Resistance during the Holocaust," in Grodin, *Jewish Medical Resistance*, p. 273. Among the famous doctors in nineteenth-century Europe were Judah (Leo) Pinsker, the author of *Autoemancipation*, the first work on modern ideological Zionism, in which the diagnosis of European antisemitism is presented as a psychopathological problem, and Max Nordau, Herzl's adviser and a member of the World Zionist organization. See Allan Nadler, "Jewish Medical Resistance during the Holocaust: Selected Papers Presented at a Conference at the YIVO Institute for Jewish Research, New York, November 1996" (unpublished manuscript), pp. 1–6. See also Avi Ohry and Amihai Levi, "Leon Pinsker, Bimlot Me'a Shana Leveidat Katovitz" (Leon Pinsker on the Centenary of the Katowitz Conference), in Samuel Kottek, ed., *Korot: Shnaton Letoldot Harefu'a Umada'ei Hateva* (Korot: Yearbook on the History of Medicine and the Natural Sciences) (Hebrew), vol. 8, (Jerusalem: The Hebrew University Magnes Press, 1984), pp. 326–329.

30 Wulman et al., *The Martyrdom of Jewish Physicians in Poland*, p. 3.

Jewish historians in interwar Poland laid the foundations of research on the history of Jewish medicine in that country, in general, and in Warsaw, in particular. One of the most prominent among them was Dr. Emanuel Ringelblum, one of the forces behind the Oneg Shabbat (or Oyneg Shabbes) Archive, the Warsaw ghetto archive documentation enterprise. In the 1930s, Ringelblum, who perished in the Holocaust, managed to write a series of studies that were published in various forums. Several of them—scientific articles on Jewish doctors' contribution to medicine in Poland—appeared in *Sotsiale Meditsin*, the Jewish periodical on social medicine affairs.[31]

Ringelblum's studies and those of other historians indicate that the activity of Jewish physicians in Poland dates back to the fifteenth century. Notwithstanding the limitations of the archive material, one may point to about 170 physicians who practiced in Poland by the end of the eighteenth century. It is evident that they were integral to the state's medical services and that they made a definitive contribution to the Polish medical profession. A list of 124 Jewish doctors who practiced in dozens of towns and districts across the country, including in at least sixteen in Warsaw, in the eighteenth century, has been preserved.

After the expulsion from Spain in 1492, Jews were barred from studying medicine at universities and from practicing other scientific professions in all European countries, including Poland, with the exception of the universities of Padua and Salerno in

31 On Ringelblum see, for example, Israel Gutman, "Emanuel Ringelblum: Historion Vezmano" (Emanuel Ringelblum: The Historian and His Times), in Israel Gutman, *Emanuel Ringelblum: Ha'adam Vehahistorion* (Emanuel Ringelblum: The Man and the Historian) (Hebrew) (Jerusalem: Yad Vashem, 2006), p. 81; Emanuel Ringelblum, "Yidishe feldsher in Amoliker Poylen," *Sotsiale Meditsin*, 9–10 (1932), pp. 128–130; Ringelblum, "Di rekhtlikhe lage fun yidishe doktoyrim in Poylen," *Sotsiale Meditsin*, 7–8 (1936), pp. 11–12; Ringelblum, "Tsveite reshime fun yidishe doktoyrim in Poylen," *Sotsiale Meditsin*, 3–4 (1933), pp. 43–47; Ringelblum, "Baitrogen tsu der geshikhte fun di yidishe doktoyrim in Poylen," *Sotsiale Meditsin*, 9–10 (1931), pp. 127–131; Samuel D. Kassow, *Who Will Write Our History? Emanuel Ringelblum, the Warsaw Ghetto, and the Oyneg Shabes Archive* (Bloomington and Indianapolis: Indiana University Press, 2007).

Italy.[32] From the seventeenth century onward, the universities of Frankfurt and Göttingen also began to open their doors to Jewish medical students. In Cracow and Vilna, in contrast, Jews were not admitted until the early nineteenth century. In defiance of the Catholic Church, which enjoined its believers against obtaining medical services from Jewish doctors, many Poles benefited from these doctors' treatments. Some actually preferred them, both because they attributed hidden power to the Jews' singularities as members of a heretic faith and a foreign race, and because Jewish doctors had acquired a reputation due to their professional attainments. Polish monarchs, aristocrats, and even high clergy employed Jewish physicians in their courts. The last of the Polish kings to do so was Stanisław Poniatowski, who wound up the independent Polish kingdom era in 1795.[33]

In the course of the eighteenth century, Jewish physicians, many of whom had been certified on the basis of examination diplomas, practiced in small communities.[34] In most communities, these doctors also attended to the health of poor inhabitants. They were required to help any patient on his or her deathbed, and apothecaries had to provide the indigent with medicines at no charge. Even as modern medicine developed, folk medicine persisted among Polish Jewry. There were rabbis who "treated" diseases by means of prayers and amulets, druggists who provided preparations based on personal knowledge, midwives who were expert in warding off the evil eye, experts in medicinal herbs, and

32 Between 1617 and 1816, the university in Padua awarded medical certification to at least 320 Jews. On the medical studies of Jewish students at this institution, see David Ruderman, *Jewish Thought and Scientific Discovery in Early Modern Europe* (New Haven and London: Yale University Press, 1995), pp. 100–117; Saul Menashe Shasha and Saul G. Massri, "Hafakulta Lerefu'a BePadova Uvogreha Hayehudim" (The Medical School of Padua and Its Jewish Graduates), *Harefu'a* (Hebrew), 141:4 (2002), pp. 388–394.

33 Natan Michael Gelber, "Letoldot Harof'im Hayehudim BePolin Bame'a Hashmone Esre" (On the History of Jewish Doctors in Poland in the Eighteenth Century), in Joseph Tirosh, ed., *Shai LeYeshayahu: Sefer Yovel Le'R' Yeshayahu Volfsberg* (A Gift to Isaiah: The R. Isaiah Wolfsberg Jubilee Book) (Hebrew) (Tel Aviv: Hapo'el Hamizrachi Cultural Center, 1957), pp. 347–371.

34 Mahler, *Yehudei Polin*, pp. 152–153.

the *rebbetzin*, who acted as a savant in women's maladies.[35] Doctors and some rabbis urged the Jewish public to beware of witch doctors[36] and criticized the practices of the feldshers [paramedics]. These seventeenth-century healers provided the royal army with medical services based on practical and theoretical training in medicine and surgery that was nevertheless inferior to those administered by the academically schooled.[37]

In the eighteenth century and increasingly in the nineteenth, as the Emancipation and the Haskalah proceeded, Jewish students began to seek medical training outside of Poland. The main characteristic of Polish statehood at this time was the loss of independence and subordination to the neighboring powers—Russia, Prussia, and Austria—which brought the development of many fields of national endeavor to a halt. The advance of higher education institutions in Poland was also heavily restricted during this time, which prompted the pursuit of studies in foreign countries. The Jewish doctors who returned to Poland brought the influence of the university schooling that they had acquired primarily in Western and Central Europe. Alongside their professional contribution to medicine, they became social leaders in their communities, serving as role models in modern Jewish

35 Gelber, "Letoldot Harof'im Hayehudim BePolin," pp. 347–371; Mordechai Lensky, "Rof'im Yehudim Mefursamim" (Famous Jewish Doctors), in Gruenbaum et al., *Entziklopediya Shel Galuyot: Varsha*, vol. 6, part 2, p. 307; Leah Aldor, "Aspektim Shel Moderna Bashtetl Hapolani: Hatatzlumim Benosei Harefu'a Vehasport Besifrei Hazikaron" (Aspects of Modernity in the Polish Shtetl: Photographs on Medical and Sports Themes in Memorial Books) (Hebrew) (Master's thesis, The Hebrew University of Jerusalem, 1995), p. 32.

36 Alexander Gutterman, "Hatza'oteihem Shel Yehudei Polin Letikunim Bema'amadam Hahuki Hakalkali Hahevrati Vehatarbuti Bitkufat Haseym Hagadol" (Proposals by Polish Jews for Corrections to Their Legal, Economic, Social, and Cultural Status at the Time of the Great Sejm) (Hebrew) (Master's thesis, The Hebrew University of Jerusalem, 1975), p. 57; John Maurice Efron, *Medicine and the German Jews: A History* (New Haven: Yale University Press, 2001), pp. 84–87.

37 On the history of the feldshers, see Edward Kossoy and Abraham Ohry, *The Feldshers, Medical, Sociological and Historical Aspects of Practitioners of Medicine with Below University Level Education* (Jerusalem: Magnes Press, 1992); Aldor, "Aspektim Shel Moderna," pp. 30, 35; Gelber, "Letoldot Harof'im Hayehudim BePolin," p. 367. According to Gelber, feldshers practiced in 197 cities in 1775.

culture, and combining familiarity with Jewish tradition with general education.

These doctors became renowned among both the Jewish and the Polish populations, devoted themselves to scientific research, and mobilized for public action to improve health sanitation in their communities. However, the Jewish doctors' success and the appreciation that they received led Polish physicians to see their Jewish colleagues as rivals and to be jealous of them. A doctrine of hatred directed at the Jewish doctors began to take shape. Tales about Jewish physicians' "nefarious schemes" against Christian patients were concocted and the litany of allegations spread to public writings.[38] This ambivalence toward Jewish doctors continued in the nineteenth century and throughout the interwar years, when Poland basked in its newly regained independence.[39]

In the course of the nineteenth century, coinciding with what Polish political history calls the "partitions era"—from the beginning of the first partition in 1772 to the recovery of independence in 1918—the general shortage of hospitals and medical schools in Poland continued, particularly in Warsaw. However, the population of Jewish doctors grew steadily since the Jews studied abroad, as previously stated. Dr. Mordechai Lensky, a physician and survivor of the Warsaw ghetto, drew up a list of eighteen doctors, most of whom had practiced in Warsaw during this time and had earned international renown for their studies and achievements in their medical specialties. They include Prof. Maurici Hirszfeld, an expert in anatomy and the nervous system; Dr. Mosze Studencki, a social-minded physician known as the "doctor of the poor"; Dr. Ludwik Natansohn, a prodigiously accomplished gynecologist, who also headed the Warsaw Jewish community, edited the medical journal *Gazeta Lekarski*, the physicians' periodical, and chaired the Polish Medical Association; Dr. Samuel Goldflam, a neurologist and Zionist, who chaired the Association of Neurologists in Warsaw; Dr. Edward Flatau, who

38 Gelber, "Letoldot Harof'im Hayehudim BePolin," pp. 347–371.

39 For an interesting analysis of the corresponding state of affairs in German society, see Friedländer, *Nazi Germany and the Jews*, pp. 73–112.

published an atlas of the human brain; Dr. Teofil Simchowitz, who researched "old-age mania"; and Prof. Mieczysław Minkowski, a world-renowned neurologist.[40]

In an effort to contend with the deficient health care system upon returning to Poland, the doctors developed the philosophy of medicine, which became a central part of a unique curriculum taught in Polish medical schools.[41] In the course of the nineteenth century and the early twentieth, Jewish doctors made a crucial contribution to the advancement of medicine in Poland. They excelled in all branches of the profession and were pioneers in research on pathogens and the struggle to defeat them. A large proportion of Jewish doctors embraced Christianity in order to overcome the barriers to the advancement of their scientific careers. Nevertheless, their work in the Jewish communities was their main livelihood. Some Jewish doctors who became renowned as successful scientists abroad emigrated from Poland.

In the early 1920s, Poland had four universities—in Cracow, Warsaw, Lwów, and Vilna—and each had a medical school. More hospitals were built and furnished with modern professional equipment. The number of physicians increased, as did the percentage of Jews among them. In Warsaw alone, according to Dr. Reuven Ben-Shem, approximately 130 Jewish doctors were practicing in the early twentieth century.[42] The proportion of Jewish

40 Lensky, "Rof'im Yehudim Mefursamim," pp. 307–323; Offer, "Ma'arach Harefu'a Begeto Varsha," vol. 2, appendix D.1, pp. 248–249.

41 Ilana Lowy, *The Polish School of Philosophy of Medicine: From Tytus Chalubinski (1820–1889) to Ludwik Fleck (1896–1961)* (Dordrecht: Kluwer, 1998), pp. 1–5. Immensely prominent in this field were the studies of the Jewish doctor and philosopher Ludwik Fleck, who researched the theory of consciousness, aspects of medical taxonomy, and sociocultural factors that influence medicine; see Arye Fleck, "Al Refu'a Bitkufat Hashoah" (On Medicine in the Holocaust Era), *Harefu'a* (Hebrew), 82:3 (1972), p. 136; Fleck, "Refu'a Umada Bitkufat Hakibush Hanatzi" (Medicine and Science during the Nazi Occupation Period), *Harefu'a* (Hebrew), 32:2 (1997), pp. 91–92; Yuval Goldbort and Avraham Ohry, "Ludvig Flek: Hoker, Rofe Ufilosof" (Ludwik Fleck: Researcher, Physician, and Philosopher) (Hebrew) (lecture delivered at the Second Nahariya Conference on Medicine and the Holocaust, May 8, 2002). I wish to thank Prof. Avi Ohry for sending me the text of this lecture.

42 Reuven Ben-Shem, "Batei Holim Yehudiyim BeVarsha" (Jewish Hospitals in

doctors rose sharply until the early 1930s. In 1926, 2,965 of the 7,310 doctors in Poland were Jewish—40.5 percent. In the early 1930s, approximately 67,000 Jews had received training in medicine, hygiene, and sanitation, and about half of them were in fact working, constituting 21.7 percent of all medical staff in Poland at the time.[43] Jews prominently represented 56 percent of private physicians. Hospitals and health care clinics employed few Jewish doctors and nurses, leaving their share in these facilities at only 11.9 percent.[44] A 1931 census counted 4,488 Jews among 7,950 private doctors in Poland—more than half of the total number. Approximately 5,000 of the 10,750 doctors countrywide that year were Jewish.[45]

In the 1930s, as antisemitism escalated, members of organizations of liberal professionals acted to purge their settings of Jews. Thus, many associations of doctors, dentists, engineers, and others, became "Jew-free" pursuant to resolutions adopted by the members at their assemblies.[46] Highly qualified professionals were expelled.[47] The antisemitic camp in the Polish medical profession fought to discriminate against Jews and thwarted their admission to medical professions at the universities.[48] From the early 1920s

Warsaw), in Gruenbaum et al., *Entziklopediya Shel Galuyot: Varsha*, vol. 1, pp. 579–585. See Offer, "Ma'arach Harefu'a Begeto Varsha," vol. 2, appendix D.2, pp. 250–256.

43 Marcus, *Social and Political History*, p. 438; Mahler, *Yehudei Polin*, pp. 47, 159.

44 Mahler, *Yehudei Polin*, pp. 56–57.

45 Ibid., pp. 166–168; Dr. Peter-Heinz Seraphim of Königsberg, an expert in research on East European Jewry under Nazi rule, wrote in *Ost-Europa Markt*, December 1938, that 45 percent of the doctors in Warsaw were Jewish. See "The Economic Role of the Jews in Poland," GFH, no. 1349.

46 "Hama'avak Haparlementari," p. 549; Mahler, *Yehudei Polin*, pp. 163–164.

47 Ringelblum, *Polish–Jewish Relations*, p. 52. At a conference of doctors in 1928, the organizers discriminated against Jews who had been invited to participate. In response, Dr. Soloveichik stood up and cried, "Jewish comrades, let's leave the party!" Indeed, the Jewish doctors walked out. See Lensky, "Rof'im Yehudim Mefursamim," pp. 320–321.

48 On the process used by antisemites to oust Jewish medical personnel in Poland, see "The Jewish Situation in Poland during October, November, and December 1937," bulletin no. 10, American Jewish Joint Distribution Committee, 1938, Archives of the American Jewish Joint Distribution Committee (JDC), AR.33-44, file 815, pp. 8–9.

onward, a numerus clausus policy in university admissions was implemented in order to reduce the number of Jewish physicians in Poland. As the quota for Jewish students was scaled back in the 1930s, the proportion of Jewish doctors in Poland shrank considerably.[49] From 1933 on, young Jewish physicians were barred from residency at Polish hospitals. This period also saw a spate of terminations of veteran Jewish doctors and residents at hospitals and public health care facilities.[50]

A "Call for Proposals" that was published in 1936, ahead of the World Congress of Jewish Physicians, powerfully expresses the deteriorating situation of the Jewish communities in Europe and the threat to the status, work, and achievements of Jewish doctors in view of the extreme political developments described above.

> The grave hardships and decrees, new ones each day, against members of our people in various countries in recent times have been particularly harmful to the status of the doctors, who even in the toughest periods in our national life have earned appreciation and respect. The proliferation of doctors in all countries has created stiff competition with the Jewish

49 Mahler, *Yehudei Polin*, pp. 172–173; Netzer, "Hama'avak Haparlementari," p. 549; Anka Grupińska, "Kah Be'emet: Bishnat 1942 Yatzati Min Habayit Ule'olam Lo Shavti Elav: Siha Im Adina Bladi-Shvaiger" (It's the Truth: In 1942, I Left Home and Never Came Back: A Conversation with Adina Blady-Szwajger) in Anka Grupińska, *Sehor Sehor: Sihot Im Lohamim Migeto Varsha* (Round and Round: Conversations with Fighters from the Warsaw Ghetto) (Hebrew) (Tel Aviv: Hakibbutz Hameuchad, 2002), p. 274n12. In this matter, see also Ringelblum, *Polish-Jewish Relations*, p. 17; M. Zillan, "Hastudentim Hayehudim Bashanim 1915–1939" (Jewish Students in 1915–1939), in Gruenbaum et al., *Entziklopediya Shel Galuyot: Varsha*, vol. 6, part 2, pp. 302–303; and Wulman et al., *The Martyrdom of Jewish Physicians in Poland*, p. 46. While conducting research on Jewish historians in the interwar period, Dr. Natalia Aleksiun consulted a catalogue of students at the University of Warsaw and found that the historian Emanuel Ringelblum had applied to medical school but had been rejected due to the numerus clausus policy. Consequently, he turned to history. See Natalia Aleksiun, "Ammunition in the Struggle for National Rights: Jewish Historians in Poland between the Two World Wars" (PhD diss., New York University, 2010).

50 Mahler, *Yehudei Polin*, pp. 166–168.

> physician. In addition, racist hatred and political animosities have deprived the families of thousands of doctors of their sources of livelihood and the possibility to subsist. Several universities have closed their doors to Jewish scholars. Opportunities for advanced training are vanishing. Medical research institutes are evicting Jewish researchers of world repute, either furtively or with vile explicitness. Thus, a decree of excommunication is being pronounced over an important area of cultural endeavor that until recently was the glory of our people and a benefit to all of humankind. This wave of savage animus, powered by those who hate us, menaces not only the economic situation of a large stratum of the Jewish people and not only the profession and knowledge to which entire generations of civilized people among us have adhered with dignity, but also the state of health of the Jewish masses, which is at risk, as a result of all the various persecutions.[51]

This discriminatory policy prompted the Jews to intensify their activities at Jewish hospitals and medical institutions, which contributed to the development of the independent Jewish medical system. On the eve of World War II, about 3,500 Jewish physicians worked in around forty Jewish hospitals in Poland.[52]

Jewish Health Care Institutions in the Interwar Period

Jewish Tradition of Medical Aid up to the Twentieth Century

Aiding the weak and the ill is entrenched in Jewish tradition. Therefore, welfare and health care activities have been focal in

51 Friedman, *Sefer Hakongres Ha'olami*, p. 10.

52 Wulman et al., *The Martyrdom of Jewish Physicians in Poland*, pp. 46–47.

Jewish community life throughout history. In the last quarter of the eighteenth century, as the Jewish population of Warsaw increased, the community's lay leaders engaged in establishing welfare and health care institutions with the assistance of all the segments and social strata of the Jewish population in Warsaw. The assimilated members founded institutions in the spirit of modern times, while the Orthodox expanded their charitable institutions in the vein of Jewish tradition.

The Jewish welfare organizations were funded by donations from the affluent members of the community and were run by public activists who joined the cause. It was within this framework that medical aid evolved. General hospitals, pediatric hospitals, and convalescent and curative homes were established—some by the community and others through the exertions of societies, synagogues, trade organizations, and so on. Some of these organizations provided basic medical care, while others developed professional caregiving services. These included the Ahim Rahmanim Confraternity, established in 1826 to aid ill members of the community; the Linas Hatzedek Society, instituted in 1882; the Bikur Cholim Association, founded in 1884; and Achiezer, inaugurated in 1901. Many others were set up in the last quarter of the nineteenth century and the early years of the twentieth as well. They assisted with rotating duty at sickbeds, the recruitment of doctors, the acquisition of medicines and food, fundraising, the administration of first aid, and other services. Over time, they set up clinics for the indigent that provided medical aid at a nominal fee. Some even developed professional laboratories, X-ray facilities, electrotherapy clinics, pharmacies, and dental clinics.

An organization named Aid to Poor Mothers, established in 1896, established a maternity home for destitute women and assisted in prenatal care and childbirth. Achiezer created a Medical Department that funded care for needy patients, a laboratory, a shelter for the ill in Otwock, and a pharmacy. A caregiving society for the mentally ill and the poor was founded in 1906. The Jewish Society for War on Tuberculosis was established in 1908 on the initiative of Dr. Josef Dawidzon. The same year saw the formation of a clinic in Warsaw, where thousands of patients would receive care each year, and of a convalescent home in Otwock. Institutions for the deaf and the blind were set up as well.[53] These aid and health care institutions operated with the assistance of American Jewish organizations, such as the JDC, HIAS—Hebrew Immigrant Aid Society—and others, along with Warsaw Jewry's own charitable institutions, which in many areas were crucial. The facilities that enjoyed American support dealt with problems throughout the country in order to help Jews and to steward them toward independent functioning. Local institutions dealt with direct relief.[54]

The Medical Situation of the Jews in Poland after World War I

During World War I and its aftermath, hundreds of thousands of refugees fled from the advancing armies. Many lost their homes and all their property in the flames of the war. Within the confines of the new Poland, about one million Jews were bereft of food and shelter. Their agonies continued through 1918–1922, until Poland's eastern border with the Soviet Union stabilized. The Ukrainians' futile struggle for independence left tens of thousands of Jews dead or wounded, and thousands of orphaned Jewish children.[55]

According to JDC reports, about half of all Jewish children suffered from illnesses, including trichophytosis (ringworm),

53 Reuven Ben-Shem, "Mosdot Ezra Vesa'ad" (Aid and Welfare Institutions), in Gruenbaum et al., *Entziklopediya Shel Galuyot: Varsha*, vol. 1, pp. 587–595.

54 Shalom Baron, "Kavim Lekoroteihem Shel Yehudei Eropa Bein Shtei Milhamot Ha'olam: Edut Bemishpat Eichmann" (Overview of the History of Interwar European Jewry: Testimony at the Eichmann Trial), in Israel Gutman and Livia Rothkirchen, *Shoat Yehudei Eropa: Reka, Korot, Mashma'ut* (The European Holocaust: Background, History, Significance) (Hebrew) (Jerusalem: Yad Vashem, 1973), p. 155; Melamed, "Hevrot Legmilut Hasadim," pp. 560–598; Ben-Shem, "Mosdot Ezra Vesa'ad," pp. 587–588.

55 Yehuda Bauer, *My Brother's Keeper: A History of the American Jewish Joint Distribution Committee, 1929–1939* (Philadelphia: Jewish Publication Society of America, 1974), pp. 6–9; Leon Wulman, "Hevrat Toz" (TOZ Society), in Gruenbaum et al., *Entziklopediya Shel Galuyot: Varsha*, vol. 1, pp. 581–582.

trachoma, skin diseases, heart conditions, rheumatism, and polio. Typhus was rife all over the country. Cholera, introduced by refugees from Ukraine, threatened to spread in the frontier areas. Chickenpox and malaria took a severe toll.[56] In addition to the rampant morbidity, the war between Poland and Russia saw the expropriation of most of the Jewish hospitals, including their equipment. Most of the doctors and nurses left their jobs and dispersed. Many were drafted into the army during the war, leaving public medical services impaired countrywide. Several hospitals were destroyed, and the pharmacies lacked drugs. The population did not receive medical care worthy of the name.

After the war, the authorities established public health care services, as well as supplemental laboratories and pharmacies. The Jewish population, however, gained little from the development of these medical services. As budget shortfalls left the medical facilities with limited resources, the health care providers set limits and barred craftspeople and merchants from membership. Therefore, interwar Jewish society developed professional medical services of its own.[57]

Despite the spread of diseases after World War I and contrary to the German fiction that the Jews carried the diseases and, therefore, their annihilation would assure the health of the rest of the world's population,[58] Jews were healthier than non-Jews were in the interwar era. Prof. Fiszel Schneerson, a well-known Jewish doctor from Poland, studied comparative morbidity of Jews and non-Jews and presented the findings of his research at the World

56 Boris Sapir, "Joint," in Gruenbaum et al., *Entziklopediya Shel Galuyot: Varsha*, vol. 1, p. 570.

57 Wulman, "Hevrat Toz," pp. 581–582.

58 The Jews were portrayed in propaganda as parasites and as a cancer in the body of the German nation. Problematic metabolism and mental illnesses were presented as examples of innate problems among the Jews. Gerhard Wagner, a doctor from Munich, became famous as a "leader in the field of health" and head of the Main Office for Public Health and the Medical Association. He termed the Jews an "ill race" and Judaism as "the disease in human form." In this matter, see Michael Hans Kater, *Doctors under Hitler* (Chapel Hill: University of North Carolina Press, 1989), pp. 20–24; Robert Proctor, *Racial Hygiene: Medicine under the Nazis* (London: Harvard University Press, 1988), p. 19.

Congress of Jewish Physicians. He asserted, "The statistical facts prove clearly that morbidity is lower among Jews than among non-Jews [because] the Jewish masses maintain a higher level of social hygiene," namely, education and strict attention to preventive medicine.[59]

Jews did contract several illnesses in high proportions—such as diabetes—but their life expectancy surpassed that of non-Jews. In 1921–1926, for example, mortality from contagious diseases was consistently lower among Jews than among their non-Jewish neighbors. In 1931–1936, the mortality rate from infectious diseases among young people in Warsaw was lower among Jews than among their non-Jewish counterparts. Mortality from tuberculosis was perceptibly lower among Jews than among the non-Jewish population. Typhus and typhoid claimed a smaller share of Jewish casualties in Warsaw than it did among non-Jews, and Jews were less predisposed to influenza and cholera than non-Jews were.[60]

In his address at the World Congress of Jewish Physicians, Dr. David Aryeh Friedman discussed the poor medical conditions that prevailed in Jewish communities after World War I and the professional medical challenges that the Jewish doctors faced.

> The legacy of the great war of nations, the changes in national life, the political economy, and the special decrees against our people caused and are causing a frightening decline in the physical resilience of [our] long-afflicted people. The Jewish doctors, whose human and national role is not only to help the ill but also to seek to improve and strengthen the future of the collective, should not only think about their

59 Friedman, *Sefer Hakongres Ha'olami*, pp. 65–66.

60 Jacob Lindenthal, "The Epidemiological Status and Health Care Administration of the Jews before and during the Holocaust," in Grodin, *Jewish Medical Resistance*, pp. 16–17. Data on Jewish morbidity in prewar Warsaw and in comparison with non-Jews appear in several statistical reports that are in the Ringelblum Archive. See, for example, Judenrat Statistics Department Bulletin, Archiwum Żydowski Instytut Historyczny (AŻIH), ARII.133; Offer, "Ma'arach Harefu'a Begeto Varsha," vol. 2, appendix A.19, pp. 93–112; and memoranda about the war on the typhus epidemic, AŻIH, ARI.85.

> personal distress at this time but also direct their attention to safeguarding the lives of the Jewish people, whose enemies have risen to obliterate them.[61]

Dr. Leon Wulman warned that even if Jews had lower morbidity rates than their neighbors in other countries, their health was deteriorating due to the persecution that they faced and the resulting situation was likely to endanger their health.

> As for the question of protecting Jewish health—at first glance, one might say that the Jewish people are the healthiest on earth because their mortality is lower, their resilience higher, their lifespans longer, their children healthier, there is no diabetes, and sexually-transmitted diseases are uncommon. However, that is not the case. We ourselves see how weak and frail the Jewish physique is… As long as the persecution of the Jews continues, as long as the Jews do not have full access to economic and social life in the countries where they dwell—all the measures that we are taking to protect our health are at risk. I know this is a death sentence for our activities in the Diaspora. It is a fact that we cannot ignore. For this reason, our work should concentrate on our youth, in particular, which are destined to lead a different kind of life.[62]

JDC Actions for the Development of Health Care and Medical Infrastructures

Despite Polish Jewry's ramified welfare activity, some harshly criticized the social activities of this population. Ringelblum pointed an accusing finger at the community leaders, finding fault with the social assistance that they marshaled. The community's welfare institutions, he said, treated their clients like beggars and used antiquated working methods. Most community activists

61 Friedman, *Sefer Hakongres Ha'olami*, p. 10.
62 Ibid., p. 64.

had scattered at the beginning of the war and had abandoned the Jewish public. Therefore, the community mechanism and its surrounding public groups lacked the strength to sustain the extensive relief work that had begun when the war ensued. In the resulting situation, only the JDC remained a source of support for all the welfare operations.[63]

The JDC was established in 1914 in order to assist Jews during the war. A nonpartisan and independent umbrella organization, it represented the relief efforts of America's most important Jewish organizations.[64] The United States government concurrently established a $100 million relief fund for Europeans. Within this framework, the JDC raised $3.3 million in aid for Jewish communities in Eastern Europe. In this manner, it was able to send its own staff members as representatives of the U.S. administration. Its American identity gave it the cachet to help Polish Jews. Thus, it became the main vehicle of relief for the rehabilitation of East European Jewish communities in the interwar years and of support during the Nazi occupation.[65]

In 1917–1918, approximately 340,000 Jews in Warsaw were in need of help. After World War I, the JDC continued to deliver relief to the Jews of Eastern Europe through welfare, health care, and social services. Unlike the philanthropic fundamental of offering relief to the poor, a "constructive assistance" approach—that is, helping communities and individuals to lift themselves out of poverty through vocational training and participation in the labor force—evolved in Poland, mainly on the initiative of the then

63 Ringelblum, *Ktavim Aharonim*, pp. 39–41.

64 Sapir, "Joint," pp. 567-568. The American Jewish Joint Distribution Committee (JDC) is an outgrowth of another entity, the American Jewish Committee (AJC), founded in 1906 to safeguard the rights of Jews wherever they may be. In World War I, yet another American Jewish aid organization came into being, the American Jewish Relief Committee (AJRC), which subsequently became a central agency for American Jews and part of the JDC. Eventually, AJRC worked with two additional associations that had basically the same goals: the Central Relief Committee (CRC) and the People's Relief Committee (PRC). The merger of these entities is reflected in the word "Joint," which is how it is commonly referred to in Hebrew. See Roland, *Courage under Siege*, p. 11.

65 Bauer, *My Brother's Keeper*, pp. 8–13.

director of the JDC, Yitzhak Gitterman.[66] JDC helped to establish institutions that employed thousands of experts in education, medicine, and social work, who had been recruited to further the advancement of the weaker strata of Jewish society. This activity, expedited in order to meet the needs identified among the Jewish population in the interwar period, created an infrastructure for activity in these areas of Jewish life in the ghettos under Nazi rule.

JDC spent $33 million on relief in 1919–1921, setting up, among other things, soup kitchens, hospitals, orphanages, feeding organizations, offices for refugee tracking and the unification of scattered families, and education systems. After delivering emergency relief, it initiated systematic vocational activities with the help of local professionals who had become leaders in welfare and health care. It mobilized the Jews in the affected countries to raise funds within their own communities, obviating exclusive reliance on money from America.[67] In January 1921, it dispatched a special medical assistance unit—comprising doctors, sanitation workers, and nurses—which established and maintained 498 facilities. Its definitive achievements were the creation of a nursing school and the eradication of trichophytosis and trachoma. JDC's principal contribution was the development of TOZ, which was assigned the task of organizing Jewish health care in Poland, following the departure of the JDC's medical mission in 1923. TOZ availed itself of the JDC until the deportations from Warsaw, which terminated all Jewish public institutions in the ghetto.[68]

TOZ—The Jewish Health Care Organization

TOZ was established in 1921 against the background of Poland's consolidation as an independent state that officially recognized its Jewish minority.[69] Dr. Gershon Lewin, a pioneer in the field

66 Ringelblum, *Ktavim Aharonim*, pp. 40–44, 54.

67 Bauer, *My Brother's Keeper*, pp. 10–13; Bauer, *American Jewry and the Holocaust: The American Jewish Joint Distribution Committee, 1939–1945* (Detroit: Wayne State University Press, 1981), p. 32.

68 Sapir, "Joint," p. 570.

69 Its founders were Dr. Samuel Goldflam, Dr. J. M. Judt, and Dr. Sara Zofia

of public medicine, was appointed its director, and Dr. Leon Wulman was named general secretary.[70] Dr. Wulman emphasized the importance of establishing an independent Jewish medical apparatus.

> The question of Jewish health care institutions is one of the most important. It is not to segregate ourselves that we wish to build these institutions. Rather, it is because a Jew who falls ill needs an environment of his own, his hospital, his people, for his convalescence. It is no caprice on the part of the Jewish community to set up special health care institutions of its own; instead, it is an innate psychological necessity. Our hospitals are the legacy of generations of our people, and we are duty bound to continue building them, supporting them, and bequeathing them to posterity.[71]

In 1921–1923, TOZ was a small-scale enterprise that operated in district branches. In 1923, when the Polish authorities approved its statutes, it convened its first national conference to discuss issues regarding the safeguarding of the health of the Jews of Poland. At the gathering, the organization elected a central committee and thereafter embarked on extensive activities throughout the country.[72] In the course of its work, TOZ cooperated with OZE—Obshchestvo Zdravookhraneniia Evreev (Society for

Syrkin Binstein, aka Sara-Zofia Syrkin-Binsztejnowa. Members included Jakob Appenszalk, Naftali Priwes, and Adv. Stawski, all from Warsaw.

70 Dr. Gershon Lewin (1868–1939) was a pulmonologist who specialized in tuberculosis. For thirty-five years he managed a department at the Jewish hospital in Warsaw. He was a member of the Zionist camp and a leading figure in Warsaw Jewry. Concurrently with helping to establish TOZ, he acted on behalf of the anti-tuberculosis association. He died shortly after the German occupation began. On this matter, see Wulman et al., *The Martyrdom of Jewish Physicians in Poland*. Dr. Leon (Lejb) Wulman (1889–1971) was one of the few who survived to testify about the activities of TOZ.

71 Friedman, *Sefer Hakongres Ha'olami*, p. 64.

72 See the *Map Showing Medical Institutions in Poland: Built, Rebuilt, and Equipped by the JDC Medico-Sanitary Department, February 1921–October 1923*, AJCD, AR.33–34; Wulman, "Hevrat Toz," pp. 581–582. The main activists were experienced and talented professionals.

the Safeguarding of Jews' Health)[73]—an entity founded ten years earlier as a medical organization for Jews in Russia and the vicinity.

JDC pledged massive budgets to medical services. In 1936, as the global economic depression battered Eastern Europe, it invested $541,500 in Poland, of which $47,400—9 percent—was allotted to TOZ medical activities and to the direct subvention of hospitals and clinics. In 1937, its investment climbed to $722,000, of which $84,000—11 percent—was earmarked for medical services.[74] TOZ organized activities in the areas of hygiene and the dissemination of information, maternal and pediatric health, medicine and hygiene in schools, and disease prevention. It also helped to provide medical assistance. In the interwar years, it sponsored 2,730 lectures on medicine and hygiene, attended by 242,227 participants; thirty-seven popular medical booklets in Yiddish; and bulletins and posters.[75] TOZ ran twenty-eight counseling stations for infant care, eleven pregnancy centers for prenatal care, fifteen daycare centers, and nineteen stations where milk was distributed for babies. Altogether, nearly 5,000 preschool children received care at these facilities.[76] TOZ also set up a far-reaching nutrition programs for needy children in the schools. In the 1938–1939 school year, as the Holocaust loomed, more than 35,000 youngsters benefited from this project. TOZ

73 Russian Jews established OZE in 1912 in St. Petersburg. Additional societies of similar nature came into being in other countries. In 1921, the Soviet authorities forced OZE to desist from its activity. In 1923, OZE relocated to Berlin and established an international association. The OZE board in Berlin was chaired by Albert Einstein. Ten years later, when the Nazis rose to power, OZE moved its activity to Paris. In late June 1940, the board relocated to the unoccupied portion of France. In early 1943, the central committee transferred the seat of its activity to Geneva. See Alain Michel, "OZE," in Gutman, *Encyclopedia of the Holocaust*, vol. 3, pp. 1,081–1,082; Mania Ostrovsky, "Zihronoteha Shel Ahot Be'irgun Oze 1916–1917" (Memoirs of a Nurse with the OZE Organization 1916–1917)" *Korot* (Hebrew), 11 (1995), pp. 65–72.

74 Roland, *Courage under Siege*, pp. 11–13.

75 There were three journals: *Folks Gezund* for the masses, *Zay Gezund* for schoolchildren, and *Sotsiale Meditsin*, a scientific periodical about medical problems; see Wulman, "*Hevrat Toz*," pp. 581–586.

76 Ibid.

invested great efforts to combat tuberculosis, trichophytosis,[77] and trachoma.[78] It established twelve modern and professional tuberculosis clinics, two convalescent homes, eight X-ray facilities for treatment of trichophytosis, and trachoma departments in general clinics in cities around the country. TOZ eradicated trichophytosis among Jews, made much progress toward wiping out trachoma, and contributed to the war on typhus.[79]

In fifteen years of TOZ's activities, 773,672 patients visited clinics and 431,847 visited dental clinics. The association supported forty-seven Jewish hospitals countrywide and helped to improve their work, established a central administration for Jewish hospitals, convened a conference of hospital officials, and established a fund for the improvement of hospital buildings and equipment. TOZ also engaged in research on the health conditions of the Jews in Poland and the spread of disease among them, and conducted statistical studies on morbidity and mortality among the community. For this purpose, it established a department of statistics and demography, and published studies in various scientific journals, including its own monthly *Sotsiale Meditsin*. It held two national conferences of Jewish doctors, attended by 561 physicians, and more than eighty lectures were delivered on topics in biopathology, anthropology, and statistics.[80] TOZ also expanded its activities among the Jews to include psychohygiene. In 1930, it established a psychohygiene counseling center that hosted educational activities on health, in-service training, and scientific seminars. The association also conducted psychological research and published several books in this field.[81]

77 A contagious disease of the scalp caused by a fungus that leads to loss of hair, particularly among children.

78 A contagious disease of the conjunctiva of the eye caused by a virus; unless treated, it damages the cornea and may cause blindness.

79 Shifra Shvarts, Penina Rotem, Yitzhak Romem, and Mordechai Shani, "Masa Hagazezet Hanishkah Shel Oze-Toz, Polin" (OZE-TOZ's Forgotten War on Trichophytosis, Poland), *Harefu'a* (Hebrew), 148 (2009), pp. 265–270. During the campaign, from the end of World War I to the eve of World War II, 27,760 children received roentgenological (X-ray) treatments.

80 Wulman, "Hevrat Toz," pp. 583–584.

81 Friedman, *Sefer Hakongres Ha'olami*, pp. 65–66.

In early 1939, 368 institutions were amalgamated under TOZ, which also managed approximately seventy branches and forty-one sub-branches in remote areas. Its main branch, located at 43 Gęsia St. in Warsaw, oversaw the countrywide system. The Warsaw branch directed far-reaching prevention activities among the Jewish population.[82] The branches were managed by 819 TOZ members, who were elected in general assemblies. In January 1939, TOZ had 15,433 dues-paying members and owned buildings, plots, and a great deal of medical equipment and other furnishings. Over a fifteen-year period, it spent nearly 19 million zlotys. JDC provided about 30 percent of these outlays. Additional funds came from fundraising campaigns abroad and from OZE. However, most of the funding—12,000,000 zlotys—was raised in Poland. TOZ had 962 paid employees, including 243 doctors, 118 nurses, 35 dentists, 265 auxiliary personnel, and 184 teachers, among others, as well as many volunteers.[83]

A close reading of the lectures that were delivered at the First World Congress of Jewish Physicians reveals the factors that powered the development of TOZ's impressive medical system. The doctors' remarks at the congress reflect the spirit behind the ramified activities of the Jewish communities and the doctors' organizations. The doctors considered themselves as having undertaken the mission of rehabilitating the Jewish communities in exile and physically strengthening the Hebrew people. In their view, two historical processes were causing Jewish medical activity to expand with gathering speed. The first was the

82 Dr. Moshe Tursz testimony, YVA, O.3/438, p. 3.

83 Wulman, "*Hevrat Toz*," p. 584. To get an impression of the extent and content of the activity, see, for example, TOZ Budget Report, April 1, 1936–March 31, 1937, JDC, AR.33–44, files 821, 840. See also Friedman, *Sefer Hakongres Ha'olami*, pp. 63–65; Leon Wulman, "OZE–Hesegeha Be'avar Vetohniyoteha Latkufa Shele'ahar Hamilhama" (OZE—Past Achievements and Plans for the Postwar Era) *Ha-rofe ha-'ivri* (Hebrew) 2 (1944), pp. 85–94; Leon Wulman, ed., *In Fight for the Health of the Jewish People: 50 Years of OSE* (New York: World Union, OSE, and the American Committee of OSE, 1968); Wulman et al., *The Martyrdom of Jewish Physicians in Poland*, pp. 118–121. Much important information about TOZ activities in Poland and Warsaw remains in the JDC archives. See, for example, Offer, "Ma'arach Harefu'a Begeto Varsha," vol. 2, appendix A.12, pp. 48–51.

grassroots movement that had developed among Russian Jewry, which varied in its ideological complexion but was characterized by pure ideology. Although the authors did not say it in so many words, they appear to have been referring to diverse manifestations of socialist ideology. The second process was the development of the Zionist movement. The resurrection of the national idea stimulated the desire to assemble the Jewish doctors under one roof, along with the centuries-old Jewish tradition that considered it the duty of the Jewish doctor to provide medical treatment to both the individual and the Jewish collective as a nation.

Against the backdrop of these processes, large Jewish health care organizations were established in the early twentieth century. The most prominent were OZE, founded in Russia before World War I, which operated many branches in Britain, Latvia, Lithuania, and Romania; TOZ, which functioned as OZE's subsidiary in Poland; the JDC Medical Department, which provided assistance in various East European countries; and WIZO and Hadassah, which focused their aid on pre-independence Israel. By dint of these organizations' efforts, the Jewish population enjoyed broader and broader medical services. In order to complement the process and meet the many needs that emerged from the challenge of providing medical care to the Jews, it was necessary to establish a world Jewish medical organization. A congress that was convened for this purpose concluded with the signing of a "World Covenant of Jewish Physicians." Although these medical societies organized professional conferences and colloquia—particularly OZE and TOZ in Poland—they had enormous shortcomings.

> The central idea of the global and international nature of the problems of Jewish biopathology, and of the professional and cultural issues confronting the Jewish doctor was absent at all these conferences....One must admit that the universal characteristic of the plight of the Jewish doctors and the distress of Jewish medical and eugenic culture became clear to many only in recent years,

as the persecutions and decrees against the Jewish doctors intensified.[84]

Thus, Jewish doctors believed that there were biopathological problems that were specific to the Jewish people, that the professional and cultural perception of the Jewish doctor and Jewish medicine was unique, and that the Jewish physicians were subject to severe international pressures. These aspects of the profession and especially the persecutions and restrictions on Jewish doctors in various countries called for the establishment of an independent Jewish medical system.

ZLRP—Association of Jewish Physicians in Poland

In 1923, as TOZ expanded its ambit and broadened its foundations, a group of noted Jewish physicians, most of whom served on the staff of the Jewish hospital in Warsaw and were active in TOZ, established a Jewish medical organization in Poland,[85] ZLRP—Związek Lekarzy Rzeczypospolitej Polskiej (Association of Jewish Physicians in Poland).[86] As demonstrated above, anti-

84 Friedman, *Sefer Hakongres Ha'olami*, p. 8.

85 Its founders included Dr. Gershon Lewin and Dr. Aharon Soloveichik (1865–1942), one of the most famous surgeons in Poland. For about forty years, Dr. Soloveichik ran the department of surgery at the Jewish hospital in Warsaw and a surgical hospital of his own, which attracted Jews from all over Poland. Alongside the department of surgery, he set up a pathological anatomy lab. He was a founding member of the Jewish nursing and caregivers' schools. Dr. Soloveichik identified with the Zionist movement. After the Nazis invaded Warsaw, he moved to Vilna but returned to the Polish capital in 1941. He died in the ghetto several weeks after his wife was taken to Treblinka. See Lensky, "Rof'im Yehudim Mefursamim," pp. 318–321. For more on the Association of Jewish Physicians, see Avi Ohry and Karin Ohry-Kossoy, "Dedicated Physicians in the Face of Adversity: The Association of Jewish Physicians (ZLRP) and the Jewish Health Organization (TOZ) in Poland, 1921–1942," *Polin: Studies in Polish Jewry*, 25 (2013), pp. 455–462.

86 Interesting remarks about ZLRP and its name were expressed in a discussion at the First World Congress of Jewish Physicians in 1936. Dr. T. Melodysta noted accusingly that the organization had not even given itself a Hebrew name. Dr. Israel Milejkowski elaborated on this, stating that Jewish doctors in Poland were in a different situation than those in *Eretz Israel* in terms of their Jewish identity. He said that the physicians' association in Warsaw had been

Jewish hostility found expression in discriminatory policies and restrictions in all areas of life. Since admission to the Polish Medical Association had become virtually impossible, the Jewish doctors decided to establish a medical association of their own.[87] In its first year, the all-Jewish entity had 288 members; by 1939, on the eve of World War II, it had 600. Its goal was to improve the scientific and professional level of Jewish doctors and to publicize their achievements in academic forums. Its members worked vigorously to set up branches in several cities throughout Poland and thus the organization expanded to become a national association of Jewish physicians within a very short period. It established a foundation that provided Jewish physicians with study incentives and scholarships. Many young Jews, who were forced to pursue their studies abroad because the numerus clausus policy had severely restricted the admission of Jews to Polish universities, availed themselves of the association's funds to cover their steep expenses. When they completed their studies and returned to Poland, the antisemitic policies raised many hurdles in obtaining recognition of the medical degrees that they had earned abroad. ZLRP also mobilized to combat the antisemitism that directly targeted Jewish doctors.

In its sixteen years of activity, ZLRP held 280 conferences on a wide variety of medical topics. As the 1930s unfolded, it began to convene scientific colloquia in which renowned experts from abroad took part. Most of its members also belonged to professional organizations in their medical specializations. ZLRP,

established in 1922–1923, when Jews were afraid to set themselves apart, and that it had sought to attract Jewish doctors who "straddled the fence." See Friedman, *Sefer Hakongres Ha'olami*, p. 60.

87 Notably, throughout Poland's medical history, Jewish physicians actively participated in developing the profession. Many belonged to professional organizations in their specializations and to the Polish Medical Association. For example, Dr. Ludwik Natansohn, an expert in anatomy and physiology, with credits to his name in gynecology as well, had been a founding member of the Polish Medical Association and had established the association's newspaper, *Gazeta Lekarska*. He served as president of the Polish Medical Association in 1863 and chaired the executive committee of the Warsaw Jewish community from 1871 until his death. See Lensky, "Rof'im Yehudim Mefursamim," pp. 308–310.

which was apolitical, worked closely with PTMS—Polish Organization for Social Medicine—which leaned sharply to the Left, and some of its members were affiliated with both entities. PTMS defined itself as an organization for social medicine that championed the establishment of a medical service system that would serve the entire population of Poland. Roughly 200 of its members labored to prepare plans to apply social medicine policies to eradicate tuberculosis, contagious diseases, and blindness; to care for the mentally ill; to provide medical care in schools; and so on. In addition, it had a clinical medicine department that served to organize conferences and to issue publications. Given that Polish medical periodicals usually rejected articles written by Jewish doctors, ZLRP published a Polish weekly journal on social medicine, *Warszawskie Czasopismo Lekarskie* (Warsaw Journal on Medical Affairs), which provided a forum for the publication of their activities and articles.

Many members of ZLRP were noted physicians and experts in their specializations. The organization's last conference took place in May 1939, four months before World War II began. Although ZLRP officially ceased to exist when the Germans occupied Poland, many of its members continued to act in its spirit and principles during the Nazi occupation. Even under the terrifying living conditions of the Warsaw ghetto, they maintained a medical system that had modern professional and social characteristics, including a medical association, as discussed in Part Two of this study.

The development of ZLRP should be viewed as part of the overall development of Jewish medicine in the late nineteenth and early twentieth centuries. As the medical studies of Jewish students in academia expanded and the number of Jewish doctors increased, it became necessary to establish local and national Jewish medical associations. Thus, for example, a doctors' association in Vilna came into being in the late 1890s. By 1910, similar entities existed in *Eretz Israel*, Russia—where OZE was established—the United States, South Africa, Germany, Latvia, Austria, and Poland. The organization in *Eretz Israel* had approximately 1,800 members at that time; the association of Jewish doctors in Austria had around 1,000; and there were hundreds in each of the others.[88]

CENTOS—An Umbrella for Organizations that Sheltered Jewish Children

In 1923, CENTOS—Centralne Towarzystwo Opieki nad Sierotami (Central Society for the Care of Orphans)—assumed responsibility for JDC's activities on behalf of indigent children. As an umbrella organization that saw to the welfare of children, it coordinated their care in the system of children's homes and orphanages in the Jewish communities in Poland, including Janusz Korczak's orphanage.[89] After World War I, there were more than 40,000 orphaned and abandoned Jewish children in Poland. CENTOS helped to create conditions that would allow thousands of them to recover and develop normally.[90]

Funded by local organizations and philanthropy,[91] CENTOS cooperated with TOZ to improve children's health by offering preventive and therapeutic health care.[92] In 1937, TOZ attended to feeding 35,514 children and CENTOS assumed responsibilty for feeding 20,590.[93] In 1938, 15,438 children received care in 195 settings under the auspices of CENTOS. This constituted only 38 percent of the children who were under the care of the organization in previous years, since at least 25,000 youngsters were functioning independently by then.[94] On the eve of World War II, CENTOS was active in 218 institutions that included orphanages, day care centers, homes for adolescents, schools, workshops, convalescent homes, and 172 children's camps. About 100,000 youngsters attended children's camps

88 Friedman, *Sefer Hakongres Ha'olami*, p. 6.

89 Bauer, *American Jewry and the Holocaust*, p. 32; Bauer, *My Brother's Keeper*, pp. 10–11.

90 Sapir, "Joint," p. 569.

91 Roland, *Courage under Siege*, pp. 11–13.

92 Zvi Parnas, "Hevrat Zentos" (CENTOS Society), in Gruenbaum et al., *Entziklopediya Shel Galuyot: Varsha*, vol. 1, p. 579.

93 Roland, *Courage under Siege*, pp. 11–13.

94 Zvi Parnas, "Hevrat Zentos," pp. 579–580.

run by CENTOS and around 20,000 attended convalescent camps. CENTOS also published professional magazines for staff training purposes: *Das Kind* (The Child) in Yiddish and *Przegląd Społeczny* (Social Review) in Polish.[95] This versatile organization continued to operate in the ghetto under Dr. Adolf Abraham Berman, who had been its chief psychologist until the German occupation, Jozef Gitler, and Rachel Stein.[96]

Czyste Hospital

The hospital for "Members of the Mosaic Faith," a large Jewish facility located in Czyste, a suburb of Warsaw, was established in 1837 by members of the Warsaw Jewish bourgeoisie at considerable expense. Representatives of this class, many of whom were assimilated, sat on the Warsaw Jewish Community Council before World War I, alongside delegates from Hasidic circles.[97] The hospital started out with 250 beds and expanded to 400 in the second half of the century. Due to the increase of the Jewish population, its doctors decided to build a new hospital, which officially opened in 1902. Designed to accommodate 500 patients and to comprise all the requisite departments, the hospital continued to grow and evolve over time. In 1911, another building that could accommodate eighty patients was erected for the mentally ill. On the initiative of the physician-researchers Jakob Szwajcer and Edward Flatau, a physical therapy department, the first of its kind in Poland, was established there. A well-equipped day clinic that served about 200 patients daily was built as well.[98] World War I halted the construction but not

95 Sapir, "Joint," p. 569. The JDC archives contain much material about CENTOS. To get an impression of its comprehensive work for children in the Jewish communities of Poland, see CENTOS in Poland report, August 1938, JDC, AR.33–44, file 822.

96 Batya Temkin-Berman, *Ir Betoh Ir* (A City within a City) (Hebrew) (Jerusalem and Tel Aviv: Yad Vashem and Am Oved, 2008), p. 61.

97 Ben-Shem, "Batei Holim Yehudiyim BeVarsha," pp. 579–580; Mordechai Lensky, *A Physician inside the Warsaw Ghetto* (New York and Jerusalem: Yad Vashem and The Holocaust Survivors Memoirs Project, 2009), pp. 21–27.

98 Ben-Shem, "Batei Holim Yehudiyim BeVarsha," pp. 581–582.

the caregiving. Once the war ended, the hospital expanded again. It earned renown in Warsaw and elsewhere for its sophisticated building and equipment, and the devotion of its doctors, even though it was short on nurses and professional caregivers.[99] In 1923, a nursing school opened next door.[100]

In 1936–1937, 14,212 patients, more than 4 percent of the Jewish population of Warsaw, were treated at Czyste Hospital. The institution's annual budget reached 2.2 million zlotys, of which more than half came from the municipality. The hospital had a staff of 483: a director, 21 administrative personnel, 43 doctors, 176 aides, including 146 nurses, 152 caregivers and technical aides, and 90 technical service and maintenance workers. In 1938, when administrative supervision passed into the hands of the municipality of Warsaw, the hospital had 1,174 beds.[101]

By virtue of their high-level professional training, expertise, and devotion to their patients, the doctors at Czyste Hospital enjoyed the admiration of the Jewish and the non-Jewish populations alike. Noted physicians worked at the hospital and Jews from all over Poland thronged to it.[102] The doctors and scientists who headed the departments were renowned in Poland and abroad. Many interns and doctors worked at their side, and large numbers of young physicians did their residencies at Czyste Hospital, because Polish hospitals had become off-limits to them.[103] This staff of Jewish doctors contributed to the high scientific level of the hospital, conducting studies and publishing them in the professional literature.[104]

99 Ibid., pp. 582–583.

100 Koren, "Hasiyud Kehelek Misherutei Habriyut," p. 12.

101 Ben-Shem, "Batei Holim Yehudiyim BeVarsha," pp. 583–584.

102 Lensky, *A Physician inside the Warsaw Ghetto*, pp. 21–27; Chaim Aron Kaplan, *Scroll of Agony: Warsaw Ghetto Diary*, ed. and tr. by Abraham I. Katsh, (Bloomington: Indiana University Press, 1999), pp. 239–240.

103 Kaplan, *Scroll of Agony*, pp. 239-240; Mordechai Lensky, "Beit Haholim Hayehudi Tzhista," p. 102; Ben-Shem, "Batei Holim Yehudiyim BeVarsha," pp. 584-586.

104 Lensky, *A Physician inside the Warsaw Ghetto*, pp. 21-27.

Bersohn and Bauman Children's Hospital

Bersohn and Bauman Jewish Children's Hospital, established in 1878, was one of four famous pediatric hospitals in Warsaw.[105] Emblematic of Jewish pediatric medicine, it had the following departments: internal medicine; surgery; ear, nose, and throat; tuberculosis; and, at certain times, infectious diseases. Children in Warsaw—Jewish and non-Jewish alike—were treated there.[106] Dr. Szymon Portner was the hospital's first chief physician. Only some of the medical specialists had tenure. Its nurses lacked prior training in professional nursing institutions and acquired their expertise on the job. In 1902–1909, Dr. Henryk Goldszmit, whose pen name was Janusz Korczak, worked there as a local physician. Bersohn and Bauman Children's Hospital admitted all children, irrespective of religion. It operated continuously as long as the Bersohn and Bauman families provided philanthropic support, but as the years passed, the families' heirs took less and less interest in the institution.[107]

In the course of World War I, the hospital, at the authorities' behest, became a military facility for the czar's army. After the war, Dr. Anna Braude-Heller[108] worked intensively to promote

105 Israel Rom (Rotbalsam), "Mahalot Hayeladim Begeto Varsha" (Pediatric Diseases in the Warsaw Ghetto), in Dworzecki, *Hama'avak Lakiyum Velabriyut Biymei Hashoah*, p. 14.

106 Ibid.; Adina Blady-Szwajger, *Yoter Mize Eineni Zoheret: Beit Haholim Begeto Varsha, Zihronoteha Shel Rof'a Beveit Haholim Al Shem Berson VeBauman, 1939–1943* (I Remember Nothing More: The Hospital in the Warsaw Ghetto, Memoirs of a Woman Doctor at Bersohn and Bauman Children's Hospital, 1939–1943) (Hebrew) (Holon: Steinbaum, 2000), p. 9. This memoir also appeared in the journal *Edut*: Adina Blady-Szwajger, "Beit Haholim Begeto Varsha, Zihronoteha Shel Rof'a Beveit Haholim Al Shem Berson VeBauman, 1939–1943" (The Hospital in the Warsaw Ghetto, Memoirs of a Jewish Woman Doctor at Bersohn and Bauman Children's Hospital, 1939–1943), *Edut* (Hebrew), 3–4 (1989), pp. 17–44.

107 Yehudit Braude testimony, YVA, O.3/2360. The testimony was given in 1962 by the sister of Anna Braude-Heller, director of Bersohn and Bauman Children's Hospital. After the war broke out, Yehudit worked as a volunteer administrator at the hospital and managed the organization TPD—Towarzystwo Przyjaciół Dzieci (Friends of Children Society), as well as three mother and child care clinics. She also worked at the TOZ clinic in the ghetto until February 1943.

108 Anonymous testimony about Dr. Anna Braude-Heller, Berson-Bauman

the resumption of its pediatric work. Renovations, which began in 1923 with subventions from the JDC and the efforts of the director of the hospital, Dr. Samuel Goldflam, were completed in late 1930. The hospital initially took in about 150 children and subsequently the number of beds increased to accommodate 250 inpatients. After contending with economic hardships, Bersohn and Bauman Children's Hospital began to enjoy economic independence, when the government health care system referred patients from the population at large for inpatient care at the hospital. The Municipal Department of Social Services also paid for each child hospitalized there, irrespective of religion.[109] Additionally, the hospital continued to avail itself of donations, including the proceeds of the annual fundraisers of its women's auxiliary.

Bersohn and Bauman Children's Hospital acquired an excellent reputation. Its doctors conducted studies, which they discussed at their staff meetings, and published articles about them in professional journals. Professional consultants participated in the ongoing medical work. The hospital's equipment, kitchen, and laundry facilities were modern, and the patients received high-quality service. Dr. Anna Braude-Heller, the chief physician, devoted herself to her hospital work, often visiting the facility in the middle of the night to attend to a sick child.[110] She also demonstrated her devotion to the task of running the pediatric hospital under the difficult conditions of the German occupation.

Children's Hospital, AŻIH, file 2947/301. Dr. Anna Braude-Heller (1888–1943) studied in Switzerland and Germany and graduated in 1911. In 1914, she returned to Poland as a pediatrician and was appointed chief physician at Bersohn and Bauman Children's Hospital. In 1916, the hospital was deactivated and shut down due to a shortage of funds. Dr. Braude-Heller did much to have it reopened. On her activities, professionalism, and devotion during the Holocaust, see the section on children's hospitals in the ghetto in Chapter 3 of this book.

109 Ibid.

110 Yehudit Braude testimony, YVA, O.3/2360. Sabina Zenderman had been a nurse at the hospital; see Sabina Zenderman testimony, YVA, M.49.E/5883; Offer, *Haluk Lavan Bageto*, appendix A.8, pp. 528–533; Esther Braude-Grodzinski testimony, YVA, O.3/392.

Friends of Children Society

During World War I, when the pediatric hospital was closed, TPD—Towarzystwo Przyjaciół Dzieci (Friends of Children Society)—was established on Dr. Braude-Heller's initiative to help administer urgent medical aid to the masses of starving and exhausted war refugees, who were crowding the Jewish neighborhoods of Warsaw. From its founding to World War II, the society organized medical and welfare projects for children that included the establishment of mother and child care clinics, an orphanage for abandoned Jewish children, a pediatric nursing school, an orthopedic clinic, a clinical psychology clinic, and a counseling and professional guidance center.[111]

Jewish School of Nursing

"My hand trembled and my eyes filled with tears as I sat down to write an account of the history, the glorious development, and the destruction of the nursing school at Czyste Hospital. I was a student in the first graduating class of this school and the director of the last one." Thus wrote Luba Blum-Bielicka (b. 1905), principal of the nursing school from 1939, shortly before World War II began, until the Nazis eradicated the institution at the time of the transports to Treblinka. She survived the Holocaust and died in Poland in 1973.[112]

After World War I, seven schools for certified nurses opened in Poland. Since the terms for admission included a certificate of baptism from the Church, Jewish girls were effectively excluded.[113]

111 Yehudit Braude testimony, YVA, O.3/2360.

112 Luba Blum-Bielicka, "Szkoła Pielęgniarstwa przy Szpitalu Starozakonnych w Warszawie, 1923–1943," *BŻIH*, 40 (1961), pp. 66–67. I wish to thank Aviva Blum-Vaks, a survivor of the Warsaw ghetto and the daughter of the director of the nursing school during the ghetto period. As a person who had grown up at the ghetto nursing school, her assistance with the testimony and the writings that she disclosed to me—articles and memoirs that her mother had written, among other materials—were very helpful.

113 D. Bridges, "Ma'amad Ha'ahayot Besherutei Habriyut BePolin" (The Status of Nurses in the Polish Health Care Services), *Ahot BeYisrael* (Hebrew), 5 (1959), p. 36; Miriam Markusfeld, "Toldot Beit Hasefer Le'ahayot Tzhista BeVarsha"

Therefore, a committee of senior physicians from Czyste Hospital initiated activities to establish a Jewish nursing school in 1921, toiling intensively for the cause,[114] along with the newly established Society for Support of the Warsaw Jewish Hospital Nursing School, whose chairman was Adolf Wajsblat, an engineer and a member of the Warsaw municipality. The municipality gave a one-time donation and the Ministry of the Interior approved the institution's statutes and program. JDC assisted by providing a $10,000 subvention and professional guidance.[115]

Amalia Greenwald and Ruth Hoffman, two highly experienced nurses, were sent from the United States to Poland by the JDC to set up the school's professional infrastructure. Greenwald, appointed as the school's first principal, began to work vigorously to prepare a suitable location for the institution. She located several rooms on the top floor of an old office building and supervised the renovations. Within four months, the preparations were completed.[116] The admission process indicated that the demand exceeded the supply.[117] The school, located at 17 Dworska St., opened on July 8,

(History of the Czyste Nursing School in Warsaw), *Ahot BeYisrael* (Hebrew), 3 (1957), p. 3; Liza Mirocznik, "Beit Hasefer Le'ahayot Tzhista BeVarsha, Toldoteha Veshitot Halimud Bo" (The Czyste Nursing School in Warsaw, Its History and Teaching Methods), *Ahot BeYisrael* (Hebrew), 9 (1963), p. 46.

114 In November 1921, Dr. Jakob Szwajcer, chief physician at the Jewish hospital, and other doctors established a society for the establishment of a modern nursing school. After persistent efforts, the group managed to find both a location for the school and to arrange financial support, which, thanks to the intervention of the municipal court, was identical to that received by the nursing school in Warsaw. See Susan Mayer, "The School that Would Not Die: The Story of the Jewish Hospital School of Nursing," p. 1. I received Susan Mayer's article from Aviva Blum-Vaks, daughter of Luba Blum-Bielicka. This paper was presented at the First International Conference on Nursing and Midwifery in the Third Reich, "Complicity and Compassion," Limerick, Republic of Ireland, June 10–11, 2004. See also Ellen Ben-Sefer and Linda Shields, "Courage under Adversity: Luba Blum-Bielicka (1906–1973) and the Nursing School of the Warsaw Ghetto," *Health and History*: *Medicine in the Shadow of the Holocaust*: *Australian Reflections*, 18:2 (January 2016), pp. 27–39.

115 Blum-Bielicka, "Szkoła Pielęgniarstwa," pp. 66–67, and Mayer, "The School that Would Not Die," pp. 3–4.

116 Mayer, "The School that Would Not Die," p. 6.

117 Ibid., p. 3.

1923, with an enrollment of twenty-two students.[118] JDC covered 75 percent of its budget until 1926, when it transferred the management of the school to the Warsaw Jewish community.[119] In 1925, pursuant to an agreement with the municipality of Warsaw, a third story was added to the Czyste Hospital administration building to serve as a dormitory for the nursing school students. The Jewish hospital, one of the largest in Poland, was short on nurses, which left the patients' care in the hands of staff who lacked training in this profession. Thus, the establishment of the nursing school was an important step toward the improvement of the hospital's medical service.

The two-and-a-half-year program of studies was patterned roughly after the American curriculum[120]—two years of practical work and academic studies at the hospital, and half a year of service in the community.[121] Since professional nursing care in Poland was in its infancy at this time, it was necessary to shape the character of the new school according to modern professional principles. This led to disagreements on fundamental issues, such as the duration of the nurses' training, the qualifications of the person who should serve as principal, and the structure of the curriculum.

Due to the shortage of nurses, the hospital administration preferred brief training and even appointed graduates of six-month crash courses to high-ranking positions. The school's first principals objected strenuously to this, insisting that they should operate according to a professional program of the highest standards. The heads of the Polish nursing school, where studies lasted two years and four months, shared this view. As for the appropriate background and profile of the principal, the American nurses who had arrived to help set up the school were supposed to go home, but the first graduates were too young to assume this

118 Ben-Shem, "Batei Holim Yehudiyim BeVarsha," p. 583; Blum-Bielicka, "Szkoła Pielęgniarstwa," pp. 66–67.

119 Sapir, "Joint," p. 570.

120 The need to translate study materials from New York University into Polish created many difficulties. See Mayer, "The School that Would Not Die," pp. 3–4.

121 Luba Blum-Bielicka oral testimony, Institute for Contemporary Jewry, The Hebrew University of Jerusalem; see Koren, "Hasiyud Kehelek Misherutei Habriyut," p. 12; Mirocznik, "Beit Hasefer Le'ahayot Tzhista BeVarsha," p. 46.

role. Therefore, it was proposed that female doctors be appointed as principals. Ultimately, it was agreed that a graduate of a two-year professional program of studies would head the nursing school. The nurses' practical training also required professional renewal. The director of the hospital wanted to disperse the students as trainees and nursing aides across all the departments of his facility. The principal of the nursing school, in contrast, thought it best to establish special teaching departments under the guidance of experienced personnel. Thanks to Greenwald's resolute determination and the support of the chair, Wajsblat, the students' training attained the quality that modern nursing schools commonly impart.[122]

The school's location inside the hospital made high-quality teaching by readily available personnel possible. It was the administration's aim that in the first stage of studies—during the first half of the first year—an opinion about the extent of each student's suitability for the profession was to be formed. In the second stage, practical and theoretical classes were given concurrently. The third stage focused only on theory.[123] The program adhered to rigid rules of discipline and a stringent daily regimen.[124] The courses included various fields of medicine, such as surgery, neurology, and ear, nose, and throat, among others. Czyste Hospital had no pediatric department, so the students were sent to Bersohn and Bauman Children's Hospital to study this area of the profession.

Those who passed their final exams, which took place before a committee of examiners and included practical testing, received the title of certified nurse. They also took national nursing tests and thus had an opportunity to join the Polish nurses' professional organization. After a year of practical work in a municipal or community hospital, they were awarded their diplomas. In return for the subsidization of their studies, they had to continue working at the Jewish hospital for five years.[125]

122 Blum-Bielicka, "Szkoła Pielęgniarstwa," pp. 66–67.

123 Ibid.

124 For example, to help realize their full scholastic potential, students were required to turn lights out at 10 p.m., make their beds meticulously, keep their sheets crisp, and so on.

125 Mayer, "The School that Would Not Die," pp. 4–5.

On October 11, 1925, a festive commencement was held for the first class of fifteen new nurses. When the community assumed responsibility for the school, JDC sent outstanding members of this class to the United States for training as principals and counselors. After completing their studies cum laude, they returned to Poland, and gradually assumed responsibility for the management of the school and for training.[126] Sabina Szindler, the assistant principal under Amalia Greenwald, became principal when Greenwald returned to the United States. After Szindler's premature death in 1938, she was succeeded by Nina Lubowska, a superb teacher of nursing who had adapted American study methods to the special conditions in Poland.[127]

Jews and Poles alike held the alumnae in high esteem for their quality and professionalism.[128] Liza Mirocznik, a member of the first graduating class, whose achievements were cited for commendation at an international conference of nurses in Geneva in 1927, undertook the task of teaching practical nursing. Luba Blum-Bielicka took charge of social nursing, a field that included infant care and advisory services in schools. In 1928, she received public health training in Paris and Brussels, and counseled students in this discipline until 1938, when she was appointed to serve as the assistant principal of the nursing school.

By 1937, 245 nurses had graduated from the nursing school. Seventy-nine were working at Czyste Hospital, forty-nine had gone into private practice, thirty-nine had immigrated to Mandatory Palestine, where they had been promised work, eighteen had left the profession, and the others had obtained positions in various medical institutions. In 1939, the nursing school requested a larger budget to expand its enrollment.[129] That year, a vacant lot next to the Jewish hospital on Dworska St. was purchased for the construction of additional facilities. Nina Lubowska went to the United States to raise funds for this

126 Sabina Szindler, Liza Mirocznik, Nina Lubowska, Ella Golomb, and Luba Blum-Bielicka were sent to the U.S.

127 Blum-Bielicka, "Szkoła Pielęgniarstwa," pp. 66–67.

128 Markusfeld, "Toldot Beit Hasefer Le'ahayot Tzhista BeVarsha," p. 5; Mirocznik, "Beit Hasefer Le'ahayot Tzhista BeVarsha," p. 47.

129 Roland, *Courage under Siege*, p. 73.

project. The outbreak of the war frustrated her plans and she did not return to Poland. Luba Blum-Bielicka became principal and fulfilled her duties with dedication, even under the Nazi occupation, when the school moved to the ghetto. On September 1, 1939, the graduates of the twenty-third class received their certificates, bringing the total alumna population to 350. On their lapels was an emblem bearing the inscription the "Jewish Hospital Nursing School."[130]

* * *

The attitudes in Jewish tradition regarding the supreme value of human life and the immense importance of healing and the preservation of health had an impact on the development of the medical profession among the Jews in Poland, in general, and in Warsaw, in particular. Influenced by the command to "choose life" in Jewish Scriptures[131] and the aphorism of the Sages, "One who sustains one life is deemed to have sustained an entire world,"[132] Jewish culture and ethics viewed medicine as a sacred vocation. This tradition, passed on from generation to generation throughout Jewish history, has produced some of the greatest physicians in history. The Torah and the Halacha (rabbinical law) spell out basic rules for sanitary precautions. Many East European Jews, including those in Warsaw, upheld these rules stringently, which helped to prevent many diseases. As they cultivated their pursuits, Jewish doctors and leaders were involved in social medicine and action for the welfare of the public and the impoverished Jewish masses. The attitude of the Jewish individual and public was key to assuring the ill that they could count on psychological and monetary support from both sources in the effort to heal them and restore their strength.

In the course of the nineteenth century and the early twentieth, as the Jewish population of Warsaw and its needs

130 Blum-Bielicka, "Szkoła Pielęgniarstwa," pp. 66–67. The inscription was revised in 1935: "Nursing School in Warsaw."

131 Deut. 30:19.

132 Mishna, Tractate Sanhedrin 4:5.

burgeoned, the Jewish welfare and health care activities kept apace with the establishment of multiple organizations and institutions to provide professional health care services to the Jewish population at large. They acted to stanch the spread of contagious diseases, safeguard personal hygiene, and disseminate basic medical knowledge among the Jewish masses. The Jewish public in Poland and Warsaw mobilized to create this array of medical organizations by virtue of the aforementioned characteristics and the Jewish collective consciousness that had evolved in Poland. Although the resulting medical institutions received assistance from American Jewish organizations, the contribution of Polish Jewry, despite the dire economic situation, was decisive. The Jewish medical institutions, old and new alike, were known for their high quality. Czyste Jewish Hospital and Bersohn and Bauman Children's Hospital stood out among them.

The proportion of Jews in medical schools and the medical industry in Poland and their crucial contributions to all fields of medicine in the country were perceptibly large and disproportionate relative to the population. In the 1930s, as antisemitism in Poland surged, deliberate actions were taken to rid the profession of its Jewish practitioners. Consequently, they became more active in Jewish medical institutions. Their mistreatment, after the fact, resulted in the creation of the infrastructure for the development of an independent Jewish medical system. Another salient characteristic from the standpoint of medical science is the lower morbidity rate of the Jews in interwar Europe. Even though the Jews contracted several illnesses at high rates, they had a longer life expectancy and they were healthier than the non-Jews were. However, in the years following World War I, morbidity in Poland rose and the Jews' medical needs multiplied due to war-related injury, antisemitism, and the grim economic conditions.

JDC, established in 1914 to provide relief to Jews during World War I, became the central purveyor of aid for the reconstruction of the Jewish communities after the war. In 1921, JDC sent a special delegation to Poland to provide medical aid. Its main contribution was the establishment of TOZ, headquartered in Warsaw. The surviving documentation indicates that this organization's activities in the areas of hygiene, information, and war on diseases among hundreds of thousands of Jews throughout Poland were impressive in terms of scale, professionalism, and the social concepts that guided them.

There were more than 400,000 Jews in Warsaw, including about 800 doctors, at the beginning of the war. From the onset of the Nazi occupation until the liquidation of the ghetto, they struggled to confront the medical disaster that the Nazis' decrees had inflicted, and the German authorities did nothing to help them to cope with the morbidity and mortality that became their lot. However, they were not alone in this struggle. The medical legacy—scientific, ethical, and organizational—that had characterized their modus operandi in the interwar years was put to the test during this fateful period, just as they were. The sanctity of life, the values of safeguarding health and of healing, the professional personnel in medical science and health care, the array of institutions and organizations that delivered medical and preventive services, the social perception of and commitment to public health, and the collective ethnic identity—all of these influenced the practices that they adopted in their attempt to maintain health and offer succor under impossible conditions. These practices will be investigated in Part Two of this book.

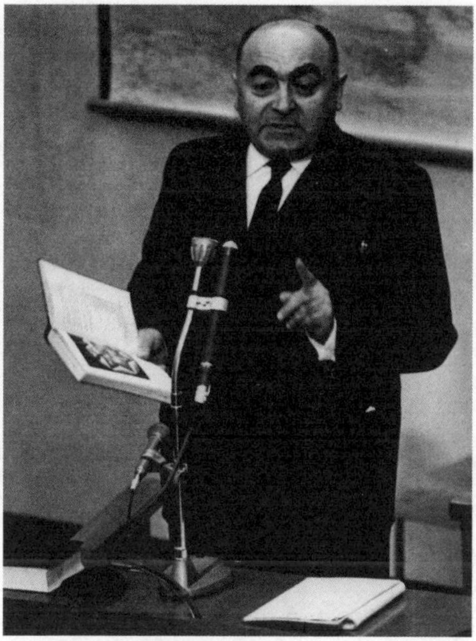

Dr. Mark Meir Dworzecki (1908–1975), physician in the Vilna ghetto and a pioneer of the study of medicine during the Holocaust, particularly of Jewish medical activity, testifying at the Eichmann trial, Jerusalem, 1961. Photo Archive, GFH, no. 26186.

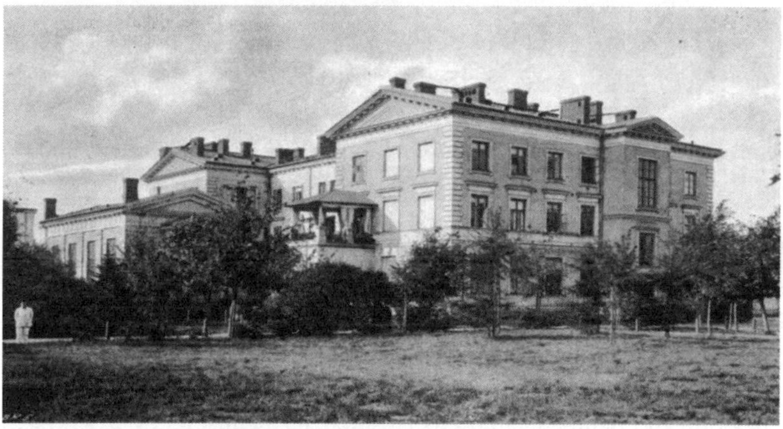

Czyste Jewish Hospital, circa 1900. *Księga Pamiątkowa*: *Sprawozdanie Komitetu Budowy*, Biblioteka Narodowa, sygn. 2.010.599 A.

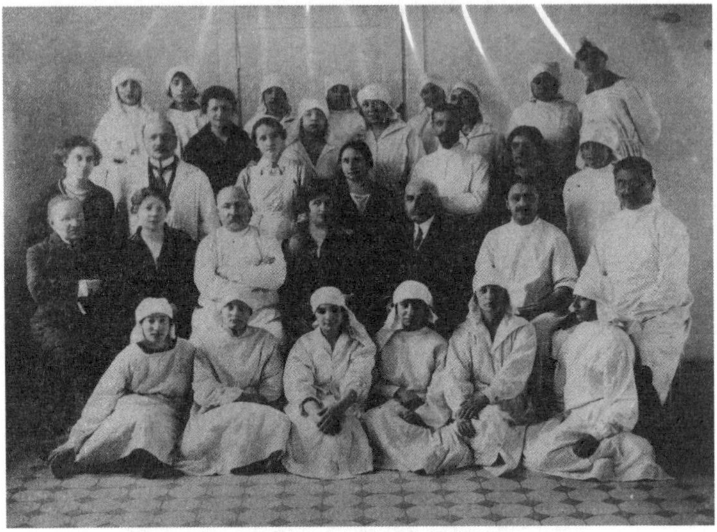

Medical and administrative staff at Czyste Hospital; Dr. Aharon Soloveichik, (1865–1942), seated, second row from the front, third from the left; Dr. Miszurski, standing, second row from the back, third from the right; Warsaw, 1930s. Photo Archive, GFH, no. 46729.

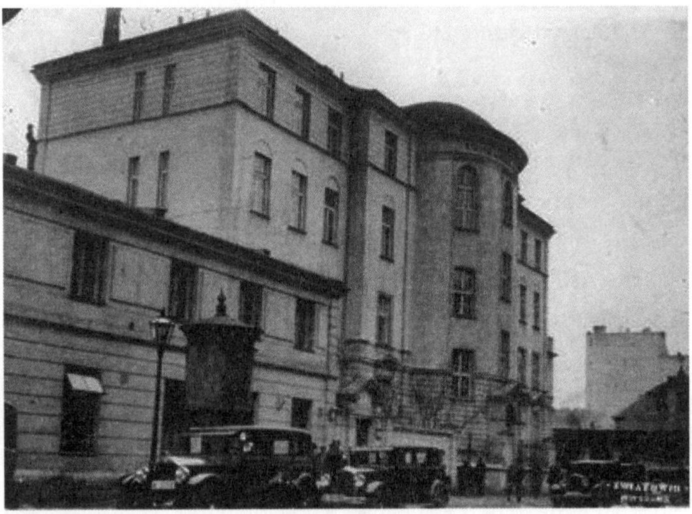

Bersohn and Bauman Children's Hospital, 60 Sienna St., 1930. Krzysztof Bielawski / POLIN Museum of the History of Polish Jews.

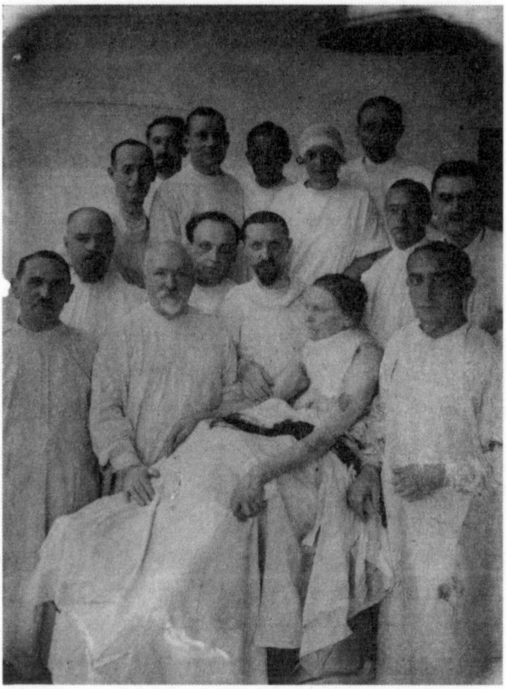

Medical staff with a patient at Czyste Hospital, Warsaw. Photo Archive, GFH, no. 46728.

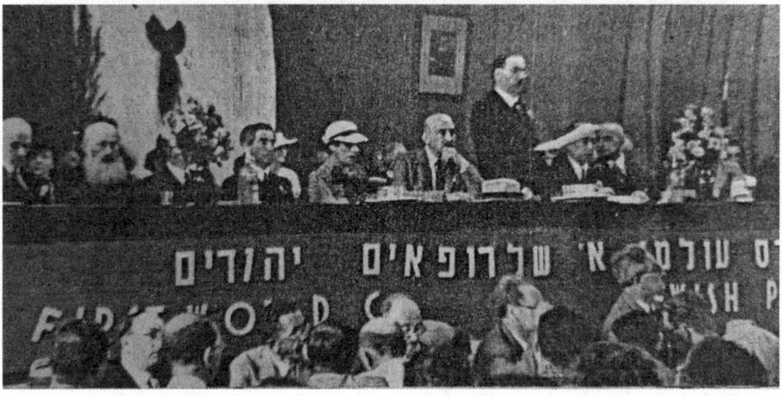

First World Congress of Jewish Physicians, Tel Aviv, 1936. Courtesy of the Israel Medical Association.

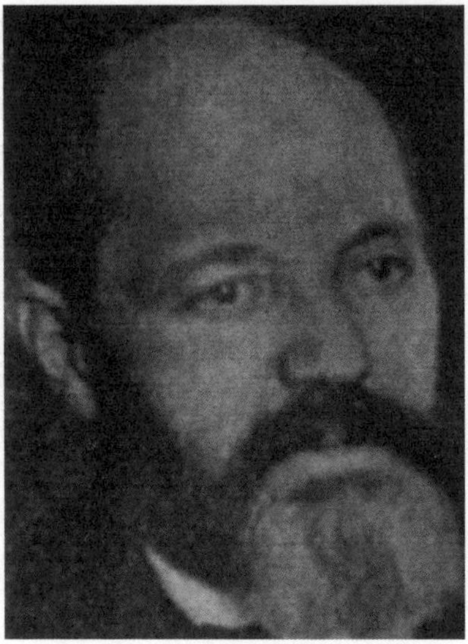

Dr. Gershon Lewin (1868–1939), Zionist activist, physician, author, director of a department at Czyste Hospital, and a TOZ cofounder. Photo Archive, GFH, no. 53941.

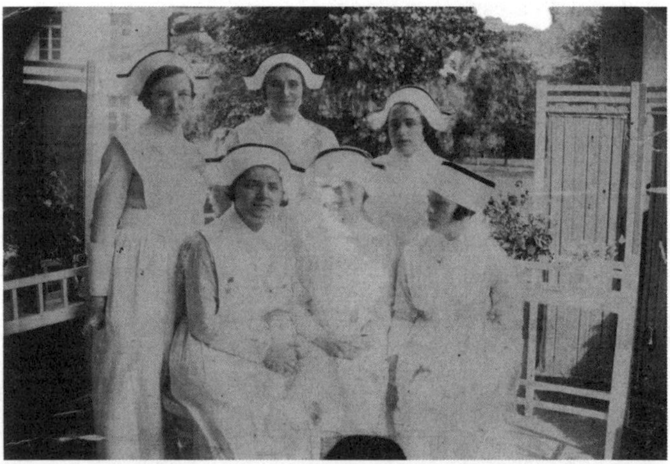

Graduates of the Jewish nursing school in Warsaw, 1927; Uka (Rachel) Bliach (1907–1942/1943), head nurse in the maternity ward at Czyste Hospital before the war and in the ghetto, back row, first left. Courtesy of her niece Hamutal Bar-Yosef.

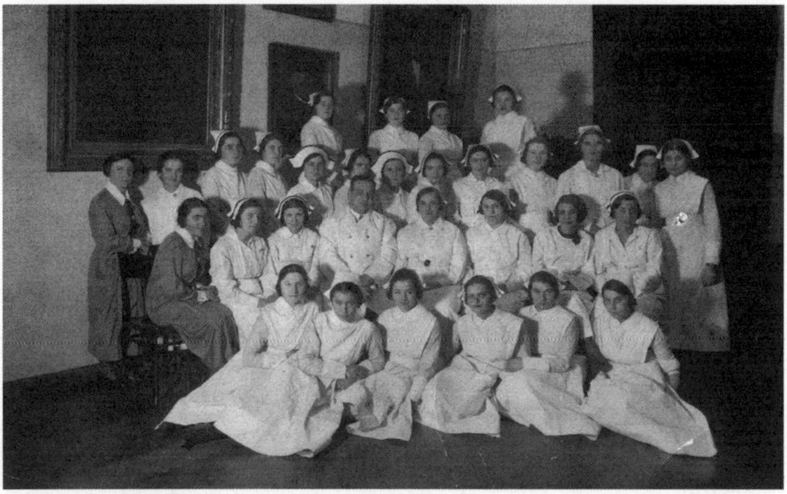

Class photo of the graduates of the Jewish nursing school in Warsaw, October 1935. Photo Archive, GFH, no. 13189.

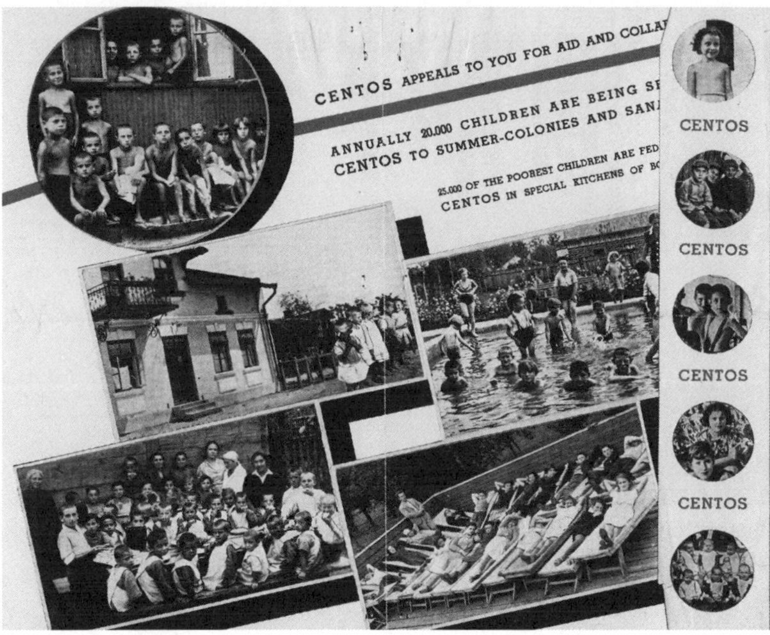
CENTOS APPEALS TO YOU FOR AID AND
ANNUALLY 20.000 CHILDREN ARE BEING
CENTOS TO SUMMER-COLONIES AND
25.000 OF THE POOREST CHILDREN ARE FED
CENTOS IN SPECIAL KITCHENS OF
CENTOS
CENTOS
CENTOS
CENTOS

Leaflet in a report by CENTOS, an umbrella organization of institutes for sheltered Jewish children, 1937–1938. JDC, AR.33-44, file 822.

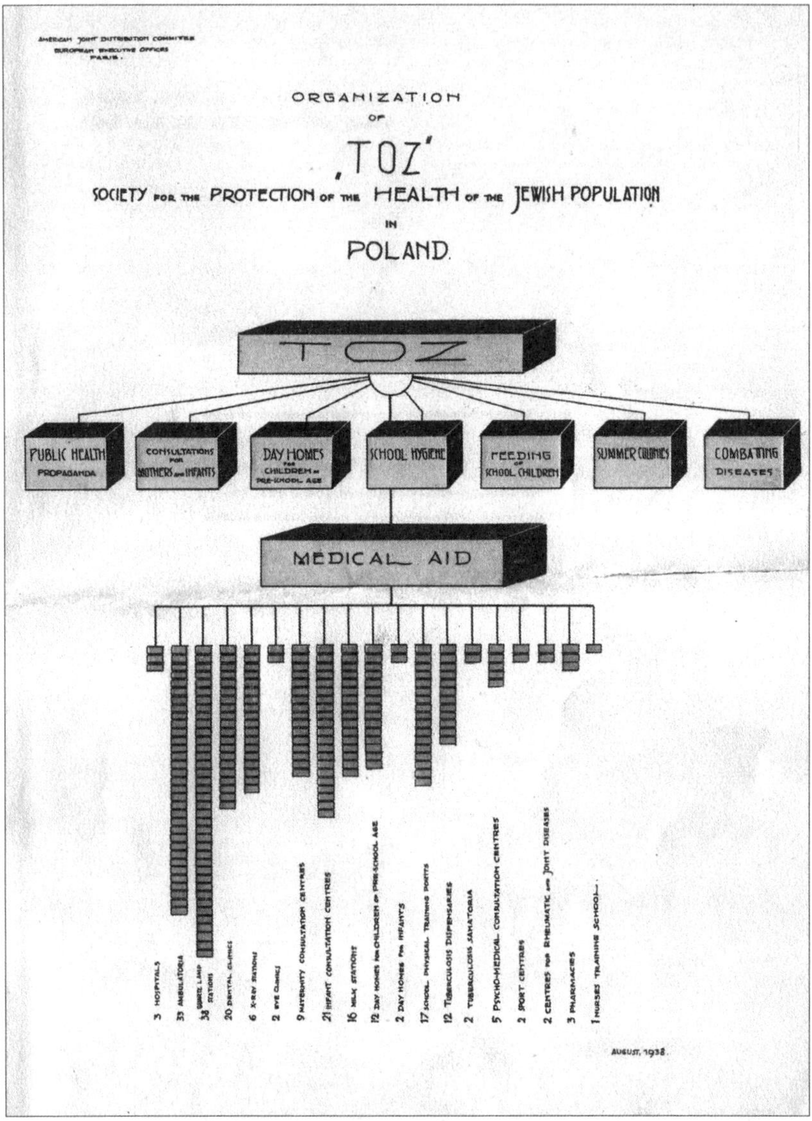

Illustration in a thirty-page report of TOZ in Poland, August, 1938. JDC, AR.33–44, file 840.

Chapter Two

The German Occupation Authorities' Policy on Jewish Medicine in Warsaw

> *Our tormentors' age-old animus toward our people has found new attire in the question of race and a falsified theory that is geared also to humiliate the dignity of other peoples and races of ancient culture. The Jew-haters have found a poisoned weapon with which to abuse us. It is the Jewish doctors' role to unmask the lie of the simpletons and ignoramuses who occupy the thugs' camp.... We are confident that the entire enlightened world, those of true human civilization, will also take our side and help us.*[1]

An additional factor—a central and definitive one—that influenced the Jews of Warsaw in their struggle to cope with the medical challenges under Nazi occupation was, of course, the Germans' policy concerning the health of the Jews. This policy influenced the conditions that caused the health crisis and left the Jews with little room to respond. The health policy that the Germans applied in the *Generalgouvernement* (General Government) was prompted by widely held views about health in Nazi Germany and the racist–nationalist antisemitic theory that served as the ideological foundation of Nazi rule.

1 Friedman, *Sefer Hakongres Ha'olami*, p. 10; Dr. David Aryeh Friedman's remarks at the First World Congress of Jewish Physicians, 1936.

At the World Congress of Jewish Physicians in 1936, Dr. David Aryeh Friedman and Dr. Ben Zion Hirshovits issued a scientific challenge to the racist views that the German health care system had adopted.

> It is our duty to awaken the conscience of the eminences among the world's nations, people of culture, thinking people, against the racial hatred that is targeting us and destroying values of generations in medicine, to awaken the conscience of the countries and institutions where the luster of knowledge has not been dulled by fanatic hatred of the eternal people.[2]

The Jewish doctors' anguished attempt to stir the conscience of those countries "where the luster of knowledge has not been dulled" fell on deaf ears.

Anti-Jewish Policy in the General Government

Germany invaded Poland on September 1, 1939, and the city of Warsaw surrendered on September 28. The Red Army immediately moved into Eastern Poland following the August 1939 Soviet–German Non-Aggression Pact and the frontier between the countries was demarcated on September 28. At the end of October 1939, the Germans deployed to extend their dominion over Poland by partitioning the country into three zones. The Soviets took control of the eastern portion; the Reich annexed the western and northern areas; and Hitler renamed Central Poland the General Government and placed it under the rule of Hans Frank,[3] a member of the Nazi elite.

2 Ibid., pp. 27–31.

3 Dr. Hans Frank (1900–1946) was a lawyer, a sworn Nazi of long standing, and a close associate of Hitler. He served as minister of justice and minister without portfolio, a member of the Reichstag, and even president of the German Academy of Law. He was noted for his ambition and fanaticism in anything pertaining to his powers in the General Government, and his adherence to his decision-making prerogatives where the Jews in his purview were concerned. The historian Raul Hilberg wrote the following about him: "In

The General Government was divided into four districts—Cracow, Radom, Warsaw, and Lublin—and a commander was appointed for each. When the Germans entered Poland, the country had a population of 33,000,000, of whom 3,300,000 were Jewish—10 percent of the total population.[4] The General Government, which was established in the center of the country on October 26, 1939, was intended to be an administered territory with a population of 11,835,510, including 1,457,376 Jews. The fate of this population was determined mainly by Hitler, General Governor Hans Frank and his staff, Heinrich Himmler, and the SS.[5] Himmler, who was considered the second most important person in the Reich, headed the SS, the Gestapo, and the Waffen-SS, and even served as the Reich minister of the interior.

The oppression of the population, which targeted Jews in particular, began at the onset of the Nazi occupation. On September 21, 1939, Reinhard Heydrich, chief of the RSHA—Reichssicherheitshauptamt (Reich Security Main Office)—who would be appointed to serve also as the Acting *Reichsprotektor* (Reich Protector) of Bohemia and Moravia in September 1941, promulgated an order to concentrate all Jews in large cities located near railroad lines.[6] Hitler and his high officials designated Poland to serve as a source of food, raw materials, and forced laborers for the Reich. As a direct consequence of this policy, the Polish

his castle…in Kraków, Frank behaved like a cultured ruler who entertained the guests by playing Chopin's piano music. In the conference room, however, he was one of the principal architects of the destruction process in Poland." The Nuremberg tribunal sentenced Frank to death by hanging. Raul Hilberg, *The Destruction of the European Jews* (Chicago: Quadrangle, 1967), pp. 133, 706; Gutman, *The Jews of Warsaw*, p. 12; Nava Cohen, "Harefu'a Besherut Ha'idiologiya Baraih Hashlishi Vehelka Bamediniyut Ha'anti-yehudit Bageta'ot Uvemahanot Harikuz," (Medicine in the Service of Ideology in the Third Reich and Its Role in the Anti-Jewish Policies in the Ghettos and the Concentration Camps) (Hebrew) (PhD diss., The Hebrew University of Jerusalem, 2003), p. 42.

4 Hilberg, *The Destruction of the European Jews*, p. 126.

5 Gutman, *The Jews of Warsaw*, pp. 13–14; Friedländer, *Nazi Germany and the Jews*, pp. 36–37.

6 Yitzhak Arad, Israel Gutman, Abraham Margaliot, eds., *Documents on the Holocaust* (Jerusalem: Yad Vashem, 1981), pp. 173–178; Leni Yahil, *The Holocaust: The Fate of European Jewry, 1932–1945* (New York: Oxford University Press, 1991), p. 297.

population was given food rations that barely sufficed to keep them alive, and most of the Polish output was sent to Germany. The Jews were even worse off.

During a discussion with the heads of the General Government in April 1940, General Governor Frank stated, "The Jews don't interest me one bit. Whether they have what to eat or not is a question that I relegate to the margins."[7] About half a year later, his remarks took a more radical turn. "Obviously all the lice and all the Jews cannot be destroyed within a year; it will have to be done farther on."[8] The General Government turned down requests to increase the Jews' food rations, even when Heinz Auerswald, the *Kommissar* responsible for the administration of the Warsaw ghetto, made the requests. "It is impossible," Frank stated in October 1941, "to provide additional food to the Jews." Auerswald ordered increases in food rations, mainly for essential workers. In practice, they received starvation rations that fell short of even one-tenth of normal consumption and, consequently, the mortality rate among Jews escalated.[9]

The General Government was defined as an autonomous administrative unit that was not annexed to the Reich. On February 12, 1940, about half a year after the occupation began, General Governor Frank and Hermann Göring met and integrated the General Government in the Four Year Plan. From then on, the administration's policy of mobilizing the territory for the war effort intensified. This economic trend clashed with the "*Volk*" policy that Hitler was eager to impose.[10] In March 1940, Frank

7 Stanislaw Piotrowski, *Hans Frank's Diary* (Warsaw: Państwowe Wydawnictwo Naukowe, 1961), pp. 98–109. For more on the Germans' policies toward Poland, see Götz Aly, *"Final Solution": Nazi Population Policy and the Murder of European Jews* (London: Arnold, 1999).

8 Piotrowski, *Hans Frank's Diary*, p. 242.

9 Ibid., p. 253; Gutman, *The Jews of Warsaw*, pp. 74–75; Ringelblum, *Polish–Jewish Relations*, pp. 81–82.

10 Cohen, "Harefu'a Besherut Ha'idiologiya," p. 50. One of the central myths in the Nazi regime was that of the *Volk*, literally translated as "people." This concept acquired enormous emotional baggage and an ideology of its own in Germany. It consisted mainly of romantic thinking that emphasized the roots, the folklore, and the "organic" aspect of the German people to the exclusion of foreign elements. In *völkisch* ideology, the German people is not only a people or a

declared a moratorium on executions in an effort to quell violence among police and individual Germans, and to underscore his authority. Henceforth, death sentences were carried out only with his approval. At this time, he attempted to turn Poland into an occupied zone in order to incorporate it into the Reich.[11] Toward the end of the General Government's first year, plans were drafted to integrate Poland into the Reich by turning it into a settlement area.[12] Within this framework, the idea took shape of banishing all Jews from Poland and settling *Volksdeutsche* (ethnic Germans) in their stead. In July 1940, Frank announced that Hitler had ordered a moratorium on the transport of Jews to the General Government. The Jews already living there would be dealt with as required by the new plan—the General Government would be *Judenrein* (cleansed of Jews).[13]

In practice, Frank's policy toward the occupied population was one of exploitation that combined moderate measures with discrimination, murder, and oppression. On September 12, 1940, about two months before the establishment of the Warsaw ghetto, Frank explained his attitude toward the occupied population. He considered the Ukrainians a friendly people, who admittedly were not close to the German people, but with whom good, distant relations should be maintained. The Polish population should be treated as second-class citizens whose basic needs had to be met, while maintaining their inferior status without cruelty.

At this stage, Frank announced his decision to enclose the Jews of Warsaw in a ghetto in accordance with the policy of segregation of the Jewish population, but noted that he would

nation but also a *Volksgemeinschaft* (united community), a unified organism based on purity of blood and connection to the common soil—a consciously exalted people that abounds with historical missions under the leadership of the führer. The concept of *Volk* in the *völkisch* state stressed the supremacy of the Aryan race and the preservation of its historical and traditional values that are endangered by foreign elements.

11 Piotrowski, *Hans Frank's Diary*, pp. 216, 226.

12 For a summary of this concept, see Aly, "*Final Solution*," pp. 4–9. This became part of a larger reorganization project for the east under the *Generalplan Ost* (General Plan East).

13 Piotrowski, *Hans Frank's Diary*, pp. 237–239.

exploit the labor of the Jewish professionals until the Poles could replace them.[14] Indeed, from the onset of the German occupation, Frank had been issuing regulation after regulation to isolate and to exploit the Jews.[15] His purpose was to implement a plan that would concentrate the Jews of the Reich and of the annexed countries in the city of Lublin—the Nisko–Lublin Plan.[16] However, the initiation of the transports of the Jews from the Warthegau,[17] the transfer of approximately 80,000 Jews within two weeks in December 1939, and Eichmann's announcement of the deportation of 550,000

14 Cohen, "Harefu'a Besherut Ha'idiologiya," pp. 58–60.

15 Ibid., pp. 62–63. For example, the promulgation of the institution of forced labor among Jews, aged 12–60, on October 26, 1939, see Polish Ministry of Information, *The German New Order in Poland* (London: Polish Ministry of Information and Hutchinson & Co., 1942), pp. 227, 558–560; the decree of the compulsory marking of Jews, from the age of ten and up, with a white armband bearing a Star of David, promulgated on November 23, 1939, see Arad et al., *Documents on the Holocaust*, pp. 178–179; the decree of the establishment of the Judenräte, issued on November 28, 1939, see Arad et al., *Documents on the Holocaust*, pp. 191–192; an order concerning the confiscation of Jewish property, promulgated on January 24, 1940, see Hilberg, *The Destruction of the European Jews*, p. 157; a statement on the need to evict the Jews from Cracow, published on April 12, 1940, see Arad et al., *Documents on the Holocaust*, pp. 197–198.

16 In late September 1939, the Germans drew up a plan to deport the Jews from Germany and from the countries that the Reich had occupied and annexed to a *Reservat* (reservation) that would be established in the Lublin district. The plan, named for its destinations, Nisko and Lublin, was part of a more comprehensive scheme for the "racial" reorganization of Eastern Europe. The Nazis wished to expand the border of the Reich eastward by deporting Jews, Roma, and Poles from the annexed territories and settling in their place *Volksdeutsche* (ethnic Germans of non-German provenance), who had been transferred from areas annexed by the Soviet Union. Thousands of Jews were sent to the "Lublin reservation," where they were housed under harsh conditions. However, technical difficulties and conflicts of interest among high Nazi decision makers brought the transports to a halt and defeated the plan. In March 1940, when Hitler expressed doubts about this solution, attention shifted to the possibility of deporting the Jews of Europe to distant territories overseas, particularly Madagascar.

17 The Warthegau was an administrative district in the western part of Poland that included the areas of Poznań and Łódź, among others, which the Germans established after the conquest of the country and annexed to the Reich. The formation and annexation of this district created territorial continuity between Germany and Eastern Prussia. The Nazi authorities, headed by Arthur Greiser, intended to purge the area of Jews and Poles.

additional Jews in January 1940, made it clear to Frank that the Lublin Plan was unviable. Therefore, he came out against these transports. According to Frank, Hitler was willing to stop shipping Jews out of the General Government in July 1940, because a new scheme—deporting them to Madagascar—had been formulated.[18] On September 12, 1940, Frank announced the sealing of the Warsaw ghetto due to the ostensible danger that its Jewish inhabitants posed.[19] The next day, he issued an order placing limits on areas where Jews could reside, which served as the legal basis for the establishment of ghettos.[20]

The SS and the police implemented the principles of the Nazi worldview through cruel acts of coercion. Himmler appointed Reinhard Heydrich, chief of the SS Sicherheitspolizei (Nazi security police), SIPO, and the Sicherheitsdienst (SS security service), SD, as the director of deportations from the annexed areas, and Ulrich Greifelt as the coordinator of resettlement activities. Himmler assumed responsibility for the implementation of the policy toward the Polish Jews—their deportation from villages and towns, and their concentration in large cities and at railroad junctions, a population census, and the establishment of the Judenräte (Jewish Councils). These measures constituted one phase toward the attainment of the "final goal" and the continuation of the policy previously implemented against the Jews of Germany and Czechoslovakia.[21]

Christopher Browning wrote that Frank's administration treated the Jews brutally for the first twenty months, because they

18 Arad et al., *Documents on the Holocaust*, pp. 216–218.

19 Cohen, "Harefu'a Besherut Ha'idiologiya," p. 64.

20 Piotrowski, *Hans Frank's Diary*, p. 90.

21 On Heydrich's instructions regarding policy and actions taken against the Jews in the occupied territories, see Arad et al., *Documents on the Holocaust*, pp. 173–178. See also Dan Michman, "Why Did Heydrich Write the Schnellbrief? A Remark on the Reason and on Its Significance," *Yad Vashem Studies*, 32 (2004), pp. 433–447. On the deportation plan, see Christopher Browning, "Nazi Resettlement Policy and the Search for a Solution to the Jewish Question, 1939-1941," in Christopher Browning, *The Path to Genocide: Essays on Launching the Final Solution* (Cambridge: Cambridge University Press, 1992), pp. 3–27; Yehoyakim Cochavi, "Göring, Hermann," in Gutman, *Encyclopedia of the Holocaust*, vol. 2, pp. 596–598.

saw no interest in exploiting them for the war. In May 1941, a group of Nazis who advocated "productivity," arguing that the health of the Jews should be preserved to help the war effort, determined policy. At this time, the establishment of factories in the ghetto prompted representatives of German firms to seek ways to lower production costs there. In any case, most of the Jews in the ghetto had no source of livelihood.[22] At a meeting of senior officials of the General Government convened on December 16, 1941, about a month before the Wannsee Conference on January 20, 1942, Frank said that the Jews had to be annihilated in order to assure the cohesion of the Reich. Shooting or poisoning 3,500,000 Jews was out of the question, but actions leading to mass annihilation could be taken, which would be discussed in the Reich. The General Government, like the Reich, had to be *Judenrein*.[23]

In the course of 1942, the Germans realized that the war in the East would be protracted and that they would have to mobilize labor to assist the army. In March 1942, the administration of the concentration camps was transferred to the WVHA—SS-Wirtschafts-Verwaltungshauptamt (SS Economic and Administrative Main Office)—so that the exploitation of the inmates' labor for war exigencies could begin. However, Himmler continued to apply the "total cleansing" policy directed at the Jews in the General Government. In mid-1942, fierce disagreements concerning the expulsion of the Jewish labor force from the General Government broke out between the Wehrmacht's armaments and logistics authorities in the General Government and the heads of the SS. Fritz Sauckel, tasked with mobilizing foreign labor for the

22 Christopher Browning, "Nazi Ghettoization Policy in Poland, 1939–1941," *Central European History*, 19:4 (1986), p. 355.

23 For excerpts of Frank's remarks on December 16, 1941, concerning the annihilation of the Jews, see Arad et al., *Documents on the Holocaust*, pp. 247–248. The Nazis' policy on Jewish labor was definitely ambivalent. Frank himself expressed conflicting views on this subject. In the course of 1941, he stated in his diary and in lectures at the University of Berlin that the Germans should employ Jewish artisans. However, in the autumn of 1941, he spoke of the need to expedite the Jews' death. In December 1942, he reverted to his view of the importance of the Jewish labor force to the Reich and the damage caused by the annihilation of the Jews. See Gutman, *Sugiyot Beheker Hashoah*, p. 165.

Reich, pressed for an increase in transports of Polish forced laborers to Germany.

By then, more than 1,500,000 Poles from the General Government had been sent to the Reich, creating a shortage of workers in this area. The Wehrmacht planned to fill the vacancies by increasing the number of Jewish workers. Suddenly, however, reports arrived about the ousting of Jews from factories in several locations. The military authorities protested the removal of these essential Jewish workers without warning and without replacing them. The SS gave the Wehrmacht a three-day notice about the mass deportation of the Jews of Warsaw. In late 1942, the Wehrmacht's authority in matters concerning the Jews was curtailed and the treatment of this population was transferred to the SS.[24]

Health Policy in the General Government

As noted above, German health policy in the General Government was predicated on the principles of the racist and antisemitic theory that leading personalities in the Reich health care system had adopted. Doctors, biologists, and anthropologists identified with the Hitlerite ideology and helped to implement it. Various trends that had emerged in medicine were integrated into the ideology of the National Socialist Movement. Genetic studies conducted at the beginning of the twentieth century emphasized biological and hereditary inequality among humans, classifying humanity into superior groups and worthless groups, and indicating the health risks that the existence of inferior groups posed to the German nation. After Hitler's rise to power, the government health care system embraced and helped to promote pseudomedical notions that the Nazi regime fostered.[25]

24 Gutman, *The Jews of Warsaw*, pp. 515–516.

25 Wolfgang U. Ecrart, *Medizin in der NS-Dictatur: Ideologie, Praxis, Folgen* (Köln: Böhlan, 2012); Paul Julian Weindling, *Health, Race, and German Politics between National Unification and Nazism, 1870–1945* (Cambridge: Cambridge University Press, 1989), pp. 339, 515–516. For a descriptive summary of the central role of physicians, scientists, and research institutes in advancing

The physicians sought to establish a scientific basis for their worldview of inequality among humans and, therefore, the danger that the non-Germans would sap the German people's strength. The recourse of the doctors to Nazi ideology resulted in the drafting of "professional" health policies in the spirit of racist ideology. The doctors developed scientific theories that recommended the exclusion of foreigners and the chronically ill from society. On July 14, 1933, already at the onset of Hitler's rule, a law was enacted to prevent breeding among persons with hereditary illnesses, the congenitally mentally retarded, and alcoholics.[26] The new statute allowed the sterilization of anyone identified as suffering from an illness surmised to be hereditary, such as feeblemindedness, schizophrenia, and severe alcoholism. The law was inspired by processes that had begun in the Weimar era, particularly the development of eugenics.[27]

Eugenics draws on a socio-biological philosophy that studies the influence of heredity on mental and behavioral characteristics among humans and seeks ways to "improve" the human species. This school of thought divides humanity into individuals with good, normal heredity and those with impaired heredity. Pursuant to the racial theory that evolved in the course of the nineteenth century and continued to expand in the twentieth, complementary schools of thought developed in some of the world's preeminent democracies—the United States and the countries of Western Europe. The most prominent among them were the schools of "racial hygiene" and of

bioracial ideas and antisemitism, and in supporting, initiating, and executing the crimes of the Nazi regime under the mantle of medicine and science until they became full collaborators in the murder of patients and helpless people with disabilities, in general, and of the Jewish people during the Holocaust, in particular, see Daniel Nadav, "Was There a 'Medicalization' of the Holocaust? SS Doctors as the Executive Arm of the German 'Biocracy' and the Perpetrators of Medical Murder," *Moreshet: Journal of the Study of the Holocaust and Antisemitism*, 16 (2019), pp. 403–459.

26 Benno Müller-Hill, *Murderous Science: Elimination by Scientific Selection of Jews, Gypsies, and Others, Germany, 1933–1945* (New York: Oxford University Press, 1988), p. 30; Roland, *Courage under Siege*, pp. 124–125.

27 The word eugenics derives from the Greek *eu* (good) and *genes* (congenital), denoting good origin, i.e., offspring of healthy, "valuable" parents. Eugenics lacks solid scientific grounding and even though it resonates in various ways today, the scientific community views it with revulsion and contempt.

eugenics. The goal of racial hygiene[28] was to breed those most highly valued and to diminish the numbers of the less valued. Eugenics developed organizational avenues for the application of these ideas and the "ongoing maintenance" of the race, e.g., counseling and intervention to promote mating among the "most valuable" and to prevent it among the genetically flawed. The consolidation of eugenics in the democracies included the sterilization of suspected carriers of hereditary diseases for the "public weal." In 1900–1933, about 27,000 sterilizations were performed in fourteen American states. In Nazi Germany alone, in contrast, approximately 400,000 such procedures were conducted in 1934–1939. German eugenics, which was developed with unparalleled radicalism, served the national-socialist racial and national goal of purging the German people of "worthless" individuals.[29]

The advocates of eugenics split into two main currents: the supporters of "positive eugenics," who favored racial improvement through positive interventions, such as encouraging births among the members of the healthy and pure race, and the proponents of "negative eugenics," who stressed the removal or sterilization of those with hereditary illnesses. After World War I, racist ideological rationales served to consolidate the trend of negative eugenics. The arguments stressed the growing need for genetic balance, primarily because the Great War had claimed so many lives among the members of the superior race. The claim was made that the maintenance of the disabled and the ill in hospitals imposed a heavy burden on a society that was in dire economic straits to begin with. Although the original statute, presented to the Prussian government in July 1932, affirmed that in the event of hereditary defects sterilization should be voluntary, the idea of forced sterilization gained strong support. An element of coercion was included in the formulation of the new law enacted in July 1933.[30]

28 Alfred Plötz coined the term "racial hygiene" in 1895. This school of thought proposed to base anthropological findings about interracial differences on the examination of the facial features of different races.

29 Nadav, *Medicine and Nazism*, pp. 12–13; Michael Burleigh, *The Third Reich: A New History* (New York: Hill and Wang, 2000), pp. 377–381.

30 Friedländer, *Nazi Germany and the Jews*, pp. 39–40.

When World War II broke out, Germany's negative eugenics policy took on a new form. The sterilization campaign ended and a decision was made to "purify the Aryan race" by killing those rendered "unfit" by disease, chiefly the mentally retarded and the severely mentally ill. Aided by members of the medical profession who lacked any restraint, a "euthanasia" campaign got underway. Here the term euthanasia, denoting mercy killing, served to mask the execution of hundreds of thousands of Germans who suffered severe illness. In this program, grounded in the Nazis' racist ideology and the principles of racial improvement, Germany murdered approximately 90,000 of its own citizens in various ways, including gas chambers. The operation was code-named T4, an abbreviation for its headquarters at 4 Tiergartenstrasse in Berlin. In the wake of the protests of the Church and of German public opinion, the program was formally halted in August 1941, but it was continued surreptitiously thereafter.[31]

Many researchers identify a connection between the policy of sterilization and euthanasia and the policy of extermination, claiming that the euthanasia process and the methods used to implement it were eventually replicated in the annihilation of the Jews. Indeed, from the onset of the sterilizations to the ostensible cessation of euthanasia in August 1941 and the beginning of the Final Solution at approximately this time, the policy toward persons with disabilities and mental disorders, on the one hand, and the Jews, on the other, evolved concurrently and along parallel paths. Friedländer, however, sees a distinction between these processes and notes the uniqueness of the Final Solution.

> If sterilization and euthanasia were meant only to enhance the purity of the national community [*Volksgemeinschaft*] and rested on cost-benefit calculations, the segregation and extermination of the Jews—although these, too, were a process of racial purification—were aimed principally at an active and daunting enemy that was perceived as a menace to the very existence of Germany and the Aryan world.

31 Nadav, *Medicine and Nazism*, pp. 32–40; Burleigh, *The Third Reich*, pp. 382–404.

> Therefore, apart from the objective of purifying the race, common to sterilization and euthanasia, and in contrast to it, the war on the Jews was perceived as a confrontation of apocalyptic magnitude.[32]

Jewish medical associations around the world decried these racist views adopted by the German health care system. Thus, the First World Congress of Jewish Physicians, held under the shadow of the Nazi accession to power, issued a statement of condemnation and protest.

> The World Congress of Jewish Physicians, held in Tel Aviv on April 23–27, 1936, hereby affirms that all human beings have the right, irrespective of their race and origin, to equality of rights in their countries of residence, and states that the upholding of this fundamental is considered a respected virtue of the culture of nations. The disentitlement and expulsion of the German Jews due to their race and origin, akin to the expulsion from medieval Spain, mark a retreat from human development and progress in this country. The desecration of elementary human rights cannot be explained on the grounds of racial contrasts between Jews and other peoples in Europe, which cannot be defined scientifically. The exploitation of this scientific falsehood for lowly political ends requires this congress to appeal to ensuing congresses and international scientific organizations and to request repeatedly that they place the question of race and racial ideology on the agenda and show it in its proper light.[33]

However, "The exploitation of this scientific falsehood for lowly political ends" expanded steadily. The application of Darwin's theory to human affairs gained broad acceptance among physicians in Germany, leading to the replacement of the humane approach,

32 Friedländer, *Nazi Germany and the Jews*, pp. 39–40.

33 Friedman, *Sefer Hakongres Ha'olami Harishon*, pp. 81–82.

which called for assisting the weak and the ill, with a different one—the cultivation of the healthy Aryan population and selection to weed out the weak. The Jews and the Roma–Sinti would later undergo this selection process.

Doctors and scientists played a role in Hitler's regime and abetted the racial improvement policy. The Aryan doctors helped to ban Jewish counterparts and scientists from research institutes, and to establish rules to murder the ill in the euthanasia program. In their implementation of the racist demographic policy, German authorities instituted the mass murder of groups of citizens with the cooperation and support of the medical practitioners. After having conceived of euthanasia years earlier, the doctors devised methods of selection and murdered thousands of patients to realize a biological, social, and national vision. Hitler and his high officials decided to annihilate the Jews. Doctors and professionals in the natural sciences established the theory that the Jews were a source of mental and physical illness, and helped to reinforce racist antisemitic arguments by invoking theories of genetics. They determined who was a Jew for selection purposes and affirmed the need to banish the Jews.[34]

With the development of medical research at the universities at the turn of the twentieth century, German society attributed social and political importance to doctors and medicine as the guardians of the nation's health. This is a concept rooted in Romantic nationalism, in general, and in Germany, in particular.[35] The doctors believed in the potential of science to solve social problems in the unified German nation–state.[36] The country's universities and research institutes received lavish state support. The nexus of state and university, along with the conservative Weltanschauung that pervaded intellectual circles, prompted a commitment to national partnership among doctors and scientists. The health care

34 Cohen, "Harefu'a Besherut Ha'idiologiya," pp. 540–544.

35 Weindling, *Health, Race, and German Politics*, pp. 158–161.

36 Walter Zwi Bacharach, *Gizanut Besherut Hapolitika: Min Hamonizm El Hanatzizm* (Racism in the Service of Politics: The Way from Monism to Nazism) (Hebrew) (Jerusalem: Magnes, 1984), pp. 413–418.

system and the political system formed strong interrelations.[37]

The doctors in the General Government also harbored Nazi medical views. They regarded the Jews as carriers of epidemics who also spread them to non-Jewish society. As early as 1933, the theory that Jews constituted a disease-prone race was taught in medical schools, universities, and the education system, which helped to create the antisemitic image of the Jews and to substantiate the idea that the Jewish problem should be solved by taking medical measures. The belief that Jews carried typhus gained acceptance, easily and rapidly, and dictated practical policy in the General Government. For example, the Nazis ordered the staff at Czyste Hospital in Warsaw to perform autopsies on Jews who died in the ghetto in order to confirm the number of deaths from typhus and to prove the theory that Jews were carriers and spreaders of the disease.

The Nazis forbade public worship in the Warsaw ghetto, arguing that public gatherings might spread the epidemic more quickly. For the same reason, Jews were banned from traveling on trains. Fear of epidemics also justified murder. In Kutno, for instance, a German policeman received a commendation for having prevented the spread of the epidemic to the German population by murdering five Jews who had left the ghetto. The German physicians in the General Government considered the Jews a race that carried disease in their blood and a source of contagion, hence, deserving of isolation from the rest of the population. This view was widely affirmed in the traditional antisemitic argument, but the proposal of medical solutions in the spirit of the racist ideology provided a new angle.[38]

The superintendent of the health offices in the General Government, Dr. Werner Kroll, described the Jews as an influential force in Poland, akin to estate owners and the Church. Against this background, Jewish physicians were depicted as being associated with the wealthy, making a great deal of money, and taking over

37 Much literature exists on this topic. See Weindling, *Health, Race, and German Politics*; Proctor, *Racial Hygiene*; Cohen, "Harefu'a Besherut Ha'idiologiya," pp. 535–536.

38 Roland, *Courage under Siege*, pp. 128–130.

jobs that rightfully belonged to Polish, Ukrainian, and German doctors—a greedy type who benefited from the Poles' money due to their commercial aptitude and despite their professional ignorance. The doctors' expertise was also suspect. Kroll claimed that when the Jewish physicians were segregated from the Aryans in the General Government and had to treat their own patients, they proved to be unskilled in surgery and therefore in need of Polish experts. In addition, while Jewish doctors could diagnose illnesses, they exploited their patients for profit. These are only a few of Kroll's charges against the Jewish doctors.[39]

In October 1939, as part of the civil administration that the Germans established in the General Government, an autonomous Public Health Care and Medical Services Department was set up. It was placed under the authority of the governor general and the Reich minister of health, Dr. Leonardo Conti,[40] who appointed Dr. Jost Walbaum[41] to head the health care system. Dr. Walbaum's goal was to create a health care system in the General Government that would consolidate all authority over the health care of the

39 Cohen, "Harefu'a Besherut Ha'idiologiya," pp. 124–130.

40 Conti (1890–1945) studied medicine in Berlin. He joined the SA in 1923 and helped set up this organization's health care services. In 1929, he cofounded the National Socialist Medical Association and headed its Berlin branch. He joined the SS in 1930 and represented the Nazi Party in the Prussian Parliament in 1932–1933. In 1939, upon the death of Dr. Gerhard Wagner, head of the Medical Association and of the Nazi Party's Main Office for Public Health, Dr. Conti replaced him in these capacities and also became the Reich Minister of Health. In July 1942, his powers were transferred to Hitler's personal physician, Dr. Karl Brandt. In 1945, he killed himself in prison in Nuremberg. See Michael Hans Kater, *Doctors under Hitler* (Chapel Hill: University of North Carolina Press, 1989), pp. 19–25; Cohen, "Harefu'a Besherut Ha'idiologiya," p. 101.

41 Dr. Walbaum (1889–1972) specialized in dermatology and roentgenology, among other fields, after World War I. In 1930, he joined the Nazi Party. In 1933, after Hitler became chancellor, he was appointed to serve as a doctor at the Berlin Health Bureau and as a municipal physician. He was among the instigators of the forced sterilization of the mentally ill, the mentally retarded, epileptics, and sufferers of other hereditary conditions. He was posted to Cracow in September 1939 to help meet the needs of the health care system in the occupied areas. When the General Government Civil Administration was set up, he was placed in charge of the health care system in that area. See Cohen, "Harefu'a Besherut Ha'idiologiya," p. 101.

German and non-German populations alike.[42] In June 1941, Dr. Walbaum and his colleagues published their policy in a special pamphlet. Poland was described as a primitive country that lacked proper sanitation services, and Poles were designated "half-citizens" who were unable to provide adequate medical services. Walbaum and his medical staff professed to have overcome this dire situation by installing an efficient medical administration that would serve the Reich and the Germans. They claimed that although they were not required to provide medical care to the Poles, the German health policies in the General Government benefited them as well.[43]

After the fighting in Poland ended, the Germans' fear of the spread of epidemics from the Polish population to their own soldiers and civilians prompted them to overhaul the Polish health care system in order to fight plagues and stanch their dissemination.[44] The German doctors at the General Government Health Department blamed the Jews for the spread of typhus, which was caused by the Rickettsia bacterium that infected humans via body lice. Dr. Ernst Georg Nauck wrote about "typhus and ethnic identity," emphatically singling out the Jews as carriers of this contagion. He claimed that typhus was rife in areas densely populated by Jews, because they were of lowly culture and lacked good hygiene. Most of Nauck's colleagues favored measures that would restrict the mobility of the Jews and, consequently, the doctors in the General Government supported the idea of ghettoization. From the physicians' standpoint, it was in the Germans' interest to protect the Polish population against epidemics and, therefore, it was necessary to quarantine the Jews to keep them from spreading their diseases.[45]

The Germans' health policies in the General Government were clearly enunciated at a conference held in Poland in October 1941 under the direction of Dr. Walbaum. Approximately 100

42 Ibid., pp. 101–103.

43 Christopher Robert Browning, "Genocide and Public Health: German Doctors and Polish Jews, 1939–1941," *Holocaust and Genocide Studies*, 3 (1988), p. 22.

44 Cohen, "Harefu'a Besherut Ha'idiologiya," p. 109.

45 Weindling, *Epidemics and Genocide*, pp. xv–xxi and particularly pp. 271–322; Browning, "Genocide and Public Health," pp. 22–23.

German public health physicians from all parts of the General Government attended it. The speakers reiterated the basic assumption that the spread of typhus was due to the undisciplined comportment of Jews, particularly those "wandering around," and expressed their support for more intensive disinfection and delousing, even among patients who were not contagious and had no lice. Some—the minority—asserted that the spread of epidemics could not be fought without addressing the causes, and since the Jews were fleeing the ghetto because of the lack of food, more food should be provided. The majority maintained that the Jews should be sentenced to death by starvation in the ghetto or by firing squad, and that the Health Department should be responsible for ensuring that the Germans were not at risk of being infected by the parasitic Jews.

Some claimed that Jewish money had thwarted the efforts to disinfect the ghetto and, therefore, authorization should be granted to shoot any Jew caught outside the ghetto without a permit. Since food shortages were part of war, it was better that the Jews starve in the ghetto than die dispersed throughout the town.[46] When Frank and his officials convened in Cracow in December 1941 to discuss typhus, the governor general took the opportunity to approve the order to shoot Jews and expanded the powers to implement this more rapidly. Apprising his associates of the Final Solution, he declared that he had always favored the idea of the disappearance of the Jews. He reported that he had participated in negotiations to deport the Jews to the East, but that no one was interested in receiving them. He added that he did not yet know how the Jews would be annihilated, but that there were plans for this in Germany and he would inform everyone present later.[47]

According to directives from the central government in the Reich, the Polish population was to be denied medical services, except for the treatment of contagious diseases. In 1939, Dr. Ernst Wetzel and Dr. G. Hecht, senior officials at the Nazi Party's Office of Racial Policy, elaborated on these guidelines

46 Browning, "Genocide and Public Health," pp. 26–28.
47 Ibid.

in a document bearing their names.[48] On July 23, 1942, in a confidential letter to Alfred Rosenberg, the leading ideologue of the National Socialist Movement and minister for the occupied territories in the East, Martin Bormann, one of Hitler's closest aides, ordered Rosenberg to implement the racist policy in these areas in a manner that would deny medical services to non-German populations and would prevent the growth of the Polish population. Nevertheless, Dr. Walbaum, director of the General Government Health Department, believing that the health of the Polish population would serve German interests, made sure that the level of health care in the General Government would match the prewar level there. The Health Department's goal was to eradicate contagious diseases among the population at large in order to prevent infecting the Germans.

Dr. Walbaum appointed Dr. Werner Kroll to set up the health system in the General Government. Acting from the perspective that the supervision of public health must be in the hands of the government, Kroll established a system in which there was a total separation between the Jews and the Aryans. A special health bureau for Jews, headed by a Jewish physician, was set up. In addition, a special office was established at the Central Health Bureau of the General Government to deal with Jewish affairs and racial testing in order to maintain strict physical separation between the Jews and the Aryans, and to act in accordance with the special definitions adopted by the General Government to determine who is a Jew. Strict separation in the medical services applied only to the Jews—only Jews treated Jews and Jews were not allowed to treat non-Jews. In the hospitals and all other medical services, physical segregation was the rule.

Frank excluded the Jewish population from the remit of the General Government and the Polish governing apparatus. Jews had to set up a self-governing system of their own. The chairs and members of the Judenräte, appointed at the Germans' behest, were

48 Mark Dworzecki, *Eropa Lelo Yeladim: Tohnit Hanatzim Leheres Biyologi* (Europe without Children—The Nazi Program for Biological Destruction) (Hebrew) (Jerusalem: Yad Vashem, 1958), pp. 37–39, 44–46; Cohen, "Harefu'a Besherut Ha'idiologiya," p. 110.

responsible for addressing the needs of the Jewish population, including health care. In the first half of 1940, before ghettoization, contact with the Polish population was still possible. However, the Jews had to provide independent medical services in Jewish facilities. This also applied to the war on epidemics. The German health authorities established a health care system that served Germans, Poles, and Ukrainians, leaving the Jews to their fate.[49]

German Health Care System in Warsaw

The health care policy applied to the Jews in Warsaw was the product of Walbaum's "vision of health," as described above. The core premises of racial and "redemptive" antisemitism—a term proposed by Friedländer[50]—were its underpinnings. Dr. Wilhelm Hagen, the director of health care in Warsaw from the establishment of the ghetto until the deportations, was primarily responsible for imposing the directives and decrees derived from this policy.[51] The following case study substantiates the Jewish adage, which may be translated as "judge the beginning by the end," and offers an edifying example.

In the middle of December 1942, Max Sollmann, SS officer and chief of police in Warsaw, placed a letter on the desk of his

49 Cohen, "Harefu'a Besherut Ha'idiologiya," pp. 107–117.

50 See Friedländer, *Nazi Germany and the Jews*, particularly Chapter 3.

51 Wilhelm Hagen (1893–1982) served as a public health physician. In 1919, he was a member of the Union of Socialist Academics. Due to his involvement in student demonstrations in Munich in the spring of that year, he was sentenced to three months in prison. He then served as chief physician of Frankfurt. He was not an ideological National Socialist. After Hitler rose to power in 1933, he was dismissed from his post for political reasons and turned to private practice. He claimed that he was forced to join the Nazi Party in 1938, as a condition for receiving a labor permit. A shortage of public health physicians in the occupied areas and his friendship with Dr. Walbaum led to his appointment as a public health physician in Warsaw and superintendent of the health of the Jewish inhabitants of the ghetto from 1941 to 1943. Thereafter, he served on the Russian front. After the war, he served as president of the West German Ministry of Health from 1956 to 1958. See Browning, "Genocide and Public Health," p. 24; Cohen, "Harefu'a Besherut Ha'idiologiya," p. 138; Weindling, *Epidemics and Genocide*, p. 409.

superior, SS General Friedrich Wilhelm Krüger, supreme police and SS commander in the General Government in Cracow. By then, almost two years had passed since Dr. Hagen had taken up his post as supervisor of the health of the inhabitants of Warsaw, including the half-million Jews confined to the ghetto. Chief of Police Sollmann submitted a complaint against Hagen for applying an ideology inconsistent with "German health policy." The reader of the document might think momentarily that Dr. Hagen was being charged with helping the Jews, but it was another matter altogether.

At this time, in December 1942, only around 60,000 Jews remained in the ghetto. Approximately 300,000 had been transported to Treblinka in the *Grossaktion* (Great Deportation) of July–September, three months before the aforementioned letter was written.[52] Hagen had not written letters of protest and had not defended the Jews of Warsaw, neither during the time that the medical tragedy was being inflicted on them in the ghetto nor during the brutal deportations to Treblinka. If so, what was Sollmann, an SS officer and a sworn supporter of the Nazi ideology, complaining about? At the same time that the Jews were being "evacuated to the East," their health care institutions were also being "evacuated," as patients were massacred and the non-bedridden were cruelly sent to the extermination camps. Since Hagen considered himself loyal to the principles of health care, as well as to professional and human ethics, he came up with the idea of waging a war on tuberculosis, which was spreading among the Poles in Warsaw and threatening to escalate into a disastrous epidemic. His plan included converting the evacuated Jewish health care facilities into tuberculosis treatment centers at an expected cost of 18 million zlotys.

Officer Sollman accused Hagen of taking an egalitarian view of his responsibilities with respect to the Polish and German patients. Where the Jews were concerned, there was no dispute

52 Havi Dreifuss (Ben-Sasson), *Geto Varsha—Hasof: April 1942–Yuni 1943* (Warsaw Ghetto—The End: April 1942–June 1943) (Hebrew) (Jerusalem: Yad Vashem, 2011).

as it was obvious that they should not receive any assistance. Moreover, the proper solution of waging war on their diseases was underway: the vast majority of the Jews of Warsaw had already been sent to Treblinka in thundering silence on the part of Hagen and his fellow health officials. However, for the Poles, Hagen was willing to act by actually taking genuine health measures, as Sollman's letter implies.

> Below is my reference to the remarks of Dr. Hagen in regard to the Jewish medical institution for the treatment of tuberculosis, Brijus:...the highest priority is to assure that the measures taken by the Poles in the war on tuberculosis remain on the same scale and quality....It is none of the Germans' business to intervene and to help in this regard; on the contrary...due to the ideological stance of Dr. Hagen who wishes to treat Germans and Poles equally, since there can be no political attitude toward the treatment of tuberculosis, he says....It should not be the Germans' job to establish a serious, active entity that would safeguard the health of the Polish people or see to the convalescence of Polish patients and the establishment of additional facilities for the treatment of tuberculosis, something that would entail a major outlay in resources and staff that would be justified only if we wish to sustain the Polish nation.
>
> **...A fundamentally different view appears here, one that aims to treat Germans and Poles equally and to preserve their health. If an institution for the treatment of tuberculosis has not been set up for the Germans to date** [emphasis in the original], it demonstrates a misreading of the situation, at the expense of treating Poles only. The goal cannot be to enhance the Poles' welfare but the contrary: to erode it down to a certain limit. The practical conclusion should have been drawn long ago: a convalescent institution for the few Germans from the Reich and for the *Volksdeutsche*, who are also not numerous, should be set up....If the German administration has an interest in sustaining the Polish nation—for whatever reason—

> then this scheme is justified. If the German administration has no such interest—then this scheme is madness!!...According to credible reports, Dr. Hagen visited Berlin recently and tried to prevail upon the director of the Reich Ministry of Health. Afterwards, Dr. Hagen traveled to Munich....In this state of affairs, Dr. Hagen and his "Polish tuberculosis scheme" should be opposed by all means.[53]

Indeed, "judge the beginning by the end." The health care policy toward the Jews in Warsaw was derived from the racist antisemitic view as described below.

When the occupation began, Warsaw had a population of around 1,300,000, including 400,000 Jews. Two separate health bureaus were established there: one for Poles, where 1,014 people—doctors, nurses, and white-collar and sanitation workers—were employed by the German health care system—and another for the Jews, employing 399 people.[54] German doctors were responsible for health policy and its administration. A supervisory medical apparatus was set up to oversee medical care and the health of the citizens in Warsaw. Dr. Kurt Schrempf was named chief physician of the city of Warsaw. In January 1941, Dr. Wilhelm Hagen was appointed to a subordinate position and charged with combatting mortality in the ghetto and typhus, which was spreading in the city.

Unlike most doctors in the General Government, Hagen did not clearly identify with Nazi ideology. However, where typhus was concerned, he subscribed to the racist antisemitic view that the disease was endemic to Jews. He maintained that the Jews had to be segregated, but also that the typhus epidemic had to be fought among them in order to stanch the plague on both sides. Other German authorities decried this policy. When

53 In the letter from Max Sollmann, SS officer and police and SS commander in Warsaw, to Wilhelm Krüger, supreme police and SS commander in the General Government, concerning tuberculosis in the General Government, Sollmann blamed Hagen for the plague, December 18, 1942, GFH, no. 7783; Offer, *Haluk Lavan Bageto*, appendix A.5, pp. 516–520.

54 Cohen, "Harefu'a Besherut Ha'idiologiya," p. 137.

66,000 refugees were transported to the Warsaw ghetto in the spring of 1941, he demanded that they be placed in quarantine for fourteen days. The German administration opposed this, arguing that fighting typhus in the ghetto was not its concern. Nevertheless, because of the attendant suffering and inefficiency, the Jews did not comply with the public health rules that Hagen had handed down.[55]

In July 1941, Hagen advised his superiors that, in his opinion, the Jews who had left the ghetto were responsible for the spread of typhus and only timely measures would keep the epidemic from worsening. Hagen criticized the lack of cooperation among the German administrative officials in the ghetto and the Jews' intransigent objections to his anti-epidemic measures. In his opinion, more supervision and control, more experts, and more medical equipment were required of the Germans. He argued that monetary considerations and principles should not prevail at such a time, and demanded that the Jewish police and Jewish medical personnel who refused to comply with the orders, as well as the Jews who were caught leaving the ghetto, should be punished by flogging, whereas any Jews found "wandering around" outside the ghetto should be shot. Hagen demanded an increase in the ghetto's food supplies to meet the required minimum. Otherwise, he claimed, the Jews would attempt to flee the ghetto in order to avoid the alternative of starving to death.

Hagen opposed Heinz Auerswald's scheme to constrict the boundaries of the ghetto in order to prevent smuggling, due to a concern about the terrible overcrowding this would cause and the inability to fight the typhus epidemic. Failing to convince Auerswald to revise his plan, Hagen wrote to Ludwig Leist, the Nazi plenipotentiary governor of the Warsaw District and the mayor of Warsaw,[56] warning that such measures would severely

55 Browning, "Genocide and Public Health," p. 25.

56 The first two mayors were Helmut Otto and Oscar Rudolf Dengel. From April 1940 to July 1944, Ludwig Leist held the post. He was appointed to the highest-ranking position in the municipal apparatus and he served as a plenipotentiary district governor on behalf of the civil administration. See Hilberg, *Horban Yehudei Eropa* (The Destruction of the European Jews) (Hebrew) (Jerusalem:

exacerbate the epidemic. Auerswald admitted that the shortage of food was causing starvation and epidemics, and condoned smuggling at first, because it alleviated the food shortage. Still, he was concerned that such activity was helping to spread typhus. He supported Hagen's proposals to increase the food supply and to shoot Jews "wandering around," and decided to defend the ghetto boundaries more stringently. Although he rescinded the idea of cutting off the southern part of the ghetto, the ghetto borders were revised, displacing 60,000 persons from their homes. In October 1941, Frank rejected Auerswald's requests to increase food supplies in the ghetto and approved the death penalty for any Jew who left the ghetto, and not just those caught "wandering around."[57]

Hagen's reports to his superiors indicate that the Jews of Warsaw were healthier than the Poles on the eve of the war. The Jews' mortality was lower and their birth rate was higher than they were among the Poles, and the Poles' mortality was higher than their birth rate. Hagen explained this by invoking an antisemitic argument concerning the Jews' preference for urban settlement. Once the war was underway, the health of the population of Warsaw, in general, and of the Jews, in particular, took a turn for the worse. In 1941, mortality declined among the Poles but increased radically among the Jews. In 1939–1941, Hagen wrote that the situation of the Poles had improved but that of the Jews had deteriorated. He described the Poles as a vibrant people and the Jews, in contrast, as a "declining race" that had lost its will to procreate.[58] Hagen considered himself responsible only for the health care services of the German and Polish populations.

Yad Vashem and Ben-Gurion University of the Negev, 2013), p. 204n174; Adam Czerniaków, *The Warsaw Diary of Adam Czerniaków: Prelude to Doom*, ed. by Raul Hilberg, Stanislaw Staron, and Josef Kermish (New York: Stein and Day, 1979), p. 131.

57 Judenrat report to Dr. Auerswald on the Warsaw Jewish quarter under the *Kommissar*'s rule, May 15, 1941–May 15, 1942, GFH, no. 3909. See Hagen's proposals concerning the shooting of roving Jews, and the fining and flogging of those leaving the ghetto, GFH, no. 5214; Offer, "Ma'arach Harefu'a Begeto Varsha," vol. 2, appendix A.6, pp. 32–33.

58 See Offer, *Haluk Lavan Bageto*, appendix B.5, p. 540; Cohen, "Harefu'a Besherut Ha'idiologiya," pp. 142–144.

He deemed that his responsibility for the Jewish population was limited to contagious diseases and excluded them from receiving treatment.[59] In early 1943, Hagen and Walbaum were removed from their posts in the General Government due to disagreements with the SS on matters that were unrelated to their attitude toward the Jews.

The crux of the dispute between Hagen and his superiors, as previously mentioned, had to do with his professional conviction that it was his moral duty to extend medical care to the Poles. That he felt no similar obligation to the Jews sharply reflects his antisemitic and inhumane attitude toward them.[60] While Hagen attempted to uphold professional principles in his treatment of the non-German population, his policy toward the Jews was influenced by antisemitic motives. In fact, his policy fanned the spread of typhus by supporting the total quarantine of the ghetto, the killing of Jews who escaped from it, and the adoption of coercive and cruel tactics in the war against typhus. He was willing to take risks to save thousands of Poles who had contracted tuberculosis but was indifferent to the lives of Jews.[61] The debate over the extent of his responsibility for the health tragedy that befell the Jews in the Warsaw ghetto took a more mordant turn after the war, when Dr. Hagen sued the historian Josef Wulf,[62] a Holocaust survivor, who had included

59 Cohen, "Harefu'a Besherut Ha'idiologiya," p. 161.

60 Letter from Max Sollmann, SS officer and police and SS commander in Warsaw, to Wilhelm Krüger, supreme police and SS commander in the General Government, concerning tuberculosis in the General Government, December 18, 1942, GFH, no. 7783; Offer, *Haluk Lavan Bageto*, appendix A.5, pp. 516–520. In Walbaum's case, a combination of factors brought about his dismissal: his argumentative nature, his support for Hagen's "tuberculosis plan," which clashed with the racial policy of the SS, and his failure to transfer health care facilities to the SS for its own use. See Browning, "Genocide and Public Health," p. 29.

61 Offer, *Haluk Lavan Bageto*, appendix A.3, pp. 505–507.

62 Nicolas Berg, "The Invention of 'Functionalism': Josef Wulf, Martin Broszat, and the Institute for Contemporary History (Munich) in the 1960s," *Search and Research: Lectures and Papers*, 4 (2003), pp. 7–38. Regarding the affair of Dr. Hagen versus Josef Wulf, see documentation related to the trials of war criminals in YVA, O.4/515. For the Hebrew translation of some of the correspondence

Hagen on his list of collaborators.[63] Hagen, then a professor at the University of Bonn, sued Wulf and demanded that he apologize. The extensive correspondence between him and Martin Broszat, head of the Institute of Contemporary History in Germany, concerning this matter has been preserved.[64]

Even before the decision to annihilate the Jews was taken in 1941, the doctors in the General Government knowingly took measures that caused the deaths of thousands of Jews. Browning considers the medical system a prime factor in the radicalization of the antisemitic policy. The health care system's demand to seal the ghetto influenced the decision to do so and converged with additional factors that prodded the central authorities to isolate the Jews from their surroundings. This policy resulted in the sealing of additional ghettos in the General Government and high mortality among the Jewish population.[65]

Medical Aspects of the Anti-Jewish Strictures in Warsaw before the Sealing of the Ghetto

In retrospect, some of the administrative decrees and orders that the Nazis promulgated in the autumn of 1939 may indicate plans for the future that were latent from the outset of the occupation to isolate the Jews from the rest of the population for hygienic and political reasons, and even to establish a ghetto later. Many of these restrictions stemmed from aspects of health and sanitation, which is how they were explained when the orders were issued. Some of them had a direct and immediate

between Hagen and Wulf, see Offer, "Ma'arach Harefu'a Begeto Varsha," vol. 2, appendices A.4–A.10, pp. 29–40.

63 Josef Wulf, *Das Dritte Reich und seine Vollstrecker: Die Liquidation von 500,000 Juden Im Ghetto Warschau* (Berlin: Arani Verlag GmbH, 1961).

64 Berg, "The Invention of 'Functionalism'"; Dr. Chaim Einhorn testimony against Hagen, GFH, no. 5214; Blumental article, "Dr. Hagen's Sin," GFH, no. 5214; extensive correspondence concerning Hagen's suit against Wulf, YVA, O.4/515; Paula Zofia Sanek's deposition against Hagen and press items in Poland and Germany contemporary to the trial, YVA, M.21/1-17; Offer, "Ma'arach Harefu'a Begeto Varsha," vol. 2, appendix A.5–A.10, pp. 31–44.

65 Browning, "Genocide and Public Health," p. 23.

impact on the health of the Jewish population, while others had indirect effects.

A German edict concerning forced labor, signed by Frank, was issued on October 26, 1939, along with an implementation order bearing the signature of SS and Police Commander Krüger. On December 12, 1939, forced labor was introduced for Jewish men aged fourteen to sixty.[66] Many of those who were abducted to perform this labor did not survive, and numerous others returned ill and physically and psychologically depleted. Due to these abductions, carried out irrespective of the age and health of the men, the Jews refrained from walking in the streets. They were afraid to resume trade and many lost their jobs[67]—to the detriment of both their economic and their physical health.

On October 26, 1939, an order prohibiting Jewish ritual slaughter was posted.[68] This may have impaired the health of those who observed the Jewish dietary laws by depriving them of meat products from the very first stages of the war.[69] On December

66 On January 13, 1940, the order was published in the Warsaw German newspaper *Warschauer Zeitung*. The length of the period of labor was set at two years, with the possibility of an extension "if the educational goal is not attained." Accordingly, Krüger, the supreme police and SS commander in the General Government, ordered the Judenrat to register all men, aged 12–60. The Jews called this registration "signing up for the camps."

67 See, for example, Dr. Moshe Tursz testimony, YVA, O.3/438, p. 4; Gutman, "Warsaw: Jews during the Holocaust," in Gutman, *Encyclopedia of the Holocaust*, vol. 4, p. 1,602–1,603; Noemi Szac-Wajnkranc, *Halaf Im Ha'esh: Reshimot Al Geto Varsha Shenihtevu Bamahvo* (Gone with the Flames: Writings about the Warsaw Ghetto Produced in Hiding) (Hebrew) (Jerusalem: Yad Vashem, 2003), p. 8.

68 Shloyme Mendelsohn, *The Polish Jews behind the Nazi Ghetto Walls* (New York: Yiddish Scientific Institute—YIVO, 1942), p. 29; Czerniaków, *The Warsaw Diary*, p. 84.

69 Regarding this matter, see the remark by Dr. Israel Milejkowski at the First World Congress of Jewish Physicians, held in 1936: "The Jewish doctor in Poland was among the first ranks of fighters against the ritual slaughter decree. We explained that Jewish ritual slaughter was one of the most humane ways of killing animals, and we set up a special committee alongside the Hebrew community in Warsaw, which worked relentlessly to explain it. It is proposed that the Congress adopt the following resolution: Now that the question of slaughter has become current again, the Congress affirms that in the current medical situation, Jewish slaughter is one of the most humanitarian and hygienic ways of killing animals." See Friedman, *Sefer Hakongres Ha'olami Harishon*, p. 66.

11, 1939, an order was issued to close the Jewish pharmacies. This decree had a direct impact on the medical services that they targeted.[70]

The ban on the use of public transport was explained on pseudomedical grounds. From January 1940 onward, any Jew who wished to use the railroads had to present written proof of having been treated for lice.[71] In February 1940, special passenger cars were allocated for Jews, who were required to carry this document with them in order to travel. Each document was valid only for ten days.[72] Signs bearing the words "For Jews Only" and a large Star of David were posted in the special sections of the railroad cars.[73] An order was published in the Warsaw newspaper to the effect that due to smuggling and the spread of epidemics, Jews were forbidden to travel on trains, unless they had a special permit from the authorities.[74] In August 1940, cars on trams designated for Jews only appeared for the first time in Warsaw and its suburbs.[75] In November 1940, an order was issued banning all Jews from traveling by train on pain of severe punishment, spelling the destruction of commerce and assets, and the restriction of freedom of movement. The rationale that the

70 Czerniaków, *The Warsaw Diary*, p. 98. On March 26, 1939, Jews in the Reich were prohibited from managing pharmacies; from January 31, 1939, they were not even allowed to work in a pharmacy. This ban was also introduced in the General Government. When the "Jewish residential quarter"—the ghetto—was established, Jews were allowed to manage several pharmacies under the supervision of the Judenrat.

71 Emanuel Ringelblum, *Yoman Vereshimot Mitkufat Hamilhama: Geto Varsha September 1939–Detzember 1942* (Diary and Writings from the War Era: Warsaw Ghetto, September 1939-December 1942) (Hebrew) (Jerusalem: Yad Vashem, 1993), p. 70. See the regulation of January 26, 1940, concerning the use of trains by the Jews in the General Government in Arad et al., *Documents on the Holocaust*, p. 182; Mendelsohn, *The Polish Jews*, pp. 26, 146.

72 Emanuel Ringelblum, *Notes from the Warsaw Ghetto* (New York: Ibook, 2006), p. 16.

73 Jonas Turkow, *Hayo Hayta Varsha Yehudit* (Warsaw Jewry that Was) (Hebrew) (Tel Aviv: Tarbut V'chinuch, 1969), p. 15.

74 Ringelblum, *Notes from the Warsaw Ghetto*, p. 17; Peretz Opochinsky, *Reshimot Migeto Varsha* (Sketches from the Warsaw Ghetto) (Hebrew) (Tel Aviv: Hakibbutz Hameuchad, 1970), p. 11.

75 Mendelsohn, *The Polish Jews*, p. 26; Turkow, *Hayo Hayta Varsha Yehudit*, p. 15.

German newspaper offered for this was that the Jews were dirty and caused contagious diseases to spread by traveling in a crowd of passengers. This edict intensified the Jews' isolation and repulsive image and helped to undermine their economic situation.[76]

Decisions to close and open schools were based ostensibly on medical grounds. According to Chaim Aron Kaplan, an order to close all schools in Warsaw was issued in mid-November 1939, because of the spread of infectious diseases, particularly typhus.[77] On December 11, 1939, Adam Czerniaków wrote that the opening of Jewish schools had been forbidden.[78] On March 29, 1940, Emanuel Ringelblum reported the closure of schools, purportedly due to an epidemic. Only five months later, on August 31, 1940, did the authorities allow the Judenrat to reopen the elementary schools. On October 11, 1940, Czerniaków remarked on the circulation of rumors that there would be no schools for Jews for fear of epidemics.[79] Not until April 1941, about five months after entering the ghetto, did the Judenrat receive permission to open schools, but for only 5,000 children.[80] The rationale for this was health related.

The Nazis continued to issue more restrictions and orders. The German physician Kurt Schrempf forbade the Jews to work in scientific and research fields[81]—to the detriment of medical

76 Chaim A. Kaplan, *Megilat Yisurin*: *Yoman Geto Varsha Chaim Aron Kaplan* (Scroll of Agony: The Warsaw Diary of Chaim A. Kaplan) (Hebrew) (Tel Aviv and Jerusalem: Am Oved and Yad Vashem, 1966), pp. 170–171.

77 Kaplan, *Scroll of Agony*, p. 71.

78 Czerniaków, *The Warsaw Diary*, p. 98.

79 Ringelblum, *Yoman Vereshimot*, p. 100; Czerniaków, *The Warsaw Diary*, p. 206.

80 Czerniakow, *The Warsaw Diary*, p. 157. In the Warsaw ghetto, Jews were forbidden to attend school. In 1941, efforts by Czerniaków yielded permission to begin the school year. In the course of the only regular school year in the ghetto, which began in October 1941, 6,700 youngsters attended nineteen schools of various affiliations. Most educational activity took place secretly. Vocational studies were permitted and vocational courses were offered through the ORT network from 1940. In mid-1941, 2,454 youngsters attended these vocational courses, including some in medicine. See Gutman, "Warsaw: Jews during the Holocaust," in Gutman, *Encyclopedia of the Holocaust*, vol. 4, pp. 1,613–1,614.

81 Ludwik Hirszfeld, *The Story of One Life* (New York: University of Rochester Press, 2010), p. 200. The original version in Polish *Historia jednego życia*

research. In January 1940, Prof. Wilhelm Richter, head of the Wehrmacht's sanitation service, ordered the closure of houses of worship, synagogues, and ritual baths on sanitation grounds.[82] Although violators faced imprisonment, there were approximately 600 underground prayer quorums in Warsaw.[83] From the beginning of 1940, entire streets were blocked off with barbed wire, due to fear of epidemics. It was forbidden to enter and to exit Grzybowska St.[84] The closure of streets exacerbated the poor economic situation of their inhabitants. In early 1940, Jewish hospitals were placed under quarantine, because of the fear of epidemics. The doctors and nurses at Czyste Hospital and at Bersohn and Bauman Children's Hospital were not allowed to leave.[85]

From the beginning of the occupation, the Jews were depicted as enemies who were liable to imperil the Polish and German inhabitants' health and resilience. Dr. Chaim Einhorn wrote that German propaganda flooded the world at large with false reports that the Jews were spreading epidemics, acting as carriers without being ill themselves.[86] In March 1940, the German newspaper in Warsaw issued a general warning against contagious diseases, stating among other things that one should beware of negotiating with the Jews, who spread infectious diseases.[87] In late October, less than a month before the Jews entered the ghetto, Ringelblum reported severe incitement against the Jews, propagated by means of loudspeakers, to the effect that the Jews were a plague that

(Warsaw: Czytelnik, 1950) was translated into German and published under the title *Die Geschichte eines Lebens* also in 1950.

82 Czerniaków, *The Warsaw Diary*, p. 105; Mendelsohn, *The Polish Jews*, p. 29.

83 Czerniaków, *The Warsaw Diary*, p. 211.

84 Ringelblum, *Yoman Vereshimot*, pp. 50, 66.

85 Ibid., p. 50; Lensky, *A Physician inside the Warsaw Ghetto*, p. 24. See also Chapter 3 in this book.

86 See the lecture series on health problems in the ghettos, concentration camps, and forests, Chaim Einhorn, "Harofe Begeto Varsha" (The Doctor in the Warsaw Ghetto), in Mark Dworzecki, ed., *Hama'avak Lakiyum Velabriyut Biymei Hashoah* (The Struggle for Survival and Health in the Holocaust) (Hebrew) (Jerusalem: Israel Administration of the World Jewish Congress and Association of Holocaust Survivor Physicians—Ghettos, Camps, Forests, 1958), p. 11.

87 Kaplan, *Megilat Yisurin*, pp. 198–199.

must be rooted out. This incitement continued in 1941, after the establishment of the ghetto.[88]

On September 19, 1940, approximately two months before the Jews entered the ghetto, an order was issued forbidding Jewish doctors to treat Aryans and vice versa. The ostensible grounds for this decree were that contagious diseases were found mainly among the Jews. If Aryan physicians were to treat Jewish patients, there was a risk of transmitting the diseases. Therefore, it was necessary to separate the two environments.[89] Economic decrees impeded the daily functioning of the Jews and even deprived them of their livelihood to the detriment of their health.[90] The municipal welfare institutions stopped granting benefits to elderly Jews, the disabled, and widows, which directly affected the situation and the health of this vulnerable population.[91] Several suffered from starvation and illness, and many died. Almost half of the dictates described above had a direct effect on the Jewish population's state of health. The Germans justified more than one-third of them on grounds related to public health.[92] The ghettoization decree, however, was

88 Ringelblum, *Yoman Vereshimot*, pp. 169, 247, 289; Lensky, *A Physician inside the Warsaw Ghetto*, p. 48.

89 Kaplan, *Scroll of Agony*, p. 197. Upon hearing about this order, Kaplan wrote that because it was customary among Jewish patients to consult Aryan doctors frequently, but not for Aryan patients to consult Jewish doctors, this decree put the Aryan practitioners of all people at a disadvantage.

90 Regarding the economic decrees and their impact on the Jews, see, for example, Arad et al., *Documents on the Holocaust*, p. 199; Gutman, *The Jews of Warsaw*, pp. 20–21, 72–77; Kaplan, *Scroll of Agony*, pp. 101–105; Ringelblum, *Notes from the Warsaw Ghetto*, p. 17; Szac-Wajnkranc, *Halaf Im Ha'esh*, p. 8.

91 "Directives Issued by the Head of the Department for Jewish Affairs on Policies Concerning the Treatment of Jews in the General Government," April 6, 1940. As stated in Section 4 of this document, "The Jews are to establish their own social insurance system and are not to pay contributions to non-Jewish insurance schemes, nor make claims on non-Jewish facilities." See Arad et al., *Documents on the Holocaust*, pp. 195–196. In a memorandum to the Germans about their economic situation at the beginning of the occupation, the Jews asserted, "Pension rights and social insurance have been withdrawn from former government officials who are Jews, and from invalids, widows, and dependents of Jews entitled to social insurance"; see Arad et al., *Documents on the Holocaust*, p. 200.

92 One of the central ideas of Nazi ideology was the "medicalization of antisemitism" or the "pseudomedical argument"—the view that Nazi doctors

the harshest blow of all. It marked a new stage in the evolution of the Nazis' anti-Jewish policy.

The Warsaw ghetto, as well as several other large ghettos that were set up in Eastern Europe, constituted until recently a representative model in historical research—"the ghetto model"—from which one might learn about "the ghettoization stage," as referred to in research on anti-Jewish policy during the Nazi era. Even before the Holocaust ended, there were historiographers and diarists in various ghettos who attempted to understand the deep meaning of the "ghetto decree period." A few of them were even aware of the historical complexity of the phenomenon. For example, Dr. Aaron Pik, an internee in the Shavli (Šiauliai) ghetto in Lithuania, expressed himself as follows:

> One man cannot possibly describe and encompass all the details of this decree, which remains in effect and on which the last word has not yet been said. Ghetto—that is to say, all our tragic lives at this time in their entire narrow scope but that branch into sundry details, require study, contemplation, investigation, and interpretation by a committee of experts, each picking out something in his own profession. Therefore, obviously, my notes will be somewhat defective and incomplete, mere chapter headings for the troubles and agonies that have befallen us. Nevertheless, it will give our offspring a picture, albeit a blurry one, of everything we have gone through in the Shavli ghetto.[93]

In his study on the ghettos,[94] Dan Michman stresses that the main characteristic of the so-called ghettoization stage is the difference—rather than the similarity—among the more than 1,100 ghettos

developed about the Jews being a "diseased race," which called for "medical measures" to solve the Jewish problem. See Proctor, *Racial Hygiene*, pp. 194–195. On the issue of "medicalizing" the Holocaust, see Nadav, "Was There a 'Medicalization' of the Holocaust?" pp. 403–459.

93 Pik, *Reshimot Migai Hahariga*, p. 106.

94 Dan Michman, *The Emergence of Jewish Ghettos during the Holocaust* (Jerusalem: Yad Vashem, 2011).

that were established across the Nazi-occupied realm. Michman contends that the phenomenon of the "Nazi ghetto," which occurred only in Eastern Europe, developed in an unsystematic, inconsistent, and protracted manner that began to peak in 1941. The ideological infrastructure of the establishment of these ghettos was not new. It was based on an understanding of the ghetto as a dense concentration of Jews in a given city, as in the large Jewish centers in Eastern Europe. These concentrations, the "ghettos," were perceived as formative sources of power and as inexhaustible demographic springs of "Jewry" and, therefore, as a threatening phenomenon that had to be confined.

According to Michman, the ghetto phenomenon developed from its inception in Eastern Europe as a response to the encounter with the "*Ostjuden*," the East European Jews, during the invasion of Poland in 1939. The racial antisemitic concepts, which intensified during the Nazi era, found practical expression at that time and were carried into the field by the local German commanders. These views induced a sense of threat and fear of the encounter with the East European Jews, who inhabited overcrowded neighborhoods that could not be controlled and, according to the Nazis, spawned not only real diseases, such as epidemics, but also racial ones. Namely, the Jews were perceived as a "disease" and as a source for the formation of Jewish traits that would erupt and seek to take over the world. "Pushing back" against the Jews and "accommodating" them in ghettos were responses to danger—albeit an imagined danger. However, these responses did not follow a rational course in the bureaucratic planning that led to the Final Solution. Local commanders, who held traditional and Nazi antisemitic opinions, took local initiatives to round up the Jews, who were dispersed in and around the cities, and confined them in ghettos that had existed for years! This banishment to old places of Jewish concentration, which the Jews themselves called "ghettos" in their internal discourse in interwar Poland, gave rise to a series of intricate problems in the daily management of urban life systems. This too usually defied all bureaucratic organizational logic. Accordingly, the ghettos that were created in each locality differed in nature.

The historian Israel Gutman states that although there is no evidence of a clear directive concerning the establishment of ghettos as part of a comprehensive German policy and no proof that the ghettos were intended ab initio to facilitate the physical obliteration of the Jews, ghettoization was a camouflaged political maneuver that required the Nazis to concoct a litany of excuses. There is no doubt that the living conditions that the Germans imposed in the ghettos were so dire that they led to death from starvation and disease. In this respect, the ghettoization process launched in late 1939 constituted a deteriorization in their attitude toward the Jews, because of the intrinsic aspect of dehumanization.[95] The ghettos in the occupied parts of Poland were not established at the same time, and the methods used to segregate the ghettos from the rest of their surroundings and in the internal regimes that were introduced were not uniform.[96]

One may assume that the initiative behind the establishment of the ghettos was in the hands of the local authorities. For example, it was Hans Frank, governor of the General Government, who gave the order to establish the ghettos in his zone. Browning claims that the concentration of Polish Jews in the cities as an initial step toward their deportation was part of the central policy that Berlin established in September 1939, but the confinement of the Jews in ghettos was an initiative of the local echelons. Due to the policy failures surrounding the deportations to Lublin and Madagascar, the fate of the Jews was subject to local decisions and initiatives until the implementation of the Final Solution.[97]

95 Yehuda Bauer argues that the term "dehumanization" is misused when used to describe the plight of the victims in the camps and the ghettos, and stresses that the word specifically applies to the Nazis themselves, because they brought on their own dehumanization. After all, the few survivors among the victims reverted to their cultural ways of life after the war. See Bauer, *Rethinking the Holocaust*, pp. 51–52.

96 Gutman, "Ghetto," in Gutman, *Encyclopedia of the Holocaust*, vol. 2, pp. 579–582; Trunk, "Epidemics and Mortality," p. 98; Gutman, *Sugiyot Beheker Hashoah*, p. 119.

97 Christopher Browning, "Nazi Ghettoization Policy in Poland," in Browning, *The Path to Genocide*, pp. 52–53; Christopher Browning, *The Origins of the Final Solution* (Lincoln and Jerusalem: University of Nebraska Press and Yad Vashem, 2004), pp. 111–138.

Those in charge of health offered a pseudoscientific explanation for the political measure of establishing the ghettos. They alleged that even though the Jews were relatively immune, they endangered the non-Jewish population, because they were carriers of pathogens. The German doctors and authorities knew that ghettoization would not prevent epidemics and that the ghetto living conditions would in fact cause the spread of epidemics, which would lead to the deterioration of the Jewish population. The Jews pointed out the absurdity of the health officials' claims. The fact that an ostensibly medical measure was meant to annihilate the Jews was manifested in the methods that the Germans employed to fight epidemics—methods that Prof. Ludwik Hirszfeld[98] called "worse than the epidemic itself."[99]

Trunk alleges that in their annihilation campaign against Polish Jewry, the Nazis used bacteria in addition to deportation to extermination camps. The calculated planning of the German

98 Ludwik Hirszfeld (1884–1954) was born in Warsaw. He studied medicine in Berlin and worked at the Cancer Research Institute in Heidelberg and subsequently at the Institute of Hygiene in Zurich. A world-renowned researcher on blood groups, he also discovered the Paratyphoid C bacterium. In 1915, he went to Serbia to help fight the spread of typhus in the ranks of the Serbian Army. Continuing his research on blood types in Salonika, he was able to determine that Type A blood is common mainly among European peoples, whereas Type B is prevalent among soldiers from Asian countries. In 1919, the Institute of Hygiene in Warsaw named him director of the departments of bacteriology and serology. In 1924, he was appointed lecturer at the Free University. Hirszfeld was awarded the title of docent—the highest that a pre-World War II Polish university could award a Jewish physician—in 1926 and served as lecturer on bacteriology. After Warsaw surrendered to the Nazis, he was dismissed from his position at the Institute of Hygiene. A convert to Christianity, he was nevertheless forced to vacate his apartment on the Aryan side of Warsaw and move to the ghetto in February 1941, where he was active in many areas of medicine. After Poland was liberated, he received a professorship at the University of Lublin. Settling in Wrocław, he served as dean of the medical school and established Poland's first institute of immunology, which still bears his name. See Ludwik Hirszfeld, *The Story of One Life*, Introduction, pp. xix–xxxv; Stefan Lutkiewicz, "Hirszfeld Ludwik," *Encyclopedia Judaica* (Jerusalem: Keter, 1971), p. 530; Lensky, "Rofim Yehudim Mefursamim," p. 318.

99 Gutman, "Ghetto," in Gutman, *Encyclopedia of the Holocaust*, vol. 2, pp. 579–582; Trunk, "Epidemics and Mortality," p. 98.

authorities in the ghettos created a situation that caused epidemics to erupt. Once this happened, they fought the plagues in ways that assured their spread. Through their actions, the Germans procured the isolation of the Jews from the outside world by quarantine and the mass murder of the ghetto inhabitants. By accusing the ghettoized Jews of causing epidemics to expand, they fanned the Poles' fear of the ostensible carriers of the bacillus. There were also attempts to justify the mass murder of Polish Jewry, because this would assure the health of the rest of the population. In July 1943, at a conference of the German Medical Association in Cracow, Governor General Frank proclaimed that the annihilation of three million Jews was inevitable for reasons of public health. The ghetto, which was supposed to assist in the war on epidemics, contributed to the spread of diseases. There is no doubt that the German high echelons knew the exact causes of the outbreak of typhus in the ghettos.[100]

The researcher Charles Roland also expresses the opinion that the Warsaw ghetto was one great typhus experiment. German scientists and doctors, like the medical world at large, knew a great deal about the disease. They knew that it had nothing to do with the Jews and that the ghetto living conditions would have caused the disease to spread also among any other population living there. However, the ghettoization policy and its justification as a matter of public medicine stifled almost all opposition on their part. Many, in fact, supported this policy. Thus, the Warsaw ghetto converged with another crime: the medical experiments regarding typhus and other subjects that were carried out in the Nazis' concentration and extermination camps during World War II. By establishing the ghetto and concentrating so many people there, the Germans could establish grounds for their argument that typhus was indeed a "Jewish disease" and that it was causing numerous deaths in the Warsaw ghetto. Overcrowding and poor sanitation conditions caused the spread of lice to escalate into an essentially inescapable plague.[101]

100 Trunk, "Epidemics and Mortality," pp. 82–83.

101 Roland, *Courage under Siege*, pp. 123–126, 130–131. See also Weindling, *Epidemics and Genocide in Eastern Europe*, particularly chap. 3.

Browning writes that the German doctors advocated the hermetic closure of the ghettos. In late 1941, the very menace to public health that they were responsible for creating made it easier to justify carrying out mass murder. These physicians' public health policy was a decisive factor in the escalation of anti-Jewish measures in the General Government. The doctors' support of the establishment and hermetic sealing of the Jewish ghetto in Warsaw served as a model for emulation throughout the General Government. The ghettos produced the expected results in the manner of self-fulfilling prophecy. In the calamitous situation that the Germans had created—hunger, overcrowding, and filth—the Jews fell victim to the diseases that had served as justification for their ghettoization to begin with. Nevertheless, the doctors continued to support a more hermetic sealing of the ghetto as a medical measure against the epidemics that they themselves had caused to accelerate.

The senior officials in the General Government were not enthusiastic about the ghettoization idea proposed by the physicians. The latter thus took steps to influence the senior officials and convinced them to change their policy in order to implement the idea on an even broader scale. According to Browning, the doctors believed that they were meticulously applying medical principles.[102] The Germans realized that confining the Jews of Warsaw to a ghetto would create problems of food shortages that would inevitably cause their death by starvation. Waldemar Schön, the head of the Warsaw District Resettlement Department, detailed the reasons for the decision to establish the ghetto that reflected antisemitic views and underscored the centrality of the medical argument as a determinant of German policy. He asserted that, in any event, it was imperative to protect the German Army and the population from the Jew who was himself immune but who carried epidemic bacteria. Schön added that the segregation of the Jews in the ghetto was a political and moral necessity for the elimination of the influence of the Jews, and that this would put an end to the black market and to the price gouging caused by the Jews.

102 Browning, "Genocide and Public Health," pp. 21, 23–29.

In a consultation held in Germany on March 8, 1940, it was decided to postpone ghettoization in Warsaw due to the proposals to establish a "*Judenreservat*" (Jewish reservation) in Lublin, where all the Jews in the Lublin district of the General Government would be concentrated.[103] When Frank and his senior officials convened in Cracow for consultations in April 1940, Ludwig Fischer, the German commander of the Warsaw district, spoke in favor of the establishment of the ghetto. In addition to the political and economic argument, he asserted, "Isolating the Jews is unavoidable due to the need to maintain the sound health situation of the population and to fight the epidemic."[104] On September 3, 1940, Arnold Lambrecht, a doctor who served as the public health inspector in the Warsaw district, warned in a report to Governor Frank that typhus would certainly spread to many places in the coming winter. The authorities in Warsaw complained about the absence of a consistent and explicit policy on the treatment of the Jews in Warsaw. The city's administrative officials argued that the construction of ghettos for Jews in the district was especially urgent "for medical reasons above all." On September 6, Walbaum met with Frank and asserted that the eruption of typhus had originated in the Jewish quarter. Thus, he convinced Frank that all the Jews in Warsaw must be confined to a ghetto for health reasons.[105]

The program that the Nazis approved recommended establishing two ghettos on the outskirts of Warsaw in order to minimize harming the city's economy, industry, and traffic. The operation was scheduled to begin on July 1, 1940, in order to complete the main stages before the winter. However, the work was halted because of the dissemination of Hitler's plan to resettle the Jews of Europe in Madagascar. At the end of August 1940,

103 See Waldemar Schön's lecture on steps leading to the establishment of the Warsaw ghetto, January 20, 1941, in Arad et al., *Documents on the Holocaust*, pp. 222–224.

104 Gutman, *The Jews of Warsaw*, p. 52; Nachman Blumental and Joseph Kermish, eds., *Hameri Vehamered Begeto Varsha* (Resistance and Revolt in the Warsaw Ghetto: A Documentary History) (Hebrew, with an introduction and synopsis in English) (Jerusalem: Yad Vashem, 1965), p. 354n8.

105 Browning, "Genocide and Public Health," p. 23.

roughly eleven months into the occupation, the ghetto proposal was relaunched on the initiative of the Health Department, due to the massing of more and more army units in the Warsaw district and the need to protect the army and the population. The decision now was to establish open ghettos—Jewish "residential quarters"—that would allow the inhabitants to maintain commercial relations with the Aryan population and thus support themselves.

The district physician argued that the "resettlement" work, which entailed the relocation of about 600,000 people, had to be completed by November 15, at the latest, due to concerns about the spread of epidemics in the winter. Given this time constraint, it was decided to establish the ghetto in a part of town that had already been closed off, because of epidemics.[106] On September 12, Frank responded affirmatively.[107] The order that he issued the next day, restricting the Jews' residence under administrative supervision, created a basis for the Jews' ghettoization.[108] On October 2, 1940, the head of the Warsaw district ordered the initiation of the requisite evacuations and demanded, per recommendation of the district physician, that they be completed by November 15, 1940.[109] The Warsaw ghetto was sealed on November 15, 1940, and the other Jewish communities in the district were ghettoized at the same time. The following spring, ghettos were established elsewhere in the General Government.[110]

Frank also raised the professed health argument as a rationale for the establishment of the ghetto. On the basis of a report published in the German newspaper *Krakauer Zeitung* on October 18, 1941, Czerniaków noted in his diary that at a meeting with Governor General Frank, the latter had explained the establishment of the Jewish residential quarters as a means to prevent the asocial behavior of the Jews from disrupting German economic and administrative consolidation. Moreover, it was a way to eliminate the constant risk of epidemics caused by the Jewish population,

106 Arad et al., *Documents on the Holocaust*, pp. 222–224.

107 Browning, "Genocide and Public Health," p. 23.

108 Piotrowski, *Hans Frank's Diary*, p. 90.

109 Arad et al., *Documents on the Holocaust*, pp. 222–224.

110 Browning, "Genocide and Public Health," p. 23.

which was known to transmit extremely dangerous illnesses. According to Frank, experience with Jewish residential quarters confirmed how essential such quarters were. In Warsaw, for example, the Germans had managed to keep typhus from infecting the rest of the town's population in this manner. He argued that rigorous control of relations between the Jewish residential quarter and the rest of the city could in the future minimize the health hazards occasioned by the half a million Jews living among millions of Germans and Poles.[111] When Jürgen Stroop, the SS commander and police general who managed the suppression of the Warsaw Ghetto Uprising reported his successful quashing of the uprising, he repeated the health argument as a reason for the establishment of the ghetto.[112]

In the autumn of 1939 and in early 1940, the Warsaw Judenrat was ordered to post signs in the area where Jews had lived before the war, alerting "Caution! Danger of Epidemic!" These signs marked the borders of the Jewish quarter that, at that time, was not enclosed by walls, since it had not yet been decided how to organize the ghetto.[113] The order to erect the walls was issued in March 1940. Dr. Kaminski of the Warsaw district and Dr. Walbaum, director of the General Government Health Department, explained that this measure was an absolute necessity brought on by the Jews' alleged disregard of the department's regulations, as specified by the Health Department.[114]

In April–May 1940, at the authorities' command, the Judenrat began to build walls around predominantly Jewish neighborhoods, creating what was termed a "closed epidemic zone." At the entrances to the zone, notices warned, "Danger of epidemic! Do not cross!" In early June, a decree signed by Ludwig Leist, the governor of the city of Warsaw, was promulgated, requiring the Jews of Warsaw to

111 Adam Czerniaków, *Yoman Geto Varsha: 9/6/1939–7/23/1942* (Warsaw Ghetto Diary: September 6, 1939–July 23, 1942) (Hebrew) (Jerusalem: Yad Vashem, 1970), pp. 235–236. See the remarks in the same vein that appear in Frank's diaries in Piotrkowski, *Hans Frank's Diary*, pp. 221, 243.

112 Blumental and Kermish, *Hameri Vehamered Begeto Varsha*, p. 353.

113 Ibid., p. 354n6.

114 Browning, "Genocide and Public Health," p. 23.

sign up for apartments only within the residential area that had been declared as being prone to epidemics. This was yet another edict that indicated the intention of gathering the Jews in this zone as would be done in October 1940 in the "Jewish quarter"—the ghetto. Although the Germans justified the creation of the ghetto for reasons of health and sanitation, plainly this action would not diminish the risk of epidemics but would instead intensify the spread of disease. The severe overcrowding and the displacement of Jewish refugees in the ghetto created conditions that could only cause diseases to spread and become more difficult to fight.[115]

How the Jews of Warsaw Perceived Their Ghettoization

The policy of gradual repression and segregation that the Germans implemented from the beginning of the occupation in September 1939 until the sealing of the ghetto in November 1940 sowed confusion and uncertainty among the Jews of Warsaw regarding the meaning of the ghetto decree. On November 4, 1939, Czerniaków wrote that the Jewish community had been notified about a "Pale of Settlement." SS Commander Rudolf Baatz read the order in a furious tone before the members of the Judenrat. According to the edict, the danger of typhus was such that the Jewish population of Warsaw had to move to a protected quarter, whose borders would be roughly demarcated by November 7. The penalty for disobedience would be a "contribution"—stiff fines that the Germans would impose on the Jewish population—along with the confiscation of possessions and valuables. The Gestapo took the deputies of the Ältestenrat (Council of Elders) hostage and severely beat them.[116] The next day, a meeting was held with the

115 Ibid.

116 See the entries of October 16, 1939, Czerniaków, *The Warsaw Diary*, pp. 87–88. The terms used to describe the Jewish leadership in the ghettos varied from place to place and from period to period, as well as in different historical sources. Therefore, in this book, the terms used will not be uniform, but will appear as they appear in each individual source. The most prevalent terms are Jewish community, Judenrat (Jewish Council), *Ältestenrat* (Council of

military commander of the city of Warsaw, General Karl Ulrich von Neumann-Neurode, who ruled that the directives of the SS should be ignored and that, in the meanwhile, there was no need to move to the Jewish quarter. The establishment of the ghetto was postponed by one year and the ghetto boundaries established in 1940 expanded those proposed in 1939 by 30 percent.[117]

On November 7, 1939, Kaplan wrote that the order to move to the quarter did not apply to businesses and shops, which for the time being would remain in the hands of their Jewish owners, nor to professionals, such as doctors, dentists, lawyers, engineers, and so on, who would be allowed to continue practicing. However, Kaplan added, "Will they be allowed to live [there]? This has not yet been decided."[118] On November 13, 1939, Czerniaków was ordered to appear before Baatz regarding the matter of resettlement. The next day, he visited the SS offices, where it turned out that the eviction was off the table.

Although the makeshift SS and Gestapo plan had fallen through, preparations for crowding the Jews into the ghetto continued. The gradual implementation of the scheme proceeded throughout 1940, until the ghetto was hermetically sealed in November of that year. On November 18, 1939, Czerniaków wrote that the establishment of the ghetto had been postponed for several months, but that the community had been instructed to post signs forbidding entry at the boundaries of the Jewish quarter, where there were people with contagious diseases: "*Achtung*! *Seuchengefahr*! *Eintritt verboten*!" (Caution! Risk of Plague! Entry Forbidden!) Although the borders were supposed to isolate the "Jewish quarter," tens of thousands of Polish non-Jews lived there as well. The boundaries of the area, while not defined precisely, did encompass the entire territory of the future ghetto, which the Germans regarded as a "quarantine zone." Two days later, signs were posted along the

Elders). For a discussion of the term Judenrat, see, for example, Dan Michman, *Holocaust Historiography: A Jewish Perspective: Conceptualizations, Terminology, Approaches, and Fundamental Issues* (London and Portland:Vallentine Mitchell, 2003), pp. 159–175.

117 Czerniaków, *The Warsaw Diary*, pp. 87–88; Mendelsohn, *The Polish Jews*, p. 6.

118 Kaplan, *Scroll of Agony*, p. 66.

way to the "ghetto" warning about the danger of epidemics and the prohibition against entering the Jewish quarter. Next to them were notices barring soldiers from entering.[119] On January 18, 1940, the attorney Waldemar Schön, head of the Warsaw District Resettlement Department, arrived in Warsaw, where he began to elaborate plans for the establishment of the ghetto in Warsaw and would play a central role in implementing them.[120]

The construction of the walls began several months before the command to establish the sealed ghetto was issued. Orders to wall in the ghetto—that is, the area marked as the "epidemic zone"—were handed down on March 29, 1940.[121] Czerniaków met with Ludwig Leist, the governor of the city of Warsaw, and submitted in writing the community's complaints about the damage to the city that the construction of the walls would cause, such as damage to the water pipes and the electrical grid.[122] Nevertheless, on April 1, excavations for the walls began at numerous locations in the city; entire streets were closed, and barbed-wire fences were erected.[123] According to Ringelblum, the Jews saw the onset of the construction of the walls around the plague-infested area as the first step toward the establishment of the ghetto.[124] About a month later, on May 10, 1940, Czerniaków wrote in his diary that he had received a diagram of the contaminated area and found that it comprised only 4 percent of the city. "Just the same, a ghetto!" he added.[125] From the time that the order to erect the walls had been issued, Czerniaków kept it on his agenda, working arduously to have the decree abolished.

119 Czerniaków, *The Warsaw Diary*, pp. 89–91, 99; Gutman, *The Jews of Warsaw*, pp. 48–51. On December 13, 1939, the Germans summoned Czerniaków to the investigations office, where he was ordered to increase the number of street poles bearing signs with the inscription "Danger of Epidemic!" Czerniaków, *The Warsaw Diary*, p. 35; Ringelblum, *Yoman Vereshimot*, p. 66.

120 Gutman, *The Jews of Warsaw*, pp. 48–51.

121 Czerniaków, *Warsaw Diary*, p. 134; Gutman, *The Jews of Warsaw*, p. 50. According to Czerniaków, the order to establish the ghetto was issued on March 25; Gutman wrote that it was issued on March 27.

122 Czerniaków, *The Warsaw Diary*, p. 134.

123 Ibid., pp. 135–136; Roland, *Courage under Siege*, pp. 22–23.

124 Ringelblum, *Notes from the Warsaw Ghetto*, p. 28; Roland, *Courage under Siege*, pp. 22–23.

125 Czerniaków, *The Warsaw Diary*, p. 148.

The Germans told the Jews that the walls were intended to protect them from Polish rioters; they told the Poles that the Jews had to be isolated in order to protect them from the typhus epidemic that was spreading among the Jews. The Jews were required to bear the costs of the construction of the walls. Twenty segments of wall had been built already by June 1940. The rest were completed close to the sealing of the ghetto after it had been established.[126]

Dr. Moshe Tursz remembers one day seeing a brick wall begin to rise. At first, the Jews thought that the Germans were building walls for strategic reasons, such as to prepare for the possibility of a French and British invasion. Eventually, however, the terror and the tribulation intensified so massively that the Jews no longer gave the walls any thought.[127] As the walls went up in April 1940, Kaplan wrote, "The Jews' camp is tantamount to a camp of lepers and the impure…All of the occupier's repairs are futile and are meant only to intensify the distress of life for the ostracized."[128] Much uncertainty surrounded the establishment and size of the ghetto. On September 23, 1940, Czerniaków still did not believe that there would be a sealed ghetto. Four days later, it became known that the area designated for the ghetto had been severely reduced. Tłomackie St., where a synagogue and Czyste Hospital were located, was not included in this area.[129] In early October 1940, Ringelblum reported having heard that the sanitation authorities and the army opposed the establishment of the ghetto.[130]

On October 2, Ludwig Fischer, the German commander of the Warsaw district, issued an order to draw the boundaries of the

126 Gutman, *The Jews of Warsaw*, pp. 50–51. Karol Laschtoviczka, head of the Finance Department of the General Government, was to issue orders regarding who should pay for the construction of the wall. On December 1, 1941, around two weeks after the ghetto was sealed, when Czerniaków was required to submit the budget reports of the Judenrat to the *Kommissar*, he argued that the wall should be financed not by the Jews but by those who would be protected from the epidemic that emanated from the Jews. "When I buy medicine at the drugstore, the druggist doesn't pay me; I pay him." Czerniaków, *The Warsaw Diary*, pp. 134–135, 304.

127 Dr. Moshe Tursz testimony, YVA, O.3/438, pp. 4–5.

128 Kaplan, *Megilat Yisurin*, p. 214.

129 Czerniaków, *The Warsaw Diary*, p. 200.

130 Ringelblum, *Notes from the Warsaw Ghetto*, p. 63.

ghetto. The target date was changed twice, but on November 15, 1940, the ghetto was actually established.[131] The order to enter the ghetto was issued on Yom Kippur, October 12, 1940.[132] Leist's decree concerning the concentration of all the Jews in the ghetto was promulgated on October 17, 1940.[133] On October 18, 1940, the ghettoization edict was published in a Warsaw newspaper.

> According to the order of the District Chief, it is necessary to avoid epidemics, to establish secluded Jewish quarters within the Warsaw area. [Here the limits of the Warsaw ghetto are specified.] Poles who live in the Jewish quarters, as well as Jews who live outside them, must leave their apartments by October 31, 1940. Poles who move before that date are entitled to choose new apartments. Jews will be provided with quarters by the Judenrat. After October 31, 1940, evacuation will be forced.[134]

After the official ghettoization order was issued, Kaplan wrote,

> The tyrant is [too] cautious to call it by its name; instead of "ghetto," a concept drawn from the Middle Ages, he calls it a special "Jewish quarter." And since a "Polish quarter" and a "German quarter" are also mentioned in this order, it's a sign that he deems them all to be equal. A "human" rationale for creating a "Jewish quarter" is also available to him: none other than an "epidemic" that's claiming victims in the Jewish street, for which reason this street has to be separated from the camp....The rationale presented is nothing but a deception....They've sentenced us to silence—and we're being silent.[135]

131 See Ludwig Fischer's order concerning the establishment of the Warsaw ghetto issued on October 2, 1940, in Arad et al., *Documents on the Holocaust*, pp. 220–221.

132 Czerniaków, *The Warsaw Diary*, p. 206.

133 Ibid., p. 208.

134 Mendelsohn, *The Polish Jews*, pp. 7–8.

135 Kaplan, *Scroll of Agony*, p. 210; Czerniaków, *The Warsaw Diary*, p. 208.

Ringelblum wrote that the Germans' intention to establish the ghetto was primarily to isolate the Jews completely and to segregate them from the Aryan population. The Germans instituted the process of uprooting the Jews from economic and social life from the moment they arrived. Ghettoization was intended to be its climax and culmination.[136] "The real aim in creating the ghetto was to starve the Jewish population," Ringelblum asserted.[137]

According to Ludwik Hirszfeld, the creation of the Warsaw ghetto was a laboratory experiment of sorts. Hirszfeld accused the Germans of taking half a million people—Jews, whose lives were worth less than those of rats and rabbits—putting them in a cage, creating all the conditions for contagious diseases, and letting them foment. Apart from the ridiculous directives, no assistance whatsoever was provided. Starvation was the main cause of death in the ghetto and anything that the doctors did to prevent disease was futile.[138] Hirszfeld also claimed that the humiliating and repressive actions taken against the Jews in the ghetto were intended to make the Jews loathsome as would befit a race that was doomed to die. Presumably, 80 percent of the Jews would die under these conditions while 20 percent would survive. The Germans tried to exacerbate the wretched living conditions so that those who would die would perish more quickly and those who survived would suffer even more. Toward this end, they further reduced the living space in the ghetto every now and then, and crammed more people into the already overcrowded quarter. The directives were imposed on the Jews with no forewarning, which allowed them little time to vacate their dwellings.[139]

The authors of articles published in the ghetto underground press expressed the view that the establishment of the ghetto was a deliberate measure by the Germans to annihilate the Jews. The following statement appeared in the Bund and Zukunft newspaper *Biuletyn*[140] in January 1941: "The purpose of the ghetto is clear:

136 Ringelblum, *Polish-Jewish Relations*, p. 59.

137 Ibid., pp. 81–82.

138 Ludwik Hirszfeld, *The Story of One Life*, p. 222.

139 Ibid., p. 234.

140 Bund—the General Jewish Labor Bund—was a socialist, Jewish, autonomous

to wipe out the entire population and render it a collective of embittered paupers who are willing to enslave themselves to the 'master race' for a pittance."[141] Rachel Auerbach wrote that the internment of the Jews behind ghetto walls was intended to facilitate the mass murder of the Jewish population by raising the natural death rate.[142] Dr. Chaim Einhorn, a physician in the ghetto, wrote that the Germans directly destroyed the ghetto by fomenting epidemics of typhoid fever, typhus, dysentery, and tuberculosis, and inducing starvation by distributing food in a quantity that provided 300 calories per day per person—15 percent of a normal subsistence diet.[143]

Dr. Tursz, an activist with the TOZ health care organization in Warsaw, claimed that the ghetto inhabitants served as guinea pigs in an experiment to observe the predictably rapid spread of the epidemic. Indeed, 5,000–6,000 people died per month, most from starvation, tuberculosis, and typhus. At that rate, it would take three or four years to annihilate the ghetto population. Having no patience for this, the Germans decided to switch from annihilation by bacteria to annihilation by gas.[144] Dr. Emil Apfelbaum, who worked at Czyste Hospital, testified that he was firmly convinced that the German policy that established the ghetto and imposed its conditions aimed to decimate the Jews systematically by means of hunger and epidemics. However, "The enemy was disappointed. He thought that by sealing people

political party in Russia, Lithuania, and Poland, founded in the Russian Empire in 1897. In Poland, Bund was an important political force which, at its peak, won approximately 100,000 votes in the 1928 general election. Most of the members of Bund were murdered during the Holocaust. Zukunft (Future) was a socialist Jewish youth movement founded by the Bund Party that was active in interwar Poland.

141 Daniel Blatman, *Geto Varsha—Sipur Itona'i*: *Mivhar Me'itonut Hamahteret, 1940–1943* (Report from the Ghetto: A Selection from the Jewish Underground Press, 1940–1943) (Hebrew) (Jerusalem: Yad Vashem, 2002), pp. 143, 146, 164.

142 Rachel Auerbach, *Tzava'ot Varsha*: *Mifgashim*, *Ma'asim*, *Goralot*, *1933–1943* (Testaments of Warsaw: Encounters, Feats, Fates, 1933–1943) (Hebrew) (Tel Aviv: Moreshet, 1985), p. 95.

143 Einhorn, "Harofe Begeto Varsha," pp. 12–13.

144 Dr. Moshe Tursz testimony, YVA, O.3/438, p. 16.

in the ghetto he would manage to annihilate the entire Jewish population. But it didn't happen. The Jewish people's survival instinct spared it from annihilation. The enemy did not have his way."[145]

In a lecture that he delivered in 1942 in New York, Mendelsohn[146] stated that the Nazis' primary goal was the physical annihilation of the Jews in the ghetto by means of starvation, epidemics, and cold. Although the Nazis attempted to justify the segregation of the Jews on the grounds of epidemics, the morbidity rate had been relatively low before the establishment of the ghettos. The incidence of contagious diseases increased after ghettoization, and when mortality and morbidity were high, the Nazis did not offer any medical support because "Jews are immune to contagious illnesses."[147] Therefore, in the eyes of Jewish leaders, doctors, and others in the ghetto, by implication, ghettoization was a deliberate plot to annihilate the Jews.

* * *

In conclusion, it is possible to identify several salient characteristics of German medical ethics, organization, and science that found expression in the German health policies in the Reich and influenced the German health policies that were imposed on the Jews of Warsaw. These aspects are discussed in many studies, although rarely in the context of the Jews' struggle to provide medical treatment.

The ethical aspect of the Nazis' health policies underscored the diametrical contrast between the ethical and professional perception of medicine in Jewish culture and that in Nazi culture. Jewish culture fostered the values of sanctity of life and the ideal of social medicine, and, therefore, focused on the right of every individual to medical care and the inculcation of a merciful

145 Dr. Emil Apfelbaum testimony, YVA, M.49.E/4510 (Polish); see also Offer, "Ma'arach Harefu'a Begeto Varsha," vol. 2, appendix A.28, pp. 130–134.

146 Before the war, Mendelsohn had been a public leader in Warsaw and a member of the board of YIVO.

147 Mendelsohn, *The Polish Jews*, pp. 11–12.

attitude toward the weak and the needy. The Nazis' perception of hygiene, which served as the basis for their public health policies and their policy of racial purity of society, demanded sacrificing "flawed" persons in violation of the values of human rights and of life. The tendencies toward dehumanization that had evolved in science, especially in the theory of eugenics that espoused the hereditary inequality of human beings and their classification as superior or inferior long before Hitler's accession to power, was fused with the racist antisemitic ideology of National Socialism. This change in the role and value of treating the ill was accentuated in German medical culture in ensuing decades.

The warped medical rationale for the elimination of German patients in order to protect public health and the purity of the master race was systematically extended and applied to the Jewish people at large. Nazi medicine diagnosed the Jewish people as an inferior and incurably ill race, whose survival posed a threat, because it was liable to contaminate the Aryan population. Therefore, in addition to the goal of racial purification—as compared with and as opposed to the objectives of sterilization and euthanasia—the war against the Jews was perceived as a confrontation of apocalyptic magnitude.

The moral perversion of social health theories and the employment of a racist perception of hygiene to justify mass murder entailed the cooperation of thousands of German medical professionals who provided the Nazis with ideological support and practical assistance. The German medical system helped to promote the pseudomedical ideas that the Nazi regime cultivated. Within two years of Hitler's rise to power, more than 45 percent of the German doctors had officially joined the Nazi Party. These doctors facilitated the passage of the Nuremburg Laws, the ouster of Jewish doctors, forced sterilizations, and the murder of the mentally ill and the disabled under the "euthanasia" program. The Nazis' plan to exterminate the Jews was implemented with the participation and support of the German doctors, who reinforced racist antisemitic arguments by putting forward scientific theories, propped up the racist policy, and abetted the annihilation of groups of German citizens.

From an organizational perspective, it is noteworthy that the director of the General Government Health Department labored to establish a health care system for Poles in order to protect Germans from contagion. The Jews, in contrast, were abandoned to their fate, and were required to set up a separate administration of their own to deal with their health care needs under harsh conditions and without the necessary resources. Dr. Kurt Schrempf, the chief German physician in Warsaw, operated in compliance with this policy. In January 1941, he was replaced by Dr. Hagen, who considered himself responsible for the health of the Germans and the Poles, and even risked opposing German health care policy in order to save Polish victims of tuberculosis. However, his responsibility for the health of the Jews in the ghetto was limited to preventing the spread of contagious diseases outside the ghetto. Although Hagen was not a National Socialist, his policies were influenced by antisemitic views. Various documents attest that he favored totally shutting off the Jews in the ghetto and killing those who fled. In the war on typhus, he invoked cruel methods that caused the epidemic to spread.

When the Germans occupied Poland and established regimes in the General Government and the great city of Warsaw, they implemented the dehumanizing medical tradition that they had been cultivating at home, since the beginning of the twentieth century and especially after Hitler assumed power. The prevailing perceptions of German health policy, including the adoption of racial hygiene theory and antisemitic ideology, were applied in practice against the Jews of Warsaw, whom they considered members of an inferior race who spread diseases and who might contaminate the city's Aryan and Polish populations. The German doctors in Warsaw recommended locking the Jews in a ghetto for an ostensibly health-related reason—in order to prevent the spread of epidemics by the Jews. Their policies led to the sealing of additional ghettos and to the deliberate increase in mortality among the Jews before the decision to annihilate the Jewish people was made.

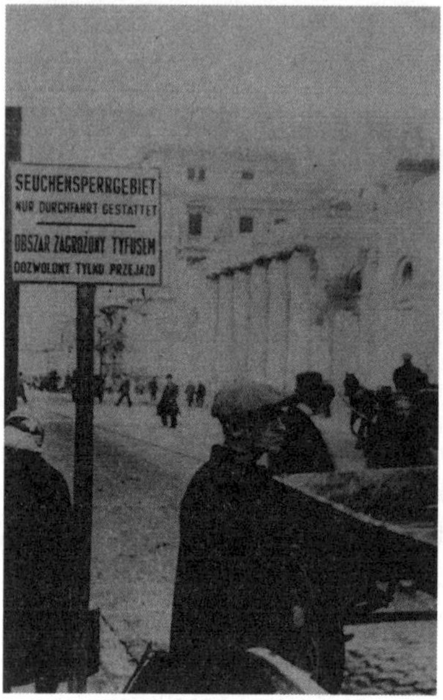
SEUCHENSPERRGEBIET
NUR DURCHFAHRT GESTATTET
OBSZAR ZAGROŻONY TYFUSEM
DOZWOLONY TYLKO PRZEJAZD

Photo Archive, GFH, no. 355.

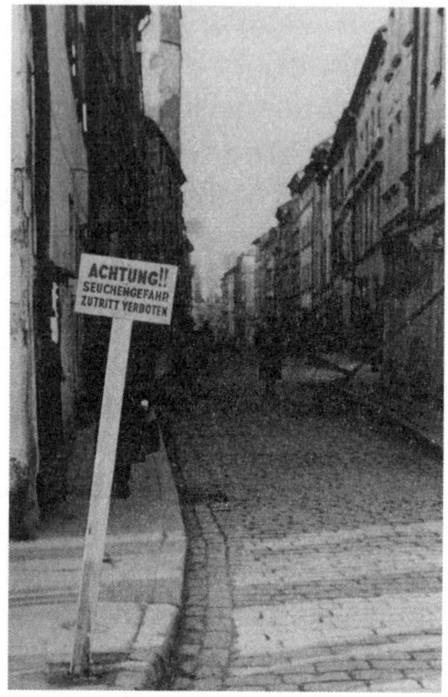
ACHTUNG!!
SEUCHENGEFAHR
ZUTRITT VERBOTEN

Photo Archive, GFH, no. 356.

Signs warning about the danger of an epidemic and prohibiting entry to the Jewish quarter, 1939.

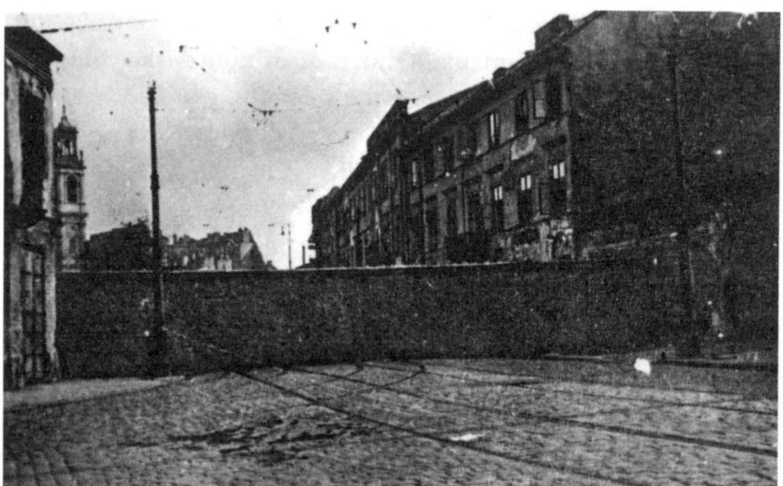

Warsaw ghetto wall. Photo Collection, YVA, 24BO4.

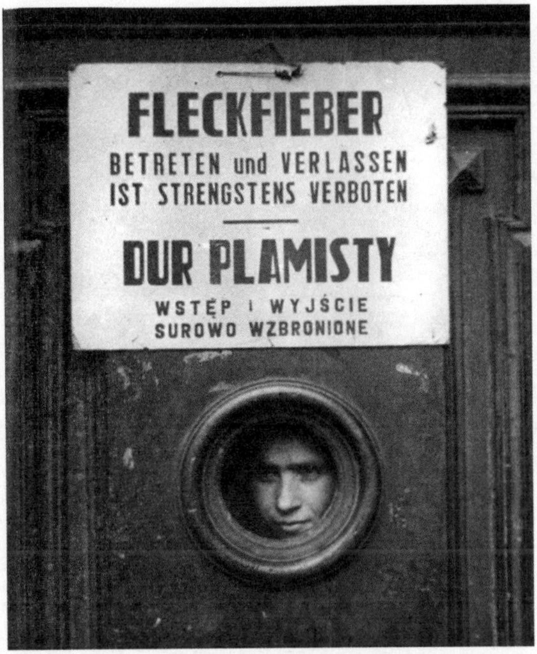
FLECKFIEBER
BETRETEN und VERLASSEN
IST STRENGSTENS VERBOTEN
DUR PLAMISTY
WSTĘP I WYJŚCIE
SUROWO WZBRONIONE

A sign in German and in Polish on a building in the ghetto prohibiting entry and exit due to an epidemic, which necessitated isolation and disinfection. Photo Collection, YVA, 1605/904.

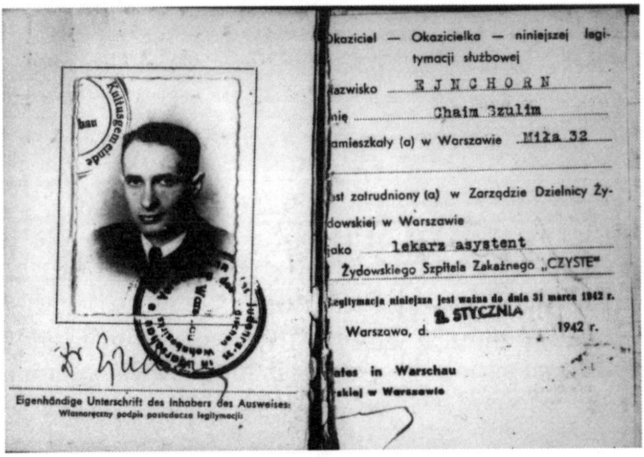

The license to practice medicine of Dr. Chaim Einhorn (1910–1978), who worked in the ghetto and at refugee centers, and participated in the hunger study. Photo Collection, YVA, 70904.

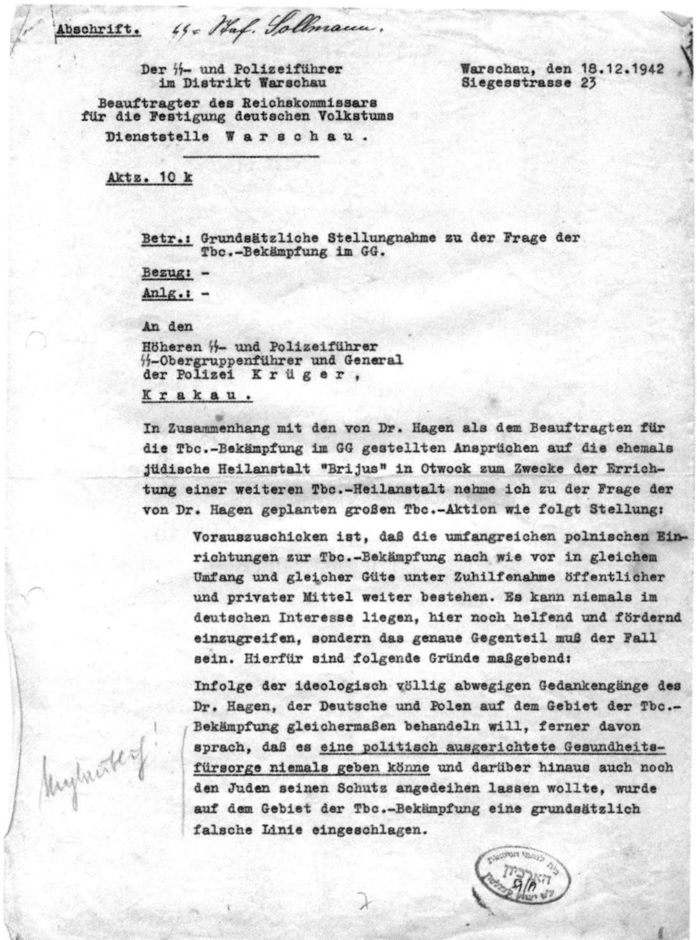

Abschrift. SS-Stubaf. Sollmann.

Der SS- und Polizeiführer
im Distrikt Warschau

Beauftragter des Reichskommissars
für die Festigung deutschen Volkstums

Dienststelle W a r s c h a u .

Warschau, den 18.12.1942
Siegesstrasse 23

Aktz. 10 k

Betr.: Grundsätzliche Stellungnahme zu der Frage der Tbc.-Bekämpfung im GG.

Bezug: -

Anlg.: -

An den
Höheren SS- und Polizeiführer
SS-Obergruppenführer und General
der Polizei K r ü g e r ,

K r a k a u .

In Zusammenhang mit den von Dr. Hagen als dem Beauftragten für die Tbc.-Bekämpfung im GG gestellten Ansprüchen auf die ehemals jüdische Heilanstalt "Brijus" in Otwock zum Zwecke der Errichtung einer weiteren Tbc.-Heilanstalt nehme ich zu der Frage der von Dr. Hagen geplanten großen Tbc.-Aktion wie folgt Stellung:

Vorauszuschicken ist, daß die umfangreichen polnischen Einrichtungen zur Tbc.-Bekämpfung nach wie vor in gleichem Umfang und gleicher Güte unter Zuhilfenahme öffentlicher und privater Mittel weiter bestehen. Es kann niemals im deutschen Interesse liegen, hier noch helfend und fördernd einzugreifen, sondern das genaue Gegenteil muß der Fall sein. Hierfür sind folgende Gründe maßgebend:

Infolge der ideologisch völlig abwegigen Gedankengänge des Dr. Hagen, der Deutsche und Polen auf dem Gebiet der Tbc.-Bekämpfung gleichermaßen behandeln will, ferner davon sprach, daß es eine politisch ausgerichtete Gesundheitsfürsorge niemals geben könne und darüber hinaus auch noch den Juden seinen Schutz angedeihen lassen wollte, wurde auf dem Gebiet der Tbc.-Bekämpfung eine grundsätzlich falsche Linie eingeschlagen.

The first page of a seven-page letter from SS Officer Sollmann, chief of police in Warsaw, to SS Officer Krüger, chief of police in Cracow, regarding the war against tuberculosis in the General Government and Hagen's attitude toward the issue. GFH, no. 7783.

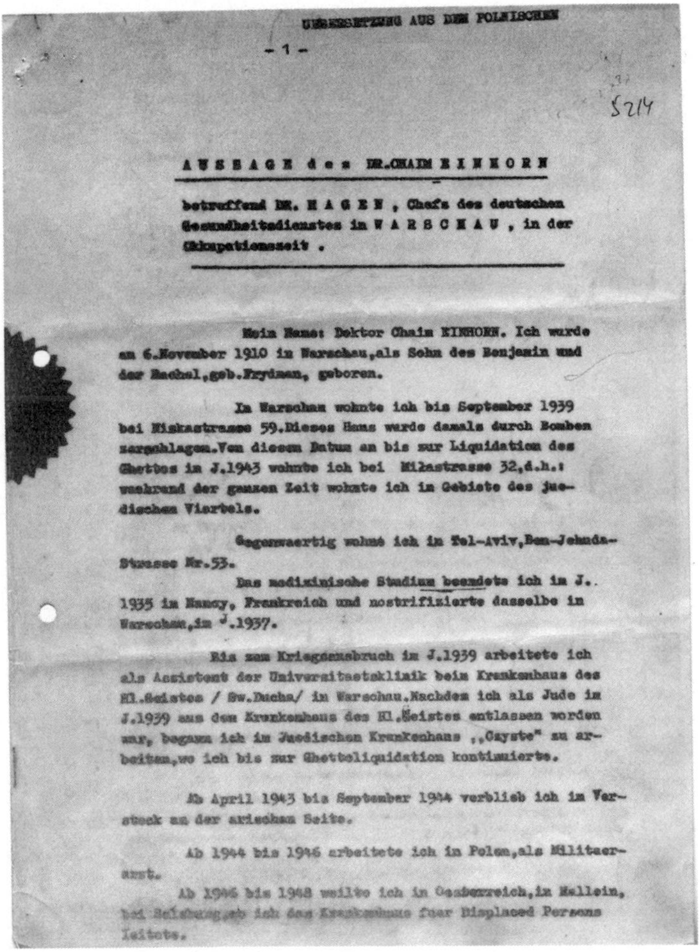
UEBERSETZUNG AUS DEM POLNISCHEN

- 1 -

5214

A U S S A G E des DR.CHAIM E I N H O R N

betreffend DR. H A G E N , Chefs des deutschen Gesundheitsdienstes in W A R S C H A U , in der Okkupationszeit .

Mein Name: Doktor Chaim EINHORN. Ich wurde am 6.November 1910 in Warschau,als Sohn des Benjamin und der Rachel,geb.Frydman, geboren.

In Warschau wohnte ich bis September 1939 bei Miskastrasse 59.Dieses Haus wurde damals durch Bomben zerschlagen.Von diesem Datum an bis zur Liquidation des Ghettos im J.1943 wohnte ich bei Milastrasse 32,d.h.: waehrend der ganzen Zeit wohnte ich im Gebiete des juedischen Viertels.

Gegenwaertig wohne ich in Tel-Aviv,Ben-Jehuda-Strasse Nr.53.

Das medizinische Studium beendete ich im J. 1935 in Nancy, Frankreich und nostrifizierte dasselbe in Warschau,im J.1937.

Bis zum Kriegsausbruch im J.1939 arbeitete ich als Assistent der Universitaetsklinik beim Krankenhaus des Hl.Geistes / Sw.Ducha/ in Warschau.Nachdem ich als Jude im J.1939 aus dem Krankenhaus des Hl.Geistes entlassen worden war, begann ich im Juedischen Krankenhaus ,,Czyste" zu arbeiten,wo ich bis zur Ghettoliquidation kontinuierte.

Ab April 1943 bis September 1944 verblieb ich im Versteck an der arischen Seite.

Ab 1944 bis 1946 arbeitete ich in Polen,als Militaerarzt.

Ab 1946 bis 1948 weilte ich in Oesterreich,in Hallein, bei Salzburg,wo ich das Krankenhaus fuer Displaced Persons leitete.

Dr. Chaim Einhorn's testimony about Dr. Hagen, the director of health care in Warsaw during the German occupation, May, 15, 1963, first page of three. GFH, no. 5214.

PART TWO

The Jewish Medical System in Warsaw in the Face of Unprecedented Conditions

Its Organization and Challenges

Chapter Three

Organizing the Ghetto Medical System

My ramified and highly intensive work in the area entrusted to me, the health board and in hospitalization for the Jewish community in the ghetto, takes up all my waking hours.... Here in the ghetto, we must make every attempt to outlast this horrific period of time....Endurance and survival—must be our current slogan....To help clarify my meaning, I will borrow two concepts from medicine: endogenous and exogenous. Internally, we must do everything possible to permit endurance and survival. But externally the oppressor's whip cracks forcing us to perform tasks and deeds beyond the ability of our frail strength...the fundamental cells of organized Jewish life where the true Jewish qualities of mercy and charity find realization.... public kitchens, medical courses, as well as other studies in order to equip the younger generation to grow up with skills. Intensive medical research being carried out on death through starvation and typhus...We simply want...to show the world that even these terrible trials could not break us....The result of this work will later be published and will be, I hope, of great interest the world over.[1]

Dr. Israel Milejkowski, Director, Judenrat Health Department in the Warsaw Ghetto

1 Joseph Kermish, ed., *To Live with Honor and Die with Honor! Selected Documents from the Warsaw Ghetto Underground Archives "O.S."* (Oneg Shabbat) (Jerusalem: Yad Vashem, 1986), pp. 741–746.

The complex Jewish medical system in the Warsaw ghetto that was swiftly organized did not sprout ex nihilo. Although Jewish society in Warsaw had been persecuted from the first day of the German occupation, the Jews had previously established medical and health care institutions and organizations. In early October 1939, the Germans foisted a new organizational framework on the Jews, the Judenrat. The activity set in motion by this combination of factors is discussed below.

Judenrat Health Care Services

According to Israel Gutman,

> Paradoxically, the Judenrat [Jewish Council], which the Germans established as an instrument to execute their orders and implement their policy regarding the Jews, had broader authority and dealt with more areas of activity than the prewar kehilla [the institutionalized leadership of the Jewish community] had.[2] This situation was already apparent at the beginning of the occupation, but it developed even further during the existence of the ghetto period.[3]

During part of its lifespan in the ghetto, the Judenrat had about thirty active divisions, comprising sundry departments, desks, and offices.[4] The most prominent were the economic, budget, social

2 The term kehilla has different meanings in the primary sources. Sometimes it refers to the institutionalized leadership of the Jewish community and at other times to the Jewish society living within geographical Jewish communities. In the latter case, each community is a kehilla, from the Hebrew word *kahal*, meaning "congregation."

3 Gutman, *The Jews of Warsaw*, p. 77; Gutman, *Sugiyot Beheker Hashoah*, pp. 80–81.

4 Different sources and studies haphazardly use the terms "divisions," "departments," "desks," and "offices," ruling out precision. Therefore, we will refer to them as the sources do and steer clear of rigid definitions. See Batya Dvir,

welfare, and burial departments. The members of the Judenrat who ran them engaged mainly in general oversight, while the heads and managers did the practical work. Gutman writes that they accomplished a great deal, and sanitation and health care improved over time in several respects. When the organization ŻSS—Żydowska Samopomoc Społeczna (Jewish Social Self-Help)[5]—found it difficult to continue funding the welfare effort, the Judenrat mobilized to take charge of the work of health care and welfare, and made perceptible progress following this change.[6]

The ghetto's medical needs were so immense and complex that no attempt to meet them was likely to succeed under the grim

"Adam Czerniaków: Yoshev Rosh HaYudenrat Shel Yehudei Varsha" (Adam Czerniaków: Chairman of the Judenrat of the Jews of Warsaw—1939–1942) (Hebrew) (Master's thesis, The Hebrew University of Jerusalem, 1993), pp. 227–229.

5 The Jewish Social Self-Help institutions in the German-occupied General Government, operating legally or quasi-legally, went by different names as the German authorities commanded and are defined differently in the primary sources in Polish, German, Yiddish, and Hebrew. Therefore, the expression "Jewish Social Self-Help" is rendered differently, as presented in each of the sources. The main names used in this context are Jüdisches Hilfskomitee (JHK), Żydowska Samopomoc Społeczna (ŻSS), Jüdische Soziale Selbsthilfe (JSS), Żydowskie Towarzystwo Opieki Społecznej (ŻTOS), and Jewish Relief Office (JUS). These institutions operated in conjunction with Naczelna Rada Opiekuńcza (NRO), an umbrella relief organization, which included the Polish Rada Głowma Opiekuńcza (RGO), Ukrainska Rada Opiekuńcza (URO), and Żydowska Samopomoc Społeczna (ŻSS). These organizations operated with the authorization and under the supervision of the German regime. Throughout the entire period of occupation, the Jewish Social Self-Help underwent different phases of administration. On relief activity in the General Government, in general, and in Warsaw, specifically, see, for example, Gutman, *The Jews of Warsaw*, pp. 40–47, 102–106; Turkow, *Hayo Hayta Varsha Yehudit*, pp. 20–21; Czerniaków, *The Warsaw Diary*, pp. 107, 126–127, 154, 157, 168, 180–181, 185, 198, 293, 314, 329, 333–335, 375; Ringelblum, *Yoman Vereshimot*, p. 93; David Ben-Shalom, *Ha'ezra Ha'atzmit Hayehudit Kemisgeret Lepe'ilut Va'adei Habatim Begeto Varsha* (The Jewish Self-Help as a Framework for Activity of Tenement Committees in the Warsaw Ghetto) (Hebrew) (Master's thesis, The Hebrew University of Jerusalem, 1995), pp. 29, 35; Aleksandra Bańkowska, "Jewish Social Welfare Institutions and Facilities in the General Government from 1939 to 1944: A Preliminary Study," *Studia z Dziejów Rosji i Europy Środkowo-Wschodniej*, 53 (2018), pp. 129–167.

6 On the change in Czerniaków's involvement in welfare and health care institutions, see Dvir, "Adam Czerniaków," p. 108.

living conditions. The Health Department, which was set up as part of the constellation of Judenrat departments, had to provide many services that the city of Warsaw had previously furnished. In addition to the many long-standing medical institutions that continued their prewar work in the ghetto, new entities were founded in response to the needs occasioned by ghettoization, including hospitals of various kinds—general, children's, psychiatric, and tuberculosis, as well as several private hospitals and clinics.[7]

The Judenrat and the Jewish Social Self-Help, with its set of institutions, received legal recognition from the Germans. They implemented budgets and had hundreds of employees in their various departments. Many members of the Judenrat in Warsaw, appointed to their posts by the Germans, had held public and political positions before the war.[8] Adam Czerniaków, chair of the Judenrat from its establishment until his suicide during the *Grossaktion*, the mass deportation of the Jews of Warsaw that began in July 1942, had been a member of the kehilla board of directors before the war. During the siege of Warsaw, he was a board member of the Jewish Civilian Committee that had been set up at that time. On September 23, 1939, Stefan Starzyński, the mayor of Warsaw, placed him in charge of the Jewish religious community.[9] Czerniaków's appointment to the helm of the Judenrat ten days later, on October 4, 1939, was almost a natural matter of course for a public activist who had been serving the Jewish population. Once in office, Czerniaków often spoke critically of the Jewish leaders who had fled for their lives during the German invasion of Poland.[10]

7 Roland, *Courage under Siege*, pp. 53–54.

8 Ibid., pp. 57–59; Gutman, *The Jews of Warsaw*, p. 37.

9 Gutman, *The Jews of Warsaw*, p. 37; Trunk, *Judenrat*, p. 15.

10 Gutman, *The Jews of Warsaw*, p. 38. Adam Czerniaków was born in Warsaw in 1880 into a middle-class family that tended toward assimilation. In 1908, he completed his engineering studies in Warsaw and did an internship in Dresden, Germany. Returning to Poland, he taught school and represented Jewish craftsmen vis-à-vis the Polish authorities. He was also active in the kehilla and the Warsaw Municipal Council and even served in the Polish Senate for a certain time. For an outline of Czerniaków's activities and controversial persona, see Gutman, *Sugiyot Beheker Hashoah*, pp. 92–117. Notably, Gutman

The community council—the Judenrat—was comprised of twenty-four active members from a litany of fields, including activists in welfare institutions, public organizations, and political parties. The members of the Judenrat board who were appointed along with them were people of impressive public experience who had remained in Warsaw. The Judenrat was tasked with satisfying all the needs of the Jewish population in the ghetto. During the ghetto period, the number of employees working in the various Judenrat departments, including welfare and medical staff, swelled from 1,741 to 6,000.[11]

The divisions that operated as part of the Judenrat included the one for hospitals, headed by the counselor Edward Kobryner; another for social welfare, chaired by Dr. Gustaw Wielikowski; a division for health, under Dr. Israel Milejkowski; and a supply division—Zakład Zaopatrywania (ZZ)—overseen by Abraham Gepner and Shmuel Winter. The latter controlled 601 food rationing distribution centers, including orphanages, hospitals, public kitchens, and refugee shelters; 273 soap distribution sites; and 70 bakeries.[12]

On September 18, 1939, even before the establishment of the Judenrat and the Health Department, and as medical problems worsened and the numbers of dead and wounded surged, the aforementioned Jewish Civilian Committee convened to tackle the Jewish community's most urgent problems. Its members appointed Dr. Israel Milejkowski, a physician and public activist, to coordinate medical assistance during the siege. They also declared the intention of establishing a 100-bed hospital under the auspices of the kehilla and of providing it with bandaging supplies

winds up the chapter that discusses Czerniaków with a July 1945 letter from Dr. Felicja Czerniaków, Adam's wife, to Adolf Abraham Berman, protesting their banishment of her husband's memory and their erasure of his name and persona, whereas she considered him "the first rebel." Gutman's choice of this conclusion may signal a tendency to assess Czerniaków's actions more favorably than the tendency that dominated research until then.

11 Trunk, *Judenrat*, p. 51.

12 Turkow, *Hayo Hayta Varsha Yehudit*, pp. 18–19; Trunk, *Judenrat*, pp. 102–103; Gutman, *The Jews of Warsaw*, p. 83.

and medicines.[13] About two and a half months into the German occupation, on December 16–17, 1939, Czerniaków inaugurated a hospitals department and named Ignacy Fliederbaum, former administrative manager at Czyste Hospital, to run it.[14]

Dr. Milejkowski assumed responsibility for the health of the Jewish population.[15] In January 1940, when the Judenrat Health Department came into being, he was tasked with setting up an authority that would consolidate all municipal powers related to health. The department established six health care centers where welfare and medical teams operated under the supervision of chief physicians. The department supported the operation of two hospitals, which were deployed in six buildings during the ghetto period; three outpatient clinics; a sanitation committee composed of doctors; eight disinfection teams from September 1941 onward; four public baths, three quarantine points for carriers of contagious illnesses; and sundry public health facilities.[16] It is important to note two Jewish health care

13 Czerniaków, *The Warsaw Diary*, p. 75.

14 Ibid., p. 100.

15 Dr. Israel Milejkowski (1887–1943) completed his dermatology studies in 1914 and practiced in Warsaw. Before World War II, he was the highly esteemed chair of the Jewish Medical Association. On September 18, 1939, in the midst of the siege of Warsaw, he was named chair of the Medical Aid Desk of the civilian committee that public representatives had set up in the kehilla building. During the occupation, he headed the Judenrat Health Department in the Warsaw ghetto. He strove prodigiously to set up the underground medical school in the ghetto and headed the team that performed scientific research on hunger. He is described as a man of noble bearing and courage. As the liaison between the Judenrat and the German health authorities, he dared to criticize the occupation authorities' cruel edicts and stayed in his post until the end. In an *Aktion* that began on January 18, 1943, members of the *Ordnungsdienst* (Jewish police) entered courtyards and ordered the residents to come out of their apartments. Jews who held "life numbers," particularly those Judenrat officials, trusted that these documents protected them and did as told. Many doctors who held important posts in the community institutions, including Dr. Milejkowski, were snared in the trap that the Nazis had set. See Czerniaków, *The Warsaw Diary*, p. 75; Wulman et al., *The Martyrdom of Jewish Physicians in Poland*, p. 419.

16 Trunk, *Judenrat*, pp. 159–160. After the occupation began, the Jewish quarter was divided into four sanitation inspection precincts, each headed by a doctor who answered to a Polish medical coordinator and who had to report weekly on the state of sanitation and on the status of contagious illnesses. When

entities run by the Judenrat that operated outside the ghetto—Brijus, a tuberculosis sanatorium, and Zofiówka Psychiatric Hospital—both situated in Otwock and supported by the JDC until July 1942.

Among all the doctors in the Warsaw ghetto, Dr. Milejkowski bore the heaviest medical burden. Before the war, he had chaired the Jewish Medical Association. As head of the Judenrat Health Department, he was personally responsible for all aspects of sanitation and medicine in the ghetto. He endured a living nightmare every Friday, when he met with the German authorities. Devoted to the Jewish population and seeing his role as his mission, he had no fear that the Germans might put him to death during one of these encounters. Those on the team who worked with him but did not know him well were amazed at how this slender man endured the Sisyphean burden that he had assumed and how he maintained the mental fortitude to survive the weekly Friday ordeal. Even those who knew him well could not fathom this and could only appreciate him immensely for it.

One Jewish doctor or another faced the threat of death daily, accused by the Germans of not doing enough to combat epidemics. The doctors felt that they could divulge forbidden details only to Dr. Milejkowski, who always assumed responsibility for them. He was characterized by his courage and dignity throughout his term of activity in the ghetto. As head of the Judenrat Health Department and together with Prof. Hirszfeld, Dr. Owsiej Bielenki,[17] and Czerniaków, he presented the German authorities with a courageous memorandum on the war on epidemics in the ghetto in which he accused the Germans of spreading typhus.[18] Dr. Milejkowski enabled a group of scientists and doctors in

the Judenrat and its Health Department came into being, the neighborhood physicians ceased to be subordinate to Polish institutions. See Dr. Chaim Einhorn testimony, YVA, O.3/1836.

17 Dr. Owsiej Bielenki (b. 1884), an internist who specialized in pulmonary conditions and one of the most prominent figures in his field in Warsaw, headed the tuberculosis department at Czyste Hospital. He perished in the Trawniki camp in February–March 1943.

18 See Miriam Offer, *Haluk Lavan Bageto*, appendix A.2, pp. 497–504.

the ghetto to set up a clandestine medical school, and initiated lectures and in-service activities for physicians. A determined man with a passion for social work, even in hopeless situations, he had the power to persuade the doctors at the hospital to engage in research.[19]

Dr. Milejkowski was a Zionist. Prof. Hirszfeld writes that he believed that although the Jewish people would never be numerous, and that those who did not identify with Judaism would be assimilated, the remainder would hoist the national banner proudly and aspire to a homeland of their own. His personal aspiration was to be a leader of his people in his professional field. His devotion and integrity impressed everyone, allowing him to attain achievements in the area of sanitation through his contacts with the occupation authorities and to help many pro bono. The gentle, slightly-built man was also strong and bold. When advised to go into hiding after the Germans arrested his deputy, Dr. Milejkowski refused, stating, "I'm waiting for the gentlemen." During the final *Aktion*, he could have saved himself but he refused, marching to death at the head of the oppressed.[20]

Dr. Milejkowski did not work in a vacuum, of course. He was directly associated with the Judenrat and its chairman, Czerniaków. During most of the period, he maintained contact with the German physician who oversaw public health in Warsaw on behalf of the civil administration. Dr. Wilhelm Hagen, who took up this post at the same time that the ghetto was established in November 1940, held this position for most of the relevant period. Dr. Milejkowski depended on German budgets, decrees, and policies to conduct his activities. His responsibilities and connections in high places helped very little to improve the Germans' treatment of him. In April 1940, for example, despite his impeccable conduct, he was arrested while crossing the street and was ordered to perform forced labor—hauling bricks—for the rest of the day in the pouring rain.[21]

19 Dr. Moshe Tursz testimony, YVA, O.3/438, pp. 21–22.

20 Hirszfeld, *The Story of One Life*, pp. 198–199.

21 Roland, *Courage under Siege*, p. 53.

As the typhus epidemic spread, the Germans threatened to liquidate the ghetto and forced Dr. Milejkowski to reorganize the medical services. As a result, Dr. Mieczysław Kon, an apostate Jew and a former military physician, and Dr. Tadeusz Ganc, who had arrived in Warsaw from the Łódź ghetto, were appointed to head these services. The ghetto was divided into precincts, and the blocks situated within each precinct were entrusted to the doctor responsible for it.[22] Dr. Milejkowski continued faithfully at his post as head of the Health Department in the ghetto until his deportation. According to Prof. Hirszfeld, this division of labor was complicated, and the role and authority of each was unclear.[23] He testified that the numerous appointments at the managerial level, some at the Germans' behest, generated friction.

The Ringelblum Archive contains a weekly newsletter, no. 1, signed by Dr. Kon, which was circulated on March 8, 1942, to all the Health Office staff. The author of the newsletter explained its purpose: "To share information on all health-related matters with all workers at the Health Office and to keep [them] abreast of all developments." The information included reports on work and payments, procedures concerning the disinfection teams and the operation of public baths, events for the children of the Health Office staff members, and a eulogy for an employee. Nowhere in this document does Dr. Milejkowski's name appear.[24]

In addition to the war on epidemics, the Health Department was active in other areas. The Judenrat strained to keep the large Czyste Hospital functioning. A report from the Judenrat statistics department in February 1942 sheds light on many of the Health Department's activities. For example, almost all the schoolchildren in the ghetto underwent three medical checkups that month. Checkups of 897 youngsters revealed 13 cases of typhus, also known as spotted fever, and 27 cases of other contagious diseases. One hundred forty-two children were referred to specialists. A hundred free medical consultations and several others at discounts

22 Einhorn, "Harofe Begeto Varsha," p. 11.

23 Hirszfeld, *Die Geschichte eines Lebens*, p. 146.

24 Health Office Weekly, no. 1, to all Health Office workers, March 8, 1942, AŻIH, ARI.260.

were arranged for schoolchildren who were under the care of the Social Welfare Department. The pharmacies department supplied twenty aid kits for immediate response treatment at the schools, and the Health Department reserved a public bathhouse near a school for the children's use several times a week. However, regular baths for children remained unfeasible due to the bitter cold.[25]

The Germans' fear of contagious diseases and their supervision of measures to prevent their spread continued throughout the various stages of the ghetto's existence, and the Health Department was required to present monthly status reports on sanitation and morbidity. In February 1942, the Judenrat submitted to the German authorities for approval the procedures it had established in compliance with the sanitary directives and the binding sanitary arrangements. A request by the Judenrat to extend the period of inoculation against bloody diarrhea to March 31, 1942, was approved.[26] Hospitalization and observation procedures changed frequently.

In March 1942, the number of typhus patients declined and restrictions on transporting people to the hospitals were repealed. Special sanitary inspection committees were set up; each included a doctor from the Health Department, a neighborhood physician, an expert in hygiene, a nurse responsible for the population, and a representative of the residents who had received training in disinfecting buildings. They inspected all the apartments in every building, exempted clean apartments from further attention, and disinfected the others using a mechanical procedure or gas.[27]

The Judenrat established additional medical committees to examine Jews destined for forced labor. At the beginning of the occupation, on February 22, 1940, the Judenrat was ordered to recruit doctors to examine 35,000 people who had been summoned to register for forced labor. Czerniaków had to present 53 doctors with letters, summoning them to examine patients during

25 Judenrat Statistics Department Report, no. 29, March 17, 1942, GFH, no. 11250, p. 6; Offer, "Ma'arach Harefu'a Begeto Varsha," vol. 2, appendix A.15, pp. 58–64.

26 Judenrat Statistics Department Report, no. 29, March 17, 1942, GFH, no. 11250, p. 29.

27 Ibid.

registration.[28] These medical committees conducted medical exams in August 1940, prior to transport to the labor camps.[29] The Judenrat also had to send physicians to the labor camps. When the doctors refused to accept this task, which subjected them to the harsh conditions in the camps, many difficulties ensued.[30] On May 24, 1941, about half a year after ghettoization, Czerniaków made efforts to release the ill from transport to the camps after medical checkups confirmed their conditions. He discussed this with the ghetto *Kommissar*, Heinz Auerswald.[31]

On January 17, 1942, about a year after the establishment of the ghetto, Czerniaków was instructed to set up a committee of doctors, composed of five Jewish physicians and one SS doctor, to examine the fitness of Jewish prisoners from the ghetto who were being punished for smuggling food. It was determined that those capable of labor would be sent to the Treblinka camp. About two days later, at the behest of the *Kommissar*, a committee of doctors became operative in the Jewish prison. Among the 250 adults whom it vetted, the panel found 54 fit for labor. An order was issued to treat some of them for scabies and to send them to perform forced labor.[32]

In response to the spread of illness and the challenges that the Judenrat faced in its attempts to deal with the mounting medical exigencies, Czerniaków initiated the formation of a professional Jewish Health Council alongside the Health Department, and invited Prof. Hirszfeld to chair it. During a discussion about the chances of surmounting the typhus epidemic, he explained to Czerniaków,

> This epidemic is like a volcano. It is difficult to catch the lava with bare hands and direct its flow, as we want it. Under the prevailing social and political conditions, I will not promise that I will defeat the epidemic. However, if I succeed in

28 Czerniaków, *The Warsaw Diary*, pp. 120–121.

29 Ringelblum, *Notes from the Warsaw Ghetto*, p. 45.

30 Czerniaków, *The Warsaw Diary*, pp. 190, 193, 196.

31 Ibid., p. 242.

32 Ibid., p. 260.

> defeating the delousing, you will have good reason to be thankful to the Health Council.[33]

It was important to Hirszfeld, as an apostate Jew, to know that the public wanted to see him at the helm of the Health Council. He was encouraged by the appearance of a delegation of Orthodox Jews who favored his candidacy, and after much vacillation, he acceded to Czerniaków's request, on condition that the council undertake to implement its decisions.[34]

Hirszfeld's personality and actions sparked controversy and criticism among the doctors and public figures in the ghetto. The main reason for this, presumably, was the fact that he was an apostate who was punctilious about attending church even in the ghetto. In addition, his expertise and his strong personality naturally generated tension between him and his colleagues, and various health care officials in the ghetto. Concerning this matter, Ringelblum wrote in March 1941 that when the Judenrat organized a lecture by Hirszfeld for doctors, many gathered in protest because, according to them, Hirszfeld had made the Institute of Hygiene, which he had headed before the war, *Judenrein* (free of Jews) and had applied an explicitly antisemitic policy.[35]

According to Hirszfeld, the Health Council was a comprehensive and central entity in the ghetto's medical community. Its membership represented all groups that engaged in the medical care of the Jewish population: physicians from the Judenrat, the Jewish Social Self-Help, and the hospitals. Dr. Józef Chajn Gołębiowski, a TOZ executive, wrote that the council had three goals: to work on scientific theories to combat infectious diseases, to study diseases in the ghetto, and to formulate sanitation rules.[36]

33 Hirszfeld, *The Story of One Life*, p. 217.

34 Ibid.

35 Ringelblum, *Yoman Vereshimot*, p. 254.

36 Roland, *Courage under Siege*, p. 69; Hirszfeld, *Die Geschichte eines Lebens*, p. 146; Dr. Józef Chajn Gołębiewski testimony, YVA, O.3/2355. The members of the council included Prof. Ludwik Hirszfeld; Dr. Israel Milejkowski, director of the Judenrat Health Department; two members of the organization Jewish

At the beginning of its activities, the council encountered difficulties concerning its powers. To mitigate these problems, it was decided that sanitation and health inspection in the ghetto would be subordinate to the Health Council and to the director of the Health Department, Dr. Milejkowski, who represented the council vis-à-vis the German administration. The Health Council became operative in October 1941, but it took a long time to get organized. By the time its status was recognized and its working procedures consolidated, the destruction of the ghetto had begun and its activities were no longer relevant. Nevertheless, some continued to work within the framework of the council without official authorization.

Another adjunct to the Health Department was a medical committee headed by the dedicated director of the children's hospital in the ghetto, Dr. Anna Braude-Heller. Dr. Henryk Makower, a virologist and head of the department of infectious diseases at this hospital, served as the committee's secretary. Although he reported that the committee was dealing with the problems of the ghetto's health care system, it was not clear to what extent it had the ability to implement its decisions.[37]

The Judenrat's income did not suffice to cover the expenses of managing ghetto life and meeting its welfare and health care needs. To overcome the deficits, it levied new taxes. Most of the revenue was obtained through indirect taxes: a fee for food ration cards; payment for exemption from forced labor—60–100 zlotys per month; a tax to maintain a "labor brigade" to meet its payroll

Social Self-Help, Dr. Szymon Wyszewiański and Dr. Józef Chajn Gołębiewski; two hospital directors, Dr. Josef Stein and Dr. Anna Braude-Heller; two hospital inspectors, the attorney Waclaw Brockman and the manufacturer Michal Friedberg; Dr. Owsiej Bielenki, chief physician for tuberculosis at the hospital; Dr. Tadeusz Ganc, an administrative director with the Health Department; and Dr. Mieczysław Kon, a former colonel and a specialist in bacteriology, who was appointed by the Germans to replace Dr. Syrkin Binstein to manage the health services alongside Dr. Milejkowski.

37 Roland, *Courage under Siege*, pp. 69–70. Judenrat report to Dr. Auerswald on the Warsaw Jewish quarter under the *Kommissar*'s rule, May 15, 1941–May 15, 1942, GFH, no. 3909. The members of the committee were Dr. Akiwa Uryson, Dr. Aleksander Werthajm, and Dr. Anna Margolis.

and support members' families; burial taxes to pay for those unable to afford them—the house committee paid in their stead or buried the deceased in a collective grave; and dozens of additional indirect taxes that the Judenrat imposed. Operating under the slogan "Everyone is equal," it made no attempt to prescribe differential taxation based on the ghetto residents' material resources.

Rent brought in 60 percent of the Judenrat's income. The community tax and the hospital tax are the only direct taxes mentioned in the sources. The hospital tax was determined according to the recommendations of the house committees, which were aware of the residents' financial means. The ghetto inhabitants incurred major expenses for welfare and inpatient medical care. In February 1942, a new 40 percent tax on every prescription filled by the Judenrat's pharmacies was imposed to the benefit of the community chest.[38]

Warsaw Judenrat Main Income and Expenses, 1940
Total Budget: 10,680,000 Zlotys[39]

Expenses	
Forced Laborers' Salaries	3,811,000
Hospitals	3,059,000
Welfare and Medical Care	920,000
Vocational Courses	113,000
Miscellaneous	2,777,000
Total Expenses	**10,680,000**

Income	
Burial Fees	1,193,000
Exemptions from Forced Labor	2,603,000
Community Tax	634,000
Hospital Tax	541,000
Population Registration Fee	423,000
Ration Card Fee	325,000
Total Income	**5,719,000**

38 Trunk, *Judenrat*, pp. 236–243; Ringelblum, *Notes from the Warsaw Ghetto*, pp. 156, 245–246.

39 Trunk, *Judenrat*, p. 247.

The budget deficit was close to 5 million zlotys at that time. It was covered by raising indirect taxes and releasing the "frozen savings" of public funds and of individuals in Polish banks in Warsaw. The ghetto administration, aided by the Ordnungsdienst (ghetto police) and other entities, was responsible for collecting taxes and punishing the recalcitrant.[40] According to the statistics department's report of March 17, 1942, the Appeals Committee reviewed complaints about the level of the hospital tax in 1942. In addition, taxes were collected from 15,000 new residents who were required to pay taxes.

Health Department and Hospitals Department Revenues, February 1942 (Zlotys)

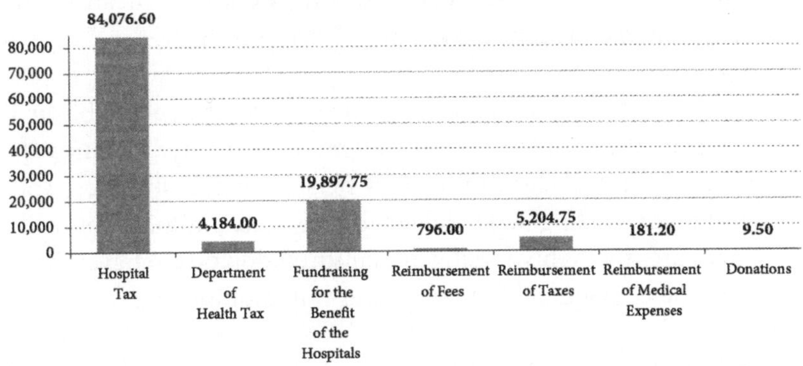

According to the data in the statistical report, the total revenue in March 1942 was 114,349 zlotys.[41] Therefore, it appears that the taxes collected in the 1942 fiscal year amounted to 1.37 million zlotys. During the fiscal year that ran from April 1941 to March 1942, the Health Department spent 5.7 million zlotys, 21.3 percent

40 Ibid., pp. 247–248. According to Trunk, the Judenrat's fiscal condition improved in 1942 for several reasons: it received a share of municipal taxes collected from Jews; it was exempt from paying forced laborers' salaries and from transferring funds to German authorities and employers; and it boosted its tax revenues, especially those derived from indirect taxes paid equally by the rich and the poor.

41 Ibid., pp. 247–248.

of the Judenrat budget that year.[42] In other words, the revenue covered 24 percent of the Health Department's expenditures and the Judenrat and others had to come up with the remainder—at least 4.37 million zlotys.

Despite the harsh reality of the ghetto, it was imperative to grant those covered by medical insurance their entitlements. In February 1942, the Public Insurance Office vetted those entitled to health coverage and found that about 60,000 were eligible for medical insurance.[43] A document written after June 25, 1942, several days before the deportations began, indicates that the collection of national insurance funds continued. Only some of the money that was collected was transferred to the ghetto in accordance with the instructions of the Jewish quarter *Kommissar*.[44] The Judenrat's activities in the area of health care were not spared criticism. Kaplan noted in his diary,

> A perfect example of this is the Health Department established under the auspices of the Judenrat to maintain standards of sanitation, cleanliness, and health. In this instance, you are not dealing with vulgar, dull-witted janitors, but with apparently highly intelligent, cultured doctors. Yet even here money purifies all filth and covers all iniquities.[45]

Czerwony Sztandar (Red Banner), the Trotskyists' underground newspaper, reported,

> In the unemployed and starving ghetto, the Judenrat has managed to operate a total system of payments, fees, duties, and contributions.... This money covers the construction of the ghetto walls but does not suffice to run the kitchens for the

42 Ibid., pp. 159–160.

43 Judenrat Statistics Department Report, no. 29, March 17, 1942, GFH, no. 11250, p. 17.

44 A document relating to social insurance in Warsaw, 1942, AŻIH, ARI.295.

45 Kaplan, *Scroll of Agony*, p. 342.

> masses, which have been closed, or to provide the hospitals and orphanages with vital medicines, food, and heating fuel.[46]

The methods employed by the Judenrat to fight epidemics also drew criticism. In September 1941, *Biuletyn* published a trenchant critique of "the Judenrat's criminal neglect in the war on epidemics and the protection of the population's health."[47]

TOZ—The Jewish Health Care Organization

As described in Part I of this book, before the outbreak of the War, TOZ was a well-developed Jewish health organization that provided medical aid and promoted health care services for the Jewish public as a national health service, and extended assistance in areas where the state offered none.[48] Immediately after the war broke out, the organization's branches in the Soviet-occupied territories were nationalized, and the activities of the Jewish health care institutions in Vilna, Grodno, Białystok, Lwów, and other cities ceased. In Poland, ties between the TOZ headquarters in Warsaw and the other branches were severed. Most branches were left without leadership and material resources. The only remaining branches were in major cities, such as Łódź, Cracow, Lublin, and Częstochowa, along with the headquarters in Warsaw. Masses of Jews arrived at the TOZ branches seeking assistance—medicines, bread, and shelter from the cold or from deportation.[49]

In September 1939, the outbreak of the war caused high mortality in Warsaw and left several tens of thousands wounded. Provisional sanitary stations were set up at the entrances of almost all the tenements and provided first aid to the hundreds of casualties who flooded them. In times of distress, the Jews of Warsaw had only one address: TOZ headquarters at 33 Gęsia St., where the largest medical center in the northern neighborhoods

46 Blatman, *Geto Varsha—Sipur Itona'i*, p. 193.

47 Ibid., p. 212.

48 Wulman, "Hevrat Toz," p. 584.

49 Ibid., pp. 584–585.

of Warsaw had arisen spontaneously. TOZ began to offer medical aid to those injured and to save lives. Its building was hit during the bombardments and some of the bombs that could have started fires were covered with sand, which minimized the damage.[50]

About a month after the occupation of Warsaw, Mechel Kulick wrote to his friend Matz, secretary of TOZ in Vilna, describing the activities of the organization and its staff in Warsaw during the first month of the war. This document also delivered the bitter news of the death of the president of TOZ, Dr. Gershon Lewin.

> I was wounded during the fire and had to undergo an operation that was rather complicated. I feel better now and my family is all right as well. Everything is fine with Osusky's family; I have provided them with food and fuel. A sanitary ambulatory station was set up in our house that also serves as a soup kitchen for mothers and children, and a shelter for refugees. For the time being, I am managing this work (at present more than sixty nurses, physicians, and auxiliary workers are working with us).
>
> Dr. Rozenblum and N. Finkelstein visited us today. They will provide the necessary funds, and I feel a little relieved. The following persons are working with us now: Rabinowitz, Seidengart, Gelbfisch, Judt (their homes and institutions were destroyed), Chmelnika, Liwska, Dina (their homes were destroyed by fire), Kaliska (Leiserowitch's house was burned down), Kopel, Rheinfeld (house destroyed), Tursch, Funk, Rachmilewitch, Graubart, Bernstein, Borenstein, Hirschbein, and others whom you don't know. Dr. Wulman's apartment was destroyed, as well as the entire building. Our building was perforated with bullets up to the second floor; buildings 39 and 41 were demolished by the bombs. The fabric factory across the street was burned down and the fire spread to our house. While doing rescue work, I was wounded by a stray bullet.

50 Dr. Moshe Tursz testimony, YVA, O.3/438, pp. 1–2. On TOZ activities at the beginning of the war, see, for example, a letter dated November 9, 1939, from Henrietta K. Buchman, JDC Poland to Mr. M. J. Kellner, JDC New York, JDC, AR.33–44, file 841.

This is the general overview of our work, which is conducted under the most difficult conditions. It is impossible to walk in the street. People are beaten and forced to do hard work....

We sincerely hope that you will do your best to make sure that our kind brethren will take care of us and come to see us, if possible. We cannot bear this burden for long. Do not envy us and do not expect our work...

Our work is slackening—I wish it were not true. There will be nothing left for me to do but to emigrate. However, my family's situation has made emigration impossible, since my brothers and sisters are in great distress and are depending on me.

Mr. Lin's house has remained intact. I sent somebody there to examine it. Mr. Hilkovitch is working with us. Our President, Dr. G. L. (Gershon Lewin) died last Wednesday. We buried him on Thursday, October 27. Only a few persons attended the funeral, since most people are afraid to go out. This fear has become the infirmity of the day in Warsaw. We have no electricity, no water or telephone in our "house," which has suffered considerably from bombardments, as have all the houses in this area.

Well, my dear friend, I could write you about many more things, but this is not possible. Be healthy and happy, and let us hope that we will see each other again one day.[51]

At the beginning of the war, two certified nurses named Rajnfeld and Kopel provided assistance at the TOZ medical center in Warsaw. Until the war began, they had worked at the organization's tuberculosis clinic. A doctor who lived nearby also helped. However, F. Wroński, the concierge, was the busiest person there. An especially nimble and dedicated man, he seemed to be able to be everywhere at once—one moment, neutralizing a bomb that had set fire to the roof, the next, taking a crate of bandages out of the cellar, and then running down to the street

51 Letter from Mechel Kulick, TOZ Warsaw, to Metz, secretary of TOZ Vilna, dated the end of October 1939, JDC, AR.33–44, file 840.

to extricate somebody who had been badly wounded. As long as the telephones worked, the TOZ staffers received emotional support and encouragement from Dr. Jakob Rozenblum,[52] a board member at the TOZ branch in Warsaw. From the beginning of the war, he took a keen interest in the fate of the Jewish population and in TOZ, the organization that assisted it. However, because he lived in the center of town and had a prosthetic leg, he was unable to make his way to Gęsia St.[53]

Before the war, Dr. Gershon Lewin and Dr. Leon Wulman headed TOZ in Poland.[54] Dr. Lewin, the organization's vital spirit, died during the first month of the war. Dr. Wulman, general secretary of the organization, spent the war in America. Many TOZ activists left Warsaw and Poland at the beginning of the war.[55] The TOZ board reorganized during the war. Both the board and the Executive Committee held meetings at regular intervals where reports on their activities were delivered.[56] TOZ had its

52 Dr. Jakob Rozenblum (1895–1943) completed his studies at the University of Warsaw in 1930. He continued his medical activities at the university's laboratories and at the Jewish-owned Czyste Hospital, even after losing a leg in a tram accident in 1937. Until the war, he was active in TOZ in Warsaw. In September 1939, with the war underway, he was given a senior post in the TOZ administration. On January 18, 1943, he was sent to Treblinka. See Dr. Moshe Tursz testimony, YVA, O.3/438, pp. 18–20; Wulman et al., *The Martyrdom of Jewish Physicians in Poland*, p. 443.

53 Dr. Moshe Tursz testimony, YVA, O.3/438, p. 2.

54 Jewish Social Self-Help report concerning TOZ, March 1942, AŻIH, ARII.92.

55 Report by Dr. Emanuel Patt on social service work among Polish Jews, March 1941, JDC, AR.33–44, file 814.

56 Different sources render the names and functions of TOZ personnel in different ways. Their job descriptions and their responsibilities may have changed during the war. In addition, some sources mention the general management of the TOZ organization, while others refer only to its activities in Warsaw. During the war, the TOZ board had thirteen members: Dr. M. Koenigstein, chair; Dr. M. Mesh, deputy chair; Nechemia Finkelstein, treasurer; Dr. Jakob Rozenblum, secretary; Dr. S. Wyszewiański, J. Rosnicki, L. Neustadt, Dr. Wohl, Dr. Mitz, Dr. Braude-Heller, Dr. Józef Chajn Gołębiewski, P. Czerski, and Dr. M. Szwalbe. The members of its Executive Committee included Dr. S. Wyszewiański, chair; Nechemia Finkelstein, Dr. Jakob Rozenblum, Dr. M. Szwalbe, Dr. Józef Chajn Gołębiewski, and Dr. Moshe Tursz, secretary. See the Jewish Jewish Social Self-Help report concerning TOZ, March 1942, AŻIH, ARII.92; and the report by Dr. Emanuel Patt on social service work among Polish Jews, March 1941, JDC, AR.33–44, file 814.

headquarters at 32 Złota St. in Warsaw and maintained its Warsaw branch at 43 Gęsia St. According to Dr. Emanuel Patt's report, Dr. M. Mesh ran the Warsaw branch and Dr. Mitz served as secretary. The members of the Executive Committee included Dr. Wohl, the deputy chair; Dr. M. Koenigstein; Dr. J. L. Pshitz; Dr. A. Vinower; Dr. B. Przewarski; and Dr. M. Goldenburg.[57]

According to many testimonies, Dr. Rozenblum was the de facto head of TOZ in Warsaw.[58] The scope of his work was very broad. He oversaw all of TOZ's activities, working under the threat of charges of sabotage by the Germans, if the requisite medical equipment was not delivered to the workers at the various German enterprises. Any position as important as this in a ghetto social service institution posed mortal danger to its holder. Rozenblum sent letters to the United States and to Switzerland with statistical data on the spread of typhus and tuberculosis in the ghetto, and a description of the Germans' treatment of Polish Jewry. The Gestapo often summoned him and accused him of disseminating anti-German propaganda. He claimed that he wrote these letters only to solicit medicine. Indeed, his efforts brought in large quantities of medicines from Geneva, which the Germans seized wantonly. Dr. Rozenblum took part in all the operations conducted jointly with the JDC, ŻSS, CENTOS, and the Red Cross, which maintained relations with TOZ.[59]

When the war began, TOZ redeployed to meet the new health requirements and expanded its activity immensely.[60] Before the

57 Report by Dr. Emanuel Patt on social service work among Polish Jews, March 1941, JDC, AR.33–44, file 814.

58 Turkow, *Hayo Hayta Varsha Yehudit*, pp. 23–24; Dr. Moshe Tursz testimony, YVA, O.3/438. According to Turkow, Rozenblum's stand-ins were Dr. Jakob Rubinstein and Dr. Szwalbe, assisted by Dr. Moshe Tursz, Dr. Jozef Chajn Gołębiewski, and Dr. Albert Mazor of Łódź. The administrative director was Nechemia Finkelstein, a co-owner of the newspaper *Haynt*.

59 Dr. Moshe Tursz testimony, YVA, O.3/438, pp. 18–20; Wulman et al., *The Martyrdom of Jewish Physicians in Poland*, p. 443.

60 From the beginning of the war and throughout the existence of the ghetto, TOZ in Warsaw sent detailed monthly reports to the JDC in the United States and to other free countries with comprehensive documentation of its preventive and therapeutic actions. For an example, see Offer, "Ma'arach Harefu'a Begeto Varsha," vol. 2, appendix A.20, pp. 140–141.

war, it had been active in the prevention of diseases. Amid the fighting, TOZ opened first aid stations to treat the many wounded who arrived in 1939.[61] Since the operation of pharmacies was banned at the onset of the occupation, TOZ began to distribute essential medicines.[62] When Warsaw surrendered, the number of people who approached TOZ for medical assistance grew steadily, including those with mild injuries who, until then, had been loath to risk venturing into the street, as well as others in serious condition. In addition, dozens of people came every day to have their bandages changed, which resulted in a shortage of bandaging material. The clinic's patient load overwhelmed the staff. There was no explicit work plan at the start of the war, and putting one together for the long-term was impossible, if not pointless, as new problems arose daily that required solutions. For example, the station for dressing wounds became a clinic, because the staff could not turn away the hundreds of injured people who visited it day in and day out.[63]

The shortages of medicines and personnel aggravated the harsh conditions. Each doctor saw eighty patients during a six-hour shift. Treatment was provided at no cost. In view of the grim situation and the number of patients, an office was opened to sort them and refer them to appropriate health care institutions; those in serious condition were hospitalized. A department for the distribution of medicines and disinfectants was set up.[64]

When waves of refugees who had been expelled from nearby towns reached Warsaw, TOZ mobilized to help them, providing sanitary and medical care at "refugee points" where hundreds were crowded together. A nurse was sent to each such station and a physician was placed in charge of two or three of them. TOZ also provided these locations with medicines, soap, and disinfectants. The number of stations in Warsaw, consisting of both large and small accommodations, where more than forty doctors were employed, reached ninety-two. Flexible logistics

61 Jewish Social Self-Help report concerning TOZ, March 1942, AŻIH, ARII.92.

62 Dr. Moshe Tursz testimony, YVA, O.3/438, p. 4.

63 Ibid., pp. 3–4.

64 Jewish Social Self-Help report concerning TOZ, March 1942, AŻIH, ARII.92.

and an experienced management were required to conduct these activities.[65] Dr. Sara Zofia Syrkin Binstein,[66] whose credentials included vast experience in social work and a stint as the JDC's chief physician in Poland after World War I, accepted the post of chief physician for the refugee points. Sanitary and medical services at the centers of refugee concentrations improved under her management. Doctors who worked at these locations presented her with weekly reports. The department expanded to become a mammoth enterprise that accomplished a great deal.[67]

Physicians who worked in hospitals also participated in TOZ's activities. Dr. Chaim Einhorn wrote, "These 'points' were literally hell on earth." The practitioners at these refugee centers who were asked to explain the importance of hygiene to prevent illness found it difficult to take up the matter with people who were starving and awaiting redemptive death. When the doctors arrived at a refugee point in the morning, they often found corpses unbeknownst to the inhabitants of the location. "The doctor's job at these points boiled down to writing death certificates

65 Dr. Moshe Tursz testimony, YVA, O.3/438, pp. 5–6.

66 Dr. Sara Zofia Syrkin Binstein (1890–1943) was born in Bielsko. In 1914, she completed her studies at the University of Kiev, which was then in the Russian Empire. After working in Moscow in 1915–1919, she moved to Warsaw. She specialized in internal medicine and was known as a successful physician. She was a member of the TOZ and the JDC boards of directors and the Jewish Medical Association, and served as the chair of the Organization of Jewish Women (IFO) and in other public positions. She held key health care positions in the ghetto and sometimes directed the Judenrat's Health Department. She had special organizational talent and contributed extensively to the war on epidemics in the ghetto. The German authorities removed her from her post. She may have committed suicide by overdosing on medicine en route to Treblinka. On Dr. Sara Zofia Syrkin Binstein, see Juliet D. Golden, "Show that you are really alive," Sara-Zofia Syrkin-Binsztejnowa's Emergency Medical Relief and Public Health Work in Early Interwar Poland and the Warsaw Ghetto," *Medizinhistorisches Journal*, 53:2 (April 2018), pp. 125–162; Wulman et al., *The Martyrdom of Jewish Physicians in Poland*, p. 464; Dr. Moshe Tursz testimony, YVA, O.3/438, pp. 20–21; Adolf Avraham Berman, *Bamakom Asher Ya'ad Li Hagoral: Im Yehudei Varsha, 1939–1942* (In the Place Where Fate Brought Me, with the Jews of Warsaw) (Hebrew) (Tel Aviv: Hakibbutz Hameuchad and Ghetto Fighters' House, 1977), p. 154.

67 Dr. Moshe Tursz testimony, YVA, O.3/438.

that reported the same cause of death each time, starvation," Dr. Einhorn wrote in his testimony.[68]

A Jewish Social Self-Help report for July–August 1940 provides an impressive picture of TOZ's activities amid the deterioration of the Jewish population's medical conditions.

> The medical and sanitation activities are carried out with the help of TOZ and the Department of War on Epidemics. Due to the difficult economic situation, only the most important needs are being met. Nevertheless, everything is progressing without a hitch...but in a downscaled format...an increasing number of patients are visiting the TOZ laboratories, many of whom are chronically ill and are getting worse due to the circumstances...Several patients are in a dire mental state. The children arrive in very poor condition—emaciated, weak, and starving. There are many cases of vitamin deficiency among them. More and more patients are arriving at the tuberculosis clinic, most in an advanced stage of the disease. The shortages of personnel, beds, and funding make it very difficult to offer the necessary....
>
> The Department of Hygiene must establish kitchens, secure accommodations for those who come from a distance, provide good nutrition for the ill, and distribute medicines. There are many cases of measles and dysentery. Four additional nurses have been sent to the main children's hospital at 18 Wolska St. to help fight the epidemics. In addition, large quantities of medicine have been sent there, as well as foodstuffs, such as cheese, cocoa, and soup powder, which the Jews of Switzerland sent. Several kitchens have been opened to prevent the spread of epidemics and for the benefit of the younger generation. Most of the children are the offspring of refugees who have come from far. Their lodgings lack reasonable living conditions. The children receive a little sugar, groats, fish, and a very small amount of chocolate.

68 Einhorn, "Harofe Begeto Varsha," p. 13. See also Offer, "Ma'arach Harefu'a Begeto Varsha," vol. 2, appendix A.25, pp. 122–124.

> The Department of War on Epidemics is continuing its activities as planned to limit the harm and to prevent contagion, but its budget is insufficient to cover everything. Therefore, workers, including some doctors and nurses, have been fired and many of the operations have dwindled. Nevertheless, enormous efforts are being made to offer assistance to those in the greatest need. More people are being sent to the bathhouses…Many people are coming to the showers voluntarily.
>
> Much emphasis is placed on disinfection. The goal is to help the population to maintain a reasonable level of cleanliness, including keeping the ill and the apartments clean. Many groups are working in this area…but due to the resource constraints, the number of these important activities is decreasing. Those in charge of these operations regularly lecture the population in order to raise their concern for cleanliness…A "cleanliness week" has been introduced to accustom people to staying clean. Thanks to the multiple efforts of the Department of War on Epidemics, such as sealing contaminated dwellings and sending the inhabitants to the bathhouse, the department has managed to help a little. It works in cooperation with the house committees.[69]

In May 1940, Dr. Rozenblum, chief secretary of TOZ in Warsaw, reported that his association was carrying out sanitation, medical, and nutrition activities in two-thirds of the cities and towns of German-occupied Poland—195 urban localities with a population of more than 1 million Jews. The organization was helping 25 hospitals, 24 isolation rooms, 40 clinics and sanitary institutions, and 70 bathhouses and disinfection units. TOZ had hired 120 doctors and 18 surgical assistants, in addition to numerous nurses and technical staff at all the facilities. In Warsaw alone, TOZ employed 200 doctors, 100 nurses, 65 pharmacists, 14 dentists, and 8 lab technicians. In addition to the institutions that it had owned before the war, TOZ acquired

69 Jewish Social Self-Help report on the doctors' activities in the war on the typhus epidemic in Warsaw, July–August 1940, July–August 1940, AŻIH, ARII.17.

2 surgical facilities, 3 maternity hospitals, infant care centers, and Zofiowka Psychiatric Hospital and Brijus Sanatorium in Otwock. Additional sanitation and disinfection facilities were opened. In May 1940, TOZ provided 26,000 daily lunches for children aged 7–14 and 1,500 food parcels for children up to age three in Warsaw.[70]

A report by TOZ in Warsaw on its activities in Poland between September 1939 and June 1940 indicates that it focused on providing medical assistance and information on the prevention of diseases and on child welfare. In September–October 1939, public places in Warsaw that were populated by newly arrived refugees and local inhabitants who had lost their homes in the bombardments received aid. During these months, it provided food and clothing to the refugees and undertook 4,200 surgical procedures, mainly for casualties of shelling. Due to an eruption of typhus, around 4,600 people were vaccinated in October, and 10 sanitation stations were set up in November. More than 150 people were treated for tuberculosis. About 4,000 children received hot meals and 900 were provided with clothing. That month, TOZ began to reach out to additional Jewish communities that required medical aid. By December, it had assisted 30 towns.

The typhus epidemic began to spread in Warsaw—the winter cold only exacerbated the situation. Undernourished children received special relief in the form of fish oil. In January 1940, cases of mental illness, typhus, and tuberculosis began to escalate—1,013 adults and 918 children were treated for tuberculosis. In February 1940, many illnesses spread with the increasing frost and hunger. Seventy-one TOZ centers distributed food to 30,000 people. About 10,635 children received food and the 628 infants who were under its supervision received milk and sugar. That month, the number of communities that availed themselves of TOZ increased to 135, some for medicines and others for food as well. In March 1940, TOZ conducted thorough disinfection operations and vaccinated 24,663 people. With the war on epidemics at its peak, 30 doctors

70 TOZ activity report, May 1940, JDC, AR.33–44, file 840.

and 25 nurses formed mobile squads that circulated among approximately 700 refugees. Thousands of items of clothing were disinfected and laundered, and the indigent were given soap. About 60,000 people received food relief, including 348,730 meals for 11,250 children at 23 centers.

In April 1940, TOZ activated 10 branches in major cities that served 185 small communities in various ways. Under its auspices, 15 epidemic treatment stations and 25 hospitals and clinics operated in several localities. In May, the typhus epidemic in Warsaw waned somewhat, prompting a supreme effort to eradicate it, despite the financial difficulties. Thus, about 50,000 people were vaccinated in Warsaw; 17,630 in the district of Warsaw; 26,819 in Lublin; and 42,469 in Radom. A comprehensive distribution of information on the prevention of illness and epidemics was undertaken as well. In June 1940, although the situation appeared to have stabilized to some degree, numerous difficulties and needs persisted. Clothing, medicines, milk, and other staples were in short supply. The number of doctors and nurses declined due to budget constraints. Without further resources, the activities could not continue.[71]

In conclusion, TOZ's activities in Warsaw and 195 additional localities across Poland were intensive, professional, and impressive. Its staff delivered medical, social, and sanitary relief to the Jewish population in the first months of the occupation, helping to eradicate the typhus epidemic. They worked in conjunction with local aid committees, the Judenräte, and doctors in the organization's service. The ill were hospitalized and isolated from their surroundings, homes were disinfected, and their inhabitants bathed. Despite the glaring shortage of disinfection materials, laundry detergent, and clothing, the number of typhus patients decreased to only a few, largely because of the vaccinations administered at all the TOZ clinics.

The extent of activity in the towns and cities in effect indicates the development of a network of TOZ-sponsored medical activities across occupied Poland. The deployment of

71 TOZ activity report, September 1939–June 1940, AR.33–44, file 840.

this network in the first months of the occupation enabled the Jewish community to establish a professional medical system, upon ghettoization and in response to the growing medical needs as the living conditions deteriorated. Medical teams mobilized around TOZ and spared no effort to alleviate the Jews' distress. The Jewish Social Self-Help and the JDC acted to raise the funds that were required for urgent medical assistance.[72] TOZ workers were deployed in many areas in the ghetto: the distribution of medicines; sanitary–medical treatment in refugee locations and bathhouses; medical services for all the inhabitants in various parts of the ghetto; feeding and hygienic care of school-age children; clubs for children whose parents were being treated for tuberculosis in clinics; and soup kitchens for convalescents.

When the United States entered the war and the JDC became illegal in Poland, TOZ assumed responsibility for the following institutions: Friends of Children Society, Bersohn and Bauman Children's Hospital, and Brijus Sanatorium and Zofiowka Psychiatric Hospital in Otwock. It managed inpatient admissions at Bersohn and Bauman Children's Hospital and other institutions. TOZ was also in charge of the private surgical institutions of Dr. Aharon Soloveichik[73] and Dr. Miszurski, which relocated to 1 Mariánské St. after the ghetto was sealed, and of two gynecology and obstetrics facilities. In addition, in late 1940, the Germans ordered TOZ to assume responsibility for providing social insurance to workers employed in the ghetto, and in the shops and in German factories in or near the ghetto; to the staff of the social service institutions; and to others. The tremendous expansion of the scope of TOZ's activities and responsibilities emptied the organization's coffers, and its staff was not paid for months.[74]

The November 1941 report of the Jewish Social Self-Help describes the extent of TOZ's medical services.

72 Wulman, "Hevrat Toz," p. 585.

73 Dr. Soloveichik's clinic was turned over to TOZ when its founder left Warsaw for Vilna at the beginning of the war. Letters on this topic between TOZ and JDC officials in the United States, which include discussion of payments to his clinic, have survived; see JDC, AR.33–44, file 840.

74 Dr. Moshe Tursz testimony, YVA, O.3/438, pp. 18–19.

Visits to the TOZ Clinics in the Ghetto, September–November 1941[75]

TOZ Clinics	September 1941	October 1941	November 1941
Internal Medicine	906	501	445
Ophthalmology	304	304	195
Ear, Nose, and Throat	255	190	162
Neurology	81	75	111
Gynecology	174	106	83
Urology and Surgery	551	1,758	2,143
Dermatology Clinics			
Patients	221	63	—
Treatments	675	395	—
Diagnostic Clinics			
Patients	433	149	—
Dentistry	707	511	361
Pediatric Clinics	292	157	136
Pulmonology	1,249	1,254	1,257
Dermatology	1,827	1,824	1,281
Laboratory: Tests	3,624	2,963	2,440
Home Visits: Doctors	442	536	494
Home Visits: Nurses	357	192	193
Medicines Distributed	3,624	2,963	2,440
For Payment	1,585	1,157	1,141
At No Charge	2,039	1,806	1,299

75 Jewish Social Self-Help, Statistics Department Report, no. 6, November 1941, AŻIH, ARI.32, see also Offer, "Ma'arah Harefu'a Begeto Varsha," vol. 2, appendix A.16, pp. 64–67.

The report demonstrates the breadth and diversity of TOZ's medical services in the ghetto. Many professional clinics operated under its auspices in various fields of specialization: surgery and urology; neurology; internal medicine; ophthalmology; ear, nose, and throat; gynecology; pediatric medicine; pulmonology; and dermatology. Specialized clinics provided additional medical services, such as skin and dental care. TOZ also oversaw a medical laboratory and sent doctors and nurses to patients' homes, averaging 738 visits per month in September–November 1941. Medicines were distributed for a fee or at no charge. Most patients—57 percent—received them at no cost. Less medicine was distributed in November.

In September–October 1941, there was a downward trend in the number of treatments at TOZ's clinics, with the exception of the clinics for surgery, urology, and neurology. The surgery clinics bandaged 1,244 wounds, treated 638 cases of frostbite, and performed 75 other surgical procedures. The internal medicine clinic saw 182 patients with pulmonary conditions, 52 with digestive illnesses, 37 with heart disease, and 29 with urinary disorders. The highest number of patients at the TOZ clinics were treated for skin conditions, followed by pulmonary ailments. Lung diseases were much more prevalent than other internal medicine: 60 percent of the population suffered from various lung conditions. While there was a decline in the incidence of skin diseases, pulmonary conditions showed no improvement.

In November 1941, the Jewish self-help organizations referred 3,139 patients to the ghetto clinics for treatment, including 1,423 referrals to TOZ facilities. Payment for care was waived for 798 patients and discounted for 625 others. Altogether, TOZ's medical institutions served 9,301 ghetto residents that month. Thousands of lab tests were performed each month. However, the dermatology and diagnostic clinics did not operate in November, because there was no electricity.[76] In January 1942, the TOZ health insurance covered medical

76 Jewish Social Self-Help, Statistics Department Report, no. 6, November 1941, AŻIH, ARI.32, pp. 18–19.

consultations in clinics and doctors' visits to the homes of 1,050 patients, treatments for 280 patients, medicines for 538 patients, 73 lab tests, and 85 hospital referrals.[77] As epidemics spread throughout the ghetto, TOZ acted in several ways to stem and eradicate them.

At this time, Dr. Sara Zofia Syrkin Binstein turned her attention to another field of medicine. After having dealt with sanitary conditions at the overnight facilities, her department focused on the war on epidemics. Its information and prevention activities in this regard included lectures, vaccinations, disinfection, delousing, cleaning of dwellings, setting up a public sanitation system, encouraging good personal hygiene, one-shot information projects, and assistance in doing laundry, and more.

In November 1941, when TOZ was still responsible for the medical care of the refugees, it sent 19 doctors and 24 nurses to 88 shelters affiliated with ŻOS—Żydowskie Opieki Społecznej (Jewish Social Welfare)—a Jewish social relief organization that housed 6,614 refugees. That month, 1,580 treatments were administered; 15 patients were referred to hospitals; medical kits were distributed and 1,535 portions of medicine were dispensed; and more than one-third of their charges visited bathhouses.[78]

TOZ moved mountains to help children in the ghetto. Approximately 80 percent of the 100,000 youngsters there required the assistance of the community welfare institutions.[79] In 1940, before ghettoization, doctors and nurses on the TOZ payroll treated 1,800 children per day. In August 1941, a team of 11 physicians and 23 nurses tended 12,063 youngsters. Checkups of 30,816 children revealed that only 13 percent had a proper diet, 35 percent received reasonable nourishment, and 52 percent suffered from malnutrition; 7,040 of these children were clean, 2,863 were not clean, and 2,260 were infested with lice and sundry parasites. Free baths at bathhouses were arranged

77 Judenrat Statistics Department Report, no. 29, March 17, 1942, GFH, no. 11250, p. 17.

78 Jewish Social Self-Help, Statistics Department Report, no. 6, November 1941, AŻIH, ARI.32, pp. 21–22.

79 Kermish, *To Live with Honor*, p. 390.

for 6,049 children, and scalp disinfection for 2,485. About 4,130 youngsters were frail and one-third of the children had illnesses that warranted medical care. The situation worsened with each passing month.[80]

The Jewish Social Self-Help documented TOZ's medical and sanitation work among the thousands of children who received food at the child nutrition centers in September–November 1941.

TOZ Sanitation and Medical Work at Thirty Child Nutrition Centers, Serving 20,649 Children, September–November 1941[81]

Sanitation Work	September 1941	October 1941	November 1941
Inspections	11,521	10,317	6,704
Baths	4,572	1,903	722
Haircuts	2,432	1,646	972
Medical Work			
Observations	2,803	3,207	5,381
Checkups	1,253	1,729	1,351
Referrals to Specialists	507	393	427

In November 1941, the Jewish Social Self-Help fed 20,649 children at 30 nutrition centers, and TOZ provided them with medical and hygienic care. There was a significant drop in the number of children treated between September and November 1941, and hygienic treatments, including baths, checkups, and haircuts, plummeted. In contrast, the doctors' work—observations, checkups, and referrals to specialists—increased by 57 percent. It may be assumed that as bathing and sanitation materials ran out, and as autumn and winter approached, the means to heat with

80 Roland, *Courage under Siege*, p. 175.

81 Jewish Social Self-Help, Statistics Department Report, no. 6, November 1941, AŻIH, ARI.32, p. 22.

coal for bathing and similar practices dwindled. The resulting decline in hygienic care caused more children to fall ill than before, which explains the increase in the doctors' work.[82]

In January 1942, doctors in the service of TOZ examined 1,861 children and found only 3 percent in good health. Approximately 65 percent were in poor health, and most were dirty and infested with lice. CENTOS attempted to feed and care for many abandoned children and orphans, but only a few received help, despite all the organization's efforts, mainly due to the lack of funds.[83] In addition to the medical service provided to the children at the food distribution points, attention was given to certain aspects of their education with the aim of raising their awareness of good hygiene and of ensuring their sound intellectual and emotional development, as evidenced in a document entitled "Educational Workplan at Food Distribution Points."

Our work objectives:

1. We wish to transform the food distribution points into centers of educational success and influence on children.
2. Primarily concerned for the children's health, we seek to develop in them a sense of good hygiene and aesthetics.
3. Mindful of the existing situation with its many dangers, we strive to immerse the children in spiritual activities.
4. To create the appropriate conditions for any educational impact, we aim to convert the food distribution group into a children's collective. This may be achieved through dialogue.
5. We endeavor to offer children the possibility of having a positive experience at the distribution points, since it is our particular desire to create for them as many happy experiences as possible.
6. We will attend to each child's social and ethical development—to instill in him or her feelings of friendliness and social responsibility, with a special emphasis on discipline.

82 Ibid.

83 Roland, *Courage under Siege*, p. 175.

7. We wish to enrich the child's intellectual development as much as possible.
8. We wish to inculcate in children a love of and a connection with the Yiddish language and culture.[84]

TOZ cooperated with the Judenrat, even though the two institutions sometimes competed with each other. The Judenrat, the official authority designated by the Nazis to manage the ghetto, operated a Health Department and a Social Welfare Department, along with others. The organizations that had predated the war, such as TOZ and CENTOS, operated independently, sometimes as rivals. Their status was reinforced by their strong and ongoing relationship with the JDC and the public's awareness of these bodies—factors that assured them a stronger financial base than that of the Judenrat.[85]

Managing sanitation in the ghetto was a very difficult task. In order to ensure the fulfillment of duties, such as keeping records of the ill, taking people to bathhouses, and conducting hygienic inspections of the blocks in the ghetto by the physicians assigned to them, it was necessary to impose sanctions, which TOZ alone could not carry out. Although TOZ remained a social institution that was independent of the Judenrat, these two institutions cooperated with each other.

In 1941, the Department of War on Epidemics, operating under the TOZ umbrella and headed by Dr. Sara Zofia Syrkin Binstein, amalgamated with the Judenrat Health Department. In fact, it is not widely known that this female physician admirably co-ran the Health Department with Dr. Israel Milejkowski, its chair, until January 1942.[86] At this time, due to an unsuccessful disinfection campaign carried out at the Germans' behest, the German chief physician Dr. Wilhelm Hagen demanded her replacement. Dr. Mieczysław Kon, an apostate Jew and a former Polish Army officer, was appointed to the post, to the Germans'

84 Educational Work Plan at Food Distribution Points, YVA, M.10.AR.1/204.

85 Roland, *Courage under Siege*, pp. 56–58.

86 Dr. Moshe Tursz testimony, YVA, O.3/438, pp. 13–14.

satisfaction. Dr. Tadeusz Ganc, also a former Polish military officer, was tasked with conducting the war on typhus. Prof. Hirszfeld described Dr. Syrkin Binstein as an industrious woman who was well versed in academic medicine but unfit to manage a health system under the harsh conditions that had arisen. Moreover, the Germans did not recognize her authority because of her gender.[87]

In fact, TOZ retained responsibility for the bathhouses and the overnight facilities for refugees. The former Department of War on Epidemics became the Hygienic Sanitation Department, headed by Dr. Józef Chajn Gołębiewski. Dr. Gołębiewski and Dr. Szymon Wyszewiański represented both the Jewish Social Self-Help and the Judenrat Health Council, which was established in 1941 and directed by Prof. Ludwik Hirszfeld.[88]

On December 4, 1940, TOZ was ordered to transfer the activities in its children's kitchens to CENTOS, which coordinated the care of orphans. TOZ was piqued by this demand. Prompted by the ban on Jewish children attending school, CENTOS had obtained permission from the Germans to provide instruction to the children before and after feeding them. Since only CENTOS received this authorization, it was decided to make this change in order to teach the children as much as possible. Professional teachers, men and women who stayed with the children in the CENTOS houses, were entrusted with providing instruction. TOZ resented losing full responsibility and overall concern for the children's nutritional and medical needs, and was neither reassured nor appeased by the decision.[89]

As time passed, the Judenrat gained increasing leverage in all the areas of activity in which TOZ engaged—especially after December 1941, when the United States entered the war and the possibilities of legally assisting Jewish organizations in the Nazi-

87 Hirszfeld, *The Story of One Life*, p. 216.

88 Dr. Moshe Tursz testimony, YVA, O.3/438, pp. 13–14.

89 Roland, *Courage under Siege*, pp. 56–57. On disagreements over authority for feeding children in the ghetto, see cables and letters between the JDC in the U.S. and elsewhere and representatives of TOZ in Poland, December 4, 1940–October 7, 1941, JDC, AR.33–44, file 840.

occupied territories dwindled. The Judenrat provided support for the care of refugees, children, and the elderly, drawing from its meager budget to finance the expenditures. In late 1941, TOZ and CENTOS were forced to merge with the Jewish Social Self-Help, apparently in order to allow the ghetto *Kommissar*, Auerswald, to control the money and commodities going into the ghetto.[90] TOZ's responsibilities were limited to medical matters and CENTOS was responsible only for the care of the children. In mid–1942, the Nazis canceled the activities of two self-help organizations, Jewish Social Self-Help and ŻTOS—Żydowskie Towarzystwo Opieki Społecznej (Jewish Society for Social Welfare). They liquidated them altogether when the Jews of Warsaw were deported. Some time later, the Nazis allowed the Jewish Relief Office (JUS) to resume operations as a self-help institution.[91]

According to a TOZ activity report, March 1942, TOZ enjoyed official legal recognition and operated as such until July 1940. On August 1, 1940, the German authorities demanded that it cease its activities, but it persevered. In October 1940, it became an official organization and continued working for the health of the Jews in the ghetto with the approval of the Germans. To this end, TOZ was supposed to receive 10,000 zlotys per month. Patients paid 20 or 30 grosz for medical care. Until September 1941, TOZ had no active connection with the Judenrat and received no money for operating the public bathhouses. On September 1, 1941, the Judenrat began to provide TOZ with a monthly allotment of coal to heat the showers and to forward payments to support the doctors' work. At the time that the aforementioned report was written in March 1942, TOZ was working with the Jewish Social Self-Help in Warsaw at 43 Gęsia St.[92]

TOZ received most of its budget from the JDC and operated in conjunction with the ŻSS. TOZ pledged most of its resources

90 Gutman, *The Jews of Warsaw*, pp. 40–41; Wulman et al., *The Martyrdom of Jewish Physicians in Poland*, pp. 202–206; Roland, *Courage under Siege*, pp. 55–57.

91 Roland, *Courage under Siege*, p. 64.

92 Jewish Social Self-Help report concerning TOZ, March 1942, AŻIH, ARII.92.

to disadvantaged population groups, neighborhood clinics, health care centers, and refugee facilities. However, its funding sources dwindled steadily and with the entry of the United States into the war, the JDC's difficulties in Poland increased. In 1940, JDC transferred 14.73 million zlotys to aid Polish Jews; in 1941, the sum contracted to 8 million zlotys. In early 1940, several months into the German occupation and about a year before ghettoization, the TOZ budget was around 1 million zlotys (about $20,000) per month, much of it from the JDC.

In early 1940, representatives of TOZ in Warsaw and of the JDC held a meeting in Amsterdam, where they reported on TOZ's activities and the needs created by the dire state of the Jews in occupied Warsaw, and drew up an emergency relief program for that beleaguered population. The plan included Medem,[93] a pediatric tuberculosis sanatorium, and Zofiówka, a psychiatric hospital, both in Otwock; the nursing school at Czyste Hospital, the hospital itself, and the research institute; Bersohn and Bauman Children's Hospital; and, of course, TOZ and its payroll. The Judenrat also set aside 10.5 million zlotys in its 1940 budget for TOZ's activities, including 6.5 million for food, 1.5 million for medical activity, and 1.3 million for child care in CENTOS institutions.[94] The Jewish self-help organizations attempted to raise funds from any possible source. TOZ, for example, reported that during six months, from April–October 1941, it collected 228,581 zlotys from patients themselves—one-fourth of its revenues at the time. If so, the fees at that stage of ghetto life were steep but still collectible.[95]

93 The sanatorium, named after Vladimir Medem, one of the socialist Jewish leaders and theorist of the Bund, was founded in January 1926 by the Central Yiddish School Organization in Poland (TSYSHO). It served as both a sanatorium and a successful, innovative, and democratic educational institution for children. See, for example, Magdalena Kozłowska, "'In Sunshine and Joy'? The Story of Medem Sanatorium in Miedzeszyn," *East European Politics & Societies*, July 2013, doi: 10.1177/0888325413494772; see also http://www.yivoencyclopedia.org/ article.aspx/Medem_Sanatorium (accessed March 17, 2019).

94 Gutman, *The Jews of Warsaw*, pp. 103–104; Roland, *Courage under Siege*, p. 56.

95 Roland, *Courage under Siege*, p. 64.

In the spring of 1942, TOZ's branches in the rural towns closed one after another, and the center in Warsaw shut down late that summer.[96] On August 4, 1942, in the course of the *Aktionen* in the ghetto, everyone at the TOZ central office in Warsaw on Gęsia St., including the doctors and medics, was deported to the Treblinka extermination camp.[97] By then, sanitation efforts had become irrelevant, and the disinfection teams served to remove corpses from the Umschlagplatz, where the Jews of the Warsaw ghetto were assembled for deportation. According to Dr. Tursz, the rescue point and station for dressing wounds at the Umschlagplatz that had been set up on the initiative of TOZ played a crucial role in providing medical assistance and rescue. When the mass transports were halted on September 13, 1942, only 10 of TOZ's 580 staff members in Warsaw were still alive. TOZ had ceased to exist and its patients were expelled. One other clinic continued to operate with the equipment and materials that it had managed to retain, but its work no longer mattered.[98]

When all the members of the TOZ staff and their remaining patients were sent to the Umschlagplatz, the TOZ building at 43 Gęsia St. remained deserted. During the 1943 uprising, it was blown up and torched, along with the rest of the ghetto. Of more than 2,000 TOZ employees in 10 cities in Poland, only 50 or 60 survived.[99] After the war, those still alive continued the organization's legacy by reestablishing medical services for Polish Jews and other survivors.[100] In the first postwar

96 Wulman, "Hevrat Toz," pp. 585–586.

97 Kaplan, *Scroll of Agony*, p. 398.

98 Dr. Moshe Tursz testimony, YVA, O.3/438, pp. 16–17.

99 Wulman, "Hevrat Toz," pp. 585–586.

100 Dr. Józef Chajn Gołębiewski testimony, YVA, O.3/2355. As for how large TOZ was immediately after the war, it is noteworthy that a postwar list of 458 doctors who were members of the association has survived; see Abraham Adolf Zylberstajn Collection, GFH, no. 223. Dr. Gołębiewski, a TOZ physician during the war who had taken part in establishing the Scientific Council and Anti-Tuberculosis League that operated in the ghetto, fled to the Aryan side in February 1943 and was sheltered by his patients. Due to extortion by Poles, he had to flee to another hideout. After TOZ was reactivated, he served as its secretary and eventually as its president. In 1963, he immigrated to Israel and practiced medicine in Rehovot.

months, TOZ resumed its activity wherever Jewish survivors gathered, establishing a network of clinics, childcare centers, a tuberculosis sanatorium, a hospital, and other institutions, which the authorities nationalized in 1950.[101]

Czyste Hospital

Czyste Hospital, the largest and most important medical institution that served the Jews of Warsaw, saw its operating conditions and services change during the war under the impact of the events that befell the Jewish population under Nazi rule. During the ghetto era, it went through five distinct phases,[102] corresponding to the ghetto's own periodization.[103]

Period 1: From the Outbreak of War in September 1939 to Ghettoization in Early 1941

When the bombardment of Warsaw began, the medical staff at Czyste Hospital were requested to remain on the premises in order to receive the many casualties of the German onslaught.

101 TOZ branches in postwar Poland began to be opened in August–September 1945, as the need arose. A provisional committee was set up under Dr. Herszenhorn, who also served on the Central Committee of Polish Jews. In January 1946, the TOZ committee convened in Geneva under the auspices of OZE, which was headed by Dr. Boris Tschlenoff. The first TOZ conference after the war took place in Warsaw in 1948; see Dr. Józef Chajn Gołębiewski testimony, YVA, O.3/2355.

102 Trunk identifies three periods during the relevant years; see Trunk, "Epidemics and Mortality," p. 99. However, in view of the documentation and the sources, we find it more appropriate to define additional periods that reflect the specific difficulties that arose in each stage.

103 Dr. Henry Fenigstein testimony, "Varshever yid. Shpitol betn nazi-rezhim, aroysgegebn durkh farlag *Ibergang* bey der federatsiye fun poylishe yidn in daytshland, amerikaner zone, 1948," YVA, O.33/1074. On Henry Fenigstein, see also Charles Roland, the Oral History Interview of Dr. Henry Fenigstein, https://digitalarchive.mcmaster.ca/islandora/object/macrepo%3A81178#page/1/mode/2up; Offer, "Ma'arach Harefu'a Begeto Varsha," vol. 2, appendix A.21, p. 113; Dr. Chaim Einhorn testimony, YVA, O.3/1836.

Dr. Henryk Stabholz,[104] director of the hospital, informed Dr. David Amsterdamski, head of the surgery ward, that the Germans were bombarding the Wola district, without declaring war. As the staff began to prepare, multiple bombs fell near the hospital. Several damaged the building, and one struck a surgical ward and demolished all the operating rooms. The three remaining surgical wards were merged, sharing a common operating theater that was set up on the ground floor.[105] The bombardments continued, wiping out additional departments, the heating system, and the kitchen. The staff carried on without electricity, gas, or water. The men had to haul water from the river, and the medical instruments were disinfected in the laundry facility.

The hospital filled with casualties—soldiers and civilians, Poles and Jews. Thirty to forty surgical procedures were performed each day. The entire hospital became a surgery ward. Its staff worked without respite, sometimes twenty-four hours at a stretch. The first operation was the amputation of the leg of a victim of the bombardment of Warsaw on September 1.[106] The staff discharged many patients who had been admitted before the war in order to make room for the newly injured.[107] The air raids terrified the wounded and the ill, who sought to escape every time the hospital or its environs were attacked. Even leg amputees responded with outbursts and attempts to flee. The nurses helped to calm them each time.[108]

104 Dr. Henryk Stabholz (1882–1941), a surgeon in Kielce and Warsaw, was fundamental in the establishment of social medicine. Before the war, he was a member of the Health Bureau in Warsaw, vice president of the Jewish Medical Association, a board member with the Relief Committee for the Victims of World War I, and a consultant for the infectious diseases department of the Jewish hospital. Admired as a doctor and a human being, he died in the Warsaw ghetto, while performing his duties at the hospital in April 1941. See Wulman et al., *The Martyrdom of Jewish Physicians in Poland*, p. 460; Weisz, Grzybowski, and Albury, "Henryk, Thaddeus, and Ludwik Stabholz," pp. 363–372.

105 Sabina Gürfinkel-Glocer, "Goralo Shel Beit Haholim Tzhista," (The Fate of Czyste Hospital) in Gruenbaum et al., *Entziklopediya Shel Galuyot: Varsha*, vol. 6, part 2, pp. 587–590.

106 Ibid., pp. 586–587; Dr. Emil Apfelbaum testimony, YVA, M.49.E/4510.

107 Roland, *Courage under Siege*, p. 77.

108 Gürfinkel-Glocer, "Goralo Shel Beit Haholim Tzhista," p. 587.

Dr. Henryk Stabholz, the famous Warsaw surgeon who ran the hospital, left his post when the war began and joined the people leaving the city eastward, after the government of Poland urged the men to leave town and assist the army to fight the Germans. Many members of the medical staff did the same. On September 26, 1939, with Warsaw on the brink of surrender and in view of the many difficulties that were interfering with the hospital's functioning, the doctors held an urgent meeting. The elderly Dr. Julian Rotstadt,[109] who had taken over as director of the hospital after Dr. Stabholz had left, had become ill due to overwork. Consequently, the participants at this meeting appointed Dr. Adam Zamenhof,[110] a well-known ophthalmologist in Warsaw, to run the institution. The department directors, Dr. Werthajm and Dr. Amsterdamski, bolstered the staff's morale and urged the doctors and staff to hold on. At this time, both patients and physicians were suffering from hunger.[111] After twenty-seven days of battle and bombardments of Warsaw, hospital occupancy reached its peak. About 5,000 ill and injured patients—soldiers and civilians—occupied all the beds and floor space.

109 Dr. Julian Rotstadt (1871–1942) completed his neurology studies in 1902 and practiced this specialty in Dr. Edward Flatau's department at Czyste Hospital. He was named director of the physical therapy department. Tremendously knowledgeable, he was active in neurological societies and published articles on neuropathology. He organized fortnightly assemblies at the hospital, irrespective of the tempests that battered the institution. He and his colleagues published a quarterly journal that presented medical case studies and documentation of conferences at the hospital. An assimilated Jew and a Polish patriot, Rotstadt was known for his honesty, kindness, and erudition. In December 1939, he was placed at the helm of Czyste Hospital in lieu of Dr. Zamenhof, whom the Nazis had sent to his death. In August 1942, he was selected and transported to Treblinka. See Wulman et al., *The Martyrdom of Jewish Physicians in Poland*, pp. 444–445; Dr. Shmuel Stanisław Waller testimony, YVA, O.3/2358.

110 Dr. Adam Zamenhof (1888–1940), the son of Dr. Ludwik Eliezer Zamenhof (1859–1917) and creator of Esperanto, completed his studies in Switzerland and passed his exams in Warsaw. A celebrated ophthalmologist, he headed the ophthalmology department at Czyste Hospital and published extensively in medical journals. See the entry of May 8, Czerniaków, *The Warsaw Diary*, p. 146; Wulman et al., *The Martyrdom of Jewish Physicians in Poland*, pp. 492–493.

111 Gürfinkel-Glocer, "Goralo Shel Bet Haholim Tzhista," p. 587; Roland, *Courage under Siege*, p. 77.

At 2 A.M. on September 28, word arrived that the Germans had entered the city. Despite their fear and anxiety, the hospital staff continued to work devotedly and unrelentingly. During the first days of the occupation, the staff encountered many difficulties. The fate of their relatives who had been drafted into the Polish Army and of the children who were waiting for their parents in their homes was uncertain. The staff also feared that the Germans would go to their homes and deport their families, while they were at work. In addition, the depletion of provisions and the shortage of money weighed on them, since the German administration in Warsaw did not cover the Jewish hospital's payroll.[112] The Jewish doctors who worked at the general hospitals were forced to leave their jobs. The Polish municipality, which owned these institutions, transferred them to Jewish hospitals.[113] The Gestapo arrested several doctors, obviously to the grave detriment of the work of the medical staff.[114]

Immediately after the onset of the occupation, a German military physician visited the hospital accompanied by two officers. He ordered the hospital director to convene all the doctors and to advise them that the Wehrmacht had occupied Poland and that the hospital would be under its auspices. He said that he did not wish to harm anyone and that he would not meddle in the management of the institution. Two hours later, Gestapo agents arrived to take away the director of the hospital, Dr. Zamenhof, and sent him to his death. They also arrested his wife and sister, both of whom were physicians.[115] The Germans appointed Dr. Rotstadt to replace Zamenhof, forcing him to assume the heavy burden once again.

Two months later, in December 1939, Dr. Kurt Schrempf, the German chief physician of Warsaw, set up quarantine and isolation services at Czyste Hospital to contend with the spread of typhus. Upon inspecting the hospital, he found the care and services provided there to be less than perfect and, consequently, Rotstadt

112 Gürfinkel-Glocer, "Goralo Shel Beit Haholim Tzhista," pp. 588–589.
113 Lensky, *A Physician inside the Warsaw Ghetto*, p. 22.
114 Gürfinkel-Glocer, "Goralo Shel Beit Haholim Tzhista," p. 591.
115 Ibid., p. 588; Czerniaków, *The Warsaw Diary*, p. 146.

and other physicians were arrested and dismissed from their posts.[116] According to Dr. Shmuel Stanisław Waller, after the Nazis had deported Dr. Zamenhof, Dr. Rothaupt, and not Dr. Rotstadt, managed the Jewish hospital very professionally.[117] Following the dismissal of Dr. Rothaupt, Dr. Josef Stein filled the position[118] until the liquidation of the hospital and the ghetto.

Before the war, Dr. Stein had specialized in pathological anatomy and had headed the pathology department at Święty Duch Hospital. Considered an expert in his field, he held the title of professor, despite his youth.[119] He was not popular in the ghetto, because of his prewar conversion to Christianity[120] to advance his scientific career and in response to the obstacles that the Jews faced at the time.[121] The Polish authorities, who trusted him because he had converted, chose him for this post.[122] Apparently, the involvement of Piątkowski, a service worker at Święty Duch Hospital before the war who had declared himself a *Volksdeutsche* and received managerial positions in the health

116 Czerniaków, *The Warsaw Diary*, p. 100; Roland, *Courage under Siege*, p. 77; Dr. Shmuel Stanisław Waller testimony, YVA, O.3/2358.

117 Before the war, Dr. Rothaupt had directed a Jewish hospital in Włocławek. During the war, he was deputy director of the surgery department at Czyste Hospital, serving under Dr. Werthajm. He perished in 1943 on the Aryan side of Warsaw.

118 Dr. Josef Stein (1904–1943) completed his studies in 1927. He was a teaching assistant and lecturer at the University of Warsaw. His research work on the micropathology of typhus was well known among German pathologists, who visited the ghetto to study it. In the ghetto, Stein researched the pathological anatomy of hunger and helped to set up the ghetto medical school. In a display of immense courage, he refused an opportunity to be rescued from the ghetto and participated in the April 1943 uprising. See Wulman et al., *The Martyrdom of Jewish Physicians in Poland*, p. 461.

119 Roland, *Courage under Siege*, p. 77; Lensky, *A Physician inside the Warsaw Ghetto*, p. 22.

120 Roland, *Courage under Siege*, p. 77. On the issue of Jewish converts to Christianity in the ghetto, see, for example, Miriam Malwist, "Assimilationists and Neophytes at the Time of War Orations and in the Closed Jewish Quarter," in Kermish, *To Live with Honor*, pp. 620–621; Havi Ben-Sasson, "Christians in the Ghetto: All Saints' Church, Birth of the Holy Virgin Mary Church, and the Jews of the Warsaw Ghetto," *Yad Vashem Studies*, 31 (2003), pp. 153–173.

121 Lensky, *A Physician inside the Warsaw Ghetto*, p. 22.

122 Ibid., p. 22; Dr. Shmuel Stanisław Waller testimony, YVA, O.3/2358.

care system during the occupation, influenced the selection of Stein.[123]

Some of the Jewish doctors felt that Dr. Stein preferred to employ apostate Jews, although most of those employed by Dr. Stein were excellent and decent professionals who upheld the rules of ethics. However, in Dr. Shmuel Stanisław Waller's opinion, Dr. Stein's personal preferences regarding certain doctors were manifested when the *Aktionen* in the Warsaw ghetto began. Dr. Waller alleged that Dr. Stein gave his Christianized colleagues priority over Jewish physicians during the distribution of the "life numbers."[124] Just the same, Dr. Stein was described as a courteous, modest man, who did not turn people away when they approached him with requests.[125]

Dr. Moshe Tursz, a senior member of the TOZ staff, remembered Dr. Stein as a good-hearted man and a well-educated scientist who carried out his duties with distinction. Setting an example of unbounded self-sacrifice, he was among those who were murdered along with their patients, caring for them until their last breath.[126] Dr. Waller testified that the last time he had seen Dr. Stein in the ghetto was in February 1943, when Dr. Stein was preparing a hideout in anticipation of another *Aktion*.[127] Sent to Treblinka with his wife, Dr. Stein was murdered in the gas chambers in May 1943.[128]

Several days after the occupation had begun, the Germans decided that the Jewish hospital, which until the war had served

123 Lensky, *A Physician inside the Warsaw Ghetto*, p. 22.

124 Dr. Shmuel Stanisław Waller testimony, YVA, O.3/2358.

125 Lensky, *A Physician inside the Warsaw Ghetto*, p. 22; Dr. Shmuel Stanisław Waller testimony, YVA, O.3/2358.

126 Dr. Moshe Tursz testimony, YVA, O.3/438, p. 16.

127 Dr. Shmuel Stanisław Waller testimony, YVA, O.3/2358.

128 Wulman et al., *The Martyrdom of Jewish Physicians in Poland*, p. 461; Dr. Israel Rom (Rotbalsam) testimony, YVA, O.3/2357. Dr. Rom (Rotbalsam) testified that he sat next to Dr. Stein on the train to Treblinka. Shot by Ukrainian guards on the train, Stein bled to death. According to Dr. Adolf Polisiuk, at a certain stage of the uprising, Dr. Stein was unable to find a hideout and was captured by the Germans while attempting to enter a bunker. See Adolf Polisiuk, "Hamatzor Ha'aharon" (The Final Siege), in Blumental and Kermish, *Hameri Vehamered Begeto Varsha*, p. 314.

soldiers and civilians alike, would henceforth treat civilians only. They sent cars and soldiers to the facility and started removing wounded soldiers and replacing them with ailing civilians. A week later, when the transfer was complete and the hospital civilianized, they issued a new order, claiming that the other hospitals were full: Czyste Hospital would become a military facility. Again, to their immense suffering, the patients were moved. After this second transfer, a new order was issued: Czyste Hospital would become a hospital for Jews only. All Aryans who were ill or injured, as well as those on the staff, were ordered to leave, and were replaced by ill and injured Jews from other hospitals. This initiated the effective isolation of Czyste Hospital from corresponding institutions in Warsaw and its detachment from the municipal hospitals department.[129]

A typhoid fever epidemic broke out in the autumn of 1939,[130] ushering in a harsh winter. The Germans now declared Czyste Hospital an institution for infectious diseases. Dr. Schrempf was appointed as the German administrator of the hospital and Dr. Henryk Sikorski, a Polish physician from Poznań, was installed as its *Kommissar*.[131] Dr. Schrempf, the German chief physician of Warsaw, believed that the Jewish doctors were carrying the epidemic to the city from the hospital, which was full of patients with typhoid fever. Therefore, he issued an order forbidding these doctors to leave the hospital and banning contact between them and the population.[132] On December 19, 1939, he informed Czerniaków of his demand to quarantine the hospital. That day, Czerniaków and Schrempf discussed problems related to inpatient care and an attempt was made to exempt the doctors from the quarantine.[133]

129 Gürfinkel-Glocer, "Goralo Shel Beit Haholim Tzhista," pp. 588–589.

130 Trunk, "Epidemics and Mortality," p. 85.

131 Gürfinkel-Glocer, "Goralo Shel Beit Haholim Tzhista," p. 490. Dr. Henry Fenigstein noted that the Polish commissioner was habitually inebriated and, evidently, this explains why he took little interest in the hospital. Dr. Henry Fenigstein testimony, "Varshever yid," YVA, O.33/1074, pp. 6–7.

132 Lensky, *A Physician inside the Warsaw Ghetto*, pp. 99–100.

133 Czerniaków, *The Warsaw Diary*, p. 101.

In early 1940, both Jewish hospitals were placed under quarantine, and their doctors and nurses were not allowed to leave. The community organized the collection of underwear, linens, and pillows for them.[134] Czyste Hospital was unprepared to accommodate the growing population of the ill. Before the war, it did not have an infectious diseases ward. Therefore, it is no wonder that relatives of the ill objected to strict isolation and smuggled patients out through the fences surrounding the hospital. Isolation at Czyste Hospital, which applied to the entire staff, lasted more than six weeks. It was canceled only after disinfection and bathing facilities were installed. However, when typhus, also known as spotted fever, resurged—there had been an initial wave of the disease in the first half of 1940—the hospital was placed in isolation again, this time for nearly three months.[135]

The quarantine requirement caused the staff and the physicians to feel humiliated and ineffective. Dr. Mordechai Lensky[136] thought it a foolish and burdensome way to fight the disease, which only made it harder to eradicate the epidemic. Instead of improving the nutrition of the Jewish population and easing control to allow the community authorities to feed the ill, the Germans issued an order stamped with hatred and contempt for the Jewish physicians, who remained in the hospital for

134 Ringelblum, *Notes from the Warsaw Ghetto*, p. 9. On the quarantine, see Adina Blady Szwajger, *I Remember Nothing More: The Warsaw Children's Hospital and the Jewish Resistance* (New York: Pantheon, 1990), p. 25.

135 Trunk, "Epidemics and Mortality," p. 100; Dr. Henry Fenigstein testimony, "Varshever yid," YVA, O.33/1074.

136 Dr. Mordechai Lensky (b. 1890 in Warsaw) studied medicine at the University of Moscow, and received his MD in 1917. He then served as a physician in the Russian Army until the end of World War I. Returning to Warsaw in 1923, he continued to practice medicine, edited and published the journal *Der Doktor* (1929–1933), and wrote a book titled *The Modern Family Doctor*. He served as a physician with the Palestine Office in Warsaw, and taught anatomy and physiology in schools affiliated with Tarbut, a network of Hebrew-language educational institutions in Poland. From 1933 to 1939, he practiced internal medicine at the hospital in Włocławek. In 1939, he returned to Warsaw. In the ghetto, he served as a physician at Czyste Hospital, at refugee points, and at the Judenrat's clinics. Before the final liquidation of the ghetto, he and his family went into hiding on the Polish side of Warsaw. Lensky, Epilogue, *A Physician inside the Warsaw Ghetto*, pp. 200–201.

several days until the Judenrat prevailed on Schrempf to remove the quarantine.[137]

According to the nurse Sabina Gürfinkel-Glocer, the Germans, who had declared Czyste a hospital for infectious diseases, isolated it precisely to enable contagion to spread. To enforce the order scrupulously, police patrols threatened violators with punishment. It was easier for male doctors and staff members to obey the decree than it was for women, because almost all the latter were also homemakers and mothers who could not leave their children unsupervised for long periods. They coped with the edict in various ways. One jumped out of a small window facing the street every day, others slipped out through the morgue, and a few secretly took off their nurses' uniforms and posed as Aryan Poles.[138]

In late 1939 and early 1940, Czyste Hospital had to contend with the damage caused by the bombardments of the war. Although it was not badly hit compared with other hospitals, the damage that it sustained disrupted its work. Wounded soldiers and injured civilians were still there—2,400 patients in all—competing for 1,200 beds. At first, some lay on the floor in their clothing, suffering from the cold and rarely fed. Laundry facilities were unavailable, coal was in short supply, and the heating system collapsed. Frostbitten toes and fingers were common.[139] Food was generally inadequate and the staff suffered from hunger as did everyone else. Initially the staff were shorthanded, because many had left for the Soviet zone, including several doctors and department directors. Their assistants stepped in and diligently managed the departments, allowing medical care to continue unimpaired. A new influx of medical personnel, including medical students, improved the hospital. Fourteen young doctors joined the staff in 1939 and their numbers climbed to fifty by the end of 1940. These men and women were an important part of the hospital staff.[140]

137 Ibid., pp. 99–100.

138 Gürfinkel-Glocer, "Goralo Shel Beit Haholim Tzhista," p. 590; Roland, *Courage under Siege*, pp. 79–80.

139 Trunk, "Epidemics and Mortality," p. 99.

140 Roland, *Courage under Siege*, p. 79; Lensky, *A Physician inside the Warsaw Ghetto*, p. 22.

Dr. Schrempf ordered all hospital personnel to bathe every day and to hand over their clothing for disinfection. This order was superfluous, since the patients were isolated in the infectious diseases ward, where only staff members were in contact with them. Nevertheless, the enforcement of this order was strictly supervised. Every employee was registered in a special book and was given a certificate of compliance after bathing and disinfection. The concierge, who checked the permits, would not allow a staff member to leave the hospital grounds without such certification. Since no such regime was introduced at the Polish hospitals, the Jewish doctors felt that the Nazi doctors had instituted the bathing and disinfection regimen to humiliate them and their subordinates.[141]

A report from the Judenrat statistics department gives an indication of the patient turnover at Czyste Hospital in the first few months of 1940. At the end of February, there were 604 inpatients; 283 of them had infectious diseases. In March, 335 of the 744 patients were hospitalized in the infectious diseases ward and in April, 437 of 833. In May, of 881 inpatients, 315 had typhus, 110 patients were under observation, and 456 had other illnesses. Ninety-five patients remained hospitalized for injuries in February and the numbers continued to decline from March.[142]

About a month and a half after the German occupation, the Germans took over Czyste Hospital and ordered the community, through the Judenrat, to pay 5,000 zlotys for repairs caused by the bombings at the beginning of the war, for renovations, and for supplemental equipment, including 500 beds, blankets, pillows, and sheets. Otherwise, some of the equipment would be confiscated. On November 12, 1939, Czerniaków consulted with leading members of the community concerning the acceptance of Judenrat authority over the hospitals.[143] While the Judenrat did much to restore control of the hospitals and the public welfare institutions to the community, the actual transfer of the hospitals,

141 Lensky, *A Physician inside the Warsaw Ghetto*, p. 24.
142 Judenrat Statistics Department Bulletin, May 1940, AŻIH, ARII.133.
143 Czerniaków, *The Warsaw Diary*, p. 88.

the orphanages, and the old-age home to the Jewish authorities was postponed until December 31, 1939.[144]

Czerniaków was in contact with Dr. Schrempf, the chief physician and head of the Sanitation Department at the office of the mayor of Warsaw. However, whether or not Dr. Schrempf had the authority to determine policy or to implement the policies set forth by the central health authority is not clear.[145] Czerniaków, who labored tenaciously to reestablish the Judenrat's control of the hospital, confronted Prof. Richter, head of the Military Sanitation Service, to settle disagreements on this account. Dr. Schrempf referred the decision to the mayor of Warsaw, Dr. Oscar Dengel,[146] but Czerniaków thought this insufficient and asked the SS to allow him to meet with the mayor.[147] Several days later, the problem appeared to have been resolved. A representative of the municipality invited the entire Judenrat to the hospital on December 5, 1939, "in regard to the transfer of the hospital [to the Judenrat]." However, the municipal official did not show up at the appointed time. The minutes on this matter were sent to the SS.[148]

Conflicts of interest among authorities appear to have influenced the disagreements about the hospital's status. The municipality adamantly objected to handing the institution over to the Judenrat. It should be borne in mind that until the war, the municipality had covered 60 percent of the hospital's annual budget.[149] When the war began, the municipal subsidy plummeted to only 5 percent. The community raised enough to cover 35 percent of the expenses; patients had to make up the remaining

144 Ibid., pp. 90–91.

145 Czerniaków, *The Warsaw Diary*, p. 91. Dr. Wilhelm Hagen succeeded Dr. Schrempf as *Stadtpräsident* (mayor) of Warsaw in January 1941.

146 Ibid., p. 94. Dr. Dengel served as mayor of Warsaw from November 6, 1939, to March 15, 1940. Legally, the city was subordinate to the district governor. Dengel was his agent. In September 1941, when Warsaw was redefined as a provincial capital, he received the title of *Stadthauptmann* (municipal governor), who was also in charge of the Warsaw city administration.

147 Ibid., p. 94.

148 Ibid., pp. 96–97.

149 Ben-Shem, "Batei Holim Yehudiyim BeVarsha," p. 584.

60 percent out of pocket.[150] The matter of forwarding payments to the city was evidently of crucial importance in the dispute between the municipality and the Judenrat.[151] At a meeting on December 9, 1939, the Germans stepped in. It was agreed that the municipality would cover the expenses for December, but the Judenrat would have to repay this loan. The Judenrat's coffers had 20,000 zlotys at the time, and Czerniaków had to raise funds for the payroll of the workers, which totaled 40,000 zlotys, as well as for the Judenrat's own payroll.[152]

In mid-December, the Judenrat secured direct responsibility for the hospital and began to organize acquiring funds by means of a special fundraising campaign.[153] On March 9, 1940, about half a year into the German occupation of Warsaw, Kaplan wrote that the Jews had ceased to receive medical aid from the municipality. A Jew could not be admitted to any hospital, except the hospital on Czyste St., even if his or her life depended on it. The hospital, in turn, had stopped receiving its annual municipal subvention, and subsisted solely at the community's expense.[154]

This struggle with the Warsaw municipality over possession of Czyste Hospital raises the question of how the Polish municipal leadership conducted itself when it came to collaborating with the occupier. To what extent was the struggle for control of Jewish public assets, such as the hospital, in the initial stage of the occupation a local initiative or a German directive? Such power struggles between municipal players and representatives of the ghetto would beset relations between representatives of the Polish municipal authority and the city's Jewish inhabitants in the future as well. Yehuda Bauer claims that the entire apparatus that was established—mayors, local officials, chiefs of police, etc.—was intended to induce surrender, enslavement, and similar responses

150 Roland, *Courage under Siege*, p. 79.

151 Czerniaków, *The Warsaw Diary*, p. 97.

152 Ibid., p. 98.

153 The sources are not clear about the exact date that the Judenrat took over the institution. It was probably somewhere between December 6 and December 9, 1939. Czerniaków, *The Warsaw Diary*, pp. 98–104.

154 Kaplan, *Megilat Yisurin*, p. 198.

among the Poles; only the Jews were targeted for total physical annihilation. Most of the non-Jewish overseers in occupied cities did not resist overtly or refuse to obey orders, even when they could have done so without risking their lives. If so, why were the Judenräte held to a different standard?[155]

On December 16–17, 1939, several days after the Judenrat had reclaimed the hospital, Czerniaków established a hospitals department in the Judenrat, appointing Ignacy Fliederbaum, the former director of the hospital, to manage it.[156] On January 1, by order of the Germans, the hospital received exclusive rights to treat Jewish residents in conjunction with Bersohn and Bauman Children's Hospital. In this manner, the Judenrat set out on one of the paths of struggle: an attempt to run a hospital—as morbidity skyrocketed and the Jewish population faced a medical disaster—with a limited budget and few possibilities of raising funds.[157] The hospital was subordinate first to the German Health Department and only then, indirectly, to the Judenrat Health Department headed by Dr. Milejkowski.[158]

In the early stages of the war, the hospital staff accounted for a large majority of the Judenrat employees. In February 1940, about eight months before ghettoization, Czyste Hospital had about 496 employees and 32 others worked at the two hospitals that were reserved for patients with infectious diseases—in all, 528 of the 782 people who were on the Judenrat's payroll.[159] The difficulties of operating Czyste Hospital as a central medical institution in the ghetto occupied Czerniaków throughout the occupation. On

155 Bauer, *Rethinking the Holocaust*, pp. 90–94.

156 Czerniaków, *The Warsaw Diary*, p. 100.

157 Judenrat Statistics Department Bulletin, May 1940, AŻIH, ARII.133.

158 Dr. Shmuel Stanisław Waller testimony, YVA, O.3/2358.

159 On December 9, 1939, Czerniaków was instructed to make 500 beds available for a new hospital for which the Judenrat would be responsible. This order may have referred to a hospital for isolation patients. See Czerniaków, *The Warsaw Diary*, p. 98. According to the Judenrat Statistics Department Bulletin of May 1940, there were three hospitals for patients in isolation: on Železná St., at 109/111 Leszno St., and at 53 Złota St.—which together accommodated 1,118 inpatients that month; see the Judenrat Statistics Department Bulletin, May 1940, AŻIH, ARII.133.

December 24, 1939, when the hospital was in the midst of its quarantine, he wrote, "I decided to devote my time today for a visit to the hospital in Czyste, and the hospitals for the convalescents… at a delousing facility in Czyste, I had to take special precautions."[160] Three days later, he tried to talk the Gestapo into releasing the Czyste workers who were still under quarantine. On December 28, 1939, he began his day with a visit to the hospital. On December 29, he convened the hospitals committee, apparently to consider how to end the quarantine.[161] In addition to imposing a quarantine on the hospital, the Gestapo had arrested several of its doctors in early 1940, causing a personnel shortage and hard feelings among the remaining medical staff.[162]

Czerniaków showed great concern for the team of doctors. In the course of January 1940, he tried to effect the release of the prisoners of "the Kott affair," the Jews who were captured after Andrzej Kazimierz Kott, a member of the PPS—Polska Partia Socjalistyczna (Polish Socialist Party)—and of a resistance group, had attempted to murder a Gestapo man.[163] Despite Czerniaków's

160 Czerniaków, *The Warsaw Diary*, p. 102.

161 Ibid., p.103.

162 Gürfinkel-Glocer, "Goralo Shel Beit Haholim Tzhista," p. 591.

163 Czerniaków, *The Warsaw Diary*, p. 109; Gutman, *The Jews of Warsaw*, pp. 33–34. The Kott incident was one of several affairs involving the collective punishment of the ghetto population for the "sins" of individual violators of Nazi decrees. On January 20, 1940, a notice informing the public that "the Jew Andrzej Kazimierz Kott" was wanted for manslaughter was posted. It included a photo of a young man and an offer of a bounty of 2,000 zlotys to the person who would capture and turn him in. Kott was the offspring of an apostate family and the founder of the Polska Ludowa Akcja Niepodległościowa (PLAN) underground movement, which sought to reinstate Polish independence on foundations of social justice. Kott headed the organization's armed wing, which was active in the first few months of the occupation. The plan was uncovered and its members arrested, but Kott managed to break out of prison. Although he had no special connection with the Jews, the fact that he was of Jewish origin sufficed to blame the entire Jewish population. The Germans ordered the Judenrat to surrender Kott within forty-eight hours. In the aftermath of the affair, as collective punishment, they arrested several Poles and approximately 250 Jewish intellectuals and professionals, including many doctors. The Judenrat's efforts to have them released were futile and most of them were murdered.

exertions, a delegation of families visited him on February 10. They bluntly accused the Judenrat of having given the Gestapo the names of 100 doctors, because of the assassination attempt by the member of the underground Kott.[164] The efforts to secure the release of the prisoners continued for three months.[165] In addition to these problems, information was received about the future appointment of a *Kommissar* for the hospital, causing uncertainty and fear about the possible effects of this move. In response, Czerniaków held meetings in his home to discuss the hospital's affairs.[166]

Apart from dealing with the Germans, ongoing internal problems arose in the operation of the hospital under the difficult conditions. The institution's needs escalated, while the possibilities to address them dwindled. On February 23, 1940, Dr. Stein, director of the hospital, met with Czerniaków and set forth his facility's troubles. Delegations from the hospital visited him to demand corrective actions in various areas. On April 9, 1940, for example, around eight months after the war had begun, doctors from Czyste Hospital, headed by the chief physician, met with Czerniaków to discuss the criticism of the institution's superintendent. A month later, on May 6, rabbis protested the serving of non-kosher food at the hospital. Czerniaków responded by convening the hospitals committee to discuss the matter.[167]

Internal labor disputes at the hospital also were brought to Czerniaków's attention for him to address. For example, members of the hospital staff, who had been terminated, informed on the hospital administration for supposedly hiring members of the intelligentsia to obtain certificates of exemption from forced labor for them at the expense of the professional workers

164 Czerniaków, *The Warsaw Diary*, p. 116.

165 Ibid., p. 138. From January 20, 1940, when Jews were arrested for the Kott affair, the Gestapo did not provide Czerniaków with a list of those being held until mid-August of that year. During these months, he tried to help representatives of the families to free their loved ones. For example, on April 8, 1940, he described his efforts to release Dr. Owsiej Bielenki. Czerniaków, *The Warsaw Diary*, p. 138.

166 Czerniaków, *The Warsaw Diary*, p. 107.

167 Ibid., pp. 121, 138, 146.

required by the hospital. A delegation from the hospital, including doctors, nurses, and ordinary workers, visited Czerniaków on June 21, 1940, and had a very heated meeting with him.[168] Czerniaków does not explain exactly what they discussed, but one may infer that the delegation demanded various changes in the hospital's procedures, and discussed the difficult work conditions and the hospital budget. Despite the efforts of Czerniaków and the staff, little appears to have changed at the hospital, which prompted the beleaguered workers to threaten a hunger strike on July 7. They continued their demands and threats to strike for two days.[169]

At a Judenrat meeting in late December 1939, it was reported that 150,000–200,000 zlotys were needed each month for the maintenance of the hospital[170]—a huge sum compared with the meager budget. Inevitably, the budget hardships impaired the institution's functioning. The German authorities did not provide any assistance to operate the hospital. Even though he raised funds and gathered materials for the hospital, Czerniaków had to obtain bank loans to keep it running. In mid-December 1939, he applied for a loan for the hospital from the Warsaw branch of a Jewish bank in Łódź that had operated until the war. The bank was required to obtain the authorization of the head of the Finance Department of the German authority that oversaw the Polish administration of the municipality of Warsaw.[171] SS approval was necessary to obtain bank loans.[172] On January 9, 1940, after the population had spent four months under war conditions, the JDC lent the hospital 50,000 zlotys.[173]

168 Ibid., pp. 159, 164. On the strike that took place at Bersohn and Bauman Children's Hospital, see Chapter 4 of this book.

169 Ibid., p. 171.

170 Ibid., p. 103.

171 Ibid., p. 89. The head of the Municipal Finance Department in Warsaw under German auspices was Karol Laschtoviczka, a *Volksdeutsche* who had managed a private bank in Warsaw before the war. He was transferred to Cracow after becoming a *Reichsdeutsche* (German citizen).

172 Ibid., p. 100.

173 Ibid., p. 106. The JDC executives in Warsaw were David Guzik, Yitzhak Gitterman, and Leib Neustadt. During the occupation, JDC in Warsaw borrowed

On January 17, 1940, 100-zloty and 500-zloty banknotes were removed from circulation, temporarily paralyzing commercial life so severely that Czerniaków could not even buy coal and basic foods for the hospital.[174] The Judenrat received significant assistance in February 1940, when the German mayor, Dr. Dengel, ordered the liquidation of all the securities held by Jews in banks in Warsaw and the transfer of the cash to the Judenrat to support Czyste Hospital.[175] During 1940, the Judenrat became increasingly worried about its budget. It was amassing debts, the value of its securities had fallen, and the hospital continued to go through enormous sums of money. Czerniaków stood helpless in the face of the hospital's expenses: "The coffers are empty. The salaries remain unpaid. The hospital services...are eating up their resources." The Judenrat was unable to pay the wages of the Czyste Hospital staff at the end of the month.[176] "We're on the brink of bankruptcy...the hospital is failing," Czerniaków wrote.[177]

From July 1940 onward, Czerniaków imposed a special tax on the population to raise funds for the hospital.[178] Kaplan described the nature of the hospital tax in his diary.

> Where would the impoverished Judenrat find the money to support it? But—seek and ye shall find. In order to supply its budgetary requirements, a special tax was imposed on us, whereby every householder would contribute what he wished and could afford. Every month the courtyard collectors come to receive it, but what with the general poverty, they don't collect even half. And so from time to time, the *Judenrat* is forced to issue calls for linens, pillows, blankets, spoons, and forks. Under these conditions, the sick are not to be envied.[179]

funds from Jews who had cash and were afraid of being robbed, promising to pay them back after the war. This enabled granting the loan to the hospital.

174 Ibid., p. 109.

175 Roland, *Courage under Siege*, p. 78.

176 Czerniaków, *The Warsaw Diary*, pp. 125, 130–132.

177 Ibid., p. 140.

178 Ibid., p. 169.

179 Kaplan, *Scroll of Agony*, p. 240.

Even so, the budget did not suffice to cover the payroll and the hospital staff went on strike. A year after ghettoization, on January 11, 1942, a fundraising rally for the hospital was held.[180] In addition, the Judenrat established a special department to mobilize additional resources for Czyste Hospital. Ajzyk Ber Ekerman, head of the department, attempted to obtain beds, linens, underwear, and cloth.[181]

Period 2: From Ghettoization in Early 1941 to the *Grossaktion* in July 1942

On September 25, 1940, about a year into the occupation and with ghettoization imminent, it was not clear if the Czyste Hospital building would be included within the ghetto confines. Hardly a day passed that Czerniaków did not concern himself with the institution's survival and functioning in the expected ghetto.[182] That month, Dr. Konrad Orzechowski, director of the municipal hospital services, visited Czyste Hospital and reported that the facility would be transferred to the ghetto. Several days later, a contingent of Nazis visited the ghetto area and inspected in particular Leszno St.—the seat of the Judenrat—as the intended site for Czyste Hospital.[183] On Rosh Hashana, October 3, 1940, Josef Bühler, secretary of state of the General Government and Governor Frank's deputy, visited the ghetto area accompanied by Waldemar Schön, *Kommissar* of the residential quarter in Warsaw and director of population evacuation and resettlement in the Regional Office. There they scouted the courthouse on Leszno St., with a view to relocating Czyste Hospital there.[184]

On October 15, 1940, Dr. Schrempf, the German administrator of the hospital, quoted Schön as saying that Czyste Hospital had to be evacuated to the ghetto and that Czerniaków's efforts were

180 Czerniaków, *The Warsaw Diary*, p. 314.
181 Roland, *Courage under Siege*, p. 89.
182 Czerniaków, *The Warsaw Diary*, p. 201.
183 Roland, *Courage under Siege*, p. 80.
184 Czerniaków, *The Warsaw Diary*, p. 204.

now directed at finding an appropriate building for the institution. Schrempf decided that the hospital would be transferred to the courthouse, on October 15, 1940. However, this did not happen, because the German authorities decided a day before the deadline that the courthouse would not be included in the ghetto.[185] Lensky wrote that the Poles opposed these exchanges.[186] About a week and a half after the order to move to the ghetto was issued, Czyste Hospital remained outside the ghetto limits.[187] A few days after the closure of the ghetto, the Judenrat still did not know whether the hospital would have to relocate to the ghetto or would remain where it was[188]

About two weeks after the ghetto was sealed, Czerniaków became increasingly concerned about finding a suitable building for the hospital, because even if the date of the relocation was unknown, it was clear that it was destined to move to the ghetto.[189] A week later, Ringelblum wrote that the Jewish hospital would be relocated by April 1941. In fact, the move took place four months sooner, in late December 1940 and early January 1941. The hospital was in a state of uncertainty and confusion at the time. Left to their own devices during the relocation, the patients did not receive adequate care.[190]

In the first two weeks of ghettoization, the doctors and the rest of the staff were unable to get to work, since the hospital was still outside the ghetto and crossing permits had not been issued. Patients suffered on this account. It sometimes happened, for example, that a doctor who had treated a patient with a brain disorder could not return to the hospital the next day to provide further treatment and, consequently, the patient died.[191] Patients

185 Ibid., p. 207.

186 Lensky, *A Physician inside the Warsaw Ghetto*, pp. 37–38.

187 Ringelblum, *Notes from the Warsaw Ghetto*, pp. 80–81.

188 Czerniaków, *The Warsaw Diary*, p. 217.

189 Ibid., p. 222.

190 Ringelblum, *Notes from the Warsaw Ghetto*, p. 108; Kaplan, *Scroll of Agony*, pp. 239–240; Lensky, *A Physician inside the Warsaw Ghetto*, p. 37; Dr. Shmuel Stanisław Waller testimony, YVA, O.3/2358; Gürfinkel-Glocer, "Goralo Shel Beit Haholim Tzhista," p. 591.

191 Czerniaków, *The Warsaw Diary*, p. 217; Ringelblum, *Yoman Vereshimot*, p. 199.

who had to go to the hospital for treatment were taken from the ghetto in carts, for lack of an alternative.[192]

In December 1940, only 75 crossing permits were issued to the hospital staff of 1,000 members; the number then rose to 200. These documents, approved by Dr. Schrempf in coordination with the SS headquarters, allowed daily trips from the ghetto to the hospital and back. Those who lacked them had to report to the gate at 6 Twarda St. every day at 7 A.M. Wearing their Jewish armbands, they then had to march in ranks to the hospital on Czyste St.,[193] often harassed by Poles or Germans—bands of hooligans threw stones at them and the border police abused them. Some workers who did not receive crossing permits made the hospital their temporary home.[194] The Judenrat was responsible for distributing these permits, which cost 5 zlotys apiece.[195]

Although the Judenrat was ordered to move the hospital to the ghetto, it failed to find a suitable building, one with enough wings to accommodate its 1,000 patients.[196] Before the evacuation, the original hospital building required an overhaul. In addition, some of its furniture, kitchen appliances, etc., had been confiscated. The Warsaw municipality withheld permission to remove the equipment until the Judenrat repaired the demolished laundry facility and kitchen at an estimated cost of 200,000 zlotys.[197] The Jews were not permitted to transfer heavy equipment, including the most expensive medical equipment, to the alternative hospital in the ghetto. In contrast, Polish building officials removed everything possible, including faucets and sinks, from the building on Leszno St., which had served as a tax office before the war and had become a hospital during the fighting in September 1939.[198]

192 Dr. Henry Fenigstein testimony, "Varshever yid," YVA, O.33/1074, p. 7.

193 Ringelblum, *Notes from the Warsaw Ghetto*, p. 107.

194 Gürfinkel-Glocer, "Goralo Shel Beit Haholim Tzhista," pp. 590–591.

195 Ringelblum, *Notes from the Warsaw Ghetto*, p. 86.

196 Kaplan, *Scroll of Agony*, p. 240; Lensky, *A Physician inside the Warsaw Ghetto*, pp. 37–38; Mendelsohn, *The Polish Jews*, pp. 11–12.

197 Ringelblum, *Yoman Vereshimot*, pp. 206–207; Trunk, "Epidemics and Mortality," p. 100.

198 Ringelblum, *Notes from the Warsaw Ghetto*, pp. 80–81; Gürfinkel-Glocer, "Goralo Shel Beit Haholim Tzhista," pp. 591–592.

On April 26, 1941, the memorial plaques at the hospital building on Czyste St. were removed and the resulting holes were filled with bricks. Thus, the former Jewish hospital building was stripped of its Jewish markings.[199] The structures made available to the hospital in the ghetto were ill suited for their purpose. Those on Stawki St. had no gas fixtures, no pipes, and, due to the freezing conditions, no running water. Much equipment had been lost or stolen during the move. The Jewish hospital entered the ghetto with shortages of materials and items, such as blankets, bedding, and medical instruments.[200] Even the beds had to be left behind, which triggered an immediate crisis that was "solved" by cobbling beds together out of pieces of scrap metal.[201]

A special fundraising drive among the Jewish population, managed by the "courtyard committees" that collected the hospital tax, was launched to help relocate the hospital to the ghetto.[202] Without appropriate clothing during the coldest part of winter, the patients were moved in first aid vehicles of the Polish Red Cross. Staff members tried to take as much equipment as they could from the hospital storerooms in these vehicles. They tucked pillows under patients' heads, lined the pillows with cotton, and stashed expensive medical equipment inside them. When a German military policeman inspected the cars, the patients pressed their heads against the pillows. Warned that the patients had high fevers, the Germans maintained their distance from the cars. A great deal of equipment was salvaged by means of this tactic, among others.[203]

While the Germans allowed equipment to go through, the Poles insisted on creating obstacles. The municipality did not allow the doctors to remove the expensive instruments that the Jews had purchased, and the occupier did not meddle in this dispute. "Writers of impressions among the Jewish doctors will no doubt tell future generations all the details of the evolution of the quarrel—

199 Ringelblum, *Notes from the Warsaw Ghetto*, p. 167.
200 Trunk, "Epidemics and Mortality," p. 101.
201 Roland, *Courage under Siege*, p. 85.
202 Kaplan, *Scroll of Agony*, p. 241.
203 Gürfinkel-Glocer, "Goralo Shel Beit Haholim Tzhista," pp. 591–592.

I don't know the whole story," Kaplan wrote.[204] It took two months of hard, conscientious, and dangerous work to transfer the hospital. The hospital staff and the students allowed themselves no respite. Many workers, doctors in particular, were still living outside the ghetto and would soon have to find housing in the ghetto. Despite all the difficulties, expenses, and personal risk, the medical teams managed to transfer a great deal of equipment.[205]

Kaplan accused the municipality of Warsaw of being antisemitic and of not treating its Jewish citizens honestly. Before the war, it had supported the hospital with the large tax revenues that it had received from the Jews, most of whom were merchants and manufacturers who provided the city with a disproportionately large share of its income. When the war began, the city terminated this support, in effect robbing the Jews of the facility. In Kaplan's opinion, antisemitic Polish physicians had been coveting the costly equipment at the hospital since peacetime.[206] Lensky described the oppressive atmosphere throughout the various stages of the move, "We left the hospital feeling gloomy...mournful...distress was unbearable."[207]

Since no suitable building for the hospital was found in the ghetto, the departments and services were scattered among several buildings, all far from one another and each unfit.[208] Sometimes the departments were transferred from one building to another, according to the ghetto's changing needs. The departments of internal medicine, neurology, surgery, radiology, ophthalmology, and ear, nose, and throat were moved to a municipal building that had previously been a factory at 1 Leszno St.[209] Obstetrics and gynecology were transferred to 4 Tłomackie St. and were set up in Dr. Friszman's clinic or in Dr. Gurewicz's private hospital. Additional departments of internal medicine and of infectious

204 Kaplan, *Scroll of Agony*, p. 241.

205 Ibid., pp. 241–242; Lensky, *A Physician inside the Warsaw Ghetto*, pp. 38–39.

206 Kaplan, *Scroll of Agony*, p. 241.

207 Lensky, *A Physician inside the Warsaw Ghetto*, pp. 37–38.

208 Hirszfeld, *Die Geschichte eines Lebens*, p. 143; Kaplan, *Scroll of Agony*, pp. 239–240.

209 Gürfinkel-Glocer, "Goralo Shel Beit Haholim Tzhista," pp. 591–592.

diseases were evidently relocated to the municipal archive building, the elementary school at 6–8 Stawki St., and 80 Żelazna St., where the chemistry, bacteriology, and pathological labs were situated. Eventually, these departments were retransferred to 21 Stawki St.[210] In the winter of 1940–1941, another department for the treatment of epidemics was added to the hospital, which was located at 109 Leszno St.[211] and run by Dr. Abraham Paweł Lipsztat.[212] The pharmacy and the disinfection equipment were set up in the badly damaged Święty Duch Hospital building at 12 Elektoralna St.[213]

210 Kaplan, *Scroll of Agony*, p. 240; Dr. Shmuel Stanisław Waller testimony, YVA, O.3/2358; Trunk, "Epidemics and Mortality," pp. 100–101; Roland, *Courage under Siege*, p. 81.

211 Gürfinkel-Glocer, "Goralo Shel Beit Haholim Tzhista," pp. 591–592.

212 Dr. Abraham Paweł Lipsztat (1903–1943), who completed his medical studies in 1928 in Warsaw, ran clinics there and in nearby Garwolin, earning a reputation of being a devoted and compassionate physician. In the first year of the German occupation, he worked as a physician at the refugee disinfection unit at 109/111 Leszno St. in Warsaw. In the Warsaw ghetto, he directed the department of infectious diseases at Czyste Hospital, where he and other scientists researched ways to prevent the spread of typhus and discovered the positive effect of metallic mercury to prevent the spread of lice. He was deported to the Treblinka extermination camp during the *Aktion* of January 1943 before he could publish his findings. He and his wife may have committed suicide by swallowing poison on the train on the way to Treblinka. His son, Aleksander (Olek) Lipsztat, later known as Olek Netzer, was saved by the mayor of Garwolin, a friend of his father, Franciszek Paśniczek, who was recognized as Righteous Among the Nations after the war. Dr. Abraham Paweł Lipsztat's sister, Dr. Natalia Julia Lipsztat-Muszkat (1908–1943), completed her medical studies in 1932 and specialized in pediatrics. She worked devotedly in Sochaczew in the Warsaw district and at Bersohn and Bauman Children's Hospital before the war and in the ghetto. She died in Treblinka following the *Aktion* of January 18, 1943. Her husband, Dr. Shmuel Muszkat, who served in the Polish Army from 1939–1940, was taken prisoner-of-war by the Soviets and exiled to Siberia, thus was saved from the Nazi occupation. Their son, Aleksander (Krolek) Muszkat was saved by the Righteous Among the Nations Irena Szandler and later became a professor of chemistry in Israel. I thank Prof. Mordechai Muszkat of the Hadassah University Hospital, Mt. Scopus, Jerusalem, Dr. Lipsztat's great-nephew, for sharing this information with me. See Wulman et al., *The Martyrdom of Jewish Physicians in Poland*, pp. 409, 422; Dr. Henry Fenigstein testimony, "Varshever yid," pp. 7-8, YVA, O.33/1074; Ciesielska, *Lekarza Getta Warszawskiego*, pp. 106, 185, 188, 301, 360, 366.

213 Roland, *Courage under Siege*, p. 81.

The dispersion and fragmentation of the departments across the ghetto had a grave effect on the efficiency and supervision of the medical services. The new buildings were unsuited to the Jewish hospital's needs but, according to Dr. Lensky, it was possible to work in them, nevertheless.[214] Lensky described the X-ray facility on 1 Leszno St. as having been organized properly to serve all the departments. It was arranged in four small rooms and although cramped, relative to its previous quarters, it was well arranged, particularly after one of the doctors donated furniture from her private clinic. The physicians, like everyone else in the ghetto, feared that the Germans would dispossess them and, therefore, they preferred to donate their furniture to the hospital. The other departments were also attractively arranged, Lensky reported. Flowerpots festooned the windowsills and corridors. The staff members worked enthusiastically, even though they were apprehensive.[215]

When the hospital moved to its new quarters, it was renamed Czyste Jewish Hospital for Infectious Diseases.[216] About nine months after ghettoization, Ringelblum wrote, "The hospitals have, for a thousand reasons, lost their therapeutic character." Dr. Milejkowski, he said, claimed that the hospitals had become "places of execution." Thousands of people in need of inpatient care preferred to stay home rather than go to the hospital in view of its tragic state.[217] Two months later, as the ghetto approached its first anniversary, Czerniaków described the ongoing medical catastrophe at the hospital. "Corpses in the corridors and three patients in each bed…while leaving the hospital, I was stopped by staff members with complaints (partly justified) to the Council about their pay, coal, etc."[218]

Prof. Ludwik Hirszfeld, an activist in health care and in the war on epidemics in the Warsaw ghetto, reported in his memoirs

214 Lensky, *A Physician inside the Warsaw Ghetto*, p. 38.

215 Ibid.

216 Dr. Henry Fenigstein testimony, "Varshever yid," YVA, O.33/1074, p. 8; Dr. Chaim Einhorn testimony, YVA, O.3/1836.

217 Ringelblum, *Notes from the Warsaw Ghetto*, pp. 194–195.

218 Czerniaków, *The Warsaw Diary*, p. 288.

that the German authorities visited the hospital frequently and were well aware of its abject state—two or three patients per bed, dysentery patients together with those suffering from typhus,[219] and all of them hungry. Very few received food from relatives or had the means to buy any. Those whose relatives were destitute and were unable to feed their hospitalized kin starved.[220] Support from the community did not suffice. Sometimes the living spent several hours lying next to the dead in the same bed. There was not enough personnel and professionals were in short supply. The staff themselves were desperately hungry. The caregivers were so weak that they could not be assigned arduous tasks. When the doctors made their rounds, the ill and the dying often cried out, "We're hungry!" Hirszfeld testified,

> I went through hell at the Serbian hospitals in World War I. What I saw during a year [in the ghetto] transcended all human imagination, because in addition to the disaster of the war, the defeat, the epidemic with everything accompanying it in psychological terms and in its grave results, the ill will of the occupier, who admittedly wanted order but did nothing to bring it about, had its effect...several times, I heard the hospital's doctors say to each other, "Would you put your parents in such a hospital?"[221]

Mindful of the catastrophic conditions, people who fell ill were afraid to be hospitalized and their families spared no effort to keep them away from the facility. Those of means bribed the medical committee and the physician assigned to their block in the ghetto. For a steep fee, doctors made surreptitious house calls. Even the most conscientious physicians refrained from sending patients to the hospital, because doing so meant not only increasing the risk to the patients' lives but also the economic burden on their families and neighbors.[222]

219 Hirszfeld, *Die Geschichte eines Lebens*, p. 141.
220 Ibid.; Lensky, *A Physician inside the Warsaw Ghetto*, p. 23.
221 Hirszfeld, *Die Geschichte eines Lebens*, p. 141.
222 Trunk, "Epidemics and Mortality," p. 105.

The nutritional level in the hospital was similar to that of the ghetto at large—patients starved to death. Preferring to keep the working inhabitants of the ghetto fed, the Judenrat supply department reduced the food supplies of the ill. The German authorities did not limit themselves to withholding special support from the hospital and sometimes confiscated food sent in non-motorized vehicles, the only kind allowed under Nazi supervision, from the central warehouse on Stawki St. to the branches of the hospital.[223] Furthermore, they did not approve any supplemental nutrition for patients with special needs, such as patients with ulcers, post-operative patients, or patients recovering from typhus.[224] Malnutrition exacerbated the patients' conditions, especially of those with tuberculosis, who became increasingly gaunt with each passing day. Lensky claimed that the German doctor in charge of Warsaw and the ghetto was uninterested in providing the hospital with food. After the war, Lensky compared the feeding of Polish patients at the municipal hospital in Włocławek during the German occupation with that of the patients in Czyste Hospital, and found that those in Włocławek were very well fed.[225]

Despite the appalling conditions of the hospital, residents of the ghetto were forced to transfer typhus patients there, because people who concealed them faced the death penalty.[226] Concern about the spread of typhus was such that an order to hospitalize anyone who had a fever was issued. Those admitted underwent treatments that sometimes caused suffering and humiliation, but were necessary to prevent contagion, including shaving their heads, delousing, baths, and disinfection.[227] Marek Edelman,[228]

223 Ibid., p. 101.

224 Roland, *Courage under Siege*, p. 85.

225 Lensky, *A Physician inside the Warsaw Ghetto*, pp. 23–25.

226 Hirszfeld, *Die Geschichte eines Lebens*, p. 141.

227 Koren, "Hasiyud Kehelek Misherutei Habriyut," p. 58.

228 Marek Edelman, who was twenty years old at the time, was a member of Zukunft, the Bund's youth organization. During the ghetto uprising, he represented the Bund in the ŻOB—Żydowska Organizacja Bojowa (Jewish Fighting Organization)—command, making him one of three leaders of the uprising, along with Mordechai Anielewicz and Yitzhak (Antek) Zuckerman.

a courier at the hospital at the time, wrote that as the typhus epidemic raged through the ghetto, the hospitals were converted into specialized facilities for infectious diseases that were filled to capacity. One ward received 150 patients per day who lay two to three per mattress placed on the floor. The ill waited impatiently at the foot of the beds of the dying to expedite the surrender of the place to the next in line. Edelman wrote that there were not enough doctors, and those who were there could not keep up with the work.[229]

In a report dated June 28, 1941, the Health Department stated the following:

> The situation is extremely tragic now. At first, old people died. Now the young, our people's future, are dying as well. The greatest difficulty is the absolute shortage of beds. We are mindful of the difficulties in finding additional buildings for the patients...we may have no choice but to take beds from [people's] homes. Every house committee will have to see to it. To treat the many who have fallen ill, we need at least 700 additional beds. We are in a dire state. If we are to help the ill, the authorities must provide us with beds at once![230]

On November 7, 1941, *Awangarda Młodzieży* (Pioneering Youth), the newspaper of the left-leaning Po'alei Tziyon Party, reported a tremendous increase in contagious diseases, foremost typhus.

His job as a courier for the children's hospital allowed him the privilege of a permanent permit to leave the ghetto. After the war, he remained in Poland, studied medicine, and became a cardiologist. Edelman was active in social, political, and human rights causes. In 1976, he joined the Polish Workers' Defense Committee and enlisted in Solidarity, the Polish trade union. In 1989–1993, he was a member of the *Sejm*, the lower chamber of the Polish parliament. Edelman received Poland's highest decoration, the Order of the White Eagle, in 1998.

229 Marek Edelman, *The Ghetto Fights: Warsaw 1939–1945* (London: Bookmarks, 2013), pp. 27–28.

230 Health Department report on the fight against tuberculosis, June 28, 1941, AŻIH, ARI.214.

The author of the piece then harshly criticized the Judenrat for its inadequate treatment of the problem.

> Therefore, the Jewish hospital, which the Judenrat treats in a scandalous manner bordering on contempt (the wealthy ill remain at home), is not equal to the tasks that the tragic reality presents. Three or four patients per bed, hallways as wards, minimal and often unprofessional medical care, and starvation diets—that is what Czyste Hospital for Infectious Diseases looks like.[231]

The conditions for tuberculosis patients deteriorated in 1941, because the tuberculosis department was on Stawki St. and the X-ray facility was on Leszno St. Patients who needed X-rays were hauled to the latter location in a primitive cart drawn by an emaciated horse. When passersby saw the vehicle and its passengers, they felt that they were not in Warsaw but in a little shtetl fifty years earlier and that the ill were being taken not to a modern hospital but to a cemetery. Also in the winter, the ill who were shivering with cold were transported in light clothing and covered with a worn-out blanket. Once treated, they had to wait for hours to return to their ward, because in the meantime the "vehicle" had left to bring a new group of patients.[232]

Obtaining medicines and medical equipment was fraught with difficulty. Smuggling was the most common method, but efforts were made to create a local response as well. The Toporol firm, for example, which had been set up to encourage agriculture among the Jews, planted herbs, such as chamomile, for use in the hospital. While chamomile was, of course, not a wonder drug, it could serve as a drug, nonetheless.[233] One of the hospital's day-to-day routine concerns was how to administer large infusions of fluids to patients in serious condition. Since the requisite intravenous equipment was unattainable, medical students used

231 Blatman, *Geto Varsha—Sipur Itona'i*, pp. 154–155.

232 Lensky, *A Physician inside the Warsaw Ghetto*, pp. 23–24.

233 Roland, *Courage under Siege*, p. 85; see also the Toporol report, July 1, 1940–May 31, 1941, AŻIH, file 370.

and reused standard needles, injecting 40 milliliters each time.[234]

As dismal as the conditions of the hospital were, some ghetto inhabitants were even worse off. Helpless families began to abandon ill kin in the community institutions, hoping that someone there would pity them and provide them with what they could not.[235] In July 1941, Mary Berg recorded in her diary that she had seen a father carrying his son to the hospital gate, where he stood hesitantly for some time, until he finally placed the sick boy on the steps leading to the institution. As the youngster writhed and whimpered, a nurse dressed in white stepped out of the hospital and began to berate the father, who stood head bowed, tears gushing. A few moments later, the boy died.[236] Ringelblum mentioned a few snippets, including the criticism that only people of means, who could also pay private doctors to take care of their ill, could afford to be hospitalized.[237]

Despite the hardships described, work at the hospital at 1 Leszno St. proceeded systematically and uninterruptedly for a year and a half, from January 1941 to July 22, 1942.[238] The staff maintained work discipline, beginning at 8 A.M., when all staff members, including doctors, signed in.[239] The medical team strove to continue to provide treatment within the same framework that was customary before the war. Participants in professional staff meetings presented disease reports. Efforts were made to maintain the hospital, both as a research institute and as a dispensary of medical aid.[240]

The three surgery departments worked intensively. At this time, a new method to set leg fractures—with interconnected rods—became common procedure, and the doctors at Czyste Hospital performed many operations of this kind. The X-ray and

234 Roland, *Courage under Siege*, p. 85.

235 Ringelblum, *Yoman Vereshimot*, p. 253.

236 Mary Berg, *The Diary of Mary Berg: Growing Up in the Warsaw Ghetto*, ed. by Susan Lee Pentlin (London: One World, 2006), pp. 75–76.

237 Ringelblum, *Yoman Vereshimot*, p. 295.

238 Lensky, *A Physician inside the Warsaw Ghetto*, p. 41.

239 Ibid., p. 24.

240 Roland, *Courage under Siege*, p. 87.

bacteriology departments conducted high-quality diagnoses. The hospital also had an institute for pathological anatomy, headed by Dr. Stein, and an X-ray therapy facility. The X-ray departments maintained a rich archive of information on rare diseases and unusual cases.[241]

Apart from the challenge of treating a growing number of patients under conditions of basic shortages of hospital accommodations, equipment, and medical supplies, the hospital staff had to contend with diseases and injuries that doctors would ordinarily not encounter. The hospital was full of typhus patients. Before the end of the typhoid fever epidemic, which had erupted at the beginning of the war, a typhus epidemic began to rage, particularly after the ghetto was sealed. The magnitude of the scourge exceeded all prior estimates. Patients lay in every corner. In some buildings, all tenants contracted the disease. Dr. Milejkowski instructed all the departments at the hospital to admit typhus patients only.[242] Sanitary conditions in the typhus ward were ghastly. Sometimes sixty typhus patients were admitted on a given day. Often a patient would wake up and find a corpse at his or her side.[243]

By order of the Germans, every case of typhus had to be reported, which led to the patient's hospitalization under conditions that were grim and even worse than at home. The cramped conditions at the hospital were among the factors that caused the outbreak to escalate.[244] When the epidemic exceeded the capacity of the building on Leszno St., a reshuffling of departments took place: The children's hospital returned to Leszno St. and typhus patients were transferred to Stawki. Each relocation was torment for staff and patients alike. The epidemic claimed victims in both populations.[245]

241 Lensky, *A Physician inside the Warsaw Ghetto*, p. 23.

242 Einhorn, "Harofe Begeto Varsha," p. 11; Judenrat report to Dr. Auerswald on the Warsaw Jewish quarter under the *Kommissar*'s rule, May 15, 1941–May 15, 1942, GFH, no. 3909.

243 Lensky, *A Physician inside the Warsaw Ghetto*, p. 103.

244 Einhorn, "Harofe Begeto Varsha," p. 11.

245 Gürfinkel-Glocer, "Goralo Shel Beit Haholim Tzhista," pp. 592–593.

Patient Overload at Czyste Hospital—June–July 1941[246]

Czyste Hospital Occupancy Rate[247] **Czyste Hospital Inpatients**[248]

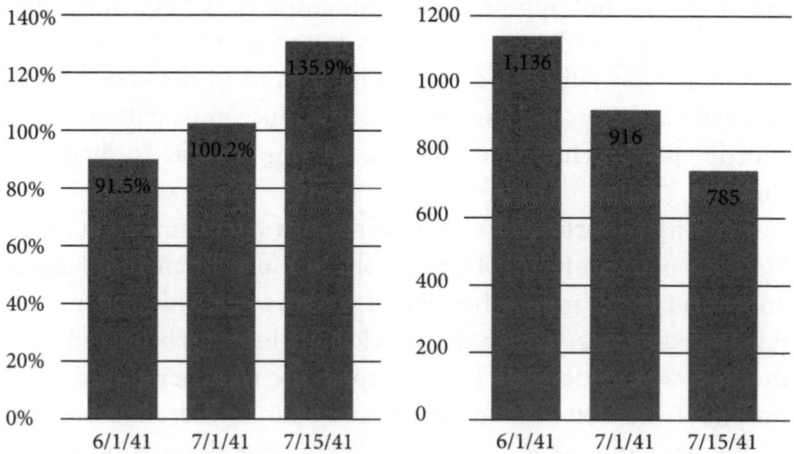

At the peak of the epidemic, Czyste Hospital was so burdened with patients that Dr. Hagen, the German physician who headed the Warsaw health care system, ordered the confiscation of half of the buildings on Prosta St. for use as isolation rooms. The ghetto had been constricted by then and this street was no longer within its confines. All departments, except for the surgery and gynecology wards, halted their work to make room for incoming typhus patients. The conditions, the overcrowding, the shortages, and the chances of contagion at the hospital were so severe that the ill would have been better off staying home.[249]

246 Trunk, "Epidemics and Mortality," pp. 102–103; report on mortality in the Warsaw Ghetto, AŻIH, ARI.223.

247 The graph was drawn from the report on mortality in the Warsaw ghetto, AŻIH, ARI.223; the data appears in Trunk, "Epidemics and Mortality," pp. 102–103.

248 Report on mortality in the Warsaw ghetto, AŻIH, ARI.223; Trunk, "Epidemics and Mortality," pp. 102–103.

249 Roland, *Courage under Siege*, p. 143.

Many typhus patients were concealed, not only from the Germans but from the Jews as well. The data that Czyste Hospital provided may have been accurate with respect to the facility, but they did not represent the situation elsewhere and offer only a general indication. There is no accurate data regarding the many who fell ill and died at home and in the streets. The hospital's statistics are also imprecise, because most patients died shortly after reaching the hospital, leaving no time to diagnose them.[250]

Trunk reported on the overcrowded conditions in Czyste Hospital in June–July 1941, when the typhus epidemic escalated and then peaked in October of that year. As the epidemic spread, more beds were required. By closing its internal medicine departments, which had become epidemic treatment wards, the hospital freed 500 beds for adults and 80 for children. However, as the epidemic spread, it was obvious that there would be a shortage of hospital beds for typhus patients. Therefore, some patients were sent home before they recovered. In June 1941, the hospital admitted 1,419 patients and discharged 947; in the first half of July, it received 1,073 and released 643. In June, high mortality—346 out of 1,419 inpatients, that is, 24.4 percent—made room for new patients.[251]

Mortality at the hospital, particularly among typhus patients, intensified severely. Of 959 typhus patients in June 1941, 176 died—18 percent. In the middle of July 1941, 153 out of 782 perished—19.5 percent. Many of those discharged died after leaving the hospital. Some were released only because of the lack of space, although their medical condition remained serious. Others died from starvation, after returning home. Therefore, the mortality rate among patients at the hospital was much higher than the aforementioned data would suggest. Among those with dysentery, death was nearly inevitable; all but 1 out of 27 died in June 1941.[252]

250 Ibid., p. 219.
251 Trunk, "Epidemics and Mortality," p. 103.
252 Ibid., p. 104.

The underground newspaper of the Bund, *Za Naszą i Waszą Wolność* (For Our Freedom and Yours), reported in August 1941 that people with typhus and dysentery had filled Czyste Hospital in such numbers that all other departments were discontinued there. Due to the lack of space, patients suffering pulmonary, cardiological, and neurological diseases could not be admitted to the hospital to receive medical care. The morbidity rate was so high that even when the entire Jewish hospital had become an infectious disease ward, it could not admit all the patients, because it lacked 2,000 beds.[253] The data from a Judenrat statistics department report provide an indication of the number of inpatients and the extent of morbidity at Czyste Hospital at the beginning and end of February 1942.[254]

At the beginning of February 1942, Czyste Hospital accommodated 1,020 patients in its various branches. By the end of that month, the inpatient load had declined by 8 percent. The number of typhus patients plunged by one-third and there were 40 percent fewer under observation. These data indicate a significant downward trend in the incidence of typhus. In contrast, the number of patients with typhoid fever quadrupled, possibly signaling the resurgence of this contagious disease, which had been quashed at the beginning of the war, before ghettoization. The group of those with other infectious diseases fell by 26 percent. Those under observation for these illnesses rose slightly by 3.5 percent.[255] This may imply that morbidity improved slightly, possibly due to the care that the hospital provided, despite the difficult conditions.

253 Blatman, *Geto Varsha—Sipur Itona'i*, p. 154.

254 Judenrat Statistics Department Report, no. 29, March 17, 1942, GFH, no. 11250, p. 10.

255 Ibid.

Patients at Czyste Hospital, 6/8 and 21 Stawki St., 1 and 109/111 Leszno St., and 4 Tłomackie St., February 1942[256]

Patient Breakdown	Feb. 1, 1942	Feb. 28, 1942
Typhus Patients	442	299
Typhus Patients, under Observation	80	47
Typhoid Fever Patients	—	—
Typhoid Fever Patients, under Observation	32	129
Patients with Other Contagious Diseases	68	50
Patients with Other Diseases	398	412
Total	**1,020**	**937**

Doctors who held senior positions in the ghetto accused the German authorities of having created, by their decrees, a lethal medical situation akin to that in the hospital and the ghetto. Prof. Ludwik Hirszfeld wrote that he himself, Dr. Israel Milejkowski, and Dr. Owsiej Bielenki had dared to draw up a document intended for the German authorities, stating candidly that the hospital could not admit all the patients in need of its services and that, under the circumstances, it would be better for the patients to be treated at home, if the conditions in their homes were reasonably adequate.[257]

Although responsibility for the medical situation and for all health-related issues, as for all matters, in fact, resided with the German authorities, harsh accusations were directed at

256 Ibid.

257 Hirszfeld, *The Story of One Life*, p. 215. See the memoranda about methods to combat the epidemic, evidently addressed to the Germans and probably written by Hirszfeld, YVA, M.10.AR.1/85. On the causes of typhoid fever in Warsaw and proposals on how to combat the illness, see AŻIH, ARI.85.

the Judenrat. In an anonymous letter to its chairman, doctors and public figures complained about the catastrophic state of the hospital: morbidity; hunger among the patients and staff; a shrinking budget; shortages of beds, linens, and underwear; poor hygiene; pilfering; staff cutbacks; appointments of people with connections; administrative and logistic mismanagement; and the failure to pay salaries. At the end of the letter, the authors proposed a set of corrective measures.[258]

> **To the Chairman of the Judenrat**:
>
> 1. **Public outcry against the frightening mortality rate among the Jewish population of Warsaw.**
> 2. **The tragic state of the hospital.**
>
> Even the statistics on funerals in the first half of this year suffice to illustrate the situation. There were 894 funerals in January of this year; 1,023 and 1,608 in February and March respectively; 2,062 in April; 3,818 in May; 4,290 in June; and more than 5,500 in July. These numbers are so significant that no explanation is required. It is necessary only to note that the main cause of this daunting mortality is a combination of hunger, the typhus epidemic, and dysentery.
>
> As for the state of the hospitals: **the mortality is a consequence of the tragic state of the hospitals under the management of the Judenrat.** Lest I be accused of exaggeration and deception, I will allow myself to quote several typical paragraphs from a letter that Dr. Stein, director of the hospital in Czyste Hospital, wrote in June of this year [1941] and forwarded to the Judenrat, under the heading "Reminders of the Current State of the Hospital." Dr. Stein wrote, "The hospital in Czyste has effectively ceased to be a hospital. It is not even a shelter, because a person

258 Anonymous public appeal from doctors and public figures concerning the state of the hospital, June 1941, YVA, M.10.AR.1/315.

who is ill and cannot afford medical assistance actually finds nothing there."

"**The feeding of patients at the hospital is a pipe dream**. The rations add up to around 700 calories per day, not even enough to sustain the body. There are inpatients who, unfortunately, must remain here for extended periods and who lack the means to obtain their own food. They become bloated due to starvation in the hospital and die very quickly. This is medical progress at the hospital, indeed[!] It is important to note that the hospital now receives 500 zlotys per day to cover all of its expenses and, even that, not every day.

"**A second pipe dream is the state of cleanliness of the hospital**. Patients often lie [in bed] without underwear, but new undergarments are not being sewn using the fabric that was purchased after encountering many problems, also because of a lack of means. There is also no money for thread. **There are not enough mattresses**; there is cloth to make mattresses, but not enough straw and material to fill them. Again, it is all due to a shortage of cash. The result: two patients lie in one bed and, worst of all, in the infectious diseases wards.

"The hospital has **few beds**. The epidemic continues and there are many cases that require surgical treatment. Beds have been added throughout the department, but **they lack bedding and mattresses**.

"Hundreds of additional new facts could be added—facts that speak for themselves. All lead to one conclusion: Our hospital today is not a hospital and it cannot continue to exist in this condition. Unless provisions are made for the maintenance of the hospital, even to a modest extent, it seems that it will be necessary to shut it down and not create pipe dreams. As it is, dozens of people are dying every day in the streets.

"If the hospital is to exist, conditions must be created so that patients will truly receive aid and care there.

Furthermore, appropriate conditions for the activities of the staff must be established because, for the time being, **the employees of the hospital are also bloated from hunger and are struggling along.**"

This is how the state of Czyste Hospital is described by its director. Is there any need for additional and more precise words to describe the tragedy of the hospital?

The description above lacks several details that cannot be ignored. First, it is worth emphasizing that the tragic reality is characterized by **the nonfunctioning of the Judenrat, the entity responsible for the hospital. The hospital's budget is in catastrophic condition**. When the Polish municipality was responsible for the hospital, the hospital received 223,457 zlotys per month. Today, under the Judenrat's management, the planned monthly budget is 209,231 zlotys, but only 50,000–60,000 have actually been disbursed, and it is no wonder that this does not suffice even for thread to sew underwear at the hospital. Moreover, the hospital staff's starvation wages have not been paid for months.

1. It is troubling that **the medical staff** at the hospital is being cut back as the epidemic is escalating.
2. As of June 1, 1940, the hospital had 389 maintenance workers. On June 1, 1941, with the hospital receiving 80–100 patients per day, 313 workers were employed, 77 fewer [than in the previous year].
3. **The management of the maintenance of the hospital is inefficient**, making the disorder at the institution all the worse. We have reliable information that the hospital director has commented about this more than once to the maintenance department. Inspectors sent by the Judenrat have found irregularities and even evasiveness on the part of the maintenance department. Nevertheless, the situation has remained the same and, if there have been any changes, they have been for the worse. Until recently, the maintenance of the hospital was entrusted to three managers, who ceaselessly

engaged in power struggles, and no one knew who was in charge of what regarding maintenance.
4. The situation in the area of **technical management** is much the same. **Those in charge of this do not work at the hospital** and are directly subordinate to the Judenrat.
5. Theft is a common phenomenon in the hospital. Underwear, linens, blankets, instruments, and medicines are being stolen. Last month, two microscopes were purloined. To this day, no one has thought about how to combat this plague. There were cases, one or two, in which the director of the hospital sued an employee for theft and, afterwards, the guilty party returned to the hospital at an even higher post.[259]
6. **Czyste Hospital is also catastrophically short of beds.** The heightened morbidity is a consequence of the epidemic. It is so steep that the Judenrat's medical committee thinks it is necessary to increase the number of hospital beds by about 3,000. According to another opinion, the isolation ward needs an additional 1,500 beds.

The problem of expanding the hospital and finding additional new buildings is currently under discussion. There is also talk of training at least 300 new nurses' aides.[260]

After describing the features of the tragedy, our consciences cannot remain silent and order us to take remedial measures. While we do not overestimate our capacity, we do not lack confidence.

Our groups of activists in the community, from ŻTOS and TOZ, have not lost faith in the Jewish population. We are building on this faith. We are aware that **the entire Judenrat is—and it is no secret—corrupt**. We do not wish to lose our faith in the **Jewish community**. Therefore, we **activists in the TOZ and CENTOS organizations have**

259 According to Dr. Lensky, hunger explained the spiraling increase in pilfering. See Lensky, *A Physician inside the Warsaw Ghetto*, pp. 23–24.

260 The letter also mentions problems at Bersohn and Bauman Children's Hospital.

decided to act on our own, and only then is there a chance for success.

In the meantime, we have prepared a basic program in three areas: (1) epidemic prevention activities, (2) the establishment of a public hospital for children and adults, including provision for its maintenance, (3) regular publication of information by the Judenrat about the hospital's problems, along with suggestions for remedial measures. We will also try to help Czyste Hospital to carry out these tasks. The first and the third points must be explained in greater depth.

The reason for the epidemic: The main cause appears to be the creation of an isolated and massively overcrowded Jewish neighborhood. The Judenrat's main role is to continue explaining to the German administration that this is the source of the epidemic and that it will only continue to get worse. Concurrently, it is necessary to demand that the German administration provide more resources for hygiene, more medicine, more bathing facilities, and to expand the hospitals. Along with these measures, community organizations should lead in taking preventive action.

Thought should be given to adding a public hospital that would engage in dealing not only with epidemics but also with internal diseases, skin diseases, and diseases of the nervous system, which is urgently needed. The departments to treat these illnesses are lacking, because most of the departments at Czyste Hospital have become infectious diseases wards. Apart from the typhus department and the pulmonology department, only two departments remain—surgery and obstetrics. There are no other departments. Should seriously ill patients, such as those with heart disease, kidney failure, and the like, remain without recourse, as is the current situation, because of the Health Department's directives?

In order to provide a better understanding of the situation, we quote several tragic statistics: the number of deaths from heart disease among the Jewish population of Warsaw was

> 1,434 in 1939; 2,309 in 1940, and 523 in the first two months of 1941—at this rate, we could expect 3,000 in 1941.
>
> We wish first **to create normal conditions at the hospital and to restore the situation that has been ruined by starvation and epidemics**. We turn to the chairman of the Judenrat and demand his assistance in attaining our goals. Our demands are based on precedents indicating that **in exceptional situations in which progress could not be made without the public's assistance, the chairman of the Judenrat turned to the public for the possibility of implementation**. Proof of this are the operations to feed the Jewish public, which rely on welfare organizations and not on the Judenrat.
>
> We will specify in precise terms the assistance that we are seeking as our activities proceed and as our needs become clearer. In the meantime, we require the following:
>
> 1. We ask the chairman of the Judenrat **to agree to the independent management of the activities of the** [Jewish self-help] organizations **ŻTOS and TOZ**.
> 2. We request authorization to receive several **buildings in order to organize a public hospital**.
> 3. We ask that **privately owned bathhouses, which are in Jewish neighborhoods and that could be made public**, be turned over to our management for our use.
> 4. We seek **the right to confiscate privately owned equipment** for the hospital's benefit.[261]

Evidently, senior physicians and public personalities who were well versed in all aspects of hospital affairs, as well as activists in the Jewish self-help organizations TOZ and CENTOS, supported by the Jewish Social Self-Help and the JDC, wrote this document. Some of them presumably worked at the hospitals. Their proposal reflects their great despair at the conditions at Czyste

261 Anonymous public appeal from doctors and public figures concerning the state of the hospital, June 1941, YVA, M.10.AR.1/315. Emphasis added by the author.

Hospital, because of the dire objective situation created by the Germans' decrees and because of the Judenrat's mismanagement. They accused the Judenrat of corruption and of inefficient and unsound management of the hospital. The writers' proposals for improvement attest to their identification with the Jewish aid and self-help organizations. However, the authors of the missive realized that without the cooperation of the chairman of the Judenrat, they would not be able to implement their alternative proposals. They requested authorization to manage their own activities on behalf of the hospitals through the offices of TOZ and CENTOS, and with the backing of the Judenrat. According to Trunk, Dr. Jakub Munwes and a group of prominent leaders signed the letter.[262]

Dr. Waller wrote that Dr. Munwes, director of the infectious diseases wards at the ghetto hospital, began to organize propaganda among young physicians directed against Dr. Stein's policy of favoring Christianized doctors in late 1941. According to Dr. Waller, the purpose of Dr. Munwes' propaganda was to induce the Judenrat to appoint new management at the hospital. Dr. Munwes did not find support for his idea among his colleagues. The doctors did not believe that such a revolt would improve the wretched situation at the hospital and they considered the staff of apostate Jews a decent group.[263]

Dr. Munwes issued another document in his capacity as a member of the hospital's Finance Committee, evidently on behalf of a large portion of the hospital staff. In a letter, written in April–May 1941, about four months after the hospital relocated to the ghetto, he censured the institution's unsound and scandalous

262 Trunk, "Epidemics and Mortality," p. 103. Dr. Jakub Munwes (1884–1943) completed his studies in 1925 and specialized in internal medicine. One of the most talented young doctors in the ghetto, he worked in the infectious diseases ward at Czyste Hospital between 1940 and 1943. He was one of the organizers of the uprising against the Germans and he maintained contact with the Polish resistance to smuggle ammunition into the ghetto. He was taken away to his death by the SS. According to Waller, he did not perish in the ghetto. He was evidently transported to Treblinka from the hospital on Gęsia St. in April 1943. See Wulman et al., *The Martyrdom of Jewish Physicians in Poland*, p. 422; Dr. Shmuel Stanisław Waller testimony, YVA, O.3/2358.

263 Dr. Shmuel Stanisław Waller testimony, YVA, O.3/2358.

conduct. He pointed out the extravagant and unnecessary number of hospital administrators, noting that while the bureaucratic headcount increased due to the partitioning of the hospital into several buildings in different locations, the real reason for this inefficiency was the desire to employ family members. Dr. Munwes charged that between thirty-five and forty families were employed for this reason. This complaint challenged a motion at a meeting of the Finance Committee to hire additional workers for the hospital administration.

Dr. Munwes proceeded to protest against what he called the injustice that took place in allocating housing to members of the hospital staff. The hospital had helped some of its employees to live on its premises. Its director, chief administrator, pharmacists, and others benefited from this assistance. Local doctors were exempted from any payment, and others were charged symbolic rent. Veteran staff had received apartments near the hospital. Since January 1940, the number of recipients of housing had increased. Some had received dwelling units within the hospital at no charge and, in return, supposedly, they were required to make renovations. Many of them benefited from the hospital's coal, gas, and electricity. Dr. Munwes considered this a public wrong in view of the ghastly conditions at the hospital—poverty, terrifying hunger, shortages of equipment and medicines, and the deactivation of departments, due to the lack of funds. He demanded an end to the phenomenon of providing housing.

He added that there was a grave shortage of linens and underwear, because the hospital had no laundry facilities and no budget for external services. The large number of inpatients and their grave condition made it increasingly necessary to procure additional undergarments and linens, and to change them frequently. There was a great deal of wear and tear, and the writer criticized the hospital administration for mishandling this objective and serious problem. The work of those in charge of laundry was inefficient and uncoordinated. The lack of control and of monitoring resulted in pilfering. When the hospital had moved to the ghetto, bedding and blankets had disappeared, and the staff members had not returned the mattresses that they had borrowed.

In half a year, about 5,000 items of underwear and linens had disappeared, and others had worn out.

Dr. Munwes complained that the heating in the departments did not work and that sanitation was not observed strictly. On the other hand, he praised the devotion of the department directors, the pharmacists, and the nurses, who had salvaged expensive equipment, bandages, and medicines, when the hospital was transferred to the ghetto. He also wrote that the X-ray equipment was not in use at the hospital building on Stawki St., ostensibly because of the lack of space and money. However, he claimed that it would have been possible to find a place for it, if one of the apartments occupied by the inflated bureaucracy had been vacated, and the renovation money had been used for public purposes. The writer emphasized that the injustices committed at the hospital were not due to objective factors caused by the occupation—hunger, poverty, and deprivation—but to insensitivity and disregard of the public's exigencies. In his opinion, it was possible to solve these problems through internal resources.[264]

Available documentation does not indicate how the Judenrat responded to the criticism directed against it with respect to the hospital. However, Ringelblum described one of the repercussions in his diary—Dr. Munwes was ordered to report to the disciplinary tribunal in the ghetto for the "crime" of publishing a memorandum containing trenchant criticism of the Jewish hospital's activity.

> Dr. Schipper's[265] defense of Dr. Munwes before the Judenrat's disciplinary tribunal made a great impression. Dr. Munwes was accused of publishing a mimeographed memorandum containing mordant criticism of the operation of the Jewish hospital. Dr. Munwes revealed only a small part of the truth

264 Letter from Dr. Jakub Munwes to the Czyste Hospital Administration Committee, May 31, 1941, AŻIH, ARI.7; Dr. Shmuel Stanisław Waller testimony, YVA, O.3/2358.

265 Dr. Yitzhak-Ignacy Schipper (1884–1943) was a noted Jewish historian, a member of the Sejm, a well-known political functionary, a member of the Po'alei Tziyon Party, and a holder of degrees in law and philosophy and a PhD in the humanities. Ringelblum, *Ktavim Aharonim*, pp. 86–95.

> about the appalling sanitary conditions in the hospital, which the inpatients were fleeing, because they could not tolerate the situation. However, his exposure of the corruption and the moral decline besetting the Judenrat's apparatus was not to the liking of the public leadership and, accordingly, legal proceedings were brought against him. Thanks to Dr. Schipper's lethal critique, Dr. Munwes was cleared of the affair unscathed.[266]

Ringelblum's remarks imply that the Judenrat had attempted to quash the harsh criticism, and the prosecution of Dr. Munwes suggests that expressing criticism involved an element of personal danger.

Along with the criticism of the Judenrat, the main problem in the hospital's functioning was the lack of funds for maintenance. Failure to meet the payroll, which sapped the staff's ability to persevere under the ghetto conditions, led to repeated threats to strike. In the middle of July 1941, about eight months after ghettoization, a delegation of about thirty hospital employees gathered at the Judenrat offices and made such a commotion in the corridors that the Ordnungsdienst (the Jewish ghetto police) had to intervene and evict them. In a meeting that Czerniaków then held with three representatives, he explained that he was trying to obtain a loan to increase payments to the staff. The hospital workers exerted so much pressure that they prevented Dr. Israel Milejkowski, director of the Health Department, from leaving the hospital offices, as long as their salaries were not paid. Senior health officials, including Dr. Stein, director of Czyste Hospital, and Dr. Braude-Heller, head of the children's hospital, stood up to Czerniaków and tried to force him to meet the payroll once and for all. Czerniaków explained that, until he knew what would be the source of the funds to make the payments and as long as he was subject to pressure and threats, he would not submit to their demands.

266 Ibid., pp. 92–93.

Czerniaków appointed and dispatched a four-person panel to continue the negotiations and settle the labor dispute: the head of the Judenrat hospitals department, Ignacy Fliederbaum, former administrative director of the Jewish hospital; Hornsztejn, veteran secretary general of the Judenrat; Nachum Remba, a senior official in the Judenrat administration; and Izrael First, who was in charge of the Economy Division in the ghetto.[267] Although they reassured those assembled, Czerniaków wrote, "Tomorrow, however, we will have to pay out over 100,000 zlotys." The next day, Czerniaków ordered a payment of 120,000 zlotys to the hospital staff, evidently at the expense of other budget items and by taking a loan from the Labor Brigade and the ZZ, the Judenrat's provision and supply agency.[268] In the course of November 1941, a delegation of hospital workers again stationed itself at the Judenrat offices; this time Czerniaków promised to pay 200,000 zlotys.[269] A week later, the workers again threatened to strike, because they had received only half of the promised funds.[270] The budget problems steadily worsened and, two months later, in January 1942, Czerniaków held a fundraising rally for the hospital.[271]

Period 3: From the *Grossaktion* in July 1942 to the Hospital *Aktion* in September 1942

Shortly before the deportations from Warsaw began, after a year and a half of efforts, all three of the infectious diseases wards in Czyste Hospital at 6–8 Stawki St. and the medical treatment facility at 1 Leszno St. resumed their mission. The wards were renovated and equipped with modern facilities and medical instruments that had been lacking until then, and the hospital became an important

267 Izrael First was the administrator of the Jewish Student House before the war. He was about thirty years old at the beginning of the German occupation. First was killed in the ghetto by the Jewish underground in November, 1942, for collaborating with the Germans. See, for example, Czerniaków, *The Warsaw Diary*, pp. 101–102.

268 Czerniaków, *The Warsaw Diary*, p. 258.

269 Ibid., p. 298.

270 Ibid., p. 300.

271 Ibid., p. 314.

medical institution, and even a scientific and teaching institute. In addition to treating the ill, a great deal of time and effort were devoted to scientific research, especially on typhus, hunger, and tuberculosis, and to training doctors and medical students.[272]

On July 22, the eve of the Ninth of Av, notices of the decree that the Jews had to leave Warsaw and travel to the eastern subdistricts, signed by the Judenrat, were posted around the ghetto. At the time, persons working for the Germans or in German-supervised workplaces and employees of community and social relief institutions were exempt from the requirement.[273] Czyste Hospital operated under ghetto conditions until July 22, 1942. According to Dr. Stein, although its staff was not evicted along with the population at large, the hospital ceased to function. All the departments and laboratories were demolished, as was the library. On July 22–23, the hospital was forced to evacuate its building on Stawki St., which became a center where Jews were concentrated ahead of transport.[274]

The underground newspaper *Wiadomości* (News) provided a detailed account of the evacuation of the Jewish activity.

> On July 21 at 1:30, at 6 Stawki St., in the absence of the director of the hospital, the administrative director of the hospital, Ignacy Stabholz, was taken hostage. On July 22 at 11 A.M., the director of the hospital was summoned by the [Judenrat] chairman, Czerniaków, and was ordered to evacuate the hospital at once, by 4 P.M. the next day…the director of Czyste Hospital was responsible for implementing the order. The hospital administration decided to transfer patients with contagious diseases to the hospital at 80 Leszno St. and all the others to 1 Leszno St. There were 761 patients at Stawki St. Because of the lack of vehicles, carts were brought in from the Aryan side and the eviction began at a crazy pace…due

272 Blatman, *Geto Varsha—Sipur Itona'i*, p. 418.

273 Lensky, *A Physician inside the Warsaw Ghetto*, p. 120; Abraham Lewin, *A Cup of Tears: A Diary of the Warsaw Ghetto* (London: Fontana-Collins, 1988), pp. 145–146; Kaplan, *Scroll of Agony*, pp. 379–380.

274 Trunk, "Epidemics and Mortality," p. 105; Lewin, *A Cup of Tears*, pp. 145–146.

> to the very tight deadline that had been imposed. The entire medical, nursing, and auxiliary staff were mobilized for the evacuation work.... The guard unit of the Ordnungsdienst and 100 people sent by the Labor Office also worked. By midnight on the first day of the evacuation [July 21], the building at 8 Stawki St. had been evacuated and the building at 6 Stawki St. was vacated by 4 P.M. the next day.
>
> In the meantime, the administration managed to obtain an extension of the evacuation deadline...the tidy and clean buildings were turned over to the authorities on July 24 at midnight. The equipment was taken to the buildings at 1 Leszno St., 80 Leszno St., 12 Elektoralna St., and 3 Dzika St. After the evacuation was completed, the hospital was reorganized under the new conditions. At 1 Leszno St., it was necessary to make room for more than 700 beds instead of 350 beds. In addition to the existing departments, three internal medicine wards were set up. At 80 Leszno St., infectious diseases wards were established. Most of the patients at the time required surgical care, chiefly due to gunshot wounds and internal diseases, e.g., severe cases of heart disease, etc. The difficult work of organization was compounded by additional orders, such as two staff cutbacks, the transfer of hospital workers to new quarters, and blockades on Leszno St., although apart from a few exceptional cases, the representatives of the authorities that had put up the barriers did not enter the hospital grounds.[275]

From that time on, Jews caught on the streets in the ghetto were held in the vacated hospital building on Stawki St., which was located near the assembly point for transport. Ghastly scenes were observed there. Desperate people stood outside the building, calling out to their loved ones as frightened, desperate prisoners pressed themselves against the windows. The detainees contracted dysentery, and there were no medicines for them. No Jew, including

275 Blatman, *Geto Varsha—Sipur Itona'i*, pp. 418–419; report from the hospital and the postal service after the *Aktion*, 1942, AŻIH, ARII.280.

members of the Jewish police, was allowed to approach the former hospital. However, a medical aid committee was set up on the Umschlagplatz and its doctors were allowed to access the building. As the number of prisoners increased, they were no longer taken inside and were left on the plaza under the open sky.

The Germans' collaborators, which included Latvians, Lithuanians, and Ukrainians, who were guarding the Jews, were taken to another building for fear of contracting the contagious diseases that had spread among the Jewish detainees on the first floor of the building. They guarded only the periphery of the former hospital, but this did not prevent them from paying the Jews surprise nighttime visits, particularly to abuse Jewish women. The bodies of those who died in the building remained among the living, who used them as "beds" so that they would not have to lie on the growing heap of filth. The fortunate few who possessed poison took it to terminate their lives. Each time a transport of Jews was led out of the building to the railroad cars, a new group of people who had arrived at the plaza was tasked with cleaning the filthy rooms and evacuating the dead—usually with their bare hands.[276]

The evacuation notice, which the Germans had dictated and the Judenrat had been forced to sign, included a detailed list of categories of people who were exempted, such as the staff of the Jewish hospitals, members of the disinfection teams, and inpatients who were unfit to travel. It appears that the exemption of the ill was intended to dupe the ghetto population into thinking that it would be treated with consideration and should not fear that the deportees would be shipped to their deaths. The exemption included the close family members of the exempt, their spouses, and their children.[277] Dr. Chaim Einhorn wrote that the doctors and the medical staff were nearly the last on the list of Jews earmarked for deportation.

Czyste Hospital continued to exist in an organized manner until the end of January 1943, although all the other public and

276 Turkow, *Hayo Hayta Varsha Yehudit*, pp. 120–122.

277 Gutman, *The Jews of Warsaw*, pp. 203–204; Lensky, *A Physician inside the Warsaw Ghetto*, pp. 123–124.

medical institutions had been liquidated. Witnesses to the Nazis' actions spent their days in the hospital, awaiting the destruction of their institutions. At night, bombardments in the vicinity of the hospital building kept them awake.[278] Even though the hospital building was not besieged until the day of the selection, September 6, many doctors were deported, as were others who were captured in the street or in private dwellings.[279] Nobody wanted to leave the hospital at this time. There were rumors that the liquidation operations had bypassed the hospital. During the six weeks of the selections, the hospital was spared, although the Germans and the Ukrainians would enter the building. For this reason, the hospital employees attempted to save others, and the beleaguered ghetto inhabitants who were aware of this put pressure on the hospital administration to save them by allowing them to pose as patients to obtain asylum in the building.[280]

The hospital had to admit to its building on Leszno St. fugitives from the *Aktionen*, as well as hundreds of patients who had been evicted from other hospitals. Dr. Adolf Polisiuk, a gynecologist at Czyste Hospital, described what transpired at 1 Leszno St., where he and his wife were staying. Along with three other colleagues and their wives, they had been given a bed in the maternity ward in the room of the physicians on duty.[281] The hospital looked more like a large camp than a medical facility. More than 1,000 people were jammed in the building, which before the deportations had accommodated 400 patients at the most.

Before the *Aktion*, the hospital at 1 Leszno was known for its therapeutic character. It had only three active surgical wards: obstetrics and gynecology; ear, nose, and throat; and ophthalmology. After the patients were evacuated from the

278 Einhorn, "Harofe Begeto Varsha," p. 9; Lensky, *A Physician inside the Warsaw Ghetto*, pp. 169–170.

279 Dr. Adolf Polisiuk diary, GFH, no. 3182.

280 Dr. Shmuel Stanisław Waller testimony, YVA, O.3/2358; Gürfinkel-Glocer, "Goralo Shel Beit Haholim Tzhista," p. 594; Lensky, *A Physician inside the Warsaw Ghetto*, pp. 169–170; Einhorn, "Harofe Begeto Varsha," p. 9; Dr. Chaim Einhorn testimony, YVA, O.3/1836.

281 Dr. Adolf Polisiuk diary, GFH, no. 3182.

building on Stawki St. to 1 and 80 Leszno St., the institution became a general hospital that had to admit patients referred to it from the children's hospital on Śliska St. and from the infectious diseases hospital on Stawki St. Contagious patients lay alongside those who had surgical and internal problems, mothers in childbirth, and women with gynecological troubles. Patients from entire wards, such as those for internal medicine, lay in the corridors, their beds placed next to each so tightly that they seriously impeded the circulation of doctors among them.

Apart from the patients, most staff members along with their near kin—about 400–500 people altogether—spent their nights in the hospital, because of the danger that lurked in the streets. They occupied places off to the side, such as doctors' rooms, offices, laboratories, operating rooms, the courtyard, and any vacant space on the floor.[282] Every family brought a few belongings in suitcases and boxes to the hospital that now served as a hotel. For lack of space, doctors sometimes could house only one family member and thus lost family members who were not granted a hideout. Some staff members and doctors sent their families out to actually work on the chance that this might save them. However, jobs were difficult to obtain, and the hospital administration managed to procure only twenty posts at Szulc's factory.[283]

Although at some point family members were no longer allowed to spend the night in the hospital, they continued to hide there during the day. Everyone attempted to hold on to the hospital building with all his might. Rumors circulated that some of the population would remain in the ghetto, albeit in a severely reduced area, and that, presumably, the hospital would have the right to exist in that area. Thus, the people maintained the delusional hope that most of them would survive.[284] In early September, after more than 200,000 Jews had been sent to Treblinka, the Nazis had not yet harmed the hospital. They evidently feared being exposed to contagious diseases and wanted to trick the Jews into imagining

282 Ibid.; Gürfinkel-Glocer, "Goralo Shel Beit Haholim Tzhista," pp. 593–594.
283 Lensky, *A Physician inside the Warsaw Ghetto*, pp. 125, 128, 136–138.
284 Dr. Adolf Polisiuk diary, GFH, no. 3182.

that they would resume their normal lives after the *Aktion*. However, there was a palpable change in the atmosphere in the hospital, as described by Dr. Mordechai Lensky.

> From the hospital, we saw long processions almost daily; hatless men, women in summer frocks holding little children in their arms...A deadly silence then fell upon the hospital... family members, devoid of any rights, just hid inside closets and lay low for hours.[285]

There were many suicides in the wards. At this time, very few new patients who were injured during the *Aktionen* arrived and the hospital had little to do. There was a prevailing atmosphere of boredom fraught with fear.[286] Ghetto life worsened with each passing day. The Germans began to abduct people from their homes—sometimes individually and at other times in groups—and to murder them in the courtyards.[287] The atmosphere in the hospital was tense and the mood agitated.[288]

As the *Aktionen* continued, the Judenrat was required to reduce the hospital staff and to revoke the family members' right to remain in the ghetto. Therefore, it was necessary to acquire certificates that would grant them the right to remain, and many attempted to secure permits to work in German workshops, thinking that only employees of these facilities would survive in Warsaw. Some doctors left the hospital to work in clinics in the Germans' factories, believing that they would be better off there. People paid thousands of zlotys for a work permit.[289]

When the staff cutbacks began, attempts were made to save the nurses and students who lost their right to remain in the hospital when they were laid off. The idea came up to arrange false marriages through mutual agreement between the single students working at the hospital and the young women. Each new couple

285 Lensky, *A Physician inside the Warsaw Ghetto*, p. 170.
286 Ibid., pp. 135–139.
287 Gürfinkel-Glocer, "Goralo Shel Beit Haholim Tzhista," p. 593.
288 Lensky, *A Physician inside the Warsaw Ghetto*, p. 121.
289 Ibid., pp. 127–128.

received an appropriate certificate bearing a rabbi's signature and, thus, as lawful wives of sanctioned workers, young women were allowed to stay in the hospital. The Germans appeared to fall for the ruse but, in the end, it turned out that a husband's permit did not protect his wife.[290]

On August 13, 1942, the authorities ordered an additional summary evacuation. The patients at 80 Leszno St. were ordered to move to the old hospital building at Stawki St., which had been serving as an assembly point for deportations since the beginning of the *Aktionen*. The pipes in the building had been damaged, and the entire building was filthy and looked like a garbage dump. When the staff members reached the Umschlagplatz, their work became exceedingly difficult and hazardous. They repeatedly had to push their way through masses of deportees, who packed the square in front of the hospital. The authorities often entered the hospital to check if any designated deportees were hiding there.[291]

According to Dr. Marek Balin, on August 15, 1942, the Germans demanded reducing the number of people remaining in the hospital building on Leszno St. to 150. This forced the doctors to carry out an agonizing selection and to send 300 patients to the Umschlagplatz. A committee of three Jewish doctors had to decide who would be included in the list of deportees. "The hospital sank into depression; everyone understood the tragic situation—Jews themselves had to expedite the process. Panic broke out among the doctors in the hospital."[292]

Period 4: From the Hospital *Aktion* in September 1942 to January 1943

A cruel ten-day *Aktion* called the *Kociol* (cauldron) began on September 6, 1942.[293] At 1:30 A.M., a cable arrived from the

290 Ibid., pp. 138–139, 141, 163, 166–168.

291 Blatman, *Geto Varsha—Sipur Itona'i*, p. 419.

292 Dr. Marek Balin testimony, YVA, O.3/441; see Offer, *Haluk Lavan Bageto*, appendix A.6, pp. 521–523.

293 Ringelblum, *Notes from the Warsaw Ghetto*, p. 312; Israel Gutman, Avraham Wein, Shlomo Netzer, Gideon Greif, eds., *Toldot Yehudei Varsha Mireshitam*

German headquarters in charge of population transfer. Addressed to all institutions, shops, and inhabitants of the Warsaw ghetto, it ordered them to leave their dwellings and workplaces, without luggage, and to report to the square formed by the buildings on the streets Gęsia-Zamenhofa, Gęsia-Stawki, and Smocza by 10 A.M. The hospital administration was instructed to vacate immediately the branches of the hospital that had not yet been evacuated at 1 Leszno St. and 12 Elektoralna St., also by 10 A.M. The patients were to move to 6 Stawki St., along with some of the staff, and some of the staff was to make its way to Zamenhofa St. All the deportees were to leave their dwellings unlocked and they were advised to provision themselves with three days' worth of food. It was announced that those found on Leszno St. after 12 P.M. would be shot on the spot. An extension of the deadline to 3 P.M. that day was obtained. Tremendous panic broke out. No one knew the purpose and meaning of the decree, and there were many rumors circulating. The most common was that there would be a general selection of the entire remaining population of the ghetto, which numbered around 180,000. After the selection, 35,000 people would remain and, presumably, that would be the end of the deportations from the Warsaw ghetto.

The doctors began to move their patients to 6 Stawki St.—approximately 1,000 people in three hours. Several doctors preferred to leave the hospital willingly and to join their families. Patients in various wards tried to consult with the staff, who did not know what advice to give. Those with relatively minor injuries or fictitious illnesses dressed and left in search of places to hide. The staff escorted ambulatory patients in groups of 50 to 100. Those who were bedridden—following surgery or in serious condition—were transported to the new location in groups of 8 to 10 in carts provided by the Judenrat. The doctors helped to load 300 people and the building was vacated quickly, leaving empty beds and clothing strewn everywhere. By 4 P.M., the remaining

Ve'ad Yameinu (History of the Jews of Warsaw from Their Beginnings to the Present) (Hebrew) (Jerusalem: Keter and Association of Warsaw Jewry in Israel, 1991), p. 229.

patients and staff members had left the hospital, leaving all the equipment behind. Doctors and their families, carrying nothing but rucksacks, formed a line and marched under a Red Cross flag to Zamenhofa St., with the director of the hospital leading the way.[294]

The next morning, there were more than 1,100 patients at the hospital building on 6 Stawki, where there had previously been 273. Space for more than 1,100 beds had to be made, and the ill lay along the walls of wards that resembled animal shelters. At 5 P.M. on September 10, the hospital was instructed to send the patients to the Umschlagplatz. By the end of the day, 156 had been transferred there.[295] Some of the staff members who marched to Zamenhofa St. arrived voluntarily at the hospital on Stawki St. to treat the ill who were lying in the street and in the mud with exposed and unbandaged wounds. All that night, they moved the sick indoors and lay them on the floor in wards that no longer had beds. The next day, the doctors and nurses prepared the operating room. Additional doctors from the assembly point on Zamenhofa St. joined the staff on Stawki St. and reported that *SS-Untersturmführer* Karl Georg Brandt, the Nazi in charge of destroying the ghetto, had given an order to leave behind a few members of the medical team to treat the laborers and workers.[296]

When the hospital staff were ordered to report for inspection, this caused a commotion. The staff members realized that those who would not receive a "life number" from Dr. Stein, director of the hospital, would be doomed to death.[297] The staff then conducted a selection that involved acute ethical dilemmas and heart-rending scenes. The fate of hundreds of medical personnel was sealed. Following the selection, a new phase of life under the constant

294 Dr. Adolf Polisiuk diary, GFH, no. 3182; Dr. Shmuel Stanisław Waller testimony, YVA, O.3/2358; Blatman, *Geto Varsha—Sipur Itona'i*, pp. 419–420.

295 Blatman, *Geto Varsha-Sipur Itona'i*, pp. 419–420; report from the hospital and the postal service after the *Aktion*, 1942, AŻIH, ARII.280.

296 Gürfinkel-Glocer, "Goralo Shel Beit Haholim Tzhista," p. 599.

297 Dr. Shmuel Stanisław Waller testimony, YVA, O.3/2358; Lensky, *A Physician inside the Warsaw Ghetto*, pp. 178–179.

threat of deportation to death began.[298] The surviving community workers, including the doctors, were forced to clean apartments, sweep streets, remove debris, and perform similar tasks.[299] At this time, many of them did not have "life numbers," meaning that they had become homeless outlaws, who feared a new *Aktion* and deportation to Treblinka.[300]

On the days that selections were conducted, the situation at Czyste Hospital, which was adjacent to the Umschlagplatz, was terrifying. On the few streets where all the remaining Jews had gathered, the Nazis administered brutal beatings and shot many people to death. In the hospital, the team of surgeons worked uninterruptedly, removing bullets, sewing lacerations, and saving lives. Those who had been evicted to this hospital—adults and children from the children's hospital—lay neglected in the unheated wards. They relieved themselves where they lay, remaining in a putrid mire of urine and feces. The staff were ordered to carry out yet another selection: one person in ten would remain in the hospital, while the others would be sent to the East. Some of the doctors could not face the ghastly task of selection. The operating room worked relentlessly; the equipment was disinfected continuously. Many casualties lay on the operating table and the stench of fresh blood filled the air. The doctors settled into a routine work mode, trying not to think about it at all.[301]

The medical teams made rescue attempts on the Umschlagplatz. They set up a clinic in front of the barbed-wire fences—two small rooms equipped with beds and clean sheets to receive the ill. In fact, there were no patients. There were only people who had been rescued from deportation at the Umschlagplatz. They tarried at the clinic until there was an opportunity to send them back to the ghetto. In most cases, they were taken in an ambulance that was made available to the

298 Dr. Adolf Polisiuk diary, GFH, no. 3182.

299 Ringelblum, *Yoman Vereshimot*, p. 419.

300 Lewin, *A Cup of Tears*, p. 185.

301 Edelman, *The Ghetto Fights*, p. 50; Roland, *Courage under Siege*, pp. 91, 212. On the medical work that took place under these conditions and its attendant ethical dilemmas, see Chapter 10 of this book.

medical crews.[302] The vehicle shuttled between the hospital for infectious diseases, near the Umschlagplatz, and the surgical wards on Leszno St. A group of nurses received permission to bring water to the detainees, who were waiting for their turn to board the train. The nurses concealed the uniforms of nurses and of other caregivers under their own uniforms, and used them to take doctors, both men and women, and, at times, other detainees, to the hospital supposedly for "surgery." The lives of these nurses, like those whom they rescued, were in constant danger.[303] Opportunities to leave the Umschlagplatz did arise but they were a drop in the ocean to the thousands in need of rescue. Marek Edelman and Dr. Einhorn wrote that the Germans themselves opened a small clinic on the Umschlagplatz for emergency cases in order to mislead the Jews before placing them aboard the death trains.

The medical teams at the Leszno St. clinic wore white smocks and held work permits. The team on duty, which had to show the SS guards a group permit, switched places with another crew each day. Noticing that the guards did not always count the people heading out, groups on their way out tried to add others who had been designated for transport. In this manner, they saved family members, friends, or public figures who had been captured. These fortunate few were dressed in white smocks and led on foot or taken in the ambulance past the SS guard. The white smock became a symbol of life. Nurses carried children and stated that they were their own. There is no doubt that they risked their lives by doing this.[304]

For unknown reasons, the Germans allowed sending the elderly from the Umschlagplatz to the cemetery or to the geriatric hospital. Thus, the Jews managed to take away living and healthy people from the plaza in the ambulance or in coffins. When the Germans began to check the ambulance and

302 Turkow, *Hayo Hayta Varsha Yehudit*, pp. 122–124.

303 Gürfinkel-Glocer, "Goralo Shel Beit Haholim Tzhista," pp. 599, 601.

304 Einhorn, "Harofe Begeto Varsha," p. 10.

the state of health of the "patients," the nursing students who were working there devised a new method of rescue. In a small room behind the clinic, using neither anesthesia nor sedatives of any kind, they broke the legs of old people by laying their limbs on a log and fracturing them with another block of wood. They did all this while wearing the white smocks of exemplary nursing students.[305]

Noemi Szac-Wajnkranc recalled being approached by two men in white smocks as she waited in a group on the Umschlagplatz. "We're from the hospital," the men told the Lithuanians who were guarding them. "We want to take a few patients away for bandaging. Why should you have to deal with them in the railroad cars?" The men in white then turned to her, "Stand up fast, wipe the blood off your face, put on a white smock, and take this document. Your name is Maria Tass. What's your name? It's Maria Tass. You're a medic." "That evening," Noemi Szac-Wajnkranc recounted, "I left the Umschlagplatz as Maria Tass."[306] Jonas Turkow called the "medical aid" that a handful of doctors and nurses managed to offer a "rescue brigade." The clinic, he claimed, was a great irony; it proved that even the steady, exacting Germans could be deceived, if only for a short while.[307]

The nurses risked their lives to rescue Jewish children from the transport plaza. Ala Gołąb-Grynberg is a case in point. Under the broad-hemmed gown of her nurse's uniform, she spirited children away from the Umschlagplatz, giving them sleeping pills to keep them from crying, aware that if she were checked, two

305 Ibid.; Dr. Shmuel Stanisław Waller testimony, YVA, O.3/2358. In her personal testimony, Shulamit Tzeder, a survivor of the Warsaw ghetto, described the attempts by doctors and medical teams to save the elderly by breaking one of their legs. Tzeder was the daughter of Dr. Maurycy Brandwein, a surgeon at Czyste Hospital before the war and in the ghetto. She had vivid memories of a dilemma that arose when she was ten years old concerning the rescue of her grandmother, who was living with her family in the ghetto. They broke one of her grandmother's legs and then took her to the hospital. Dr. Brandwein perished in the "doctors' bunker" during the uprising.

306 Szac-Wajnkranc, *Halaf Im Ha'esh*, pp. 77–78.

307 Turkow, *Hayo Hayta Varsha Yehudit*, pp. 122–124; Einhorn, "Harofe Begeto Varsha," p. 10.

Jews would be killed.[308] After each day's train departed, Dr. Adina Blady Szwajger hurriedly gathered up children whose mothers had abandoned them. Bribing the Ukrainian guards with vodka, she managed to place the forsaken youngsters in the hospital. She sent them in a carriage toward the city, not knowing who would receive them there. Several of them returned to the same place.[309]

The clinic just off the Umschlagplatz had a staff of several doctors and approximately forty nurses.[310] Ringelblum depicts the nurses' feats as acts of heroism. "The heroic nurses—the only ones who saved people from deportation without [asking for] money...Nurses' headkerchiefs saved hundreds of professionals, employees of the Jewish Council."[311] Nachum Remba, secretary of the Judenrat, and nurse Ala Gołąb-Grynberg headed this group of doctors and merciful nurses. They proved that the German annihilation machine could be resisted, and that hundreds could be rescued from the Umschlagplatz every day. This display of valor by the medical teams on the plaza was the last phase of the great Jewish medical endeavor in the ghetto—a reflection of the medical teams' devoted feats from the beginning of the war to the *Grossaktion*.[312]

The massive operation that sent most of the Jews of Warsaw to their annihilation lasted nearly two months, from July 22 to September 12, 1942. At 11 A.M. on September 12, an order to deport the patients arrived and representatives of the authorities, along with members of the Ordnungsdienst, entered the grounds of the hospital near the Umschlagplatz. Nine hundred and fifty patients and fifty staff members were deported, and the hospital was liquidated.[313] Dr. Tursz commented on the tragedy.

308 Turkow, *Hayo Hayta Varsha Yehudit*, pp. 123–124, 140–144.

309 Ibid.

310 Lensky, *A Physician inside the Warsaw Ghetto*, pp. 132–133.

311 Ringelblum, *Notes from the Warsaw Ghetto*, p. 311.

312 Turkow, *Hayo Hayta Varsha Yehudit*, pp. 122–124; Einhorn, "Harofe Begeto Varsha," p. 10.

313 Blatman, *Geto Varsha—Sipur Itona'i*, p. 420. That month, Ringelblum wrote about this matter in his diary, noting that 1,000 patients had been transferred from the hospital on Stawki St. to the Umschlagplatz. Ringelblum, *Yoman Vereshimot*, p. 418; Lewin, *A Cup of Tears*, p. 180.

> The calamitous fate in this misfortune belonged to the hospital. A separate chapter should be written on this topic, and I will not produce it alone. I lack the words to describe the immensity of the disaster, and I fear that I will not adequately capture the terror, the agony, and the sadism of the German tormentors.[314]

At the end of the *Grossaktion*, the Jewish quarter remained without a hospital. Persons who needed inpatient care due to injury at the "shops" and other workplaces, or because of illness, had nowhere to go. On September 17, a clinic was opened on Stawki St. Although it gave its patients the sense of being cared for and treated, it was a mere, two-room, temporary setup that was too cramped to accommodate all those who turned to it for aid.[315]

An additional provisional infirmary with twelve beds and a bandaging and surgery room was established at 6 Pawia St. Dr. Josef Stein, with the assistance of Dr. Kobylinski who mediated between the German authorities and the representatives of the ghetto, obtained permission to open a Jewish hospital at 6–8 Gęsia St. Two buildings that had served as textile warehouses were connected and readied for their new use. The entire staff participated in cleaning the premises, and small wards were established over a two-week period—internal medicine, infectious diseases, two surgical wards, and pediatrics—which were set up in three small rooms on the first floor. Operating rooms were installed under primitive conditions, and the staff were housed in the rear of the building and nearby at 24 Franciszkańska St. and 48 Gęsia St. Concurrently, the construction of a bunker on the ground floor and the first floor to hide patients and staff was begun. This was the third and final venue of Czyste Hospital in the ghetto. About 800 patients were accommodated there this time. Medicines were available and surgical procedures were still performed sporadically, largely in cases of emergency, but the number of people dwindled

314 Dr. Moshe Tursz testimony, YVA, O.3/438, p. 16.

315 Gürfinkel-Glocer, "Goralo Shel Beit Haholim Tzhista," p. 602; Roland, *Courage under Siege*, p. 92.

as successive *Aktionen* reduced the ghetto population. Most employees of Czyste Hospital were no longer alive.[316]

When the typhus epidemic broke out again in late October 1942, the medical staff was in a desperate situation, because nurses, sanitation people, technicians, and others had been sent to the Umschlagplatz and then to their deaths in Treblinka. During the night shift, one nurse was responsible for hundreds of patients.[317] The number of patients grew with each passing day, particularly in the surgery and the infectious diseases wards. The staff worked under the strain of intense anxiety, fearing that the SS would enter and take the patients—along with members of the staff, as sometimes happened—to the Umschlagplatz.[318] Thus, they continued to work with devotion and trepidation. "At the time of the selections," Sabina Gürfinkel-Glocer testified,

> The Germans first took away the ill. What mattered to us was to give the patients whatever we could…no one had any hope of surviving. That is how the members of the medical team spent their days, continually gripped with fear as they tended patients and their families.[319]

The nurses conferred with the chief nurse, Fried, to consider possibilities of placing ambulatory patients in hiding. These were a special type of patients. Some had leaped from trains during deportation and had sustained severe head, facial, and/or limb injuries. The SS and the Ukrainians had shot others, usually in the abdomen or the head. Most died shortly after reaching the hospital. The nurses tried to put those who were able to get out of bed to work cleaning the ward, because gangs of Germans and their collaborators who occasionally burst into the hospital murdered the bedridden first.

316 Gürfinkel-Glocer, "Goralo Shel Beit Haholim Tzhista," p. 602; Blatman, *Geto Varsha—Sipur Itona'i*, p. 420; Dr. Shmuel Stanisław Waller testimony, YVA, O.3/2358.

317 Roland, *Courage under Siege*, p. 93.

318 Gürfinkel-Glocer, "Goralo Shel Beit Haholim Tzhista," p. 602.

319 Ibid., pp. 594–595.

One day during Hanukkah 1942, the engineer Marek Lichtenbaum, Czerniaków's successor as chairman of the Judenrat, following the latter's suicide, and the historian Prof. Meir Balaban visited the hospital on Gęsia St. All the patients who could walk gathered in the largest of the rooms, where they lit the Hanukkah candles. Prof. Balaban spoke about the strength of the Jewish people, who respond to suffering not by succumbing but by emerging more steeled than ever. Even the current agonies would not extinguish them, he exhorted. The Jewish people, he concluded, are like the Jewish hospital in the Warsaw ghetto, which was reestablished each time.[320] At this time, the Germans began to allow larger food rations. Doctors even received an allotment of alcohol. A grocery store opened, where it was possible to buy canned meat and even salted fish. "Before the slaughter, they began to fatten up those who remained," Waller remarked.[321]

After the September 1942 *Aktion*, the ghetto expected to enjoy a respite until Passover. In October, it was discovered that Lichtenbaum, the new Judenrat chairman, had been summoned, along with several other representatives, to a meeting with Ludwig Fischer, the governor of the Warsaw district. Fischer gave them a cordial welcome and assured them that all the lamentable incidents were behind them. He promised that a new life would begin and, particularly, that an investment would be made in the orphanage, where the Jews' future resided. Tensions eased after the visit. However, a few days later, the Germans rounded up a large group of Jews on the Umschlagplatz. Realizing that the Germans had made false promises, several doctors tried to plan ways to flee the ghetto. Concurrently, many desperate Jews who had escaped from the ghetto returned there, because of the difficulties of hiding on the Aryan side and the false assurances by the Germans.[322]

The small ghetto was liquidated in the wake of the September 1942 *Aktion*, and the large ghetto was divided into two sections

320 Ibid., pp. 594–602. On Prof. Meir Balaban, see Władysław-Wolf Glocer testimony, YVA, O.3/398.

321 Dr. Shmuel Stanisław Waller testimony, YVA, O.3/2358.

322 Ibid.

that could be crossed only with great difficulty. Hence, it was difficult to obtain medical services at the hospital at its new location at the edge of the ghetto. It was particularly difficult to treat members of the resistance who were injured during their operations, since transferring them to the hospital was liable to put them, their caregivers, and the entire ghetto population at risk. Therefore, in such cases, a doctor and a nurse went to the bunker, where the wounded were hiding, to provide the necessary treatment. The identities and the clandestine activities of dozens of people were divulged to the teams of doctors and nurses who were chosen for this mission. The first aid equipment of the underground was distributed among the bunkers, and one bunker was set aside as a provisional hospital.[323]

Period 5: From January 1943 to the Warsaw Ghetto Uprising, April 19–May 16, 1943

During the *Aktion* of January 18–22, 1943, the hospital was liquidated again, claiming all but a few patients.[324] Gestapo men armed with handguns and truncheons entered the hospital wards, pointed truncheons at the patients, and forced the staff to lift them out of bed and place them in a cart. Those who could walk were ordered to do so. The victims were given no opportunity to dress and the staff desperately threw blankets over them and marched out with them. Staff members were taken away as well, and those left behind waited for the next *Aktion*.[325] In the course of the January *Aktion*, the Jewish policeman Bronisław Grszelak informed the hospital staff that the ghetto might be wiped out for good the following morning. Several hundred patients were

323 Stefan-Shalom Grajek, *Shlosha Yemei Krav* (Three Days of Battle) (Hebrew) (Tel Aviv: Ma'arachot, 1972), p. 121.

324 Gutman, *The Jews of Warsaw*, p. 309; Ludwik Stabholz, "Hora'at Anatomiya Bamahteret" (Teaching Anatomy in the Underground) (Hebrew) (paper presented at a conference on "The Medical Faculty in the Warsaw Ghetto and Polish–Jewish Medical Collaboration in the Holocaust," Sackler Faculty of Medicine, Tel Aviv University, May 5, 2005).

325 Gürfinkel-Glocer, "Goralo Shel Beit Haholim Tzhista," p. 595.

languishing in the internal medicine and infectious diseases wards at this time. The nurses discreetly informed the patients so that those who were able could go into hiding, but it was difficult for them to help the bedridden.[326]

About 400 patients were taken to the Umschlagplatz. Those unable to climb out of bed were shot to death. SS soldiers hurled screaming patients out of windows from all floors of the hospital. A heap of corpses formed in the courtyard.[327] Staff members went into hiding in cellars and other locations near the hospital. Dr. Einhorn testified that several doctors had built hideouts for themselves and their families in the loft of a nearby building; during the *Aktion,* he and fifteen others retreated to this location. With the help of a patient who engaged in illegal smuggling, they managed to obtain three handguns. Einhorn described the horrors that took place in the hospital, which he witnessed through a small window in the hideout. Only by miracle did those in the loft survive.[328]

About thirty Jewish doctors and their families concealed themselves in a room camouflaged as a wardrobe. Two hundred people hid in a basement on the hospital grounds. A trapdoor with a handle on the floor of a clinic in a spacious room led to the large basement. A sheet of linoleum was laid over the trapdoor and a table was placed on it. On the table were packages of sterile bandages and bottles of disinfectant, salves, and the like. Injured and ill people arrived at the clinic, but the Ukrainians and the Nazis, who often entered it in search of staff, found nothing suspicious. About ten steps led from the room down to the basement, where three rooms were crowded with fugitives who had to maintain absolute silence.

The Germans rampaged through all parts of the hospital, seizing patients and demanding that they reveal the whereabouts of the staff. Stabholz, a warehouse worker at the hospital, who was forced to accompany them, bravely explained that the others had finished working and had gone home, and that they must have already been taken away from there. Finding himself unobserved

326 Ibid., pp. 596–597. On this *Aktion*, see Dr. Shmuel Stanisław Waller testimony, YVA, O.3/2358.

327 Roland, *Courage under Siege*, p. 93.

328 Dr. Chaim Einhorn testimony, YVA, O.3/1836.

for a moment, he slipped into the shelter and apprised those inside it of the horrific news, including the abduction of the chief nurse, Fried, and many other staff members. There were many young children in the shelter and since any noise was horrifically dangerous, the doctors had them injected with morphine and there was total silence. Those in the basement suddenly heard the Germans' ponderous steps overhead and the inquiry of one of them as to where the opening in the clinic led. The warehouse worker replied that it led to the rooms for the typhus patients. The Germans fled and those hiding in the basement breathed a sigh of relief. The fugitives remained there for three days.[329]

In another room, fifty staff members in hiding stood shoulder to shoulder. Dr. Amsterdamski, one of the physicians, could not endure it and suffered a fatal heart attack.[330] As the *Aktion* continued, one of the workers asked staff members who were hiding in one of the basements to help move patients out of the hospital, on the Germans' orders. This made the extremely intense situation even worse; most of them refused. Two staff members who courageously volunteered to go out to help were sent to the camps in the transports, along with the patients. Some of the other staff members who were taken to the Umschlagplatz managed to escape.[331]

The *Aktion* that was conducted in the hospital on January 18, 1943, lasted all day. Patients in critical condition were shot in the forehead in their beds. The dead were left in their beds in the surgery department. In a ward where forty patients lay, only one young man survived, pretending to be dead. The typhus patients

329 Lensky, *A Physician inside the Warsaw Ghetto*, pp. 190–192; Gürfinkel-Glocer, "Goralo Shel Beit Haholim Tzhista," p. 597.

330 Dr. Shmuel Stanisław Waller testimony, YVA, O.3/2358; Lensky, *A Physician inside the Warsaw Ghetto*, p. 23. Lensky testified that Dr. Amsterdamski, a surgeon, died suddenly on January 18, 1943, while hiding with other doctors on the hospital premises at 6–8 Gęsia St. during the *Aktion*.

331 Shulamit Tzeder, daughter of Dr. Maurycy Brandwein, a surgeon at Czyste Hospital before the war and in the ghetto, was in a bunker in the hospital during the *Aktion*; see her testimony in Shulamit Tzeder, *Hamar'e Hara Sheli* (My Bad [Jewish] Look) (Hebrew) (Megiddo: Heshvan Publishing, 2004), pp. 22–24.

met a similar fate. When it was over, all the remaining patients, along with the doctors, nurses, and clerks, were loaded onto trucks. Several physicians and patients committed suicide by injecting themselves with morphine.[332]

In the course of this bloody *Aktion*, 800 patients and 80 staff members were murdered.[333] Some of the doctors who survived joined groups of fighters, others descended to the bunkers, and a few took shelter in hideouts.[334] Around 6,000 people were sent to Treblinka. A large number of Jews who held "life numbers," believing that their survival was assured, reported to the Umschlagplatz, as demanded by the police. There were many doctors among the victims, including Dr. Jakob Rozenblum, a leading personality in TOZ; Dr. Sara Zofia Syrkin Binstein, who had held senior positions in the medical services before ghettoization and the Holocaust; and Dr. Israel Milejkowski. The three apparently took cyanide on the train.[335] The deportation of Milejkowski had a devastating effect on the surviving doctors and the Jewish population at large. The liquidation of those who remained, including well-known figures who were active in the Judenrat and community organizations in the ghetto, was plainly imminent.[336]

After the January 1943 *Aktion*, a ghastly silence descended on the hospital. The beds were empty or occupied by the corpses of those murdered. The remaining nurses wept bitterly as they attended to the bodies.[337] Many sought ways to escape to the Aryan side.[338] Nurse Sabina Gürfinkel-Glocer wrote that a dilemma of whether or not to reopen the hospital arose after the

332 Luba Blum-Bielicka, "Vegn di 'aktsye' in varshever yidishn shpitol dem 18 Yanuar 1943," *Bleter far geshikhte* 1:3–4 (August–December, 1948), pp. 211–221; Turkow, *Hayo Hayta Varsha Yehudit*, p. 173; Gürfinkel-Glocer, "Goralo Shel Beit Haholim Tzhista," p. 597.

333 Trunk, *Judenrat*, pp. 155–156.

334 Einhorn, *Harofe Begeto Varsha*, pp. 9–10.

335 Dr. Moshe Tursz Testimony, YVA, O.3/438, pp. 16–18; Lensky, *A Physician inside the Warsaw Ghetto*, p. 192.

336 Lensky, *A Physician inside the Warsaw Ghetto*, pp. 192–194.

337 Gürfinkel-Glocer, "Goralo Shel Beit Haholim Tzhista," p. 597.

338 Lensky, *A Physician inside the Warsaw Ghetto*, pp. 194–195.

Aktion. Most hopelessly claimed that there was no point. "Should we treat patients so that the Germans can come and take them away or murder them on the spot?" However, others felt that it was their duty to reopen the hospital and to administer to the ill until their last moments. Despite everything, life had proven that there was still a need for the hospital's medical services. The day after the *Aktion*, people began to arrive at the hospital, after having leaped off the trains or been shot by the Germans. Once again, a small group of doctors and nurses stepped up to fulfill their noble duty.[339]

The Jewish resistance's armed uprising against the German Army began on the Eve of Passover, April 19, 1943. However, on April 18, the Judenrat members who remained in the ghetto were taken hostage by the Germans and, therefore, various sources testify that staff and patients began to hide in the bunkers on that date.[340] On April 20, battles raged near the hospital, which provided refuge and assistance to the wounded throughout the uprising. The hospital's bunker, which had been prepared many weeks before the uprising, contained all manner of war materials, as well as folding cots, water, and food. It offered shelter to the wounded and a place to rest to the fighters during the fighting. Several nurses and doctors were members of the resistance. The nurses took charge of first aid, bandaging the wounded in subterranean bunkers and providing the rebels with food and water. The surviving population of the ghetto suffered from the heat generated by the torched buildings and from a shortage of water. That day, the Germans burned down the Jewish hospital building on Gęsia St., taking the lives of all of its patients, as well as those of many staff members.[341]

Dr. Thaddeus Stabholz, who had helped to design the bunkers built in the area of the hospital during the uprising, went into hiding in one of them, along with the rest of the medical team and the patients. After the war, apparently during his stay in the

339 Gürfinkel-Glocer, "Goralo Shel Beit Haholim Tzhista," p. 598.

340 Havi Dreifuss (Ben-Sasson), *Geto Varsha—Hasof*, p. 392.

341 Koren, "Hasiyud Kehelek Misherutei Habriyut," p. 79; Dr. Shmuel Stanisław Waller testimony, YVA, O.3/2358; Grajek, *Shlosha Yemei Krav*, pp. 118, 121.

DP camps, he testified about the responsibility that the hospital displayed during the Warsaw Ghetto Uprising.

> Late April 1943. We're sitting deep in the cellar...more than a hundred people: women, children, and men of various ages, most of us are on the staff of the Jewish hospital in the ghetto...overhead, the thunder of hell. Explosions are heard in succession and the walls of multistory buildings collapse. Through the small window that serves as a lookout, thick smoke enters. Fires...since the uprising on April 18...Today is April 30. That means that we've already been sitting in this cellar for twelve days. We do not cook; we do not talk; we lay on the bunks and think—about what? About death... Why must we die? For lack of hope about our situation...A tremendous explosion is heard near us. A mine has gone off nearby. The candles and flashlights have gone out; whitewash and cement fall from the walls and the ceiling straight onto our heads. Hearts pound vigorously. Evidently, the hospital has blown up. Several people run to the small observation hatch. Yes, it's the hospital! The walls of the building along with all four floors collapse and fall into the courtyards, the surrounding plaza, and over our heads.
>
> The director, Dr. Stein, gives us handguns, one weapon per person, some bullets, and a few hand grenades. "If you encounter *Schwaben* [ethnic Germans]—kill them, as many as you can, but remember, comrades, our fate is sealed and hope—there's none.[342]

342 Dr. Thaddeus Stabholz testimony, YVA, O.33/648. Stabholz was the son of Dr. Henryk Stabholz, who had directed Czyste Hospital before the war. On the eve of the war, Thaddeus had been a medical student. In the ghetto, he worked as a medical assistant at Czyste Hospital during the day and, in the evening, continued his medical studies at the underground medical faculty. He was deported to Treblinka, and was transferred to Majdanek, Auschwitz, Sachsenhausen, and Dachau. Dr. Thaddeus Stabholz completed his medical studies after the war and wrote a well-documented book about the Holocaust; see Thaddeus Stabholz, *Seven Hells* (New York: Holocaust Library, 1990).

Dr. Adolf Polisiuk,[343] director of the gynecology department at Czyste Hospital, also went into hiding in the bunkers with senior medical staff and patients during the uprising. His record of the uprising was written in June 1943 in Warsaw, several days after he had managed to pull off a rare escape to the Aryan side.

> Sunday, April 18, 1943...in the past few months, the workers...have set up six subterranean hideouts on the grounds of the hospital...with room for 400 people. Our group of 130 entered the shelter...the director of the hospital, Dr. Josef Stein, and his wife, the deputy director, Dr. Anna Braude-Heller, director of the admissions department, Dr. Wertman...eight doctors...some of the nurses...some of the hospital's logistic workers...the shelter consisted of sixteen cellars...the patients, about 100, including some who were seriously ill, following abdominal surgery, were accommodated in the hideouts as well...we began our subterranean lives...echoes of gunshots and explosions reached us from outside...those two days, a manhunt was conducted at the hospital...on April 22, they set fire to the hospital. There was smoke in the shelter...on April 24, three people, including me, were sent to the surface. The sight that we witnessed...instead of the hospital...the whole area was full of debris and strewn with the workers' corpses...masses of people were wandering around...many had been killed... the ill, burned alive...our hospital had been torched three times...a week later, the "mine-laying" operation began...all the while, I kept thinking about how to get out of this hell and go to the "Aryan paradise," but there was no way...I often administered first aid, because I was the only gynecologist on the hospital grounds...I performed operations in shelters, under horrific conditions, in suffocating, filthy,

343 Dr. Adolf Polisiuk testimony, YVA, M.49.E/5061. For details about Dr. Adolf Polisiuk, his diaries, and his writings from the ghetto period, see Chapter 10, note 69, of this book.

> and unlit rooms, while everyone in the shelter looked on… until May 11…about 300 of us remained on the hospital grounds. That day…the municipal…the Germans' voices, "Out!"…I headed for another shelter…thirteen people followed me, including Dr. Braude-Heller…near the covered entrance to the shelter, a few others gathered, including the director, Stein, and Remba…they didn't let us into the shelter, because the Germans were already in the area…we heard how [the Germans] caught them…only sixty of us remained, including three doctors…with Dr. Braude-Heller. We scattered…we lost all hope…we were more willing to die than to surrender to the executioners…through an opening that we had plugged up with soil, a strong flow of asphyxiating gas filtered in.[344]

Dr. Polisiuk and a small number of medical workers appear to have been among the few survivors of the bunkers that had concealed the last of the medical team and their patients. His account, written several days after the events, is one of the few surviving documents that attest to the fate of the patients and the medical staff in the ghetto's death throes—the final chapter in the history of Jewish medicine in the Warsaw ghetto.

Bersohn and Bauman Children's Hospital

The history of Bersohn and Bauman Children's Hospital in the Warsaw ghetto, like that of Czyste Hospital, was influenced by the changes that swept the ghetto throughout its duration. Five significant periods are discernible over the course of its existence, from the beginning of the war in September 1939 to the uprising in April 1943.

344 Polisiuk, "Hamatzor Ha'aharon," pp. 310–317.

Period 1: From the Outbreak of War in September 1939 to Ghettoization in Early 1941

At the onset of the massive German shelling of Warsaw, there were around 100 children in Bersohn and Bauman Children's Hospital. Because the hospital was located near lumber warehouses, there was great concern that the building would catch fire, if the area were shelled, and the young inpatients were placed quickly with families nearby, some of them non-Jewish. At the beginning of the war, Varsovians still maintained civic solidarity and engaged devotedly in noble deeds, such as rescuing ill children, irrespective of their religious affiliation. The doctors, nurses, and hospital staff personally carried ailing youngsters to families who had agreed to receive them. Medicines and equipment, including mattresses and small beds, were transferred as well. Children with infectious diseases were housed separately.

As the shelling intensified and the number of wounded increased, the hospital also admitted adults who were rushed there, including some who were transferred from the university hospital. The admission of adults to a children's hospital created special difficulties. The beds were not suitable; shortages of equipment, medicines, underwear, and linens soon set in and worsened with time; and food supplies that should have lasted for several months ran out.[345]

When the occupation began, the Germans allowed the hospital to continue providing medical services in order to stanch the spread of epidemics. For this purpose, they demanded that the hospital concentrate on treating contagious illnesses. However, by falsifying diagnoses and reports, the doctors also managed to treat children in both internal medicine and surgical wards, and the hospital continued to treat children for as long as the Warsaw ghetto existed.[346]

Bersohn and Bauman Children's Hospital was headed by the noted pediatrician Dr. Anna Braude-Heller. Before the war,

345 Yehudit Braude testimony, YVA, O.3/2360; Sabine Zenderman testimony, a nurse at the hospital, YVA, M.49.E/5883.

346 Rom, "Mahalot Hayeladim Begeto Varsha," p. 14.

she had toiled indefatigably to advance medical services for the Jewish population. A member of the Bund Party, she had helped to found the Towarzystowo Przyjaciół Dzieci (Friends of Children Society), mother and child care clinics, an orphanage, and a tuberculosis clinic. Throughout the ghetto period, she discharged her duties with unlimited devotion.[347] Dr. Moshe Tursz described Dr. Braude-Heller as an outstanding physician and a social activist, and noted, "Her name should be written down in letters of gold as one who properly fulfilled her role in the history of the ghetto and set an example of boundless self-sacrifice."[348] Her friends offered to hide her in the Aryan side of the city, but she refused to leave her patients behind. After the *Grossaktion*, she helped to reorganize Czyste Hospital. In the Warsaw Ghetto Uprising, Dr. Braude-Heller helped to treat the wounded, until she died with the fighters in battle.[349]

Dr. Adina Blady Szwajger was about to finish her medical studies when the war broke out. About half a year into the occupation, she began to work in the internal medicine ward of the children's hospital. In her memoirs—an important testimony about the hospital's Holocaust history—she described the medical work at Bersohn and Bauman Children's Hospital as "superhuman."[350] All the staff members at Bersohn and Bauman Children's Hospital wore white armbands with a red star and the words "Children's Hospital."[351] In the second half of December 1939, the hospital was placed in isolation on the pretext of the need to avert the risk of contracting typhus.[352] A policeman

347 Blady Szwajger, *I Remember Nothing More*, pp. 37–38.

348 Dr. Moshe Tursz testimony, YVA, O.3/438, pp. 16–18.

349 On Dr. Braude-Heller and her lifework, see Wulman et al., *The Martyrdom of Jewish Physicians in Poland*, p. 322; Rom, "Mahalot Hayeladim Begeto Varsha," p. 14; Roland, *Courage under Siege*, pp. 94–95; Blady Szwajger, *I Remember Nothing More*, pp. 19, 37–38; Yehudit Braude testimony, YVA, O.3/2360; Dr. Shmuel Stanisław Waller testimony, YVA, O.3/2358. See also the testimony of Dr. Adolf Polisiuk in Blumental and Kermish, *Hameri Vehamered Begeto Varsha*, pp. 310–317. Dr. Polisiuk witnessed the final hours of Dr. Braude's life.

350 Blady Szwajger, *I Remember Nothing More*, pp. 4–7, 22.

351 Roland, *Courage under Siege*, p. 95.

352 The isolation decree that was imposed on Czyste Hospital on December 19, 1939. The isolation lasted for several weeks. Czerniaków, *The Warsaw Diary*,

stood guard at the gate to ensure that no one entered. All the staff members spent several weeks sequestered in the hospital building, sleeping side-by-side on the library floor, eating nothing but watered-down soup and showering on the premises. The proximity of the Germans, who had decreed the isolation of the staff and the patients, toughened the staff and strengthened their sense of fraternity.[353]

By January 1940, Bersohn and Bauman Children's Hospital was wrestling with tremendous difficulties. It was receiving patients with infectious diseases in large numbers and investing much of its budget in their care. That summer, even before ghettoization, the hospital asked the Judenrat for support. TOZ and JDC provided assistance, until the United States entered the war in December 1941.[354] In March 1940, the departments of the hospital functioned relatively well despite the difficulties. The internal medicine ward, for example, was properly equipped and professionally run. It had glass partitions that allowed the nurses to observe everything going on. Its beds were spotless and the walls were bleached so rigorously that they shone. The ward was crowded with young patients who had common illnesses and ordinary childhood diseases. Although it was already difficult to obtain food, special feeding prescriptions for infants were still distributed, and older children in need of more nutritious food even received eggs and cocoa. Doctors made daily rounds and Dr. Adina Blady Szwajger recalled being proud and pleased to have had the opportunity to join the pediatric profession. It was clear to her that she had to do everything possible to save human lives, or at least to provide some relief.

> …that we had our duty as human beings and that we were there to help. That is why this medicine was "superhuman" and why, although it is all like one great wound, it is the most beautiful thing of all.[355]

p. 101; Ringelblum, *Notes from the Warsaw Ghetto*, pp. 8–9.

353 Blady Szwajger, *I Remember Nothing More*, p. 25.

354 Roland, *Courage under Siege*, p. 94.

355 Blady Szwajger, *I Remember Nothing More*, p. 22.

The prevalent feeling at this time was that things would change and the situation would blow over, that reasonable possibilities of treating ill children still existed. At first, there were the usual, curable patients, but then children suffering from starvation began to arrive—at this stage, it was still possible to help them by administering glucose, egg powder, margarine, and leftover watered-down milk.

Dr. Anna Margolis, a director of a ward at Bersohn and Bauman Children's Hospital, insisted on working exactly as before the war and refused to deviate even slightly from accepted medical procedure: administering morning care, taking blood samples, making rounds, writing down instructions, and then accurately recording the medical history in patient files. The daily routine at the hospital began with a report to the managing physician, albeit only concerning the severely ill and those whose condition worsened. Whenever a death occurred, the staff had to explain the event and to prove that everything had been done to save the patient's life. The need for such explanations escalated steadily.[356] As the sealing of the ghetto approached, the number of lice-infested and starving children at the hospital grew, and the cases of tuberculosis multiplied. Under the circumstances, the likelihood of recovering from tuberculosis was nil.[357]

Period 2: From Ghettoization in Early 1941 to the *Grossaktion* in July 1942

Bersohn and Bauman Children's Hospital did not have to relocate due to ghettoization, because both of its venues, 60 Sienna St. and 51 Śliska St., were within the ghetto boundaries that the Germans had determined in 1940.[358] The hospital was required to maintain daily records on file cards and reports on typhus patients and their blood tests, and to forward them to the Germans.[359]

356 Ibid., pp. 28–29.
357 Ibid., p. 28.
358 Roland, *Courage under Siege*, p. 94.
359 Hanna Krall, *Shielding the Flame: An Intimate Conversation with Dr. Marek*

Outwardly, the condition of the medical staff seemed nearly the opposite of that of the children. Staff members wore white smocks, none suffered from distention, and their intake of the alcohol to which they had access provided a few extra calories and somewhat dulled their hunger pangs. It was their role and duty to offer assistance, to cure, or at least to assure a serene, "pleasant" death. Although the situation steadily worsened, staff members found reason and purpose in their work. If they could hold on, they believed they could save the children and themselves.[360] Workers and doctors at the hospital had to undergo disinfection twice a day, upon arriving and upon leaving. They also were inspected for lice.[361]

The young patients' conditions worsened to the point that it was difficult to distinguish four-year-olds from six-year-olds and even ten-year-olds from twelve-year-olds. Sick children stared sadly and solemnly at their caregivers. Their hands, normally in constant motion, lay still and helpless.[362] The hospital was inundated with ill and dying children. In March 1941, four months after the ghetto was sealed, two or three children occupied one bed. There were no diapers; strips of sheets served as a makeshift.[363] With no heating fuel available, children shivered in the cold and some froze to death.

At the outset of their rule, the Germans confiscated all supplies and equipment from the operating rooms. Anesthetics were continually in short supply. When staff members sought to leave some equipment behind for emergency surgeries and other crises, doctors were punished with imprisonment. It was difficult for the hospital to perform disinfections. Only after repeated pleading by the director of the hospital, Dr. Anna Braude-Heller, did Dr. Schrempf, the chief German physician before ghettoization, authorize the purchase of a disinfection machine, funded by the JDC.[364]

Edelman, the Last Surviving Leader of the Warsaw Ghetto Uprising (New York: Holt, 1986), pp. 35, 41.

360 Blady Szwajger, *I Remember Nothing More*, p. 42.

361 Ibid., pp. 40–41.

362 Ibid., p. 31.

363 Roland, *Courage under Siege*, p. 95.

364 Yehudit Braude testimony, YVA, O.3/2360; Dr. Israel Rom (Rotbalsam) testimony, YVA, O.3/2357.

About half a year after the ghetto was sealed, children were starving to death in the hospital.[365] No provisions were made for the specific kind of support required at a children's hospital. One three-year-old child weighed 4 kilograms, the normal weight of a two-month-old baby. Hunger was so acute that adults pilfered food from children. Children who could barely move their swollen legs began to appear in the wards. Staff members worked ten to twelve hours each day without a break. Doctors had very meager resources: intravenous injections and an allocation from the JDC that sufficed to provide powder equivalent to half an egg and 10 grams of margarine per person, as well as vitamin C for the starving.[366] It was forbidden to leave these treasures unguarded lest the staff members or others would consume them. Due to the onerous hunger, all members of the medical staff gave up 200 grams of half a liter of milk and 20 to 60 grams of their bread ration. At a special staff meeting, this policy was adopted and it was decided to distribute the rations thus freed among all the employees and caregivers at the hospital to enable equal nutrition—300 grams of soup and 40 grams of bread per person per day.[367]

Four months after the sealing of the ghetto, one of the nurses described the ghastly conditions in the hospital in her diary.

> My duty is from 3 until 11...When I come to my ward, it's a real hell. Children, sick with measles, lie in twos or threes to a bed...shaved little heads...covered with lice...My assistant and I have to take care of fifty children. Pressure of work drives us crazy. What first? Distribute medicines, give injections, serve food, redo dressings on the heads to keep off the lice...There are ten children waiting in the reception room...I have no beds, no linens, no blankets nor sheets. I call up the head nurse asking what am I to do....Where shall I put them, with what shall I dress them...Where I have two children, I must put three, that's all...The laundry

365 Czerniaków, *The Warsaw Diary*, p. 232.

366 Roland, *Courage under Siege*, p. 96; Blady Szwajger, *I Remember Nothing More*, p. 31.

367 Krall, *Shielding the Flame*, p. 17.

> is not working, no coal for fuel. The rooms are terribly cold, the children huddle under the blankets and the fever shakes them…In the entrance hall lies a boy of five, swollen with hunger. He is in the last stage, his life ending because of hunger…he utters for the last time "a piece of bread"…. Dead for a piece of bread.[368]

At the end of the first year of the ghetto's existence in the autumn of 1941, there seemed to be nothing but a sense of helplessness. Whenever a child recovered, there was no one to come and take him or her home from the hospital.

As the workday grew longer, the caregivers' fatigue escalated. With faltering legs, they treated pressure sores, bandaged swollen limbs, and administered "medicines." The food shortage worsened. There was no longer enough alcohol to fill the little cups, which the staff members used as a mild sedative to be able to show some expression on their faces when making contact with the children. However, the daily routine at the hospital was maintained, as doctors continued to hold meetings, make their rounds, and record patients' histories that increasingly ended with the date of death.[369]

Many children in the hospital had no guardians. This state of affairs, along with their dire state of health, imposed a physical and mental burden on the nurses. Apart from providing round-the-clock care and support, they had to cope with the deaths of children, sometimes many dozens each week. To avert contagion among the young inpatients, the nurses strove to maintain hygiene and sanitation under harsh conditions of lack of soap, underwear, linens, and water. The food shortage was a critical problem; it caused the youngsters' immune systems to collapse, exposing them to further infections that made their recovery less likely.[370] One of the nurses described the plight of the starving children at the hospital.

368 Kermish, *To Live with Honor*, pp. 403–404. For photos of Bersohn and Bauman Children's Hospital, see AŻIH, ARI.989. See also Offer, *Haluk Lavan Begeto*, appendix A.7, pp. 524–527.

369 Blady Szwajger, *I Remember Nothing More*, p. 39.

370 Yehudit Braude testimony, YVA, O.3/2360.

We're already putting four patients in a bed. They cry out from all directions, "Nurse, help!" I have to hear these cries alone. I approach the bed where four children are lying. One of them tugs the blanket toward himself. Another pulls it in his own direction. The third, who is left uncovered, wants to stretch his legs and kicks the fourth one in the stomach. The sounds and screams reach the very heavens. The other nurses do not want to hear. Everyone lying there has a swollen face or sunken cheeks, and withered arms and legs, but their eyes gleam, asking over and over only for food. They wear me out with questions, "When are they going to give us the food?" They ask such questions hundreds of times in an hour, until they hear the noise of the cart that delivers the soup. Then the real hell begins. First, I'm given a pot of water with a few dozen dumplings for eighty children, and I have to divide this up so that each one gets the same and no one gets more than another. The kitchen staff warned me that I had to hand out small portions…I stand next to the food boiler, trembling with the thought that there won't be enough for all the children. Now they come running…and ask for a little more, but it's impossible.

They go to bed with empty stomachs and have trouble falling asleep. Again, shouts are heard. What next? I approach carefully and witness the following scene: a boy running toward his bed with a parcel containing a few rolls that he filched from a child who still had them from home and had fallen asleep in the meantime. The hungry soul.…A third boy noticed this and cried out. When I got there, the little one did not move. I left one roll with him and put the others back. He promised not to steal anymore. However, the whole story repeated itself twenty minutes later. I hear shouting like this several times each night as starving children look in others' cupboards to relieve their hunger.[371]

371 Testimony of an anonymous nurse at Bersohn and Bauman Children's Hospital, YVA, M.10.AR.1/1099.

The medical staff had few options and little medical equipment. There were severe shortages of equipment, even of mattresses, which dwindled in number due to rotting occasioned by diarrhea. The children began to suffer from cold, and pneumonia spread. Even so, some recovered.[372]

One overcast autumn day about a year after ghettoization, the staff saw a boy undress at the hospital gate and, naked as the day he was born, he pleaded to be admitted to the hospital, because he was hungry and freezing.[373] The incident made a profound impression as described in the underground press.

> At the gate of the hospital, a boy, maybe twelve years old, stripped to his skin. He shouted until he was hoarse, asking to be allowed to enter, that a door should open for him, behind which [he could find] cleanliness and warmth. He cried that he was hungry, that he was cold, that he could no longer stand up....The doctor, pale with apprehension, thought it over. It couldn't be helped; we had to receive him....He seemed to have...attained only one goal, the kindness of a quiet death...not on the floor, not in a puddle of blood...not naked under the melting snow...but in a bed...a kindness that, at least in the final hour of his brief life, he felt, in the vestiges of his consciousness, not as a persecuted, excluded, and disparaged creature but almost as a human being.[374]

In addition to the attempt by sick children to be admitted to the hospital, relatives abandoned infants at the hospital entrance, hoping to save them in this way. Dr. Adina Blady Szwajger recalled that while exiting the hospital one day, she felt that she had tread on something soft. It proved to be the body of a dead baby, wrapped in paper. As time passed, more and more starving children were admitted to the hospital, mainly to the internal medicine ward, where all the beds were occupied.[375]

372 Blady Szwajger, *I Remember Nothing More*, p. 42.

373 Ibid., p. 43.

374 Blatman, *Geto Varsha—Sipur Itona'i*, pp. 233–234.

375 Blady Szwajger, *I Remember Nothing More*, p. 30.

Due to the soaring morbidity, Bersohn and Bauman Children's Hospital had to turn away many ailing children. In June 1941, several doctors who were active in TOZ and the Jewish Social Self-Help advised Czerniaków that the hospital was in tremendous distress.

> This hospital has 200 beds but, in the opinion of its management, at least another 500 beds are required. The upturn in diseases among the children is so great that 506 children instead of 200 are hospitalized there. For lack of space, they turn away 20 to 50 children who approach them every day. Therefore, a frightening number of children among the poor Jewish population is dying, particularly those from infancy to two years of age.[376]

The letters from doctors and public figures about the shortage of beds in the children's hospital may have led to a decision to search for a building that would allow more youngsters to be received and hospitalized. Thus, an additional branch of the children's hospital was established in late August and early September 1941. Some staff members moved to the new building, a former school on the corner of Leszno St. and Żelazna St.—a gloomy three-story edifice, abutting a station of the guard detail that watched over the ghetto walls. The Labor Office and a quarantine station—where people who had been in contact with typhus patients were interned—were on the other side of Żelazna St.

The new hospital facility had three wards—for infectious diseases, directed by Dr. Henryk Makower, on the first floor; internal medicine, run by Dr. Hela Keilson, on the second floor; and neonatal, managed by Prof. Anna Hirszfeld, the wife of the convert to Christianity Prof. Ludwik Hirszfeld, on the third floor. Its wards were spacious, once having served as classrooms. An operating room was set up in a large hall on the ground floor, where children shot by German gunfire were taken. In the larger halls,

376 Anonymous public appeal from doctors and public figures concerning the state of the hospital, June 1941, YVA, M.10.AR.1/315.

boys and girls lay on paper mattresses placed on straw-covered bunks. Tin pails stood in the corners of the rooms at night for children suffering from bloody diarrhea who could not reach the latrines in time. Skeletal and bloated, they sprawled on the bunks; only their eyes showed signs of life.[377]

Due to the hospital's abysmal situation, the director, Dr. Anna Braude-Heller, established a women's auxiliary for the institution that brought together women and mothers among the ghetto population. The association organized conferences in an attempt to improve the state of the hospital by soliciting funds and equipment. Its volunteer activity included the preparation of homemade soup for the hospital every Sunday. The auxiliary's efforts appear to have caused a change in the attitude of those of influence in the ghetto. By the spring of 1942, the hospital wards were equipped with beds that had mattresses, linens, blankets, and underwear. They also acquired bowls, chamber pots, cups, and the like. However, this lasted only a few months, until the deportations and the *Aktionen* at the hospital began. Despite the improvement that had occurred—the white beds and the increased food rations, paid for by the JDC—the medical profession stood helpless in the face of a rising tide of fatal tuberculosis.[378]

To get an idea of the overcrowding and diseases at the hospital, it is useful to consult a report that the Judenrat statistics department presented to the head of the Judenrat in March 1942. At the beginning of February of that year, both branches of the hospital had admitted 513 children. At the end of that month, their numbers had risen by 17.3 percent. The population of children with typhus declined by 18.3 percent in the course of February. The number of typhus patients under observation fell by 4.4 percent. In contrast, the group of patients with other contagious diseases did not decrease. More and more children with other illnesses were admitted—a 67 percent increase in one month, from the beginning to the end of the month.[379]

377 Blady Szwajger, *I Remember Nothing More*, pp. 40–42.

378 Roland, *Courage under Siege*, p. 59.

379 Judenrat Statistics Department Report, no. 29, March 17, 1942, GFH, no. 11250, p. 10.

Patients at Bersohn and Bauman Children's Hospital, 60 Sienna St. and 80 Leszno St., February 1942

Patient Breakdown	Feb. 1, 1942	Feb. 28, 1942
Typhus Patients	169	138
Typhus Patients under Observation	113	108
Typhoid Fever Patients	—	—
Typhoid Fever Patients under Observation	—	—
Other Contagious Patients	46	47
Other Patients	185	309
Total	**513**	**602**

A comparison of the medical situation at Bersohn and Bauman Children's Hospital with that at Czyste Hospital at the same time, February 1942, shows that morbidity was even greater at the children's hospital than at the adult facility. Furthermore, while the patient load at Czyste Hospital declined by 8.1 percent from the beginning to the end of February, there was a 17.3 percent increase at Bersohn and Bauman Children's Hospital. In both hospitals, the number of typhus patients fell—by 32.4 percent at Czyste Hospital and by a much lower rate of 18.3 percent at Bersohn and Bauman Children's Hospital.

The rate of typhus patients under observation fell to 41.3 percent at Czyste Hospital, while it edged downward by a mere 4.6 percent at Bersohn and Bauman Children's Hospital. The count of patients with contagious diseases dropped by 26.5 percent at Czyste Hospital but remained stable at the children's hospital. The number of those with other infectious diseases soared by 67 percent at Bersohn and Bauman Children's Hospital, but increased only slightly by 3.5 percent at Czyste Hospital. There was an outbreak of typhoid fever in late February 1942 among adult patients, but there was no evidence of one at the children's hospital.[380]

380 Ibid.

Many of the children who contracted tuberculosis were kept in isolation. Those with typhus suffered from weakness due to acute hunger, and mortality among them was high. The combination of disease and severe hunger created unusual complications. Dr. Anna Braude-Heller reported, for example, the case of an eleven-year-old boy whose autopsy revealed that he had had tuberculosis, although all the tests had been negative. Unable to detect the boy's tuberculosis, the doctors surely could not have treated it, although, under the circumstances, it is doubtful that they could have helped him, even if they had been able to diagnose his condition. Children arrived at the hospital full of lice and in spite of the strenuous efforts of the staff, it was impossible to eradicate lice and fleas. These conditions resulted in a high child mortality at Bersohn and Bauman Children's Hospital—roughly one-fourth of 724 inpatients in the last quarter of 1941.[381]

Period 3: From the *Grossaktion* in July 1942 to the Hospital *Aktion* in September 1942

The onset of the *Grossaktion* in July 1942 threw the hospital into massive disarray. The small ghetto was liquidated and the children's hospital facility on Śliska St. was transferred to the facility on Leszno St., which was also receiving children from other hospitals. At this time, Bersohn and Bauman Children's Hospital and Czyste Hospital shared the same fate. The patient load was no longer heavy, since youngsters who had parents had been taken home. Nevertheless, the staff attempted to maintain a routine work schedule.[382]

Many staff members, doctors, and nurses were sent to Treblinka during the *Aktion*. Some managed to go into hiding and flee to the Aryan side.[383] The rest of the staff continued to report to work. They often spent the night at the hospital, because

381 Roland, *Courage under Siege*, pp. 94–97.

382 Blady Szwajger, *I Remember Nothing More*, p. 48.

383 Yehudit Braude testimony, YVA, O.3/2360.

of the ongoing manhunts in the streets. They continued to care for their patients to the bitter end. Dr. Adina Blady Szwajger wrote,

> As if in a drugged stupor, we continued to keep case notes although there was no longer any order to them... Dr. Makower, who was a police doctor, came to the Umschlagplatz at five o'clock and said that all the people who had been taken there the night before had gone straight into the cattle trains. So I went to work as usual.[384]

The doctors kept up their daily rounds. Staff members continued to maintain records and files. "But we thought that if those case histories were to survive then, after the war, somebody would find them and there would be historical evidence," Dr. Adina Blady Szwajger noted.[385]

Period 4: From the Hospital *Aktion* in September 1942 to January 1943

When the *Aktion* in the hospital began on September 6, the remaining patients and the remnants of the staff—children and adults alike—were transferred to the hospital on Stawki St. near the Umschlagplatz.

The testimony of Chaya Elbaum-Dornbus reveals the fate of young children in this *Aktion*.

> As I approached the deportation square, I saw the toddlers from the children's hospital on Śliska St. Surrounded by sentries, barefoot, clad in robes, obediently going wherever they were being led. Some of the children were wrapped in a towel, while others pulled the robes over their heads to protect themselves from the irksome, dripping, light rain... their skinny blue legs trembling...leading the march—two

384 Blady Szwajger, *I Remember Nothing More*, p. 48.
385 Ibid., pp. 37–38, 49.

> nurses from the hospital, in white smocks, each with babies in their arms.[386]

On the Umschlagplatz, in a small fenced-in wooden building, was a room for babies. Nurses there organized duty rotations and gave the little ones water. The infants lay still, perhaps already enfeebled. There were twenty to thirty of them in the room. They were taken away and replaced twice daily. Each time a transport was about to set out, the nurses had to surrender them.[387]

In the September *Aktion*, the management of the children's hospital was also forced to conduct a selection among its staff, choosing those who would be granted a "life number." Some staff members left the hospital on the Umschlagplatz with such numbers in their possession. Approximately fifty doctors were ordered to remain in the hospital with the patients. Not everyone with numbers managed to avoid deportation. Those with numbers, who had been released, attempted to rescue the staff members who lacked numbers and who had been left behind in the hospital on the Umschlagplatz by passing their numbers to them via ambulances. At this time, about 200 employees at the Stawki St. hospital were designated for deportation along with the patients.[388]

Dr. Adina Blady Szwajger faced the wrenching dilemma of euthanasia when the medical team was ordered to send its patients to the Umschlagplatz, knowing, as everyone knew, that they would be transported to the extermination camps. Indeed, she carried out mercy killings of children and adults alike. In order to spare them from the death camps, she injected the hospital's last surviving children with morphine.[389]

After the September 1942 *Aktion*, the children's hospital shared quarters with the hospital for adults in a rented apartment on Gęsia St. Three cramped rooms on the first floor were allocated

386 Chaya Elbaum-Dornbus, "Hageto Biymei Hagerush" (The Ghetto at the Time of the Deportation), in Gruenbaum et al., *Entziklopediya Shel Galuyot: Varsha*, vol. 6, part 2, p. 618.

387 Dr. Shmuel Stanisław Waller testimony, YVA, O.3/2358.

388 Grupińska, "Kah Be'emet," pp. 20, 154–155, 157.

389 Blady Szwajger, *I Remember Nothing More*, pp. 53–58.

to the children. While there was a dire shortage of nurses, there were enough doctors—some of the doctors worked as physicians by day and as nurses by night.[390] The harsh winter of 1942–1943 began on the heels of the *Aktion* and there were many cases of frostbite and frost burns. However, nutrition improved and there were no longer any signs of hunger-related edema at the hospital, since it was possible to obtain bread, honey substitutes, and other commodities through smugglers who availed themselves of the ration cards left behind by the Jews who had been sent to Treblinka. Nonetheless, the medical conditions and the resources available to provide treatment were intolerable. There was almost no medical equipment, nor was there a pediatric surgery department at the time. Dr. Seweryn Wilk performed the surgical procedures of both children and adults.

> I can't remember where I sterilized the instruments…All I remember is following Dr. Wilk around the wards with a tray covered with napkins. And I understood more and more clearly that you had to bring help right up to the very end, but first you had to be made of stone…because nothing could compare to bedsores all over the buttocks, dead tissue cut away with ordinary scissors and no anesthetics. Or people who had been burned while working on the Aryan side, lying on sheets soaked in saline solution. Frostbitten feet were an everyday occurrence, fingers and toes black with gangrene, amputated on the bed without a table, even without gloves—we'd simply wash our hands. And the stench—the terrible stench…I didn't like my children's ward then. I didn't like assisting during the amputations of tiny frostbitten fingers or the bandaging of little children who had been fatally burned through lack of care.[391]

390 Ibid., pp. 59–60.
391 Ibid., pp. 61–62.

Period 5: From January 1943 to the Warsaw Ghetto Uprising, April 19–May 16, 1943

The events surrounding the January 1943 *Aktion* at the pediatric ward of the hospital on Gęsia St. were tragic for child and adult inpatients alike. Dr. Adina Blady Szwajger, who still worked in that ward, reported that they were awakened in the hospital by shouting in German. A boy came downstairs and reported that the *Aktion* had begun. Gestapo men had entered the hospital. She recalled that after hearing knocking on the door of the ward, the Gestapo men came in and glanced at the patients and the staff. As she stood there in her smock with a stethoscope around her neck, a handgun was pointed at her. Only by miracle was she not shot.

The male medical staff were ordered to go downstairs in order to help evacuate the patients.[392] Several staff members found a place to hide in the cellars, where there were several very young children. Since any sound presented an extreme danger, the doctors ordered injecting them with morphine.[393] At the end of the *Aktion*, the Nazis set the hospital ablaze and brutalized the babies. Among the thirty-six staff members, half of whom were physicians, seventeen were killed.[394]

Medical Institutions in Otwock—Brijus Sanatorium for Tuberculosis and Zofiówka Psychiatric Hospital

The medical institutions in Otwock, a suburb of Warsaw outside the ghetto, remained active during the war. Two well-known Jewish institutions operated there: Brijus Sanatorium, a tuberculosis sanatorium with 150 patients, and Zofiowka Psychiatric Hospital, with around 300. In 1942, the patients in both institutions were sent to extermination camps or were murdered on site. Many doctors and staff members committed

392 Ibid., p. 63.
393 Sabina Gürfinkel-Glocer, "Goralo Shel Beit Haholim Tzhista," p. 597.
394 Blady Szwajger, *I Remember Nothing More*, pp. 179–181.

suicide.[395] From the very beginning of the occupation, the psychiatric hospital owned by the city was threatened with closure. A perceptible stigma attached itself to psychiatric institutions, Ringelblum noted. Their property was evidently looted and instructions were issued to hand over their furniture and kitchen implements. In early February 1940, a rumor spread that hundreds of mental patients had been murdered.[396]

In February 1940, Ringelblum wrote that the number of psychiatric patients had increased considerably. Two months later, he reported that Jews who had resisted the Germans and had tried to defend themselves had also been placed in this particular hospital. In September 1940, a year into the war and two months before ghettoization, most Jewish patients in psychiatric hospitals were there for political reasons.[397] About a year and a half into the occupation, Czerniaków wrote that the institution was in dire straits because of the lack of resources and, having no choice, its managers were threatening to evict the patients. The Judenrat was unable to raise enough money to maintain the hospital.[398] Upon visiting the institution in July 1940, Czerniaków wrote that the community tried to provide assistance throughout the occupation,

395 Roland, *Courage under Siege*, pp. 72, 94. On the fate of patients with mental illness at Zofiówka Psychiatric Hospital, see Kamila Uzarczyk, "'Schluss mit der Rassenschande!' From Separation to Extermination: The Fate of Jewish Mentally Ill Patients in Germany and in Occupied Poland, 1939–1942," in S. Hildebrandt, M. Offer, and M. Grodin, eds., *Recognizing the Past in the Present: New Studies on Medicine before, during, and after the Holocaust* (New York and Oxford: Berghahn Books, forthcoming, 2020), chap. 14.

396 Ringelblum, *Notes from the Warsaw Ghetto*, pp. 11, 16, 35, 75n1; see also Stanislaw Batawia, "Zagłada chorych psychicznie," *Biuletyn Głównej. Komisji Badania Zbrodni Hitlerowskich w Polsce*, 3 (1947), pp. 91–106.

397 Ringelblum, *Notes from the Warsaw Ghetto*, pp. 21, 35, 50; Ringelblum, *Ktavim Aharonim*, p. 154.

398 Czerniaków, *The Warsaw Diary*, p. 156. The Judenrat was responsible for additional institutions in the vicinity of Warsaw, such as a Jewish psychiatric institution in Tworki. Thus, the Judenrat received a demand to pay for the hospitalization of one of the Jewish patients there in November 1941. See a bill for an unnamed Jew's stay in a Jewish psychiatric institution from the Kommissar for Jewish Affairs to the chairman of the Judenrat in Warsaw, GFH, no. 7783.

but it did not have the resources to help as required.[399] In August 1940, he visited again.

A month later, as the deadline to move to the ghetto approached, Czerniaków wrote that the Polish authorities in Otwock were about to take over the Jewish hospitals and to appropriate Brijus Sanatorium, and that Zofiowka Psychiatric Hospital was in danger as well. Later that month, he wrote that both facilities had been spared for the time being, but they were not allowed to admit new patients.[400] By the middle of September 1940, Zofiowka Psychiatric Hospital was in dreadful condition. Ringelblum described its patients, who suffered from grievous hunger.

> These people are rotting alive. They have become half-animals, including the shriveled women, spines twisted, terrifying faces. A horrible stench. Following a denunciation to the effect that the hospital had sold some of its supplies, supplies worth 60,000 zlotys have been confiscated.[401]

At the time, Zofiowka Psychiatric Hospital had 300 patients, including 200 from Warsaw. After its chain fence was stolen, some of them fled to their homes. One threw himself onto the railroad tracks. More than twenty suffered from a contagious African disease.[402] Two months after ghettoization, in the middle of January 1941, it was feared that the community might lose this institution to the occupiers. Ringelblum accused the Judenrat of not supporting it.[403]

In April 1941, five months after the Jews had been banished to the ghetto, all Jewish psychiatric patients in Poland were concentrated in Zofiowka Psychiatric Hospital. More than 100 from Tworki and 30 from Kobierzyn, not far from Cracow, were sent there. "In all, there are about 400 patients, who are dying of

399 Czerniaków, *The Warsaw Diary*, pp. 176, 177.

400 Ibid., p. 202.

401 Ringelblum, *Yoman Vereshimot*, p. 142.

402 Ibid. Ringelblum placed the name of the illness "Aquilula" in quotation marks. Such a disease is unknown in today's medical literature, and it is difficult to know what it means.

403 Ibid., p. 233n2.

hunger."[404] According to reports of November 1941 by the Jewish Social Self-Help, there were 226 patients in Zofiowka Psychiatric Hospital, in late October 1941. In November, it admitted two additional patients, and it removed thirteen people from its records, without specifying where they went and under what circumstances. Forty-one patients died in November 1941. The mortality rate nearly doubled in six months, beginning in May 1941.[405] On August 19, 1942, during the *Aktionen*, the health care institutions and Zofiowka Psychiatric Hospital, were liquidated. All the patients were shot, and the staff were sent to Treblinka.[406] At the time of the *Aktion* in Otwock, the Polish police had prior knowledge of the deportation, but most did not warn the Jews and even misled them. One Polish policeman, Pietrasz, tipped off the hospital management, allowing several people to survive. Others, having no way to save themselves or lacking the mental fortitude to attempt it, committed suicide by ingesting cyanide.[407]

Zofiówka Psychiatric Hospital Mortality Rate, May–November 1941[408]

May 1941	10%
June 1941	16%
July 1941	12%
August 1941	9%
September 1941	7%
October 1941	15%
November 1941	18%

404 Ibid., p. 269. On the concentration of these patients at Zofiowka Psychiatric Hospital, see also Cohen, "Harefu'a Besherut Ha'idiologiya," p. 153.

405 Jewish Social Self-Help, Statistics Department Report, no. 6, November 1941, AŻIH, ARI.32, p. 26.

406 Lewin, *A Cup of Tears*, p. 161n305; Ringelblum, *Ktavim Aharonim*, p. 154; Cohen, "Harefu'a Besherut Ha'idiologiya," pp. 152–153.

407 Calel Perechodnik, *Hatafkid He'atzuv Shel Hati'ud*: *Yoman Mahbo* (The Sad Role of Documentation: A Diary in Hiding) (Hebrew) (Jerusalem: Keter, 1993), pp. 48–49; Calel Perechodnik, *Am I a Murderer? Testament of a Jewish Ghetto Policeman* (Boulder: Westview Press, 1996), pp. 30–31.

408 Ibid.

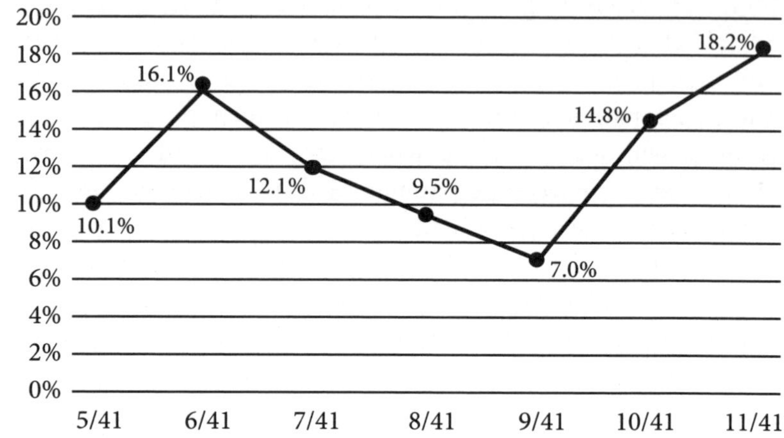

Pharmacies and Medicines

About a month and a half after the occupation began, the effects of the war and the shelling generated an enormous demand for medicines and home medical equipment that resulted in acute shortages in Warsaw. Long lines formed in front of utterly depleted pharmacies.[409] The medicine shortage was particularly problematic among the Jews, due to an order that had forced the Jewish pharmacies to close their doors. Two and a half months into the occupation, on December 11, 1939, Czerniaków reported that the Jewish pharmacies had ceased to exist.[410]

Several days before the move to the ghetto, negotiations regarding the pharmacies were conducted with the Poles. There were 21 such establishments in the ghetto area, 7 owned by Jews. When the occupation had begun, the Jewish proprietors had been ousted and replaced by Poles. After ghettoization, the Germans intended to leave 11 pharmacies there, under Jewish

409 Ringelblum, *Yoman Vereshimot*, pp. 94, 190.

410 Czerniaków, *The Warsaw Diary*, p. 98. On March 26, 1936, Jews in the Reich were forbidden to run pharmacies. About eight months before the war began, on January 31, 1939, they were no longer allowed to work in pharmacies. This prohibition was also imposed in the General Government.

ownership and supervised by the Judenrat.[411] Seeking to improve the supply of pharmaceuticals and medical equipment in the ghetto, Czerniaków discussed the issue of wholesale businesses, drug stores, and pharmacies with Dressel, an official in the German Trusteeship Office.[412]

In February 1941, after the Jews had been living in the ghetto for two months, medicines were manifestly in short supply. The non-Jewish pharmacies had totally run out.[413] In March 1941, due to the dearth of pharmaceuticals, 300,000 zlotys were raised in credit to buy out the Polish owners of 9 pharmacies.[414] Two months later, the ghetto had 14 pharmacies that employed 150 pharmacists and 120 other workers. In August 1941, there were 19 pharmacies, one of which dispensed medicines to the poor at no charge.

Moris Kohn and Zelig Heller, refugees from Łódź, were involved in the pharmaceutical activities. They collaborated with Abraham Gancwajch and Group 13 for a certain period,[415] but subsequently broke away and strengthened their relations with the Gestapo, expanding their operations in the ghetto—operating the horse-drawn carts that had replaced the trams and holding a franchise for the delivery of medicines to pharmacies.[416] Until July 1941, there seem to have been Polish factories and pharmacies in the ghetto. Polish workers entered the ghetto each day and, with their assistance, the Jews conducted many transactions with the Aryan side.[417]

411 Kaplan, *Scroll of Agony*, pp. 223–224. On the pharmacies, see also Trunk, *Judenrat*, p. 157.

412 Czerniaków, *The Warsaw Diary*, p. 219.

413 Ringelblum, *Notes from the Warsaw Ghetto*, p. 131.

414 Ibid., p. 141.

415 Group 13 comprised a network of institutions and associations in the ghetto established by Abraham Gancwajch and a group of people, most of them refugees, whom he had gathered. The "13" got its name from 13 Leszno St., where it had its offices. It had 300–400 members. The Germans supported its activities, and many in the ghetto regarded it and its members as Nazi agents and informants. Indeed, its activities were under German supervision and its members operated as German agents. See Gutman, *The Jews of Warsaw*, pp. 91–94; Bauer, *Rethinking the Holocaust*, pp. 90–94.

416 Roland, *Courage under Siege*, pp. 71–72.

417 Lensky, *A Physician inside the Warsaw Ghetto*, p. 47.

There were times when one pharmacy served 25,000 people. According to Trunk, the Judenrat supply department was authorized to buy medicines outside the ghetto through the offices of the Transferstelle, a German-run transfer bureau that was in charge of the transfer of goods to and from the ghetto, overseeing the ghetto's limited official economic relations with the outside world. The ghetto also had a wholesale shop that held a franchise for supplying the ghetto pharmacies with medicines.[418] According to the Judenrat statistics department, the ghetto had 17 active pharmacies with a turnover of 367,370 zlotys in February 1942. That month saw an increase in the number of prescriptions that the pharmacies filled at a 50 percent discount for the poor. However, the total turnover shrank due to the weakening of the epidemic, the increase in the prices of certain medications, and the shortages of others in the market. For these reasons, the pharmacies applied to the authorities for permission to raise the prices of the medicines that they prepared by 100 percent relative to their 1938 levels.[419]

The difficulties in obtaining medicines also caused the increase in prices. Since an institution received a small fee for a medical checkup by a physician, it sought to reduce expenses by limiting the provision of medicines. Patients who wanted a special new drug had to buy it at a high-priced, private pharmacy. In the end, most medicines apparently came from the Aryan side illegally and through multiple intermediaries.[420] In the context of the phenomenon of bribery that thrived in all the Judenrat departments, Edward Kobryner, the head of the Pharmacists' Association, was also a target of criticism. The Judenrat taxed medicines at 40 percent.[421] In February 1942, the Bund/Zukunft underground newspaper *Der Wecker* (The Awakener) bitingly

418 The directive to establish the Transferstelle was promulgated on April 14, 1941. Initially this body was responsible for supplying food to the ghetto. In the spring of 1941, it also took charge of production and of the ghetto factories. See Blatman, *Geto Varsha—Sipur Itona'i*, p. 156; Trunk, *Judenrat*, pp. 157, 605.

419 Judenrat Statistics Department Report, no. 29, March 17, 1942, GFH, no. 11250.

420 Lensky, *A Physician inside the Warsaw Ghetto*, p. 104.

421 Ringelblum, *Notes from the Warsaw Ghetto*, p. 166.

decried the high cost of medicines, in general, and the Judenrat's policy, in particular.

> A scandal that cries to the heavens is raging at the pharmacies. The kehilla [Judenrat] is taking an additional 40 percent on the price. Because of the exorbitant price, the poor cannot afford drugs that have been prescribed for them. The kehilla clerks are exempted from the levy.[422]

However, it is important to remember that the Judenrat allocated huge sums from its parched budget for medical care.[423] According to the Jewish Social Self-Help, TOZ, Linas Hatzedek, and other associations distributed thousands of medicines free of charge or at a discount.[424]

The efforts invested in running the ghetto pharmacies were essential for the provision of medical services, but they fell far short of the needs. Those responsible for health care and medicine issued an urgent call to Jewish relief organizations and their representatives in the free world to ship medical supplies and equipment to the ghetto to help eradicate epidemics. The issue of receiving pharmaceuticals from sources outside the ghetto, apart from its implications for alleviating the shortage of such commodities, sheds light on the procurement of relief from those fortunate enough not to be under occupation—the "observers" or "bystanders." It is possible to learn from the array of players about the tensions and the complexity of the Jewish entities that operated in Nazi-occupied Warsaw and Poland, and elsewhere as well. The sources indicate that several bodies were involved in sending medicine to the ghetto, albeit in very limited and inadequate quantities, and it is possible to identify various channels of shipments of medicines, some aided by public institutions and others as private initiatives.

422 Blatman, *Geto Varsha—Sipur Itona'i*, p. 202; Ringelblum, *Yoman Vereshimot*, p. 347.

423 Trunk, *Judenrat*, pp. 159–160.

424 Jewish Social Self-Help, Statistics Department Report, no. 6, November 1941, AŻIH, ARI.32, p. 24.

In an early 1943 report, Dr. Boris Tschlenoff, the head of OZE, described an "OZE medicine operation for the benefit of the Jewish population in Poland and other occupied countries" between November 1940 and January 1943. Already in 1940, when the OZE headquarters was still in Paris, initiatives were taken to help Polish Jewry, and budgets were set aside for this purpose. Drugs, essential instruments, and small quantities of food were sent to TOZ in Warsaw through the mediation of the International Committee of the Red Cross in Geneva. Tschlenoff wrote that with the help of the Red Cross, the shipment was expedited with no customs and freight charges, and its delivery to the correct addresses was assured through the local offices of the German Red Cross.

The TOZ parcels were distributed among the inhabitants of Warsaw and the vicinity, mainly for children, and among the hospitals and the social medicine institutions. However, the depletion of OZE's resources, occasioned by the many tasks that the international situation foisted on the organization, forced it to terminate its relief shipments. Nevertheless, OZE was able to send shipments to Poland and other occupied countries later on, thanks to the assistance of the Federation of Swiss Jewish Communities under Saly Mayer.

The first large shipment to reach TOZ in Warsaw arrived in late 1940. In 1941, as transport difficulties mounted, only four cargoes reached Warsaw and Cracow. In 1942, with Saly Mayer's assistance, more resources became available and the number of shipments, which included medicines, vitamins, bandages, and the like, increased. However, Tschlenoff claimed in a report that it was impossible to meet the tremendous needs even slightly amid such distress and that only a government agency could accomplish this. Therefore, the goal was limited to attempting to send scarce medicines that would help to fight dangerous epidemics, as well as to provide assistance to improve sanitation. In all, medicines worth 220,000 Swiss francs were shipped in 1942, and more than 10,000 Swiss francs were allocated for food parcels.[425]

425 These data pertain not only to Warsaw, in particular, and to Poland, in general, but to all other countries that interacted with the OZE.

In the course of 1941, medicines were sent directly to Warsaw. However, in 1942, large quantities were shipped mainly to Cracow through Dr. Michael Weichert, who at the Germans' behest presided over the Jewish Social Self-Help in the General Government. Thus, the Germans granted limited permission to distribute medicines among various locations in that territory, especially valuable drugs, such as typhus vaccinations, cardiac medications, vitamins, hormones, analgesics, bandages, and so on. Small quantities of food were sent as well. Dr. Tschlenoff noted, in particular, a shipment of 6,900 doses of the typhus vaccine to Cracow, expressing some misgivings.

> Even if, to our delight, several Jewish organizations, as well as individuals in Switzerland sent reinforcement measures, medicines, and more to Poland, it remains highly regrettable that we were unable to transfer enough due to a lack of funds.... Unfortunately, I must add that leading Jewish circles in Switzerland showed no particular interest in the desolate Jewish population of Poland.[426]

Alongside the OZE–TOZ activities that Tschlenoff facilitated, the virtually private initiative of Elias Sternbuch, president of the Bikur Holim Society in St. Gallen, Switzerland, is notable. The archives contain documents from Sternbuch's correspondence with Weichert, and with others from whom Sternbuch managed to procure medicines, including the International Committee of the Red Cross in Geneva, particularly Dr. Robert Boehringer, the chief of the Medical Department of the ICRC's relief enterprises, and the Institute for Hygiene at the University of Zurich, headed by Prof. Hermann Mooser.

In one of Sternbuch's letters, it appears that Sternbuch transferred funds to the Red Cross for the purchase of typhus

426 Tschlenoff report, November 1940–January 1943, GFH, no. 1194. See also the correspondence between Dr. Tschlenoff and Tropper—the purchase of medicines for TOZ Poland, letter from Dr. Tschlenoff to Lisbon—JDC, AR.33–44, file 840. On actions undertaken by the Red Cross on behalf of the Jews in the occupied countries, see Dworzecki, "The International Red Cross," pp. 71–110.

vaccines from Prof. Mooser during 1942. Sternbuch also negotiated with others at the Red Cross, and it is possible to discern a "triangular relationship" comprised of Sternbuch, the Red Cross, and Weichert's Jewish Social Self-Help organization in Cracow. At first, Sternbuch apparently tried to send the shipment directly to Warsaw and to other destinations, but the Red Cross restricted him and ordered him to transfer the provisions through Weichert in Cracow.

In the course of 1941, Sternbuch broached the idea of a humanitarian relief operation to send medical supplies—medicines, vaccines, and disinfectants—to the Warsaw ghetto. He tried to mobilize the assistance of all the organizations and people he thought would be able to help. In November 1941, with the ghetto in the throes of a typhus epidemic, Sternbuch corresponded with Dr. B. de Rouge of the Red Cross concerning the planned operation. The Red Cross demanded 15 Swiss francs per vaccine, with payment through the German Red Cross. However, according to the letter, the shipment had yet to be approved. In return for undertaking Sternbuch's shipment of medicines, the Red Cross demanded $10,000.

In January 1942, Dr. Boehringer of the Red Cross confirmed in a letter to Sternbuch that he had received 3,741 Swiss francs as an advance payment for the operation. However, he also implied in the letter that Dr. Tschlenoff, acting on behalf of OZE, operated along channels that were inconsistent with Sternbuch's work. Thus, by his account, the JDC funds, which were intended for general medical purposes and not exclusively to combat typhus, could not be allocated for Sternbuch's operation.[427] In February 1942, the Red Cross sent a postcard to Sternbuch, confirming the arrival of 306 ampules and informing him that Prof. Hirszfeld in the Warsaw ghetto had been let in on the secret. The contents of the postcard also indicated that Sternbuch had solicited donors to raise money for the typhus vaccines.[428]

427 On the reverberations of these disagreements, see JDC correspondence with the president of Agudath Israel concerning medicines for Poland, December 1941, JDC, AR.33–44, file 840.

428 GFH, nos. 21351–21356.

In April 1942, Sternbuch wrote to the Jewish Social Self-Help in Cracow, "We expedited the operation at the Red Cross and did all sorts of things to help your needy efficiently." He reported that he had sent 90 ampules for certain individuals and 240 for general use. Sternbuch hired a Swiss citizen living in Warsaw to oversee the ampules that had been delivered, and to ensure that they would reach those in need of them and would not be "put on the market." He also implored Weichert to apprise TOZ in Warsaw of these ampules.[429]

Sternbuch also described the professional discussions held in Geneva concerning ways to help typhus-ravaged communities, including their proposal to emphasize setting up a delousing facility. Sternbuch asked what instruments and chemical substances were required for the war on lice, and made it his goal to procure them. He also imparted Prof. Mooser's opinion on ways to fight typhus and asked for details about what the Jews needed to prepare for a far-reaching, anti-lice campaign in Warsaw and in other cities.

There are also six postcards sent by Dr. Weichert in Cracow to Dr. Sternbuch of the Bikur Holim Society in the archives. In April 1942, Weichert wrote to Sternbuch, thanking him for his willingness to help with the shipment of sterilization instruments and medicines, and enclosing lists of all the chemicals and pharmaceuticals needed. Another letter that arrived the next day, addressed to the supply department of the Bikur Holim Society, included a note on how the medicines were to be distributed. Dr. Weichert made it clear that all shipments to the General Government had to be addressed to the ICRC's general commissioner in Cracow, who would pass them on to the Jewish Social Self-Help. Weichert explained that if any shipments were intended specifically to help the Jews of Warsaw, the shipments should be addressed to the Red Cross representative in Warsaw on behalf of the Jewish Social Self-Help. He added that if Warsaw was the sole destination, forwarding the supplies to other ghettos would be problematic. However, if they reached Cracow directly,

429 Ibid.

he had the authority to distribute them to other communities.[430]

Sternbuch and the Red Cross continued to correspond in May 1942. From this correspondence, we learn that Sternbuch continued to transfer funds to the Red Cross for the anti-typhus campaign and the purchase of vaccines that it entailed. However, the 300 ampules, some of them earmarked for Warsaw, due to arrive from Prof. Mooser were delayed. That month, Sternbuch received a letter from the Red Cross confirming the arrival of typhus vaccines from the Institute of Hygiene of the University of Zurich. The correspondent noted that some of them would be transferred to the Jewish Social Self-Help in Warsaw.[431]

In July 1942, Sternbuch advised the Jewish Social Self-Help in Warsaw that two packages and a crate containing 500 kilograms of soap powder, three parcels containing 500 kilograms of coal oil, and five crates containing 500 kilograms of sulfur had been shipped. They were intended for a delousing campaign and instructions concerning their use would follow. Sternbuch added that Mr. Domb, a Swiss citizen living in Warsaw, had been charged with overseeing that the shipment would be used correctly, and he requested confirmation of the shipment that had been made through the Red Cross.[432]

In an August 1942 letter, Weichert explained that the Jewish Social Self-Help was responsible for the 400 Jewish communities and, therefore, he should be advised of the names of the localities if they wished to send the shipment to certain recipients. He also expressed his commitment to distributing the serums intended for specific individuals, as stated in the request on the list that had been sent. In a letter to Sternbuch in November 1942, Weichert confirmed that he had received a large shipment of serum and that the material would be used for its intended purpose and not for anything else, as promised.[433]

430 GFH, no. 1933.

431 GFH, nos. 21351–21356.

432 GFH, no. 21342. Concerning certification from Weichert, see the letter from the International Red Cross to Sternbuch, February 23, 1942, in which Weichert confirmed having received the vaccines, GFH, no. 9574.

433 GFH, no. 1933.

In August 1942, Sternbuch received a letter from W. Simon, an official from the Medical Department of the Red Cross, confirming that a shipment of 50-gram boxes of Neocid powder had been sent to the Jewish Social Self-Help in Warsaw. The boxes reached the Red Cross representatives in Warsaw as part of the anti-typhus operation. Dr. A. Grumbach of the Institute of Hygiene in Zurich contacted Sternbuch in September 1942 to express puzzlement about a piece that had appeared in a Jewish weekly concerning typhus vaccinations, implying that someone else was sending vaccines into the ghetto. He demanded an explanation, "Since we're the only ones who produce typhus vaccines, I would appreciate it if you would tell us where you're buying this vaccine." Dr. Grumbach's remark suggests that others must have been manufacturing vaccines for the ghetto population. Indeed, it was known, for example, that Prof. Rudolf Weigl, who had developed an effective vaccine against typhus, helped to smuggle this preparation into the ghetto, where it had become an important source for fighting the epidemic.[434]

In November 1942, Dr. Boehringer of the International Committee of the Red Cross advised Sternbuch that his organization could deliver 100 units of typhus vaccine to the Jewish Social Self-Help in Cracow.[435] In his efforts to obtain food and vitamins for the Jews of Poland, Sternbuch also made inquiries with the Kajotes firm in Lisbon about the possibility of shipping disinfectant, vaccines, and foodstuffs via the Polish Red Cross in August 1943.[436] As for shipments of medicines after the liquidation of the Warsaw ghetto, several letters have survived. It seems, at this stage, that the letters appear to have arrived several months apart and that communication among those involved had become more difficult.

A letter sent in June 1943 indicated that even though seven months had passed since Sternbuch had sent 100 units of

434 See Chapter 7 of this book.
435 GFH, no. 21352.
436 GFH, no. 21368.

the typhus vaccine in November 1942, confirmation of receipt had not yet arrived. In his letter, Sternbuch asked whether the shipment had reached its destination. He repeated the request in July 1943, adding that pending confirmation of the arrival of the shipment, he would not be able to send additional parcels. In June 1943, Weichert wrote about the distribution of shipments of medicine and equipment to forced labor camps where Jews had been sent. Until May 1944, there was extensive correspondence between Switzerland and Cracow that aimed to facilitate these ongoing shipments.[437]

Another avenue of activity that Sternbuch employed was through Prof. Mooser of the Institute of Hygiene at the University of Zurich. In November 1941, Mooser informed Sternbuch that he had approached the American Red Cross to request that it take action to obtain a large quantity of typhus vaccines for the Jews of Poland. He also reported that he had sent to the International Committee of the Red Cross in Geneva typhus vaccines for 100 persons, which he had personally taken part in preparing, and that Dr. Tschlenoff had promised to arrange payment for them. However, once again, the tension between Dr. Tschlenoff and Sternbuch was apparent. According to Prof. Mooser,

> Tschlenoff claimed, "As for typhus, the situation in Warsaw isn't as bad as you say. Tschlenoff doubts that we will receive $10,000 for the relief actions. How he came around to this opinion is not clear to me. Would you be willing to get in touch with him? I have the impression that he's jealous of you, but I might be wrong. I only read this between the lines.[438]

In January 1942, Prof. Mooser reported that the Red Cross had made available enough vaccines for 5,000 people at no charge, but added that he did not know when the shipment would arrive. It turns out that Mooser, who had received payment for every portion of serum, had lowered the price to 10 Swiss francs per person.

437 GFH, no. 21344.
438 GFH, no. 21339.

"Unfortunately, I cannot lower the price any further because I have to work only with mice; the use of hatching eggs is forbidden." The correspondence indicates that Mooser was in touch with Prof. Hirszfeld in the Warsaw ghetto.[439]

In yet another channel of activity, Sternbuch established a connection with members of Agudath Israel in the United States with the hope that they could influence other Jewish institutions in that country. In response, Jacob Rosenheim, president of Agudath Israel World Organization in New York, advised Sternbuch in October 1941 that the JDC in the United States had approved an allocation of $10,000 for the purchase of the vaccines. To the best of his knowledge, Rosenheim continued, $7,500 had been sent and the rest would be transferred later through the Quakers, a Christian group. In November 1941, Rosenheim advised Sternbuch that the JDC had informed him during a telephone inquiry that they had a receipt for this sum, which had been paid in Lisbon.[440]

Even after the ghetto had been razed, some Jews in Warsaw continued to receive medicines, bandages, and food from abroad. Dr. Weichert claimed that between May 2 and July 15, 1943, fifty-six ships with parcels of medicines and other medical supplies had arrived from overseas. The goods had been sent to twenty-nine camps, ghettos, and enterprises that employed Jews.[441] During this period, contacts and correspondence concerning shipments

439 Ibid.

440 GFH, no. 21338. See also JDC correspondence with the president of Agudath Israel concerning medicines for Poland, December 1941, JDC, AR.33–44, file 840; Offer, "Ma'arach Harefu'a Begeto Varsha," vol. 2, appendix A.22, pp. 114–116.

441 Michael Weichert's inquiries to the Committee for Aid to Jewish War Casualties, GFH, no. 1186; Weichert's letters to high SS and police officials in the General Government, GFH, no. 4102; Weichert's reports, May 12–June 1944, GFH, no. 1145; Weichert's letter to the SS and Police commander regarding medicines for prisoners, GFH, no. 1160. On shipments of parcels (including medicines) to the ghetto by means of Jewish welfare offices in neutral countries, see Raya Cohen, *Bein Sham Lekan: Sipurim Shel Edim Lahorban, Shveitz 1939–1942* (Between Here and There: The Story of Witnesses to the Destruction, Jewish Emissaries in Switzerland 1939–1942) (Hebrew) (Tel Aviv: Am Oved, 1999).

of medicines and medical equipment for Polish Jews by means of the Red Cross and the Jewish Social Self-Help continued.[442]

It should be noted that groups of activists from various Jewish organizations in Warsaw were mordantly critical of Michael Weichert's activities. Accusing him of serving the Germans more than serving the Jews, they found his actions repulsive, even before the *Aktionen* and the deportations, and all the more so after them. In a letter from Warsaw to London in May 1944, they wrote, "We demand that the shipping of medicines and food through Geneva and the CKM in Cracow be stopped immediately.[443] We also demand that all funds from the government be sent solely to Warsaw. We are in direct contact with…the camps."[444] Unlike this group of activists, Tschlenoff considered the support center in Cracow the only safe place for the delivery of medicines to Jews in the General Government.[445]

The few Polish doctors who stayed in touch with their Jewish colleagues were another source of medicines and medical equipment for the ghetto. Some of these doctors risked their

442 GFH, no. 21352.

443 CKM were evidently the initials of another name of the National Jewish Social Self-Help Committee, seated in Cracow, the capital of the General Government, which Dr. Michael Weichert continued to run in 1944, even at this advanced stage of the Holocaust. Weichert and his actions stirred controversy during and after the war. In the context of his role as the head of the JSS during the war, the main criticism concerned his continuing to run the organization under Nazi supervision, after the Germans had begun the systematic murder of Polish Jewry. During that time, the organization was renamed the Jewish Welfare Office (JUS) in the General Government. After the war, Weichert was tried by a Polish court on the charge of collaboration with the Germans and was acquitted. Thereafter, he was tried before a public tribunal of the Central Committee of Polish Jews. On these trials, see David Engel, "Remove the Evil from the Midst of Thee: On the Concept of Collaboration in the Trials of Michael Weichert," in Shmuel Almog et al., *The Holocaust—History and Memory: Essays Presented in Honor of Israel Gutman* (Jerusalem: Yad Vashem and The Avraham Harman Institute of Contemporary Jewry, The Hebrew University of Jerusalem, 2001), pp. 1–24. See also Engel, "Who Is a Collaborator? The Trials of Michael Weichert," in Slawomir Kapralski, *The Jews in Poland* (Cracow: Judaica Foundation and the Center for Jewish Culture, 1999), vol. 2, pp. 339–370.

444 GFH, no. 19852.

445 GFH, no. 1194.

lives doing so. They were recognized after the war as Righteous Among the Nations. Noteworthy among them is Prof. Edward Loth, who helped set up the medical school in the Warsaw ghetto. In addition to books and scholastic and scientific materials, Loth smuggled drugs into the ghetto and even helped to treat patients when called upon to do so. Loth was killed in the August 1944 Polish uprising. He was recognized as Righteous Among the Nations in July 1996.[446]

The individual and organizational efforts described above deserve our appreciation. However, it is important to note that, despite these efforts, they were unable to amass enough medicines and medical supplies to assure the survival of the ghetto inhabitants, and when shipments did reach the ghetto, the Germans often confiscated them. Dr. Józef Chajn Gołębiewski, who practiced medicine at the TOZ clinics and held additional positions in the ghetto medical system, attested that he had repeatedly visited the Transferstelle to receive the shipments of medicines that had arrived from Switzerland for TOZ. However, each time, he found that some of the supplies had been confiscated by the *Volksdeutsche* who had been appointed by the Warsaw municipality as liaisons between the German health care services in town and the Judenrat Health Department in the ghetto. Dr. Kobylinski, one of these liaisons, was tried after the war but was exonerated.[447]

The following diagram presents the entities mentioned above, describing the various methods used to attempt to send medications and other medical necessities to the Warsaw ghetto.

446 Benjamin Anolik, "Rofim Polanim Hasidei Umot Ha'olam" (Polish Doctors Righteous Among the Nations) (Hebrew) (paper presented at the Eighth Nahariya Conference on Morbidity and Medicine in the Holocaust, Western Galilee Hospital, Nahariya, May 20, 2007). I am grateful to the late Benjamin Anolik for sending me his paper.

447 Dr. Józef Chajn Gołębiewski testimony, YVA, O.3/2355.

Shipments of Medicines to the Warsaw Ghetto

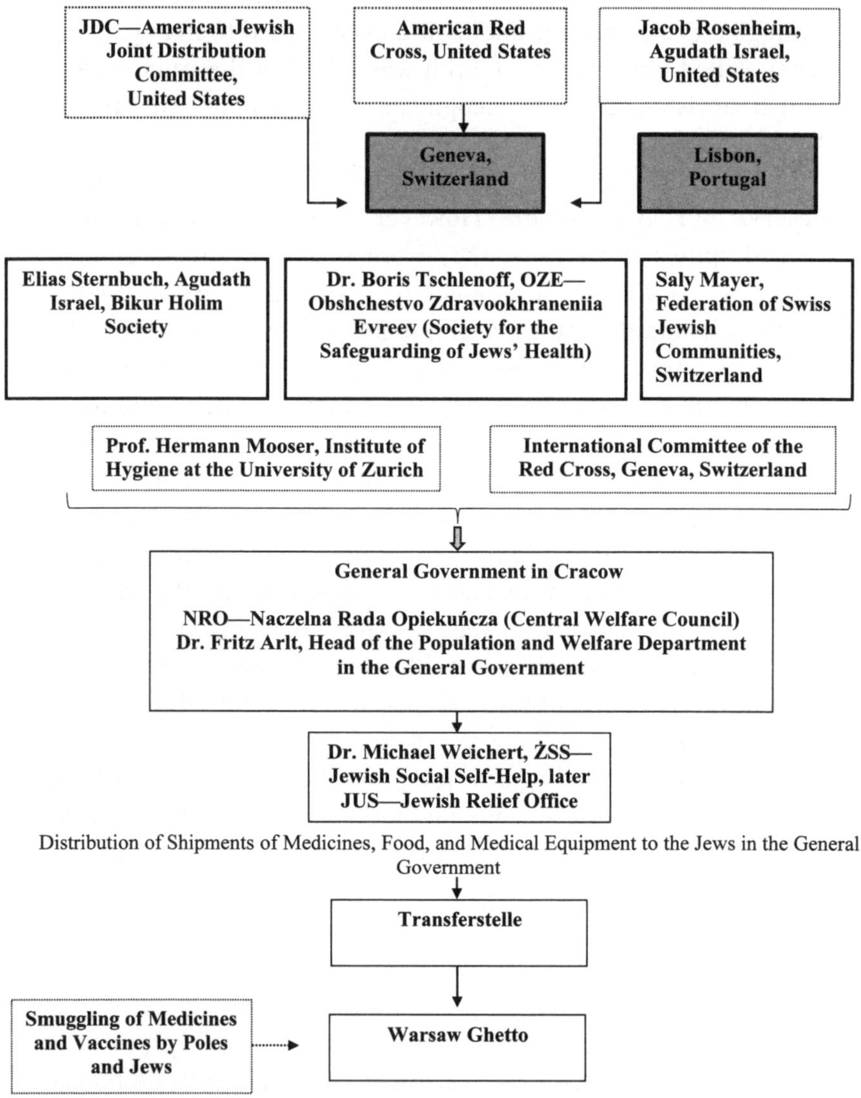

First Aid Station

After the Jews were banished to the ghetto, there was an urgent need to establish a first aid service for them. The Jews were being brutally beaten and seriously injured in the ghetto streets, and it took a long time to provide aid to the ill and the wounded.[448] Due to the urgency of the matter, an alternative first aid station was set up in the "Warsaw First Aid Building" at 58 Leszno St. in the ghetto. The building had been gradually falling into ruin after its tenants had abandoned it, and the Warsaw first aid administration agreed to hand it over to another Jewish institution that had promised to maintain it.

The Jewish Social Self-Help appointed the first aid staff in late 1941 and early 1942. At first, the team of doctors was assembled according to professional requirements. However, as the situation worsened, people with connections were allowed to join. In all, the staff was composed of around ten physicians and four aides.[449] All the hospitals in the ghetto acknowledged the station's activities and recognized its importance. The ill and the wounded who were taken to the hospitals by the first aid workers, upon the referral of the station doctors, were treated as special cases who did not have to wait in line.[450] When the *Aktionen* began, the doctors and staff of the station, along with their families, moved into vacant apartments near the facility. The area was marked with a red cross, the familiar emblem of a medical institution and, therefore, was safe and protected from abductions and deportations.

The clinic at the station operated round-the-clock. An old Citroen, painted yellow and adapted as an ambulance, served as its

448 Ringelblum, *Notes from the Warsaw Ghetto*, p. 114.

449 The initiating committee was led by a Jewish community activist and lawyer, the Jewish apostate Zundelewicz. The gynecologist Dr. Gottlieb, director of the board, served as the chief physician of the first aid station; Lichtenstein (or Lichtenbaum) was the secretary; Mr. Margulies was the treasurer; and there were two other members of the board, Mr. Rotsztajn and the lawyer Dawidowicz.

450 Jerzy Ross (Rosenberg), "Tahanat Ezra Rishona Begeto Varsha" (A First Aid Station in the Warsaw Ghetto), *Yalkut Moreshet* (Hebrew), 14 (1972), pp. 67–69.

first aid vehicle. The station also had a "sanitary rickshaw" composed of a crate and metal rails on small wheels, bearing stretchers and a seat for the physician on duty. In addition, the station used ordinary rickshaws when the doctors found it necessary to move patients from place to place. The staff of the station received special German permits that allowed them to circulate without restriction during curfew. Staff members wore standard dark blue caps decorated with a blue and white band with the Red Cross emblem. The medical equipment at the clinic included an operating table, sterilization instruments, and a set of surgical implements, among other things, and the staff members would take one of three packs of first aid supplies with them when summoned.

The worse the conditions in the ghetto became, the more critical the role of the first aid station. The station was the only entity that could move the ill and the wounded from one place to another, and its staff were summoned to all kinds of rapid-response situations—shootings, beatings, suicides, and the like. In several cases, they crawled into fields of gunfire to extricate casualties. Both the ghetto population and its German overseers called on the first aid station staff when necessary, either in person or by telephone. Nocturnal calls were usually for bowel spasms, intestinal crises, kidney stones, or gallstones. The doctors were also summoned at night to administer first aid for gunshot wounds when, for example, German police fired on smugglers who threw goods over the wall, or when people attempted to slip over to the Aryan side.

When the ill were transported, a fee was charged according to the distance, the floor level, and the patient's estimated financial wherewithal. Although the station delivered aid at no charge, patients paid for bandages and sometimes for costly anesthesia.[451] When the station first began to operate, its service included travel outside the ghetto, for a fee, mainly to the Jewish convalescent homes and the clinics in Otwock. There were also trips to shtetls, where the staff surreptitiously carried away people who had been shot by the Gestapo and had been presumed dead. This clandestine

451 Ibid., pp. 68–71.

activity was conducted by telling the authorities that a contagious patient was being moved.

When the transports began, a group of wealthy individuals in the ghetto paid the driver of the first aid station, Spiwak, to drive to Treblinka and gather information about what was taking place there. Spiwak did as he was told. Equipped with German papers identifying him as a buyer of bristles for a brush factory, he returned with the first report about what was transpiring at the extermination camp before the arrival of the first escapees from Treblinka to Warsaw in the summer or autumn of 1942.[452] The first aid workers sometimes had arguments with those around them when they refused to take people who were dying of starvation in the street to a hospital, knowing that no hospital would admit them. This also occurred when they were asked to transport persons who were severely wounded and dying.

At first, the main aim of first aid was to respond to calls for help from people enfeebled by starvation. Jerzy Ross (Rosenberg) wrote about such cases.

> We were at a loss, having no resources with which to feed or strengthen [people]. Like everyone, we were undernourished. Under pressure from the crowds, we had to give people who were dying of starvation injections of camphor, which were worthless. We sometimes gave camphor together with strychnine (a vegetable substance that stimulates the nervous system, elevates the pulse, and heightens breathing).[453]

During the *Grossaktion*, the station continued to operate, no longer as a regular public institution but as a workplace that provided its members with a minimum income and sheltered them from deportation. By now, everyone in the ghetto was working without pay, and some found a way to make a living in the first aid profession—doctors went into private practice and members of the sanitary team administered injections or performed cupping,

452 Ibid., pp. 72–75.
453 Ibid., pp. 70–71.

moved patients from place to place, and traded surreptitiously in medicines.

During the transports to Treblinka, the staff of the first aid station participated in the medical teams' efforts to rescue people. Even in this framework, as in all organizations, some individuals revealed their weaknesses. Rotsztajn, a member of the station's board, and the aforementioned driver Spiwak set up a "business" of their own, assisting anyone who could pay well for the privilege of escaping from the Umschlagplatz. Rotsztajn was ultimately captured and shot by the Gestapo.[454]

In April 1943, at the beginning of the uprising, a provisional hospital for wounded fighters and the civilian population was established on the grounds of the first aid station. Medical aid was provided in underground passageways and lofts, which the staff reached by passing through openings in cellars and attic walls without stepping onto the street. The members of the first aid team sometimes took advantage of their freedom of movement to send information and parcels of weapons and ammunition from Leszno St. to the streets Zamenhofa, Muranowska, and Miła in the ghetto. The station was unique among the ghetto's institutions. Evidently, it was also the last sanitary institution to be evacuated—on April 23 or 24, the fifth day of the uprising.[455] Jerzy Ross held the crucial work of the first aid station under the grim conditions in high esteem.

> There was never a case of refusal to go to some emergency, day or night. They took no account of their personal safety under conditions never before known in history, and set a personal example of fulfilling their duty, loyal service, and quiet heroism.[456]

The first aid facility set up by Group 13 was of a completely different nature. On May 18, 1941, about half a year after the sealing

454 Ibid., pp. 73–74.
455 Ibid., pp. 69, 72–73.
456 Ibid., pp. 75–76.

of the Warsaw ghetto, this organization established a network for the delivery of first aid under the management of Dr. Sierota. When it first became active, it made sure, among other things, to distribute a certain quantity of slices of bread to the hungry.[457] In early June 1941, its people suddenly appeared in the ghetto streets, wearing special caps with blue bands and red Stars of David.[458]

On June 7, 1941, festivities erupted on Ceglana St. in celebration of the delivery to the hospital of an ambulance wagon as a gift from Group 13.[459] The purpose of the vehicle was to gather ill people in the streets, give them first aid, take them to the hospital, and feed them bread and tea. The vehicle appeared to have dealt with emergencies and to have helped capture smugglers, until Group 13 was put out of service in August 1942. The group set up clinics that were never activated. Czerniaków managed to terminate some of its policing operations, and its members became part of the Judenrat and thus ceased to operate as a separate body.[460]

In addition to the Jewish police, volunteers from other organizations and groups participated in the deportation campaign, headed by the crimson-capped members of Abraham Gancwajch's first aid staff.

> This organization of swindlers had never given a single Jew the medical aid they promised...voluntarily reported for the assignment of sending Jews to the hereafter—and they distinguished themselves with their brutality and inhumanity. Their caps were covered with the bloodstains of the Jewish people.[461]

The ending of this organization attests to how it began and what it actually was.

457 Ringelblum, *Notes from the Warsaw Ghetto*, p. 179.
458 Ibid., p. 185.
459 Czerniaków, *The Warsaw Diary*, p. 247.
460 Roland, *Courage under Siege*, pp. 67–68.
461 Ringelblum, *Notes from the Warsaw Ghetto*, p. 332.

Clinics and Laboratories

Alongside inpatient services in the hospitals, ambulatory clinics were established in the ghetto and were visited by thousands each month. They were run by sundry institutions and organizations, foremost TOZ, the Judenrat, Linas Hatzedek, the Friends of Children Society, Brijus Sanatorium, Czyste Hospital, and private physicians. Some patients were referred to clinics that were subsidized by the Jewish Social Self-Help. For example, according to a report from this organization, in July, eight months after entering the ghetto, the organization's Medical Department referred 8,278 people to these clinics. From July 1941 to November 1941, monthly referrals plummeted to 3,152, a 62 percent drop, because of the dwindling budgetary options to allocate to the provision of treatment.

Referrals by the Jewish Self-Help Organizations to Medical Institutions, July–November, 1941[462]

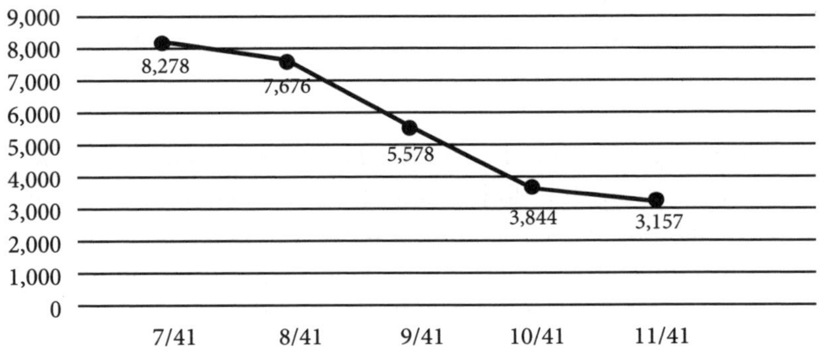

The Medical Department of the Jewish Social Self-Help referred patients to medical care providers for free or discounted consultations.[463]

462 Jewish Social Self-Help, Statistics Department Report, no. 6, November 1941, AŻIH, ARI.32, p. 17.

463 Ibid. The organizations had quite a few departments, including one for medical care. See Turkow, *Hayo Hayta Varsha Yehudit*, pp. 20–21, 23.

Referrals to Medical Institutions for Free or Discounted Care, November 1941[464]

Institution	Clinics Treatments		In-Home Treatments		Subtotal Treatments		Total
	No Fee	Discount	No Fee	Discount	No Fee	Discount	
TOZ	798	510	—	115	798	625	1,423
Judenrat Clinic	100	412	21	68	121	480	601
Linas Hatzedek	242	294	—	10	242	304	546
Friends of Children Society	107	23	—	—	107	23	130
Brijus Sanatorium	18	56	—	—	18	56	74
Czyste Clinic	—	25	—	—	—	25	25
Private Physicians	124	19	215	—	339	19	358
Total	**1,389**	**1,339**	**236**	**193**	**1,625**	**1,532**	**3,157**

TOZ received the largest subsidy: 46 percent of the total medical aid budget of the Jewish Social Self-Help. Nineteen percent of the budget went to the Judenrat clinic, 17 percent to Linas Hatzedek, 11 percent to private medicine, 4 percent to the Friends of Children Society, 2 percent to Brijus Sanatorium, and only 1 percent to the Czyste Clinic. About half of the 3,157 clients of the Jewish Social Self-Help were exempted from payment for medical services and the others received discounts.

Linas Hatzedek provided medical aid to thousands in the ghetto. In August 1941, 12,679 people were treated at its clinic. Historical research devotes less attention to this organization than it does to TOZ. According to a Jewish Social Self-Help report, relative to TOZ, which operated a broad and professional health care system in the ghetto, Linas Hatzedek was a large institution

464 Jewish Social Self-Help, Statistics Department Report, no. 6, November 1941, AŻIH, ARI.32, p. 17.

that provided medical services to a significant number of people, even in comparison with TOZ. There was actually a 40 percent decline in the number of patients treated by this organization in the ghetto between July and November 1941.

Patients Treated by Linas Hatzedek, July–November 1941[465]

July 1941	11,006
August 1941	12,679
September 1941	7,744
October 1941	7,256
November 1941	6,665

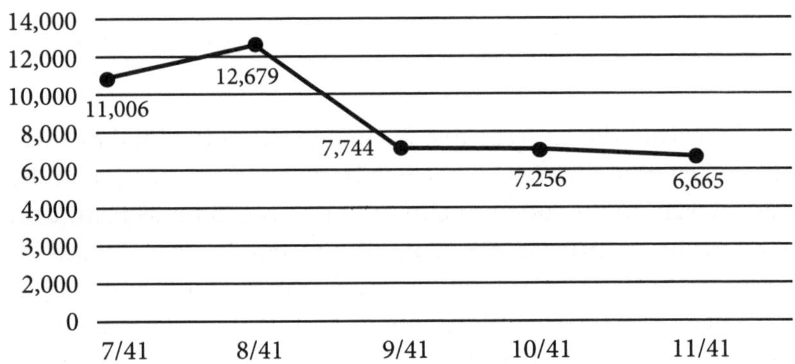

465 Ibid.

Medical Services Provided by Linas Hatzedek, September–November, 1941[466]

	September 1941	October 1941	November 1941
Ambulatory Consultations	4,775	4,166	4,207
Home Visits	424	487	488
X-rays	276	135	132
Laboratory Tests	1,159	1,225	915
Therapy	471	457	349
Bandaging	603	768	567
Other Care	36	18	7
Total	**7,744**	**7,256**	**6,665**

Compared with the figures in September 1941, in November 1941, there was a significant decrease in the numbers of laboratory tests, of patients receiving therapy, and of paramedic services. In contrast, the number of doctors' home visits increased.[467]

The vast majority of recipients of medical care at Linas Hatzedek paid full price. Only 7.4 percent received discounts in November 1941 and 4 percent were treated at no cost. The patient load fell by 38 percent between September and November, whereas those receiving care at no charge contracted by 29 percent. Just the same, the Linas Hatzedek clinic handed out 3,577 portions of medicine at no charge, in contrast to TOZ, which dispensed 2,440 portions that month, including 1,299 at no charge.

The mother and child care clinics in the ghetto were very active. This is indicative of the immense effort that the ghetto made to provide devoted care to preschool children and, no less, of the

466 Jewish Social Self-Help, Statistics Department Report, no. 6, November 1941, AŻIH, ARI.32, p. 26; on visits to doctors for payment, with discounts, or at no charge at the Linas Hatzedek clinic, September–November 1941, see Offer, "Ma'arach Harefu'a Begeto Varsha," vol. 2, appendix B.30, p. 185.

467 Offer, "Ma'arach Harefu'a Begeto Varsha," vol. 2, appendix B.30, p. 185.

population's unexpectedly high fertility rate, despite the ghastly living conditions. There were four mother and child care clinics in the Warsaw ghetto—at 28 Śliska St., 21 Nalewki St., 5 Lubeckiego St., and 11 Leszno St. The Friends of Children Society ran another large facility at 6 Elektoralna St. From July 1941 to November 1941, the mother and child care clinics saw a decrease in referrals of children for care. In contrast, there was an upward trend in the Friends of Children Society Clinic's patient load.[468]

Children Treated at the Mother and Child Care Clinics and the Children's Friends Society Clinic, July–November 1941[469]

Month		Mother and Child Care Clinics					Friends of Children Society Clinic
		28 Śliska	21 Nalewki	5 Lubeckiego	11 Leszno	Total	
July 1941		683	591	1,133	737	3,144	5,486
August 1941		654	558	991	734	2,937	5,774
September 1941		645	511	817	549	2,522	6,145
October 1941		557	478	831	577	2,443	6,390
November 1941	Beginning of Month	557	478	831	577	2,443	6,390
	New Patients	11	33	25	9	78	188
	Discharged	69	56	5	6	136	—
	Died	8	2	1	1	12	4
	End of Month	491	453	850	579	2,373	6,574

468 Ibid.

469 Ibid., pp. 24–25.

Overall, 8,630 infants and children received care at the five clinics in July 1941. Of these, 36 percent visited the four mother and child care clinics and 64 percent went to the Friends of Children Society Clinic, which had amassed a great deal of experience in mother and child health care in the interwar years. There was a 19.8 percent increase in the number of patients treated at the latter between July and November 1941, even as the number of patients of the mother and child care clinics dropped by 24.6 percent. In November of that year, 8,947 youngsters visited all five centers,[470] which distributed dry foods, milk, and, to a limited extent, food supplements. In November 1941, 69 percent of children who visited the clinics received dry foods; 13 percent, milk; and 8 percent, food supplements. In November, 6,362 youngsters visited the Friends of Children Society Clinic at 6 Elektoralna St. and 212 home visits were made. In all, 683 visits to doctors were recorded that month and 810 in October. Nurses administered treatment to 20 children in November and to 31 in October. Medicine was distributed to 97 patients and 203 children received 783 food parcels.[471]

In her testimony, Yehudit Braude attested that she ran three of the mother and child care clinics in the ghetto—at 11 Leszno St., 6 Elektoralna St., and 5 Lubeckiego St., working actively until August 1942, after the *Grossaktion* began. Sonja Lifszyc, a veteran nurse who was highly regarded by the patients, worked at the 11 Leszno St. facility. When the war broke out, the station continued its regular services, such as counseling and follow-up for pregnant women, periodic checkups, child development testing, and the like.[472]

The Friends of Children Society Clinic at 6 Elektoralna St. was opened at the beginning of the occupation in 1939. Run by Dr. Wasserman, it served youngsters aged four to fourteen. An oversight committee of sorts, which included the wife of the

470 On medical activity at the mother and child care centers and feeding clinics in September–November 1941, see Offer, "Ma'arach Harefu'a Begeto Varsha," vol. 2, appendix B.31, pp. 185–187.

471 Ibid., p. 26.

472 Yehudit Braude testimony, YVA, O.3/2360.

chairman of the Judenrat, was set up next to the clinic. A club facility was opened nearby that served about eighty children in groups who were switched every two weeks. The youngsters received breakfast and lunch, as well as medicines and food supplements from CENTOS. In the summer of 1942, when the *Aktion* to liquidate the ghetto began, appalling hunger set in and famished parents visited the clinic to plead for food for their starving children, who became weaker with each passing day.[473]

One of the clinics that operated at the direct initiative of the Judenrat was located at 6 Twarda St. Set up to provide broad medical services for the population at large, it had many rooms, which allowed quite a few doctors to work there simultaneously. Dr. Mordechai Lensky, one of these physicians, claimed that many patients sought treatment at the clinic. Doctors who were close to the Judenrat leaders through kinship or friendship received many patients, while the others received few. Doctors did not have consultation rooms of their own, which resulted in a lack of privacy during treatments.[474]

Medical Services Provided by the Judenrat Clinic, 6 Twarda St., February 1942[475]

Medical Service	Patients	Medical Service	Patients
Medical Consultations Full Fee	874	Home Visits Full Fee	54
Consultations Discount	712	Home Visits Discount	85
Consultations No Fee	3,664	Home Visits No Fee	857
Total	5,250	**Total Home Visits**	996
Treatments Fee	366	Laboratory Tests Fee	135
Treatments No Fee	1,976	Laboratory Tests No Fee	85
Total Treatments	**2,342**	**Total Tests**	**220**

473 Ibid.

474 Lensky, *A Physician inside the Warsaw Ghetto*, pp. 87–89.

475 Judenrat Statistics Department Report, no. 29, March 17, 1942, GFH, no. 11250, p. 10.

In February 1942, the Judenrat clinic offered four types of medical services: consultations, treatments, home visits, and laboratory tests. In all, 8,808 treatments were administered in February. Every day, 367 people visited the clinic. Most of the treatments, 72.6 percent, were administered at no charge; 9 percent at a discount; and only 18.4 percent for the full fee.

Additional clinics operated in the ghetto. In the early days of the ghetto, Dr. Chaim Einhorn and Dr. Owsiej Bielenki set up a tuberculosis clinic next to Czyste Hospital. Although they had an X-ray machine that allowed them to examine patients by means of X-ray imaging, they were unable to do so because they had no film. The doctors physically examined patients' phlegm to detect Koch's bacillus. The usual treatments were calcium shots, which were of limited efficacy, since the ghetto lacked what the patients really needed: good nutrition, hygiene, and fresh air. The clinic's work was terminated when the hospital moved to Leszno St. From then on, by order of the Nazis, its staff joined those of the typhus wards.[476]

Until the *Grossaktion* and the liquidation of the small ghetto in the summer of 1942, an orthopedic consultancy station operated to provide orthopedic treatment to children.[477] Another clinic in the small ghetto at 43 Pańska St., not far from Bersohn and Bauman Children's Hospital, performed emergency surgical procedures. In the course of 1941, an especially brutal German named Finkelstein was appointed to guard the gate between Železna St. and Leszno St. in the large ghetto. He shot so many people in the open that an emergency surgical clinic had to be set up in an old public school building across from the Arbeitsamt (Labor Office) and the medical school. Here Finkelstein's victims received initial treatment before being sent to the surgery ward at Czyste Hospital.[478]

In 1940, by order of the Germans, TOZ began to provide medical services at no charge to Jews employed by German enterprises in clinics set up at the workplaces. The premiums of Jews who carried health insurance reached the coffers of the

476 Einhorn, "Harofe Begeto Varsha," p. 12; Rom, "Mahalot Hayeladim Begeto Varsha," p. 15.

477 Yehudit Braude testimony, YVA, O.3/438.

478 Roland, *Courage under Siege*, p. 54.

German government. The Germans had an interest in keeping their Jewish factory workers healthy. For example, they ordered Dr. Rozenblum, the head of TOZ, to supply eyeglasses to workers who needed them. The Germans viewed any delay in providing service as willful sabotage for which Dr. Rozenblum was liable to suffer.[479]

From October 1942, after the *Grossaktion*, most Jews who remained in the ghetto worked in shops within the ghetto confines, and medical service at the workplaces was discontinued.[480] Many people in the ghetto sustained injuries every day, making it necessary to organize blood donations. Prof. Hirszfeld, a noted expert on blood groups, set up a blood bank, and a donation facility was opened next to the first aid station at 58 Leszno St. The donor file, containing approximately 200 names, was maintained at the first aid station, where donors were screened and summoned when needed.

The members of the Jewish police refused to donate blood, even though they occasionally required the station's services. Medical students and the sanitary staff of the hospital and its institutions, in contrast, were willing to donate, and thanks to them, a basic donor pool was established. The Judenrat supply department helped the donors, most of whom suffered from malnutrition, to withstand the loss of blood by giving them a little food—usually flour, oil, and honey substitutes. Sometimes donors generously gave these supplements to the injured.

Prof. Hirszfeld explained that the initial reluctance to cooperate was due to the lack of a precedent in this field, but it was not difficult to motivate the young people to donate. The staff of the first aid station also donated blood, because it was important to have a donor on site for urgent cases. Indeed, it often happened that a paramedic or caregiver from the first aid station would lie down next to a seriously injured patient who had the same blood type in order to save his or her life by means of a direct transfusion. Indirect transfusions could not be performed, because there

479 Dr. Moshe Tursz testimony, YVA, O.3/438.

480 Ringelblum, *Yoman Vereshimot*, pp. 408, 413.

was neither plasma nor a refrigerator to preserve the blood.[481]

Given the prevalence of contagious diseases in the ghetto and in the hospitals, urgent bacteriological and biochemical laboratory services were needed. A laboratory to provide them was set up on Prof. Hirszfeld's initiative.[482] In his memoirs, Hirszfeld described how it came into being: "Only one who acknowledges his slavery becomes a slave. In the medical field, the occupiers were unable to break our spirit." The lab had a staff of ten, plus several volunteers. Wages were minuscule and paid sporadically. The staff, like most inhabitants of the ghetto, suffered from malnutrition and hunger. Hirszfeld tried to arrange additional income for staff members by means of jobs on the side. With great effort, he managed to obtain the requisite equipment. At first, there were neither laboratory animals nor resources with which to buy many necessities. "I did not believe that we would manage to establish something really scientific, but we succeeded, nevertheless," he wrote.[483]

Another report described the tests performed by the chemo-bacteriological institute that was set up with the assistance of the Judenrat Health Department. According to this source, sample testing of food and sundry commodities were conducted, in addition to laboratory tests carried out for medical and research purposes.[484]

Miscellaneous Private and Clandestine Institutions

Before the war, many doctors in Warsaw had engaged in private practice and had no affiliation with public institutions. This changed in the ghetto, where almost all the doctors worked under the auspices of some public institution.[485] Due to the difficult conditions at the hospitals, the well-to-do in the ghetto sought and

481 Hirszfeld, *Die Geschichte eines Lebens*, p. 132; Ross, "Tahanat Ezra Rishona," p. 69.

482 Roland, *Courage under Siege*, p. 70.

483 Hirszfeld, *Die Geschichte eines Lebens*, p. 136.

484 Report from the Chemical-Bacteriological Institute of the Judenrat, July–December 1941, YVA, M.10.AR.1/191.

485 Einhorn, "Harofe Begeto Varsha," p. 13.

received medical care at home, where the conditions, particularly among the members of the middle class, were much better than those at the hospital in terms of cleanliness, treatment, and supplies, as well as from the medical standpoint. A patient who was treated privately could even buy new medicines from abroad, which were smuggled in from the Aryan side.[486]

A private hospital was also set up, apparently secretly. Ringelblum reported that on March 10, 1941, as the typhus epidemic was gaining strength, an undercover hospital for typhus patients was discovered in a building that had no sewage system. Eight patients received treatment there. Two doctors and a medic were involved in this affair.[487] It is possible that small underground hospitals were set up as well in various parts of the ghetto in order to avoid "regular" hospitalization, which involved reporting patients, disinfection, and isolation. A private and maternity hospital also operated in the ghetto.[488]

486 Lensky, *A Physician inside the Warsaw Ghetto*, pp. 103–104.
487 Ringelblum, *Notes from the Warsaw Ghetto*, p. 135.
488 Berg, *The Diary of Mary Berg*, p. 92.

Chapter Four

Doctors and Nurses at Work

Medical Service Personnel—Number, Composition, and Working Relations

According to a report by Dr. Wilhelm Hagen, the German chief physician of Warsaw, there were 2,111 Polish doctors, 865 Jewish physicians, 25 German doctors, and 25 physicians of other ethnic origins in the city between September 1939 and March 1942. Warsaw also had 3,848 practitioners of paramedical professions: 2,099 Polish caregivers and nurses (male and female), 311 Jewish caregivers, 1,143 Polish midwives, and 295 Jewish midwives.[1] Dr. Mordechai Lensky reported that there were 830 doctors in the ghetto, serving a population of about 400,000.[2] In December 1940, shortly after ghettoization, Ringelblum estimated the ghetto population at 460,000, including approximately 750 Jewish doctors.[3]

Considering that 100,000 Jews were on the brink of starvation and another 100,000 were desperately poor and unable to buy medicine, about 200,000 Jews were able to approach a public institution or a private physician and obtain medical care for a fee. By this reckoning, there was 1 doctor for every 250 people in the

1 Cohen, "Harefu'a Besherut Ha'idiologiya," p. 137.

2 Lensky, *Jewish Life in the Warsaw Ghetto*, pp. 37, 87.

3 Ringelblum, *Yoman Vereshimot*, p. 203.

ghetto—an exceptional ratio, as Lensky pointed out. However, due to economic problems, there were fewer medical service providers than the minimum required in the ghetto. Doctors who did not belong to the regular hospital staff filled unpaid positions and many unskilled individuals, such as students and practical nurses, worked there, which impaired the quality of medical care. The hospital provided these workers with the opportunity to acquire a license through on-the-job training, while earning a living by providing private care.[4]

Czyste Hospital accommodated 1,000 patients or more during the ghetto period. About 260 doctors were employed there, aided by students who, in many cases, had to interrupt their studies on account of the war.[5] Around 30 physicians headed hospital departments in the ghetto.[6] In February 1940, the hospital had 496 people on its payroll, and 32 others worked at the two hospitals for isolation patients. The number of Jewish physicians in Warsaw was so great relative to the city's population that in late September 1940, about two months before ghettoization, Chaim Mordechai Rumkowski, chairman of the Judenrat in the Łódź ghetto, visited Warsaw to recruit Jewish doctors for his city, where such professionals were in short supply—there were 30 physicians when 200 were required.[7]

In contrast to the surfeit of doctors in Warsaw, there was a shortage of nurses. In the summer of 1940, the nursing school had only thirty-five students—too few to meet the escalating demand brought on by the spiraling morbidity. The hospital could not hire all graduating nurses, because there was not enough food for the patients and the staff.[8] Some of the nurses who had no prior experience were young women whom the hospital had hired for odd jobs to protect them from abduction. Later, many medical

4 Trunk, "Epidemics and Mortality," p. 103.

5 Lensky, *Jewish Life in the Warsaw Ghetto*, pp. 37, 87.

6 For their names, see Dr. Shmuel Stanisław Waller testimony, YVA, O.3/2358; Dr. Henry Fenigstein testimony, "Varshever yid," YVA, O.33/1074, p. 6; Dr. Chaim Einhorn testimony, YVA, O.3/1836.

7 Ringelblum, *Yoman Vereshimot*, p. 53.

8 Roland, *Courage under Siege*, p. 73.

students from the ghetto's underground school volunteered to work there. During the first year or two of studies, they studied in the evening and helped out at the hospital during the day.[9] Despite the shortage of nursing staff, there was a tendency to arrange jobs for intellectuals in community institutions and hospitals. Therefore, engineers and lawyers also worked there and, in this manner, were freed from performing forced labor for the Germans.[10] In July 1942, on the eve of the transports to Treblinka, approximately 46,000 Jews were employed in various capacities in the ghetto, including 4,000 doctors, nurses, dentists, pharmacists, and so on, who dealt directly with matters related to health care and hygiene.[11]

When the occupation began, doctors who had been expelled from other hospitals, because they were Jewish, arrived at Czyste Hospital,[12] as did doctors who had fled or had been evicted from other cities, or had returned to Warsaw after attempting to reach the Soviet-occupied sector of Poland.[13] Some of the physicians who held positions with the Judenrat and many hospital workers, including doctors, were assimilated Jews or converts to Christianity, who had arrived at the ghetto after the Germans had identified them as Jewish on the basis of the religion of their parents or grandparents, disregarding their Christian identity. Although some of these doctors faithfully served the community, all met with resistance on the part of much of the Jewish population.[14] About a month after ghettoization, Ringelblum wrote about the problem of the apostates.

> Highly talented people from the medical world who held key positions in Polish life arrived and now had pretensions of

9 Ibid., p. 86.

10 Lensky, *A Physician inside the Ghetto*, pp. 25–26.

11 N. Rosen, "The Problem of Work in the Jewish Quarter, July 1942," in Kermish, *To Live with Honor*, p. 254.

12 Gürfinkel-Glocer, "Goralo Shel Beit Haholim Tzhista," p. 589.

13 Lensky, *A Physician inside the Warsaw Ghetto*, p. 22; Dr. Henry Fenigstein testimony, "Varshever yid," YVA, O.33/1074, p. 4.

14 Dr. Henry Fenigstein testimony, "Varshever yid," p. 4; Lensky, *A Physician inside the Warsaw Ghetto*, pp. 32–34, 37–38.

> directing the lives of Jews. The sentimental Dr. Milejkowski told me that Max [an apostate] suffers from inferiority feelings toward Christians and grandiose delusions toward Jews. We can give them bread, share [our last slice] with them, but they will not seize the helm of those who speak for the Jews' lives.[15]

Around three months later, in March 1941, Ringelblum made blunt comments about the converts to Christianity in the ghetto and at the Jewish hospital.

> The converts are behaving miserably. One of them, Dr. Szeniszer, is angry at the "filthy Jews" in the hospital. Dr. Werthajm, another convert, is said to have appealed to the authorities, stating that he had converted thirty rather than twenty years before, and his attitude toward the Jews was hostile; consequently, he was made the administrator of the Jewish Hospital.[16]

When the war began, Dr. Aleksander Werthajm,[17] who had converted to Christianity as a boy, directed the department of surgery at Czyste Hospital. Prior to that, he had worked as the deputy director of a ward at a military hospital, where he had been a candidate to head the department but had been denied the post because he was Jewish, even though he had converted. His appointment as department director at Czyste Hospital in 1938 evoked resistance among a certain group of Jews. Dr. Werthajm was proud of his relations with Polish non-Jews. An erudite man, who was noted for his remarkable personality among the directors

15 Ringelblum, *Yoman Vereshimot*, p. 206.

16 Ringelblum, *Notes from the Warsaw Ghetto*, p. 142.

17 Dr. Aleksander Werthajm (1872–1942) completed his studies in surgery in 1896. He held equity in a private hospital called Omega, which doubled as a convalescent home for non-Jews. Although he had no private practice in the prewar years, Jewish patients called on him for consultations and appreciated him as a talented doctor. Before the *Grossaktion*, he fled from the ghetto to the Aryan side with the help of his two daughters-in-law. In late 1942, he began to display signs of schizophrenia. See Dr. Shmuel Stanisław Waller testimony, YVA, O.3/2358.

of the Czyste Hospital surgery departments, he was considered the best surgeon in Warsaw, and he was too well known to find a hideout on the Aryan side.[18]

"The Jews did not like the apostates," Adina Blady Szwajger, a nurse at the ghetto hospital, recounted in an interview many years after the war. "You can be a non-believer but to change religions for a career is just a despicable thing to do. The Hirszfelds were not liked in the ghetto for that reason. They were also blatantly Catholic and it was terrible."[19] Blady Szwajger wrote that although the apostates were appreciated for their scientific achievements, they and the Jewish doctors were mutually estranged. The former Jews plainly suffered from a sense of double discrimination—deprived of their high professional status and reduced to being odd men out on the social scale. The administration of the children's hospital hesitated to hire Prof. Anna Hirszfeld, the wife of Prof. Ludwik Hirszfeld, but ultimately acceded due to her renown as a doctor and their wish to help her to cope with a personal tragedy—her only daughter, Marysia, was dying of a terminal disease.[20] Due to the human and multicultural diversity of the hospital staff, the vernacular there was Polish. Even the junior staff spoke it.[21]

Several doctors at Czyste Hospital, along with their entire families, converted to Christianity during the war. Others remained Jewish, but their children did not. All doctors who embraced Christianity for material reasons, that is, to remove obstacles to their scientific careers, did so surreptitiously. A few, while not converting themselves, were advocates of conversion. One of them, an elderly physician who ran a department at Czyste Hospital, personally chose to remain Jewish and perished in the ghetto with the rest of the Jews. Dr. Lensky wrote,

> Was his daring outcry in favor of conversion an act of protest against himself? Accusing his weak will of not daring to

18 Ibid.; Gürfinkel-Glocer, "Goralo Shel Beit Haholim Tzhista," p. 592.

19 Grupińska, *Sehor Sehor: Sihot Im Lohamim*, p. 136.

20 Blady Szwajger, *I Remember Nothing More*, p. 40.

21 Lensky, *A Physician inside the Warsaw Ghetto*, p. 25.

> approach the priest and asking to be sheltered in the bosom of Christianity? Or was he crying out to his Maker in view of the calamity that had befallen His Chosen People? Who knows another's soul and can explore the riddles of his aching mind?[22]

Many high-ranking members of the ghetto hierarchy were assimilated Jews who associated with the liberal intelligentsia or the apostate population. This social diversity intensified the interpersonal challenges of the administration of the ghetto and affected work in various areas, including in the medical field.[23] Despite the diversity and the social tensions that prevailed among the medical staff, the professional and social relationships with their colleagues at work were a source of strength and encouragement for the private physicians. The doctors conversed about events in various parts of the ghetto, shared general reports from the German press and the Polish-language underground bulletin, and discussed the situation. The discussions with their colleagues provided them with information and a support group in the ghetto.[24] Work was also a form of escape from the daily tribulations. Members of the hospital staff got caught up in their passion for their work and were able to forget the overall situation, if only a little. The doctors felt that their work was vital and useful, which offered them the illusion of being needed by the Jewish population.[25]

22 Ibid.

23 On the assimilated Adam Czerniaków and his bias in placing Jewish converts to Christianity in key positions in the ghetto, see Gutman, *Sugiyot Beheker Hashoah*, pp. 98–99. Among the apostate Jews were Prof. Ludwik Hirszfeld, who held important posts in the ghetto; Col. Dr. Moritz Kon, who directed the Judenrat Health Department for some time; Dr. Tadeusz Ganc, who oversaw the war on epidemics; Dr. Jerzy Landau, manager of and physician at a medical center; and Dr. Wilhelm Szenwic, a department director at Czyste Hospital. Even the director of Czyste Hospital, Dr. Stein, was a Christianized Jew and Czerniaków, chairman of the Judenrat, belonged to the liberal intelligentsia and was close to the assimilationists. See Roland, *Courage under Siege*, p. 31.

24 Lensky, *A Physician inside the Warsaw Ghetto*, pp. 72–74.

25 Ibid., pp. 39–40, 71–72.

Status of Doctors—Working Conditions, Livelihood, Decrees, and Special Characteristics

During the first few weeks under occupation, Jewish doctors were free to circulate in the streets. However, after December 1, 1939, when the armband requirement went into effect, their status deteriorated abruptly, because the police and soldiers disregarded the additional colored armband that identified them as doctors and subjected them to abuse.[26] In addition to the standard "Jewish armband," people with special positions in the ghetto wore colored bands that indicated their various duties—doctors, Judenrat employees, provisions staff, first aid workers, and employees of the Jewish Social Self-Help. The double marking protected them, somewhat, against disturbances in the streets. Furthermore, under a hierarchy-based regime in which anyone of importance wore a uniform, the additional armband hinted at preferential status and extra privileges.[27]

The Jews' "regular" badge was a white armband bearing a blue Star of David. Medical service staff wore a white patch displaying a red Star of David. Those at the first aid station wore standard dark blue caps with an azure stripe bearing the emblem of the Red Cross. Of course, due to the demand for armbands and badges with medical markings, special trade in these items emerged.[28] However, the special status indicated by the medical armband sometimes caused harm. In early February 1940, about four months after the occupation began, Ringelblum wrote that a doctor who had covered his Jewish armband with the red one that marked his profession had been beaten and punished.[29] As of March 1940, Jewish doctors were not allowed to wear Red Cross bands.[30]

26 Gutman, *The Jews of Warsaw*, p. 30.

27 Ibid., p. 31.

28 Roland, *Courage under Siege*, p. 33; Ringelblum, *Yoman Vereshimot*, p. 64; Ross, "Tahanat Ezra Rishona," pp. 68–71.

29 Ringelblum, *Notes from the Warsaw Ghetto*, p. 19.

30 Ringelblum, *Yoman Vereshimot*, p. 88.

On May 27, 1942, roughly two months before the deportations from Warsaw began, Auerswald, the German *Kommissar* for ghetto affairs, promulgated a new edict, prohibiting Jews from wearing any other armband than the one prescribed by law. Only the Jewish police were exempt from this decree; they were allowed to continue wearing a special armband in addition to the standard Jewish one.[31] Dr. Schrempf, the Nazi physician, issued documents to Jewish doctors that protected their property and prohibited the confiscation of furniture from their homes. Not all Nazis honored these papers, and the possessions of some doctors were confiscated from their homes as well.[32] About two months into the occupation of Warsaw, for example, German doctors visited and ransacked a Jewish physician's clinic in search of microscopes. Books were stolen from Jewish doctors' libraries.[33] In March 1940, the offices of Jewish doctors were plundered, when their owners were not at home.[34] These incidents were constant. In September 1940, around two months before ghettoization, a doctor was evicted from his apartment on ten minutes' notice.[35] In early November 1940, a German officer came to a Jewish doctor's home to arrest him, while a group of Jews, who were collaborating with the German to blackmail the Jewish doctor, stood by.[36]

From the very beginning of Nazi rule, Jewish doctors were included in a list of intellectuals and liberal professionals who were targeted for collective punishment for the "criminal act" of an individual who had evaded capture by the Germans during a manhunt. In early January 1940, numerous doctors were arrested on this account.[37] However, until the *Grossaktion* began in July 1942, doctors and nurses from Czyste Hospital who had the appropriate permits moved about in the ghetto streets with more freedom than any others. Jewish doctors served as precinct physicians who

31 Lewin, *A Cup of Tears*, p. 101.
32 Lensky, *A Physician inside the Warsaw Ghetto*, p. 39.
33 Ringelblum, *Yoman Vereshimot*, p. 72.
34 Ibid., p. 88.
35 Czerniaków, *The Warsaw Diary*, p. 198.
36 Ringelblum, *Yoman Vereshimot*, p. 175.
37 Ibid., p. 69.

dispensed medical services at no charge and were allowed to make home visits. Ordinary Jews who violated the curfew at night were shot by the Germans, while doctors and nurses were allowed to move about even then. Nevertheless, this special privilege put them in danger, because some guards shot at anyone who breached the curfew, without identifying them or checking their permits.[38] Some medical officials had a permit to cross to the Aryan side but few carried it with them. Marek Edelman, a courier for Bersohn and Bauman Children's Hospital, legally visited the other side daily to deliver the blood samples of typhus patients to the German Health Department on Nowogrodska St.[39] Prof. Hirszfeld possessed this document as chairman of the Jewish Health Council. However, these permits were revoked later.

On September 19, 1940, roughly two months before ghettoization, Kaplan wrote that the Jewish physicians were no longer allowed to treat Aryans and vice versa. He even offered a rationale for it.

> It is well known that contagious diseases are prevalent primarily in Jewish areas, of course. If an Aryan doctor serves Jewish patients, there is danger of spreading the disease from one quarter to another. And, therefore, the two areas should be completely separated. The Jews laugh heartily at this stupidity. It was common for Jewish patients to go in great numbers to Aryan doctors, but this was never so in the case of Jewish doctors and Aryan patients. The latter rarely come to Jewish doctors. So who will lose by this? Obviously the Aryan doctors. But the occupier isn't concerned about that. Nevertheless—it's making trouble here, too!
>
> This peculiar order makes no distinction between patients with contagious diseases and those with organic diseases. Jews with heart or lung trouble who have been treated by Aryan doctors must now leave the doctors who devoted themselves

38 Turkow, *Hayo Hayta Varsha Yehudit*, p. 140; Einhorn, "Harofe Begeto Varsha," p. 9; Lensky, *A Physician inside the Warsaw Ghetto*, pp. 169–170; Ringelblum, *Yoman Vereshimot*, p. 40; Roland, *Courage under Siege*, p. 63.

39 Krall, *Shielding the Flame*, p. 41.

> to their cure and go to a Jewish doctor. This ban applies to dentists and midwives as well. This is a preview of the Europe of the future. A partition between one people and the other.[40]

During the first year of the occupation, private physicians were evidently allowed to treat anyone, meaning that Jewish patients could continue to be treated by their Polish doctors. On September 17–19, 1940, Ringelblum recorded in his diary false rumors about sixteen anti-Jewish clauses that included restrictions on the practice of Jewish doctors.[41] Therefore, it is possible that the decrees may not have been issued yet and that Kaplan's report was based on rumor. It is difficult to understand from these sources exactly when the edict that restricted Jewish medical practice before ghettoization was imposed.

In the first few months of the occupation, doctors were among those abducted in the street for forced labor, since some Germans disregarded their papers, which identified them as essential workers at the hospital. About a month into the occupation, Kaplan wrote that when the Germans barged into private homes to seize Jews for labor, they came upon a doctor who was treating a patient and sent both to perform forced labor.[42] Dr. Lensky was hauled away for forced labor even though he held a certificate stating, in German, that due to his duties as a doctor, no other labor should be imposed on him.[43]

Even before the ghetto was sealed, doctors en route to the hospital found themselves under attack. Those using the tram were at greater risk than pedestrians, but the staff felt it necessary to take the tram that stopped near the hospital gate, since the hospital was at the edge of town. At the beginning of 1940, the Germans cancelled the last two stops of the tram. Polish youths attacked the doctors on their way to the hospital, hurling stones

40 Kaplan, *Scroll of Agony*, p. 197; Kaplan, *Megilat Yisurin*, pp. 337–338.

41 Ringelblum, *Yoman Vereshimot*, p. 140.

42 Kaplan, *Megilat Yisurin*, p. 71.

43 Czerniaków, *The Warsaw Diary*, p. 138; Lensky, *A Physician inside the Warsaw Ghetto*, p. 17.

and verbal abuse.[44] In the first week after ghettoization, doctors riding the tram to Czyste Hospital were forced to get off and were subjected to humiliation for an hour.[45] Staff members who received crossing permits and walked to work were often harassed by the Poles, and by the Polish and German guards who manned the crossing points, as they headed out of the ghetto.[46] Staff who lacked crossing permits faced an agonizing trilemma: Should they stay in the hospital without being able to return to the ghetto, remain in the ghetto and give up their work at the hospital, or risk walking to and from the hospital without a permit?[47]

Some doctors had privileges that most people in the ghetto lacked, including the right to have and use a private telephone. Telephones were permitted in offices of institutions and businesses, and important officials in the ghetto and practitioners of certain occupations, such as doctors, were allowed to have telephones in their homes. They could communicate with Poles on the Aryan side and, at a later stage, with Jews who had gone over and were living there in hiding.[48] This was the case concerning medicines, which were in perilously short supply in the ghetto. Therefore, in addition to official medications sold in pharmacies, pharmaceuticals were smuggled in through the black market. Doctors who were allowed to leave the ghetto occasionally for some purpose, such as to check on a patient, returned with small quantities of medicines.[49]

Although the price of the serum against typhus was exorbitant, each of the doctors at Czyste Hospital received a dose at no charge to inoculate themselves. Many forwent the vaccination in favor of relatives.[50] Under the living conditions in the ghetto, alcohol was a prized commodity. Those in charge of preventing epidemics and maintaining sanitation distributed monthly rations of alcohol to the doctors for disinfection purposes, of course, even after the

44 Lensky, *A Physician inside the Warsaw Ghetto*, pp. 19, 26–27.
45 Ringelblum, *Notes from the Warsaw Ghetto*, p. 88.
46 Gürfinkel-Glocer, "Goralo Shel Beit Haholim Tzhista," p. 591.
47 Ibid.
48 Gutman, *The Jews of Warsaw*, pp. 112–113.
49 Koren, "Hasiyud Kehelek Misherutei Habriyut," p. 50.
50 Einhorn, "Harofe Begeto Varsha," p. 11.

ghetto was sealed. Private practice was limited and doctors always had some clean alcohol left over. Since many physicians lacked a livelihood, the alcohol was a godsend, because they received a fair price for it due to the high demand.[51]

Jews in the ghetto had to perform all forms of forced labor according to Nazi orders. During the first few months of the occupation, doctors were also seized for forced labor, even though it was Judenrat policy to exempt them from it. This situation continued for quite some time. However, after the first *Aktion*, the surviving physicians were required to perform forced labor twice a week, like everyone else,[52] although it was of a different nature: providing medical services in forced labor camps. On August 25, 1940, roughly three months before ghettoization, the Judenrat attempted to send four doctors with equipment and medicines to the labor camp in Bełżec, but was unable to find candidates who were willing to undertake the mission in view of the ghastly working conditions there. About a week later, Dr. Arnold Lambrecht, director of the Sanitation Department at the Warsaw district administration, demanded that twenty doctors be sent to the camp but, again, no one agreed to go.[53] The conditions in Bełżec were indeed horrific, even though the site had not yet become an extermination camp. In any case, the doctors did not have enough medicines or equipment to provide the camp inmates with any real assistance.[54]

A few doctors received certification as specialists in their fields of study during the war. In April 1941, about five months into ghettoization, Ringelblum wrote that several dozen Jewish physicians received professional licenses, which they had been striving to obtain for years. Prof. Ludwik Stabholz,[55] who taught

51 Lensky, *A Physician inside the Warsaw Ghetto*, pp. 67–68.

52 Einhorn, "Harofe Begeto Varsha," p. 9.

53 Czerniaków, *The Warsaw Diary*, pp. 190–193.

54 Daniel Nadav, "Limed Anatomiya Begeto Varsha," p. 10.

55 Prof. Ludwik Stabholz (1911-2007) completed his medical studies at the University of Warsaw and was hired as a surgeon at Czyste Hospital in 1939. During the Nazi occupation, he continued to work at the hospital, which had been transferred to several buildings in the ghetto, and held important managerial positions in the ghetto underground medical school, while teaching

anatomy at the underground medical school in the ghetto, testified that he had been awarded the title of professor during the ghetto period.[56]

The economic situation of the doctors, some of whom had earned 1,000 zlotys per day before the war, deteriorated within a few months of the occupation, because the public could no longer afford to pay for medical care.[57] According to Hirszfeld's account, most doctors in the ghetto were starving, after having been dismissed from their jobs. Since few patients could pay a doctor for his services, most practitioners worked at community clinics, refugee points, and the like. Wages were not always paid in these places and when they were paid, the wages were too paltry to sustain life.[58] Almost a year after ghettoization, Czerniaków wrote that many doctors were unemployed.[59] The Judenrat tended to arrange jobs in community institutions for members of the intelligentsia. It is possible that some were placed in jobs that should have been given to doctors.[60]

anatomy. During his work in the ghetto, the Germans ordered him to treat an SS officer who was suffering from back pain, under threat of death if he would fail to cure him. Despite his lack of experience in the field, he developed a method of releasing the pressure on the spinal column, and the treatment helped. Ultimately, he and his wife, Miriam, a surgical nurse, were smuggled out of the ghetto by his teacher at the University of Warsaw, Prof. Edward Loth, who arranged a hideout for him on the Aryan side. Yad Vashem awarded Prof. Loth the title of Righteous Among the Nations in 1996. After the war, Dr. Stabholz served as an officer in the Polish Army and practiced medicine in Gdańsk during the revitalization of that city. He immigrated to Israel in 1950, where he practiced surgery and ran a clinic for back problems. He specialized in researching spinal diseases and problems and developed a special treatment for back pain. Inter alia he invented a revolutionary device to treat a slipped (herniated) disc and his method is implemented in hundreds of clinics throughout the world. Prof. Ludwik Stabholz was the nephew of Dr. Henryk Stabholz and the first cousin of Dr. Thaddeus Stabholz. I thank his children, Prof. Adam Stabholz, Adv. Orit Grober, and Adv. Joseph Stabholz, for sharing this information with me.

56 Ringelblum, *Yoman Vereshimot*, p. 265; Stabholz, "Hora'at Anatomiya Bamahteret."

57 Ringelblum, *Notes from the Warsaw Ghetto*, pp. 10, 30.

58 Hirszfeld, *Die Geschichte eines Lebens*, p. 135.

59 Czerniaków, *The Warsaw Diary*, p. 286.

60 Lensky, *A Physician inside the Warsaw Ghetto*, pp. 25–26. White-collar workers at the hospital complained about having been dismissed from their jobs and

The doctors made strenuous efforts to find work to support themselves. Lensky described having to work in multiple medical institutions to earn a living—in the hospital facility at 1 Leszno St. in the morning, at 18 Stawki St. in the afternoon, as well as in the Judenrat clinic at 6 Twarda St. and in the Linas Hatzedek clinic at 24 Pawia St. He found work at the Judenrat clinic only by dint of vigorous lobbying and months of waiting. "It was like chasing the wind—a heated, motivated chase, perhaps, but still largely a waste of energy." The work was not done for material gain, given the paltry wages. Indeed, the monthly income for work at a public institution could not sustain a family for even half a week.[61] Many ghetto residents arrived at the Judenrat clinic for treatment and the doctors' fees were determined by the number of patients that he or she examined. The salary was so low that it covered only the commute by rickshaw.[62]

Since there were so many doctors, many did not find work in the ghetto medical institutions and attempted to make a living in private practice. Those who worked in the public medical system also tried to augment their minuscule incomes in this manner. Private medical services entailed all kinds of dangers: denunciation, punishment for breaching the curfew to make home visits at prohibited times, and more. The hospital was overcrowded and because of the fear of contracting infectious diseases, the demand for private care increased and the doctors who needed to make a living responded accordingly.

Most doctors who worked for hospitals and in residential blocks were employees of the Jewish Health Council in the ghetto. The physicians who worked in the blocks were responsible for a specified number of buildings and were not employed in the hospitals. Most, if not all of the doctors, belonged to one of two Jewish medical associations—one for hospital physicians

replaced by the Judenrat with members of the intelligentsia in order to exempt the latter from forced labor. See Czerniaków, *The Warsaw Diary*, p. 159.

61 Lensky, *A Physician inside the Warsaw Ghetto*, p. 72.

62 Ibid., p. 89.

and another for those working elsewhere. Both were headed by Dr. Milejkowski.[63]

Lensky noted that the doctors were better off than other professionals, such as lawyers and engineers. They were able to continue practicing their profession and found work with the German authorities' consent, because contagious illnesses were so common and the spread of typhus was so acute. This professional stratum underwent a slow demise. Many in this group survived until the final days of the ghetto.[64] On February 20, 1942, Mary Berg wrote that the doctors and pharmacists were among the ghetto's most successful groups; the former, she reported, worked both in the hospitals and in their homes during private reception hours.[65]

Nurses also engaged in providing private services, such as giving injections, bandaging wounds, cupping, and administering additional treatments in the homes of well-off patients. It seems that the income earned in this manner was risky, and the nurses may have lacked official authorization. One nurse, S. Kamiński, described treating someone who suffered from recurrent boils. After the patient told a Jewish friend, who had connections with the Gestapo, that the nurse was charging for her services, Kamiński shut down her private practice for fear of punishment. The patient was transferred to the hospital.[66]

Some doctors were very well-off by ghetto standards, because their work was deemed vital or because of their connections with colleagues outside the ghetto. It was also possible for some of them to bring their possessions to the ghetto, to be given hiring preference as Christianized Jews, to take bribes from people seeking to avoid disinfection, or to treat affluent patients who could afford private care. However, most doctors exhausted their resources and became paupers. Those who had lived in the suburbs of Warsaw and had treated non-Jews lost their clientele when they moved

63 See Dr. Milejkowski's response to a questionnaire of the Warsaw Ghetto Oneg Shabbat Archive in Kermish, *To Live with Honor*, p. 60.

64 Lensky, *A Physician inside the Warsaw Ghetto*, p. 167.

65 Berg, *The Diary of Mary Berg*, p. 126.

66 Koren, "Hasiyud Kehelek Misherutei Habriyut," p. 70.

into the ghetto. The large number of doctors who were expected to serve the poor in the ghetto caused many to be unemployed. Doctors who arrived among the waves of deportees and refugees were similarly jobless and penniless. JDC tried to employ refugee physicians as sanitation workers at refugee centers, to supply them with food, and to arrange housing for them in the ghetto. Sometimes, doctors who were sent to forced labor camps lost their jobs when they returned.

Nevertheless, there were exceptional cases of doctors who became rich in the ghetto or earned almost as much as they had before the war, such as Dr. Zygmunt Fajncyn and Dr. Mejlachowicz. Dr. Fajncyn had amassed a great deal of money before and during the war. When he marched to the Umschlagplatz on his way to Treblinka, he lost his suitcase, which contained about 7 million zlotys. Dr. Mejlachowicz, a specialist in sexually transmitted diseases, assumed arrogant airs in the ghetto and even enlisted in Group 13, which terrorized the ghetto inhabitants.[67]

Matters relating to paying employees of the medical services and public medical institutions figured prominently in Czerniaków's diary. The Judenrat chairman's journal entries on this topic make it clear that these workers were not paid as required, nor on time. By and large, salaries were paid sporadically and at a lower rate than expected or promised.[68] Most doctors were better off than the average person before the war due to their higher status and greater resources and, thus, their lives in the ghetto began from a better point of departure. However, they also had to contend with the appalling economic realities of the ghetto, just like everyone else.

Medical care in Eastern Europe during World War II, with the exception of the Soviet Union, was delivered for payment, which was sometimes paid by insurance companies. In some locations, there were free clinics for the poor. Idealistic doctors charged

67 Roland, *Courage under Siege*, pp. 60–61, 64–65.

68 Czerniaków, *The Warsaw Diary*, pp. 169, 171, 258, 288, 298, 300, 314; Ross, "Tahanat Ezra Rishona," p. 73.

modest fees for their services. In health care, as in other fields, the wealthy paid more than the working class paid, and they were able to benefit from their payments to doctors for private medicine, both for hospital services and for treatments in hospitals, such as surgery.[69] According to reports from the Jewish Social Self-Help, many inhabitants of the ghetto continued to pay for medical care until a relatively late stage. In November 1941, for example, 38,259.20 zlotys were paid in monthly health taxes, and donations amounted to 6,902.90 zlotys.[70]

Bribery in the War on Infectious Diseases

Corruption among the doctors was made possible by the dysfunctional system that was charged with fighting epidemics. Within this framework, doctors were able to offer the people they examined a clean bill of health, even if they were infected with a contagious disease, thereby excusing them from the disinfection process. Every case of illness had to be reported and every patient had to be referred to a hospital. Concealing information about a patient carried the death penalty. Since people were as afraid of disinfection as they were of the disease itself, a new source of income was created: the masking of information by treating physicians and precinct doctors in exchange for a stiff fee due to the high risk involved.[71]

The doctors' involvement in systematic and extensive bribery earned them the hostility of the ghetto inhabitants. Peretz Opochinsky described the depth of the corruption.

> The house committee, through its chairman, had already worked out an agreement with the precinct physician…and had arranged the whole deal with him. He would go easy in

69 Roland, *Courage under Siege*, p. 63. On doctors who did not charge any fees, see the testimony of one such physician, GFH, no. 19765.

70 Jewish Social Self-Help, Statistics Department Report, no. 6, November 1941, AŻIH, ARI.32, p. 30.

71 Hirszfeld, *Die Geschichte eines Lebens*, p. 141.

> his report, which would ease the medical inspection....For this kindness, the doctor would receive a gift in hand. How large? Only one man knows—the chairman...Henceforth, the doctor would cost the house committee money every month and, thereafter, he would even receive a regular monthly allowance that would, of course, consume much of the committee's revenue.[72]

When buildings were inspected for cleanliness and decisions were made concerning the need to disinfect apartments and possessions, it was possible to bribe the doctor who came to do the disinfection, as well as the disinfection teams, thereby taking the bitter edge off the directive. The head of the house committee would hand the doctor a bribe of several hundred zlotys—or several thousand for a large building—and would give him a list of apartment owners who had participated in the bribe. In return, he would ease the inspections of their dwellings and would exempt them from going to the public bathhouse.[73]

The Jewish doctors were a very greedy bunch indeed, Ringelblum noted. The residents of a given tenement would take up a collection and pay them off to escape disinfection and the dreaded visit to the public bathhouse.[74] In late April 1940, for example, a person could spare a building from disinfection by paying the German in charge 2,000 zlotys. The Jewish doctor earned 200 zlotys per month.[75] In May 1940, a building where fifteen typhus patients were discovered was not quarantined, because the doctor responsible for this decision received a payoff of 800 zlotys per month.[76]

Doctors were also censured for extortion when they made house visits. They secretly treated thousands of people in their homes and charged 50 zlotys, or even 100, per visit. They also

72 Opochinsky, *Reshimot* (Sketches from the Warsaw Ghetto) (Hebrew) (Tel Aviv: Hakkibutz Hameuchad, 1970), pp. 46, 80–81, 157.

73 Lensky, *A Physician inside the Warsaw Ghetto*, pp. 105–106.

74 Ringelblum, *Yoman Vereshimot*, p. 98.

75 Ringelblum, *Notes from the Warsaw Ghetto*, p. 35.

76 Ibid., p. 42.

stipulated in advance the number of compulsory visits per day.[77] Hirszfeld wrote that doctors also took part in exploitation by looting the dwellings of the people whose apartments were disinfected.[78] Opochinsky accused the doctors of concocting a malevolent plan as soon as they were hired. The extensive bribery scheme harmed the residents' health, dispossessed them of what remained of their money, and even led to the death of entire families. "The doctors during the war were no different from any other flesh and blood who knows he has a stomach that must be filled," he stated.[79]

When faced with the plight of the Jews who were condemned to death on the Umschlagplatz, a few doctors took advantage of their status by using their connections in an attempt to rescue these wretched individuals in exchange for money. For example, Dr. Goldberg had permission to recruit several Jews to work at an airport. He employed people for 500 zlotys per person and collaborated with two German pilots.[80] Rotsztajn, a member of the board of the first aid station, also viewed the possibility of saving people on the Umschlagplatz as a personal opportunity to make a buck. He and his driver set up an operation of their own, using the first aid station vehicle to whisk from the plaza people who could pay for the privilege.[81] Trenchant criticism accused doctors involved in such activities of blatantly violating medical ethics against the background of the grim life in the ghetto. However, caution should be taken when drawing sweeping conclusions about the entire population of physicians. It is difficult to know how many of the 800 doctors who worked in the ghetto were involved in the disinfection and bribery activities. Among the doctors who were forced to take part in the disinfection process, some undoubtedly maintained their integrity. Concerning this matter, an anonymous doctor testified,

77 Ibid., pp. 217–220.
78 Hirszfeld, *Die Geschichte eines Lebens*, p. 125.
79 Opochinsky, *Reshimot*, p. 60.
80 Dr. Shmuel Stanisław Waller testimony, YVA, O.3/2358.
81 Ross, "Tahanat Ezra Rishona," pp. 74–75.

> There were cases when a sanitary physician was a decent fellow who did not take part in any "dirty business" with members of the disinfection teams.... Those on the disinfection teams worked in such a way that the doctor had no access to the documents and, therefore, could not report them.[82]

An anonymous text by a member of a disinfection crew also affirms that some doctors (and disinfection workers) had integrity: "Nevertheless, not all of them demanded a bribe and not all of them received one.... Some people released [residents] from the great humiliation of being taken to the showers and disinfection without taking a bribe."[83] According to Dr. Mordechai Lensky, most doctors honorably coped with the moral challenges of ghetto life.

> It must be noted that of the 830 doctors present in the ghetto, very few did not measure up morally. Some doctors abused their patients' trust, out of greed...but such cases were rare, and the number of doctors whose deeds would have been condemned by any society was negligible.[84]

The anonymous author of a document in the Ringelblum Archive disagreed.

> I may be accused of misanthropy and of excessive criticism, but I must denounce the doctors for the quality of care and their attitude toward the sick. Their role in the horrific ghetto is highly significant—a matter of life and death. It is as important as the problem of bread. The state of sanitation is very bad for various reasons...Many Jews studied medicine before the war and many were unemployed. Now everyone is working, even people who just finished courses, feldshers and nurses, which isn't enough, and the situation has become abnormal....

82 Testimony of an anonymous physician, July 1942, AŻIH, ARI.270.

83 Memoirs of a disinfector, AŻIH, ARI.268.

84 Lensky, *A Physician inside the Warsaw Ghetto*, p. 104.

Students who have not finished their studies work in the hospitals...They are not good enough to function as doctors. People who were not trained are giving injections and various treatments...while the doctors are getting rich....Almost everyone is taking advantage of the difficult situation for his own benefit. The doctors want money and are getting it. They offer the ill, who do not understand, all sorts of expensive tests...The doctors also refer patients from one to another and advise [them] to go to another doctor. He will help... There is no cure whatsoever without injections, regardless of the type of illness...Jewish patients believe in doctors. A doctor is God.

Every injection costs the patient 10 zlotys. (That's a lot of money in the ghetto.) Sometimes the patient has to pay for injections every day and he sells his last shirt to buy a piece of bread...but he wants to be healthy. The fact is that in the ghetto, it is better to live the way the doctors, the bakers, the high-level bureaucrats, and the smugglers do...there is no reason to envy these doctors, but they should spend more time in the hospital, where they are so badly needed. A doctor must provide fair treatment even in the difficult times of the ghetto. I have nothing against bakers, butchers, merchants. But for God's sake, who can we turn to in such dire distress...There are doctors who are kindhearted and sincerely willing to help those in need. They are few, but there are some in the ghetto.[85]

Difficulties and Hazards of the Work of Medical Staff

The hospital staff, like the patients, were starving.[86] Some came down with hunger disease but continued to treat patients. One of the nurses at the children's hospital is a case in point.

85 Report on various aspects of life in the ghetto, AŻIH, ARI.428.

86 Lensky, *A Physician inside the Warsaw Ghetto*, p. 24.

> All I know is that with superhuman strength she would stand on her swollen legs and lift...helpless bodies, wash and change them, and give them clean nappies, until, one day, she didn't come to work. Struck down by starvation, she lay on a squalid bunk and waited for death. We managed to save her then. Every day, after work at the hospital, we'd split among ourselves visits to staff who were dying of hunger. We brought them the only thing we had—intravenous glucose, which sometimes restored their strength for a short while.[87]

Adina Blady Szwajger wrote that breakfast for the staff at the children's hospital consisted of 100 grams of thinly sliced bread and about 10 grams of beet jam.[88] Staff also received a 25-gram portion of straight alcohol in order to infuse a little spirit into their work. During the *Aktionen* of July–September 1942, hunger at the hospital was particularly acute. Some doctors were starving along with their families, since it was difficult to do business on the hospital grounds for fear of *Aktionen*. Not all doctors and staff members suffered from the economic straits.[89]

The nurses had a staggering workload. They dispensed medicine, gave injections, applied bandages, administered infusions, and the like. Due to the difficult conditions that the shelling and the destruction of infrastructure had created, they also had to see to unusual basic needs, which at the beginning of the war included hauling water, setting up beds (occasionally without bedding and sometimes for two or more patients per bed), and assisting in the maintenance of the entire hospital—doing the cleaning and preparing meals from the scanty quantities of food staples available to the hospital. The nurses carried out their work under harsh physical and psychological conditions.[90] Every nurse worked both in her own department and helped out in others as well. Each was responsible for about

87 Blady Szwajger, *I Remember Nothing More*, pp. 31–32.

88 Ibid., p. 27.

89 Lensky, *A Physician inside the Warsaw Ghetto*, pp. 140–142.

90 Gürfinkel-Glocer, "Goralo Shel Beit Haholim Tzhista," pp. 594–595.

ninety patients.[91] The nurses worked weekly day or night shifts that were twelve hours long, and they often had to work overtime as well. In the evenings, they and other hospital workers returned to their apartments in organized groups, so as not to walk alone in the dark ghetto. Working conditions were abysmal. Lacking transportation, they had to walk to the hospital, dead tired, as they struggled to support their families.[92]

By the autumn of 1941, it seemed that there was nothing but a sense of powerlessness in the children's hospital. As the workday grew longer, the caregivers became increasingly fatigued. On faltering legs, they treated pressure sores, bandaged swollen limbs, and administered "medicines."[93] The onerous workload, the successive months without pay, and the acute starvation prompted the medical staff to organize strikes and protests. Doctors appeared to have been better off than the nurses and the technical staff. The Ringelblum Archive contains the minutes of a meeting in which the nurses at the children's hospital attempted to organize a strike.

> The general assembly of all hospital workers, more than 120 people, has begun. On the agenda: regular payment of salaries. This is a serious problem from our standpoint, one that pains and angers us.
>
> Mrs. Dr. K. has the floor: We have gathered again to discuss the decisions we must make, so that we may receive at least some of the wages for our hard work....
>
> The auxiliary nurse S. has the floor: In my opinion, we cannot continue to work under these conditions. All of us are owed four months of wages. Despite all the exhausting work, we cannot buy ourselves even a piece of bread. The bowl of soup, for which we wait until midday, cannot possibly sustain us to be able to stand on our feet. Every day somebody faints from hunger at a bedside. None of our requests and attempts

91 Ibid., p. 587.

92 Ibid., pp. 589–590, 594.

93 Blady Szwajger, *I Remember Nothing More*, p. 39.

to approach management has helped. How long can we endure this suffering? Therefore, I move that we stop working. We'll strike because there's no other way.

Nurse…has the floor: Finally the moment has come for us to decide, once and for all, to go on strike. All of us, in solidarity, of course, will walk off the job. Then the result that must come, will come. In other words, we must be paid for the hard work that we have done under such difficult conditions, surrounded by infectious diseases, by hungry and oppressed people. We have done our duty thus far and can no longer continue to do so.

The motion is up for a vote. Everyone is in favor of striking. We begin deliberations on how to organize the strike and to leave people on duty in the departments. When it is time to act, it seems that the male doctors begin to whisper to each other. Suddenly a motion is presented to the presidium as follows: "We group of men have decided not to strike for special reasons that we're prepared to explain. The *Kommissar* said that striking means sabotage and the punishment for that is death by gunfire." So they do not want to strike.

Passions are high among those in attendance. We women explain that such behavior is indecent and a terrible act of treachery. Another doctor explains, "We doctors are responsible for the strike and we do not want to expose our heads to the Germans' bullets." The technical staff are furious and reply, "Sure, the doctors still do not know what hunger is and what it means to be so hungry that you stumble as you work. That's why the doctors want to save their own lives, but we have nothing to lose. We're starving to death anyway, every day.[94]

According to the testimonies, despite the difficult working conditions and workload that severely impeded their work at

94 Testimony of an anonymous nurse at Bersohn and Bauman Children's Hospital, YVA, M.10.AR.1/1099.

Czyste Hospital, the staff members felt that their devotion to their patients did not flag.

> However, we doctors and nurses, for whom our work at the hospital was our life, struggled to continue to overcome all the obstacles and to do what was literally impossible. It is not possible for me to describe the supreme struggle of this small group of workers at the hospital.[95]

Under the prevailing conditions in the ghetto, members of the medical staff also fell ill, some infected by their patients. Since there were not enough vaccines for all the staff members, many died of typhus. One-fifth of the nursing staff who received patients at the medical care stations in the ghetto died of typhus, as did 8 percent of the doctors, after contracting the disease from their patients.[96] An anonymous nurse at the children's hospital described her work in the typhus department.

> As we prepared to bathe the children again, we received another phone call. The director was on the line, "Hello, nurse, be careful! The children are full of lice!" I grit my teeth and start to work. The first patient, Avreimik, five years old… one louse bite—and I'll come down with typhus. I don't have to look hard. His head is full of scabs from wounds infested with lice moving about and infecting so many people with the dreaded disease…I have to wash and clean his head… The boy's head is full of blood but I have to remove the scabs. Then I put him to bed.[97]

Dr. Lensky described how he himself became ill at the time of the deportations. He had access to a pill to reduce the fever. He evidently suffered a heart attack, combined with an acute intestinal disease that affected his large intestine, for which he was treated

95 Gürfinkel-Glocer, "Goralo Shel Beit Haholim Tzhista," p. 591.

96 Dr. Henry Fenigstein testimony, "Varshever yid," YVA, O.33/1074, p. 10.

97 Pictures from the children's hospital, AŻIH, ARI.989.

with injections. As a doctor, Lensky was able to obtain the food that he needed, albeit at a high price. These privileges were key to his recovery. However, he was left physically weak and he began to lose his teeth.[98]

The medical workers treated a severely impoverished population and their work often entailed special sacrifice. Some doctors treated poor patients free of charge and some paid for this with their lives, infected by their patients. In his diary, Michael Zylberberg described Dr. Lajb Korman, who had been a pediatrician in Warsaw before the war.

> I often furnished him with lists of people who were sick and too poor to pay a doctor, and he went fearlessly from house to house, trying to help and cure [them]. Of course, many of his patients died, but he never stopped working. Every evening, he would tell me about his visits and give me a resume of the state of his patients.[99]

In writings that have survived in the Ringelblum Archive, Regina Wajłowna, a nurse at Czyste Hospital during the ghetto period, described "one case history," in which she was summoned late one evening to help a sick boy from a poor family who was living in a cellar. The diary entry reflects the immense devotion that she evinced as she beheld the abject situation of the family and the three-year-old child. She visited the family immediately, gave the boy one injection of the vaccine, and returned the next day on her own initiative to give him another injection. Finding that the ampule had broken, she paid for another shot to replace it. Regina, herself a refugee from Łódź, worked hard to survive in the ghetto, along with her mother. Not only did she respond to the request to visit the boy at home at an unusual time of day, not only did she treat him at no cost, but she covered the cost of treatment with her own funds.[100]

98 Lensky, *A Physician inside the Warsaw Ghetto*, pp. 115–116, 120.

99 Michael Zylberberg, *A Warsaw Diary, 1939–1945* (London: Vallentine Mitchell, 1969), pp. 49–50.

100 Nurse Regina Wajłowna testimony, "History of One Case, 1941," AŻIH,

Reports from doctors who worked at refugee points reveal the unique difficulties that physicians at these centers confronted. They warned about the situation in an attempt to help and bring about improvements. For example, in January 1942, while working at the refugee point at 9 Stawki St., Dr. Einhorn wrote, "I share this information and strongly request that the appropriate authorities be advised so that they may act to correct this unsanitary situation."[101] Sometimes doctors were accused of insensitivity and behavior toward their patients, which is typical of burnout due to the grinding routine. Michael Zylberberg added the following:

> It is interesting to note that life had become very cheap in the ghetto. This is an unusual attitude for those of the Jewish faith, but death was so common, so expected, that even the passing of a child seldom evoked comment or compassion. This attitude was transmitted even to the medical men, whose task was so hopeless that sympathy evaporated in the face of disease and death. And yet, in the moments of greatest horror, there were doctors who went on believing that their duty was to strive and to save.[102]

Patients—some of whom were mortally ill and were unlikely to have been saved, even under ordinary circumstances—occasionally thrust the full burden of their pain and suffering on the doctors and accused them, unjustly, of malpractice.[103]

ARI.196. This is one of the two different writings by Regina Wajłowna that remain, which are in the Ringelblum Archive. The other is a memoir pertaining to the 1939–1941 period, AŻIH, ARI.195. See also Offer, "Ma'arach Harefu'a Begeto Varsha," vol. 2, appendix A.17, pp. 67–69.

101 Report on the medical situation at refugee points, AŻIH, ARI.84; Offer, "Ma'arach Harefu'a Begeto Varsha," vol. 2, appendix A.25, pp. 122–124.

102 Zylberberg, *A Warsaw Diary*, p. 50.

103 Roland, *Courage under Siege*, p. 65.

Chapter Five

Medical Studies and Research in the Ghetto

Nursing School

The twenty-third graduating class of the two-year Jewish nursing school associated with Czyste Hospital celebrated its commencement on a fateful day, September 1, 1939, amid the sirens and bombardments that marked the beginning of the Nazi invasion of Poland and World War II.[1] When the war broke out, the students mobilized to help treat the many wounded who had been rushed to Czyste Hospital. After the Germans occupied Warsaw, the building, which was damaged in the bombardments, was overhauled and the debris removed. The JDC administration in Warsaw raised the necessary support to ensure the continued existence of the institution.[2] In January 1940, the new authorities in Warsaw allowed the school to resume its activity.[3] Almost all nursing schools in Poland were shut down. The Jewish school was one of the few that was not closed, possibly due to the Germans' fear of epidemics.[4] Under German occupation,

1 Aleksander Blum, "The Nursing School in the Warsaw Ghetto," in Michael A. Grodin, *Jewish Medical Resistance*, pp. 173–177.

2 Blum-Bielicka, "Szkoła Pielęgniarstwa," pp. 66–77; Luba Bielicka-Blum, YVA M.49.E/4264; YVA, M.49.E/5865; YVA O.33/6403.

3 Czerniaków, *The Warsaw Diary*, p. 178. In addition to permission to reactivate the school, the Germans allowed the professional dance studio at Melody Palace to continue operating.

4 Koren, "Hasiyud Kehelek Misherutei Habriyut," p. 80; Blum-Bielicka, "Szkoła Pielęgniarstwa," pp. 66–77.

the Jewish population began to suffer from the decrees, torment, and humiliation. However, the nursing school carried on undisturbed and became an island of stability and safety.

The chairman of the institution's board, the eighty-five-year-old engineer Adolf Wajsblat, and his seriously ill wife were tormented by the Germans' edicts and were brutally evicted from their apartment. Mrs. Wajsblat was allowed to move into the school, where the students devotedly cared for her until she died in 1941. It was a tribute to the person who had dedicatedly stewarded the establishment of the facility and the realization of the vision of modern Jewish nursing in Poland. Some outstanding doctors, including a few assimilated Jews, relocated to the Jewish quarter and became lecturers at the nursing school, where they contributed to the high quality of studies. Among them were Dr. Josef Stein, Dr. Bronisława Fejgin, Dr. Żmigrider-Konopkowa, and Dr. Emil Apfelbaum. The school had all the equipment that it needed.[5]

Until the nursing school was ordered to move to the ghetto, along with Czyste Hospital, its building was well maintained. The management and staff struggled tenaciously to maintain their institution's autonomy. Part of the building was handed over to the hospital for use as housing for its doctors.[6] In 1940, under German rule in Poland, the nursing school was still operating in the hospital, when it expedited its program of studies to allow three classes to complete them with the assistance of the JDC, which provided money, food, and clothing.[7] A new class of 20 students began the program in April 1940, and 16 of its members graduated in the ghetto in March 1942. Another class of 32 students—chosen from about 300 candidates—began in October 1940. Twenty-eight completed their studies in August 1942, immediately after the *Grossaktion* was launched.[8]

The nursing school was authorized to operate in the ghetto and its principal, Luba Blum-Bielicka,[9] insisted on running it

5 Blum-Bielicka, "Szkoła Pielęgniarstwa," pp. 66–77.

6 Ibid.

7 Blum, "The Nursing School," p. 174.

8 Blum-Bielicka, "Szkoła Pielęgniarstwa," pp. 66–77.

9 Luba Blum-Bielicka, a member of the first class of the nursing school that was

according to the same professional standards as in peacetime. Thus, impeccable order was maintained, aprons were as white as snow, kerchiefs were starched, and disciplinary procedures were exemplary. Even when patients verged on death, nurses maintained the ironclad discipline that the principal had introduced.[10] When Luba Blum-Bielicka succeeded Nina Lubowska as principal, she continued to work as a nurse in the ghetto, even during the first days of the deportations that began in the summer of 1942 and in early 1943. In the final days of Czyste Hospital, she remained there in her white uniform until the final liquidation of the institution.[11]

In late 1940, after the hospital and the nursing school were ordered to move to the ghetto, the authorities allowed the school to remain on the Aryan side for three more months, until the move was finalized. During this time, staff members were not allowed to circulate in the streets without special permits; only three were issued for the entire hospital staff. Donning her nurse's cap and a scarf that masked the compulsory Star of David armband, Blum-Bielicka walked up and down the ghetto streets in search of an alternative location. Adolf Wajsblat, the chairman of the board of the nursing school, took advantage of his acquaintance with Czerniaków, the head of the Judenrat, to have an appropriate building in the ghetto allocated to the school—although only after protracted lobbying.

When the nursing school was transferred to the ghetto, it was set up in offices on Wołyńska St., which had been used by a foundation to assist the ill before the war. As time passed,

inaugurated in 1923, graduated in 1925. She also studied in Paris and taught at the Warsaw Nursing School. In 1932, she became the assistant principal and later on, during the war, from 1939 to 1943, she served as principal. In 1938, the then-principal, Nina Lubowska, went to the United States to raise funds for the school, but did not return to Poland, due to the war. In 1939, the Blums turned down an offer of Belgian passports, because of Luba's sense of responsibility for the school and for her students' fate, and the feeling that war and Nazi invasion were inevitable; see Blum, "The Nursing School," p. 174.

10 Krall, *Shielding the Flame*, p. 43; Blady Szwajger, *I Remember Nothing More*, p. 62.

11 Roland, *Courage under Siege*, pp. 73–74; Blum, "The Nursing School," pp. 174, 177.

the school was moved to Mariańska St., in an area known as the small ghetto, and became associated with Bersohn and Bauman Children's Hospital, where students could complete their training in pediatrics. They studied social medicine at the mother and child care clinic on Śliska St., under the direction of Dr. Anna Margolis, and in refugee centers.

With the assistance of David Guzik, director of the JDC Warsaw office, all its equipment was transferred to the new location. The premises were crowded but, thanks to the efforts of all the staff members and students, the school began to operate in the ghetto on January 15, 1941.[12] Young students in nurses' uniforms plied the ghetto streets to help out in emergencies, especially to aid refugees and victims of starvation. The nurses wore white clothing, smocks, and caps, and the nursing students wore pink dresses, white smocks, white kerchiefs, and blue caps. When the ghetto was in its final stage in late September 1942, the school moved to 31 Gęsia St.[13]

The nursing school offered two programs of study. One followed the regular format, and the prewar curriculum of theoretical and practical studies was taught. The staff of instructors trained the students in their practical work in the hospital wards. Classes in the ghetto were conducted as if in a cocoon. There was no lack of scholastic equipment, the dormitory had what it needed, and the classroom looked like an ideal hospital department. The second program offered 250 young women a course that covered two-thirds of the study material alongside intensive work at the hospital. The curriculum was followed so closely that even the cooking classes continued at a time when the hospital did not have enough gas, electricity, and food for its patients. Classes were held late in the evening, when the hospital's meager supply of gas could be tapped. Time devoted to clinical studies was also maintained strictly. The disparity between the classroom—where there was order, cleanliness, and proper equipment—and the reality in

12 Blum-Bielicka, "Szkoła Pielęgniarstwa," pp. 66–77.

13 Roland, *Courage under Siege*, pp. 73–74; Helena Szereszewska, *Memoirs from Occupied Warsaw, 1940–1945* (London: Vallentine Mitchell, 1997), p. 28; Blum, "The Nursing School," p. 176.

the hospital departments was immense. They seemed to be two separate and unequal worlds.[14]

During the war, approximately eighty women attended the nursing school in three graduating classes. The curriculum included all the relevant subjects, and the lecturers were among the finest in the ghetto.[15] The dormitory remained in use and clinical studies continued to be held in the various health care institutions. Nurses received advanced training and worked in all the branches and departments of Czyste Hospital, in the children's hospital, in preventive medicine, and in the psychiatric department.

The nurses' dedication knew no bounds. Even though they were starving, they traversed the entire ghetto on foot, each day, to treat typhus patients in the hospital on Stawki St. To fight the typhus scourge, they developed a meticulous procedure that concentrated on admitting new patients: A reception desk was set up where all the patients underwent delousing, bathed, and changed clothing before being admitted to the hospital wards.[16] Efforts to keep the school going persisted even after the *Aktionen* had began.

> The school was still functioning despite everything. The students' coats were hanging on pegs. One of the professors even had a lecture today. Women from the staff in white aprons milled about the corridors and asked the director for instructions.[17]

During the mass deportations, classes and regular work ceased. The principal took on a job as a sanitation worker at the Szulc

14 Szereszewska, *Memoirs*, pp. 28, 63; Koren, "Hasiyud Kehelek Misherutei Habriyut," p. 81.

15 Dr. Mieczysław Szejnman taught chemistry, anatomy, and physiology; Dr. Minc, pharmacology; Dr. Emil Apfelbaum, internal diseases; Dr. Sara Zofia Syrkin Binstein, hygiene; Dr. Aleksander Borkowski, surgery; Dr. Maria Goldman-Wilk, ophthalmology; Dr. Dawid Wdowiński, psychiatry; Dr. Emma Moscisker, ear, nose, and throat; Dr. Josef Stein, pathology; Dr. Jan Przedborski, pediatric diseases; Dr. Hermann, neurology; and Dr. Żmigrider-Konopkowa, bacteriology.

16 Blum, "The Nursing School," p. 174.

17 Szereszewska, *Memoirs*, p. 63.

workshop. "I often saw her coming back from work in a nurse's cap and a blue shawl," Szereszewska wrote. "The students at the school supported themselves, dragging a wagon with some bread or cabbage."[18] By now, many were no longer attending nursing school. Some had joined their parents in rural towns and others had accepted posts in workshops as paramedics or laborers.[19]

The nursing school facility was liquidated along with the small ghetto on August 16, 1942. SS men surrounded the building and escorted the students to Grzybowska Square, where the 4,000 remaining inhabitants of the small ghetto, including Dr. Janusz Korczak and his pupils, had been rounded up. All were designated for transfer to the Umschlagplatz and thence to Treblinka. The principal instructed the students and the staff to put on nurses' uniforms. She exploited the Germans' fear of the typhus epidemic, calling her students an "epidemic prevention team" and, thus, spared them from deportation, for the time being.

The school was transferred to a six-room apartment at 33 Gęsia St., where it was allowed to function as a *Schwesterheim* (nurses' home). Even there, underground studies continue to take place. On August 18, two days after the liquidation, the twenty-fifth graduating class completed their studies. One day during this period, the entire staff at the *Schwesterheim*, including the principal's two children, were ordered without warning to go to the Umschlagplatz.[20] The nurses marched to the plaza in their professional attire. "They looked like white birds. With their pink dresses; wide, white bibbed aprons gathered at the waist; and their stiff, white caps."[21] When the principal returned from her job at the Szulc workshop, she found the *Schwesterheim* empty. She raced to the Umschlagplatz at once, and obtained permission to release twelve of her students, her sister, and her children and to send them back to the *Schwesterheim*.[22]

18 Ibid., pp. 91, 113.

19 Ibid., p. 106.

20 Blum, "The Nursing School," p. 176.

21 Szereszewska, *Memoirs*, p. 98.

22 Blum, "The Nursing School," 176.

On January 18, 1943, SS men broke into the hospital and murdered all the patients, doctors, and nurses. The principal, Blum-Bielicka, had tipped off the staff and the patients about the impending *Aktion* through the Jewish resistance, the ŻOB—Żydowska Organizacja Bojowa (Jewish Fighting Organization). She took her children and several students away from the hospital grounds and hid them.[23] The remaining staff and students, members of the twenty-ninth graduating class, were murdered in the January 1943 *Aktion*.[24] Seven or eight members of this class, who began their studies during the war, survived. These graduates received their certification from the Polish Ministry of Health after the war on the basis of confirmation by Blum-Bielicka, who also survived.[25]

Blum-Bielicka testified that the Poles made insufficient efforts to assist the school. Nevertheless, some Polish nurses did everything possible to help their Jewish colleagues, advising them, providing information, and actively assisting them in other ways.[26] Despite the exceedingly difficult conditions and against all odds, forty-four nurses completed their studies in the ghetto. Several of those who survived joined the partisans and took part in resistance operations. In her memoirs, Blum-Bielicka wrote that the graduates of the nursing school in Warsaw were the vanguard of the nursing profession in Jewish society and that they contributed to the first steps of modern professional nursing in the Jewish community at large.

After the *Grossaktion*, Blum-Bielicka went into hiding on the Aryan side of Warsaw in the guise of a Polish nurse. The hardships of ghetto life and the tribulations of running the ghetto nursing school did not defeat her. Driven by her personality, professionalism, and commitment to her patients, she mobilized

23 Ibid., p. 177. On the distribution of "numbers of life" in the *Aktionen* by the principal, see Chapter 10, which addresses the ethical dilemmas of the work of the medical staff.

24 Nachman Blumental, "Batei Hasefer Bageto," in Gruenbaum et al., *Entziklopediya Shel Galuyot: Varsha*, vol. 6, part 2, p. 546.

25 Koren, "Hasiyud Kehelek Misherutei Habriyut," p. 82.

26 Blum, "The Nursing School," p. 176.

for the new tasks that presented themselves after the war. In 1945–1949, she ran an orphanage in Otwock and dedicated herself to attending to the rehabilitation of children who had lost their parents in the Holocaust.[27] In 1965, the Red Cross awarded Luba Blum-Bielicka the esteemed Florence Nightingale medal for her leadership, courage, and adherence to professional ethics as principal of the nursing school in the Warsaw ghetto.[28]

Underground Medical School

An order prohibiting higher education in occupied Poland was issued on November 6, 1939. Universities were shut down, and some professors and instructors were arrested and sent to concentration camps. The flames of the Nazi occupation appeared to have engulfed academia. However, immediately after the edict was promulgated, underground medical studies began at the Sżpital Dzieciątka Jezus University Hospital in Warsaw, which was made possible by a resistance movement that enjoyed support from the Polish government-in-exile that was situated initially in Paris and later in England. During the occupation, medical subjects and pharmacy were taught clandestinely in Warsaw, Cracow, Częstochowa, Vilna, and Kielce. Pursuant to a decision by the underground board of the Faculty of Medicine at the University of Warsaw, secret departments of study were set up at all hospitals in the Polish capital. Teaching ensued in an atmosphere of Nazi terror. For the next five years, lecturers and students were in continual danger. Some were murdered for the crime of illegal underground activities.

27 Sabina Zenderman was a nurse at Bersohn and Bauman Children's Hospital before the war and in the ghetto. She survived Auschwitz and, after the war, she worked at the orphanage at Otwock with its director Luba Blum-Bielicka. In 1949, Blum-Bielicka began to resurrect the nursing school in Warsaw, overseeing its construction on the ruins of the Jewish hospital, using the original 1923 blueprints. The first class began its studies in 1952. The nurses Liza Mirocznik and Huttner returned to Poland to work with her as administrators and instructors.

28 Luba Blum-Bielicka died in Poland in 1973. A plaque in her honor was installed in the school building. See Mayer, "The School That Would Not Die," pp. 15–16.

The underground medical school of the University of Warsaw was established in October 1941. Its curriculum was designed in a way that allowed a three-year program of study to be completed in two years. Clinical specialization was organized at almost all the universities in Warsaw and at clinical study centers in the hospitals. A similar program was implemented in the western areas of the Warsaw district, at the faculties of medicine, and at the professional medical school run by Prof. Jan Zaorski.[29] This ramified, covert activity influenced the Warsaw ghetto establishment to set up an underground medical school of its own. Of course, the conditions in the ghetto were far worse; they provided a kind of framework for gradual annihilation. However, it may be assumed that the extensive clandestine activity organized by the physicians of the University of Warsaw was an inspiration for the physicians and leaders who established the underground school in the ghetto. The Polish university recognized the ghetto underground medical school as a full-fledged academic institution and cooperated with it as an expression of the spirit of fraternity among scientists and doctors. According to Prof. Hirszfeld, the attempts to circumvent the ban on studies began in the Jewish quarter and spread only afterwards to the Aryan side.[30]

The mortality rate in the ghetto generated much tension among the population and the Judenrat, the ghetto's sole de facto governing authority. The chairman of the Judenrat, Adam Czerniaków, aided by the director of the Judenrat Health Department, Dr. Israel Milejkowski, worked intensively to improve the grave situation that prevailed in the ghetto. They contacted experts in the ghetto, primarily Prof. Hirszfeld, a scientist of world repute, and Prof. Juliusz (Julian) Zweibaum,[31]

29 Witold J. Rudowski, "Clandestine Medical Education in Poland, 1939–1945," *American College of Surgeons Bulletin*, 78:1 (1993), pp. 7–13.

30 Hirszfeld, *Die Geschicte eines Lebens*, p. 130.

31 The histologist Dr. Juliusz Zweibaum (1887–1959) was the moving force behind the establishment of the underground medical school in the ghetto and, once it was up and running, he became its director. Zweibaum, a judicious, pleasant man and riveting lecturer, had earned the degree of docent before the war and had lectured at the Warsaw University Medical School after completing his studies in biology in 1913. In 1924, he initiated the growth of culture tissue

and set up a committee that introduced a sanitation course to combat contagious diseases. To accomplish this, the Judenrat received a grant from the JDC, and Czerniaków personally solicited donations from residents of the ghetto. Finally, they approached Dr. Wilhelm Hagen, the German chief physician of Warsaw, who approved the inauguration of a course on epidemic prevention in the ghetto, prompted by the Germans' fear of contracting the diseases that had become common there.[32] Although the occupation authorities approved the course, they strictly limited the curriculum to practical aspects and conducted regular inspections to ensure compliance. The license for organizing the course was issued to the docent, Prof. Zweibaum, who organized the studies very successfully.[33]

About five months after ghettoization, Czerniaków presented the German security police in Warsaw with Zweibaum's program of lectures in order to obtain approval for the course. In mid-May 1941, Dr. Stein delivered the opening lecture, titled "Life and Death," on the topic of sanitation.[34] From October 1941 onward, the curriculum was taught systematically.

> The university professors [the bacteriologist] Hirszfeld and [the histologist] Zweibaum are giving medical courses in

outside of an organism. In 1935, he was among the founders of the Histology and Embryology Department. In addition to his academic activities, he was a member of the Friends of the Hebrew University in Jerusalem and the administrative council, and was among the founders of the Polish Anatomical Society. When the deportations started, a student from the underground faculty helped him to escape from the Umschlagplatz. Zweibaum refused to leave the ghetto, but after the *Grossaktion*, he moved to the Aryan side and was hidden by Polish friends. He survived the war and helped publish the book on the hunger study that had been conducted by physicians in the ghetto. He reestablished the Histology and Embryology Department in the Warsaw Faculty of Medicine, and served as a professor there until 1958. I wish to thank Zofia Perzyńska, Juliusz Zweibaum's granddaughter, for sending me her lecture about his life, which she presented at the Third European Conference on NaziMedicine, "Building Memory–Building Resilience," Warsaw and Lublin, Poland, October 3–5, 2018.

32 Stabholz, "Hora'at Anatomiya Bamahteret."

33 Hirszfeld, *The Story of One Life*, p. 201.

34 Czerniaków, *The Warsaw Diary*, pp. 225, 233.

> the ghetto, at a university level. The students work in an anatomical laboratory.[35]

Four personalities were behind the opening of the epidemiology courses: Dr. Milejkowski, Prof. Hirszfeld, Prof. Zweibaum, and Czerniaków. Zweibaum acceded to the wishes of students who were not satisfied with the epidemiology courses that they had been offered. Having studied medicine before the war and wishing to continue their studies and to complete them after the war, they urged Czerniaków to establish medical courses.[36] Zweibaum planned a medical school in the ghetto, where the coursework of the first years would be taught. Hirszfeld undertook to set up the fourth and fifth year classes.[37] According to Hirszfeld, the initial teaching faculty included Zweibaum and himself, both of whom had taught at the medical school in Warsaw, as well as Prof. Mieszysław Centnerszvwer, who taught chemistry, and Prof. Hilai Lacks, who taught physical chemistry. Thus, they were able to improvise an academic curriculum that covered the first two years of medical studies. Czerniaków provided all the support that he could. After some time, it became possible to open another course and, a year later, yet another.[38] About fourteen doctors taught at the clandestine ghetto medical school.[39]

In order to examine the possibility of establishing an underground medical school in the ghetto, the policy of the University of Warsaw administration regarding this matter had to be clarified. For this purpose, contacts were pursued

35 Ringelblum, *Notes from the Warsaw Ghetto*, p. 225.

36 Stabholz, "Hora'at Anatomiya Bamahteret."

37 Roland, *Courage under Siege*, pp. 187–188.

38 Hirszfeld, *The Story of One Life*, p. 201; Prof. Adam Drozdowicz testimony, YVA, O.3/3647.

39 Additional teachers included Josef Stein, Władysław Sterling (1876–1943), Henryk Lewenfisz-Wojnarowski (1894–1956), Mieczysław Centnerszwer (1874–1944), Henryk Stabholz (1882–1941), Ludwik Stabholz (1911–2007), Henry Fenigstein (1913–1993), Bernard Waksman (1909–2009), Henryk Makower (1904–1964), and Paul Borenstein. See Roland, *Courage under Siege*; Prof. Adam Drozdowicz testimony, YVA, O.3/3647; Dr. Thaddeus Stabholz testimony, YVA, O.33/648.

with representatives of the university senate, which had gone underground. Prof. Ludwik Stabholz, who before the war had been an assistant to Prof. Edward Loth, a world-renowned researcher in anatomy, was asked to explore with Loth the possibility of recognizing the ghetto's clandestine school as an extension of the University of Warsaw. Loth saw this as an opportunity to exploit approval for the epidemiology courses to set up additional courses in medicine. The senate agreed to recognize the ghetto's two-year medical school as a full-fledged academic institute for medical studies.

Under Polish law, at the end of each academic year, a certificate signed by a professor confirming the completion of studies in basic medical subjects was required. Since Dr. Stabholz would become a lecturer in anatomy and there would be another lecturer for physiology, and since neither of them held the title of professor, Loth granted this rank to Stabholz and his colleague with the senate's consent. Thus, they could sign off on all the students' grades, as required by the University of Warsaw.[40] The university and many of its instructors cooperated with the medical school, both professionally and administratively. For example, lists of students were sent out of the ghetto to the offices of the university, which recognized the nurses in training as its own students, and exchanges of lecturers and study materials took place, as long as this was possible.[41]

The underground medical school was located at the western end of the ghetto in a building that belonged to the Labor Office. It had served as a high school and had chalkboards and a laboratory equipped to teach biology and chemistry.[42] The coursework was based on lectures and on

40 Stabholz, "Hora'at Anatomiya Bamahteret."

41 Shaul Menashe Shasha, "Harefu'a Bageta'ot Bitkufat Hashoah" (Medicine in the Ghettos during the Holocaust), *Harefu'a* (Hebrew), 141:4 (2002), pp. 320–322.

42 Prof. Adam Drozdowicz, Prof. Makower's assistant, stated that there was no permanent location and that the lectures took place in various sites that were not concealed, because the talks had been authorized in the guise of sanitation lectures. Some lectures were held in rooms inside the Judenrat building on Grzybowska St., while experiments were conducted at the bacteriology-chemistry lab on Muranowska St. Prof. Drozdowicz also worked in the ghetto

only a few laboratory experiments, because the lab facilities were outdated. All the basic courses taught at the Faculty of Medicine at Warsaw University were taught there. Students who had studied in Warsaw and elsewhere before the war joined first-year students and participated in the clinical studies. Lectures were given in Polish, and the Germans were told that they covered basic material in anatomy, hygiene, and public health. In fact, full-fledged medical studies were taught. The curriculum included entry-level pre-clinical and clinical work. The two-year pre-clinical program comprised physics, biology, histology, anatomy, and organic and inorganic chemistry. Despite the high mortality, anatomical specimens were scarce. Skulls, histological and pathological materials, and other supplies were smuggled into the school by colleagues at the University of Warsaw and were passed from hand to hand among the students. Most anatomy studies took place in the hospital morgue. In addition to attending formal classes in the evenings, the students worked during the day in the hospital departments and clinics, where they served patients and gained hands-on experience in medicine.

The four-year clinical studies program was conducted at Czyste Hospital, the children's hospital, small hospitals, clinics, and health care services that operated in the ghetto. The practical training was even more intensive than that of students at other medical schools. Medical students in the ghetto learned to give injections, write prescriptions, and make diagnoses. They also participated in doctors' home visits and conducted visits under supervision. From time to time, there were lectures for doctors during the day and, on these occasions, students alternately covered for members of the medical staff. They also assisted by doing the work of nurses.[43]

The studies were conducted under the guise of sanitation courses. Classes typically began by addressing topics related to

lab, where they studied chemistry and anatomy. See Prof. Adam Drozdowicz testimony, YVA, O.3/3647.

43 Roland, *Courage under Siege*, pp. 188–192.

epidemics, vaccinations, and contagious diseases. These topics had been authorized and were the basis of the consent to conduct the courses. They then segued to the forbidden subjects of medical study and research: physiology, pathology, and biochemistry. The students and staff made sure to maintain strict secrecy. They left papers and books about infectious diseases on the table in the lecture room to create the impression that these were the topics, and they sprayed the rooms with an antibacterial agent to give them the distinctive odor.[44] Lectures were delivered between 5 P.M. and 8 P.M. When the electricity went out, they took place by candlelight and carbide lamps. Now and then, gunshots were heard as soldiers standing guard near the building fired at Jews. The students were used to this and continued to listen to the lectures, finding a measure of solace in their studies.[45]

Prof. Hirszfeld described the dilemma that he faced in choosing study topics and teaching methods. He noted that Prof. Zweibaum took a formal approach to his work, believing that the courses taught would be recognized for credit in the future. Hirszfeld himself tried to create a scientific and spiritual experience in his classes. "What was I to talk about….I felt that my main task was to keep up their morale….I would capture their imagination with lofty ideas and alleviate their pain."[46] For example, he chose to lead his students to the banks of the Ganges to teach them about blood types.

> "Look," I said, "I am here with you behind the wall, and any old soldier can kill you or me to suit his whim. But no one can prevent me from roaming through distant countries, in my thoughts, and this I can do because I have loved science above all." Thus, I gave them a vision of strong experiences, distant travels, and intense thoughts. I took those poor children by the hand and led them to the summits where the air was pure, where people prayed in ecstasy at sunrise, and

44 Ibid., p. 190; Shasha, "Harefu'a Bageta'ot," p. 322.

45 Hirszfeld, *The Story of One Life*, p. 202.

46 Ibid.

> no one despised them, and where, in the glory of mankind, they could build, think, and dream....[47]

Prof. Hirszfeld wished to compensate his students for their adolescence and the love that had been taken from them. He strove to combine emotion and spirit with professional knowledge, "Did I reach the Jewish soul? I do not know; I only know that I reached very, very unhappy people." Hirszfeld had converted to Christianity years before he was forced into the ghetto. After earning his students' trust, he decided to lecture on the most dangerous topic of all: racial theory and antisemitism. "I wanted to absolve them of the curse of being held in contempt, because even hatred is easier to bear than contempt." The class on this topic was fraught with peril and, in the case of denunciation, Hirszfeld was liable to pay for it with his life.[48]

Study conditions were harsh. The classrooms, which were bitterly cold, were lit with oil lamps that gave off a vile stench. However, it was even worse in the students' homes. Because of the curfew, the students could not move about at night and had to study in groups each night in someone else's room. Fearing a surprise inspection by the Nazis, they stopped all activity whenever a car was heard in the dark streets. Getting to school, which was outside the ghetto, was one of the most difficult tasks. Until a bridge was built, the students had to get past the Polish, German, and Jewish security guards at the ghetto gate. In addition to the usual documents that all ghetto inhabitants had to carry, students were required to have student cards. They became anxious each time they passed through the gate, due to the violence of the police. The female students were afraid of being raped in the guards' kiosk. The men were also at risk and some were beaten on their way to class.[49]

There was a severe shortage of textbooks and other educational equipment. Prof. Edward Loth brought books, materials, bones, and tools for Dr. Stabholz's classes from the Aryan side. On the pretext of assisting in the approved epidemiology

47 Ibid.

48 Ibid.

49 Roland, *Courage under Siege*, pp. 190–191.

courses, Prof. Loth instructed Dr. Stabholz on how to teach under ghetto conditions. He visited the ghetto every week, bringing materials for the various courses each time. He did so at great personal risk, since the SS murdered well-known professors who visited the ghetto to perform surgical procedures.[50] In an effort to acquire the supplies and equipment that was lacking, secret contact was established with Dr. Witold Orlowski and Dr. Konopacki of the University of Warsaw.[51]

After the first two years of medical studies and pharmacology, it became necessary to look after approximately thirty veteran students who were working at the ghetto hospitals. Unable to pursue advanced training in their specializations, they were at risk of accustoming themselves to slipshod work. They did not report to work regularly, they sometimes left the doctors' room dirty, and they failed to keep up their studies. There was concern for their professional future. In response, Prof. Hirszfeld submitted a request for approval for continuing studies for this group, which Wilhelm Hagen, the German chief physician of Warsaw, authorized. Hirszfeld then recruited several senior physicians at the hospital, organized advanced medical studies, and set up a laboratory. Czerniaków approved the requisite funding.

A department for clinical experiments was established on the first floor of the ghetto hospital building, alongside a bacteriology and biochemistry lab. The facility also had a lecture hall, where the advanced medical studies took place. Dr. Julian Fliederbaum[52] and Dr. Emil Apfelbaum conducted the scientific studies in the physiological chemistry lab. A talented painter produced charts of academic quality. In due course, the walls were covered with

50 Stabholz, "Hora'at Anatomiya Bamahteret."

51 Roland, *Courage under Siege*, pp. 189–190.

52 Dr. Julian Fliederbaum, who was born in 1898 in St. Petersburg, Russia, studied medicine in Warsaw, served as a municipal physician, worked at the university clinic under Prof. Orlowski, and was a member of the Czyste Hospital medical staff. From 1933 to the beginning of World War II, he also worked at the University of Warsaw. He published approximately 100 scientific articles on galactosemia. At the beginning of the German occupation, he evidently moved to Vilna, but then returned to Warsaw and worked at the Jewish hospital in the ghetto, where he perished.

these tables and graphs. The floors of the lab were sparkling clean. Flowerpots stood on the windowsills. Eventually, the essential instruments were acquired. The first implements needed were microscopes and a cabinet to keep cultures, but these items were too expensive to even think about buying. To solve the problem, an engineer named Kurowski who lived on the Aryan side provided the means. Several doctors brought their microscopes with them, while other expenses were partly covered by the Judenrat, and the lab received support from the JDC. As Prof. Hirszfeld noted, "It was typical of the Jews. Science was important to them even in the greatest distress."[53]

The laboratory was impressive. Those entering it saw heads bent over the microscopes. The sight evoked amazement and a sense of a return to civilization. Lectures in the laboratory took place every day from noon to 2 P.M., distracting lecturers and students from day-to-day worries as they focused on the topic of study.[54] The medical students' achievements were measured by means of ordinary exams. Efforts were made to forward the tests to the medical school in Warsaw for certification. One of the doctors at the school recalled that it had been necessary to hand the exams over to Prof. Hirszfeld, whose job it was to relay them to Prof. Franciszek Czubalski, the supervisor of the ghetto medical school at the medical school on the Aryan side. Some exams were given orally; others were in writing. Prof. Stabholz tested his anatomy students orally. Final exams for the first year were held on January 20, 1942, and the results were announced about two weeks later.[55]

Ongoing issues relating to the medical profession in Jewish society and the encouragement of new medical students were discussed at the First World Congress of Jewish Physicians in 1936, when many universities were already excluding Jewish students.

53 Hirszfeld, *Die Geschichte Eines Lebens*, pp. 132–133.

54 Ibid.; Hirszfeld, *The Story of One Life*, pp. 204–205; Prof. Adam Drozdowicz testimony, YVA, O.3/3647.

55 Roland, *Courage under Siege*, p. 192.

> Heaven forbid that we sever the holy strand of scientific endeavor, work in public medicine, and the commandment to heal the ill for posterity....The gates of teaching in Central Europe are closed; hundreds of scientists have been exiled from their places of work and are impatiently waiting to continue to use their talent in research and teaching. The question of establishing a Jewish university in the Jerusalem of Lithuania or in some other Diaspora center is off the table. The place is here and the time is now. Let us create the possibility of medical studies for a small group among the thousands of young people who thirst for this knowledge—a small number but in a safe place, for the benefit of our people and our country.[56]

Dr. Milejkowski, who attended the conference, surely shared this sentiment, which reflected the sense of concern and responsibility for the training of the next generation of Jewish doctors. His activities on behalf of the clandestine medical school is a quintessential expression of the fulfillment of the responsibility that he and his fellow physicians in the ghetto assumed in order to impart the profession to future generations of young Jews.

The underground medical school operated from May 1941 to July 1942. Charles Roland wrote that elements of the motivations of anyone who enrolled in medical studies or who taught in medical schools in normal places in normal times could be perceived in the aspirations of Prof. Zweibaum and his colleagues to establish the school and of the students to enroll in it. The ghetto abounded with talent and with patients. There also may have been a sense of the need to replenish the doctors' ranks. This project also reflected the will to continue leading ordinary lives amid the abnormality of the ghetto. There were students who had almost completed their studies and wished to do so. It was an ordinary, albeit underground, school.

Some survivors regard the establishment of the school as a form of rebellion and believe it may be defined as such. The

56 Friedman, *Sefer Hakongres Ha'olami*, pp. 29–30.

ban on setting it up was a natural factor in the motivation of the students and lecturers alike, as evidenced in the way the school organized its daily work. There were additional and more prosaic reasons for the establishment of the school and for its allure to teachers and students. For example, Dr. Henry Fenigstein claimed that he joined the teaching staff because he enjoyed teaching and being involved in the underground school. He found it interesting, challenging, and satisfying. Several students considered enrollment a way to solve problems related to staying at home and to the perils of the streets. Other students signed up to please their parents, who wanted their children to become doctors.

Roland wrote in the conclusion of his book that the Warsaw ghetto abounded with modest and great examples of self-denial, self-sacrifice, and devotion to others amid the terror in the ghetto. The establishment of the underground medical school is a good case in point. The courses were organized professionally and humanely, and were recognized and highly respected in the ghetto. He added that, in retrospect, the establishment of the Warsaw ghetto medical school appeared to have been futile. However, it was possible that until 1942, most inhabitants of the ghetto believed that many, if not all, of them would survive. There was no precedent that would induce them to think otherwise. They thought that this "big pogrom," as the ghetto was viewed, would pass and life would return to normal.

Such optimism in response to highly difficult and dramatic events is not unusual among Jews. In addition to the school's general contribution to ghetto morale, it was perceived as an example of the triumph of the human spirit, and its organizers deserve credit for its concrete achievements. About 500 students participated in its courses, although only about 50 survived. After the war, those who had attended the ghetto's underground medical school were directly admitted, without exams, to third-year university studies on the basis of their coursework and grades. Several became professors and doctors of worldwide repute.[57]

57 Roland, *Courage under Siege*, pp. 195–196, 226–227; Stabholz, "Hora'at Anatomiya Bamahteret."

Library, Lectures, and Courses for the Medical Community

The ghetto had one medical library, which was located in Czyste Hospital. Some of the books from the hospital's original library had survived and others had been donated by doctors or smuggled into the ghetto. The library, which was in Szpital Dzieciątka Jezus Hospital, occupied a large room that was burned. Dr. Szwatzowa oversaw the library, but it was usually closed. It contained new journals and old books, since the new books at the original Czyste Hospital had been stolen or defaced when the library was transferred to the ghetto.[58]

In the General Government, scientific discussions were prohibited and scientific journals were shut down. Dr. Schrempf forbade Jews to engage in research. Even the sale of books was forbidden to Jews. Prof. Hirszfeld worked with Czerniaków and Dr. Milejkowski, and following a discussion among them, they decided to take action in three domains: organizing professional lectures, fighting epidemics, and establishing a scientific laboratory at the hospital.[59] The physicians assigned to blocks in the ghetto vaccinated the Jewish population against typhus at this time. Nevertheless, the Germans occasionally summoned them, reprehended them, and accused them of failing to prevent the spread of the epidemic in the ghetto. Hirszfeld suggested offering these doctors lectures on vaccination and measures to fight epidemics, and since this did not require the authorities' approval, a series of lectures for these doctors were initiated.

Hundreds of doctors attended the first lecture, given by Prof. Hirszfeld, at the Judenrat offices with Czerniaków in attendance. The lecture dealt with the subject of "the bacterium cell," as described by Hirszfeld.

> I had noticed that Jews did not like popular lectures...So now I also delved into difficult matters, such as the complex

58 Roland, *Courage under Siege*, p. 71.
59 Hirszfeld, *The Story of One Life*, p. 199.

> structure of the bacterial cell and recent biochemical research. I saw eyes opening wider and wider in amazement: so there was still a world of ideas; the night has not yet devoured everything! When I finished, there was stormy applause, and the chairman expressed his hope that this was the beginning of a whole series of lectures. I saw that I had struck the right chord, that these people were yearning for meetings, lectures, exchanges of ideas, and everything else that resembled their normal prewar life.[60]

It was also decided to open a course on contagious diseases—a two-month series of twice-weekly, two-hour classes. Dr. Hagen, the German chief physician of Warsaw, allowed the course to take place, believing that it might be useful in the war on typhus. Some of the doctors at the Jewish hospital, including a few bacteriologists, gave lectures. A summary of the lecture was distributed after each class. At the end of the course, the summaries of all the lectures were compiled for publication. This was the only scientific text published during the war. Following the course on infectious diseases, another course on general pathology, which addressed the problem of vitamins and nutrition, was organized on the initiative of the dentists. This initiative prolonged the lecture program by several months.[61]

During a discussion on how to assist doctors who worked in non-hospital settings in the ghetto, it was decided to begin a course on typhus that would take place every two weeks. Although it was approved, attendance was nil because the doctors did not want to create the impression that their knowledge about typhus was deficient. Therefore, it was decided to hold the course in a format of weekly, two-hour clinical discussions. The doctors attended en masse. Mary Berg wrote that the public in the ghetto heard about these meetings and knew that the lectures were having an impact on medical practice. The doctors at Czyste Hospital sought to create a kind of "privileged aristocracy." After winding up the discussions

60 Ibid., p. 200.

61 Ibid., p. 201; Hirszfeld, *Die Geschichte eines Lebens*, p. 129.

about typhus, they moved on to other topics, such as tuberculosis. Since the lecture hall could not hold them all, additional courses were set up. Because they were for the physicians in the ghetto, no further request for permission was required.[62]

Dr. Adina Blady Szwajger reported that fortnightly scientific meetings at the children's hospital were held to discuss exceptional cases, including proposals for curative methods and brief academic lectures.[63] Dr. Chaim Einhorn, a staff member at Czyste Hospital, stated that the medical scientific work in the ghetto, which was very dynamic, ended only when the ghetto was liquidated. The work was conducted at three centers: Czyste Hospital, under Dr. Stein; Bersohn and Bauman Children's Hospital, under Dr. Braude-Heller; and TOZ, where all the other doctors were concentrated.

Czyste Hospital hosted regular scientific meetings once a week—sometimes even twice a week—with the active participation of the department directors. On these occasions, cases were discussed and original scientific lectures were read, followed by vigorous debate. Summaries of the hunger disease studies that the scientists had begun to conduct under Dr. Milejkowski's influence were also presented. These meetings, undertaken despite the tragic situation in the ghetto streets, helped the participants to forget, if only for a fleeting moment, what was happening in the ghetto, and gave them the strength to keep up the struggle.[64]

Typhus Research in the Ghetto

Many typhus patients in the ghetto were treated in the department of infectious diseases at Czyste Hospital, which was run by Dr. Jakub Penson.[65] Defying the Nazis' injunction, about twenty

62 Hirszfeld, *Die Geschichte eines Lebens*, p. 129; Berg, *The Diary of Mary Berg*, p. 111.

63 Blady Szwajger, *I Remember Nothing More*, p. 37.

64 Einhorn, "Doctor in the Warsaw Ghetto," p. 13. Dr. Fenigstein described at length the ramified scientific activity and range of courses for the nursing and medical teams in the ghetto. See Dr. Henry Fenigstein testimony, "Varshever yid," pp. 11–12, YVA, O.33/1074.

65 Dr. Jakub Penson was born on April 23, 1899, in Poland. He completed his

doctors there performed scientific studies on the clinical progression of typhus, giving special attention to hyperazotemia, blood urea, and renal complications. The results of the study were presented at clinical meetings at Czyste Hospital in 1941–1942 and published in a Polish journal in 1946.

From 1939, Dr. Penson headed the department of internal medicine at Czyste Hospital, where he and his colleagues observed 1,500 patients in the course of the "small epidemic" that erupted after the war had begun. It became a department of infectious diseases in 1940. When a second typhus outbreak ensued as Czyste Hospital was being forced to move to the ghetto, the department was transferred to a smaller building in the sealed Jewish quarter. Despite the harsh conditions there, it was possible to continue the research on typhus that was initiated at the onset of the first epidemic, because the staff had managed to transfer the laboratory and the department of pathology to the ghetto. More than 6,500 patients were included in the study. The research team was composed of 20 doctors and medical students, but only 4 doctors, including Penson, survived.[66] Penson and various neurologists and pathologists jointly described the course of the two epidemics that broke out among the Jews of Warsaw under the Nazi occupation. The organic and systemic changes that occurred in the course of the illness are discussed in minute detail in various articles, based on the observations and records noted in the ghetto, and the recollections of the colleagues who survived. As mentioned, Penson presented his conclusions at the clinical discussions held

primary and secondary studies in Plock, served as a volunteer soldier in the Polish–Soviet War from 1918 to 1921, and studied medicine at the University of Warsaw. After surviving World War II, Penson was named head of the internal medicine department at the Medical University of Gdańsk and became a pioneer in clinical nephrology in Poland. See Joanna Muszkowska-Penson, "Prof. Dr. Jakub Penson (1899–1971) Część I. Okres Przedwojenny I Okupacji," *Annales Academiae Medicae Gedanensis* 32 (2002), pp. 321–330, http://pbc.gda.pl/publication/4123 (accessed March 17, 2019).

66 Penson's name appears on a list of doctors who survived the Holocaust in Poland and were members of the Jewish health care organization TOZ, which resumed its activities immediately after the war to assist Holocaust survivors. See Abraham Adolf Zylberszajn Collection, GFH, no. 5223.

at Czyste Hospital in 1941–1942, which he wrote up in 1946.[67] In the introduction to his series of articles, he wrote,

> I would like to dedicate this work to all who collaborated with me in such a dreadful period; heroes and martyrs who died during the uprising in the Warsaw ghetto or were humiliated in gas chambers in Treblinka, Majdanek, and other places of terror and death.[68]

Prof. Hirszfeld also attempted to investigate typhus and possible ways to eradicate it. It was known that the scientists Edmund Weil and Arthur Felix had successfully isolated the typhus pathogen found in patients' urine during World War I and had developed the Weil-Felix Test to detect typhus and other illnesses caused by the Rickettsia bacterium. However, the doctors in the ghetto did not have any instruments, such as a centrifuge, to isolate the pathogen in the patients' urine. Therefore, Hirszfeld and his colleagues drew their conclusions on a theoretical basis only and applied them to typhus. Nevertheless, they discovered important and hitherto unknown findings. They hoped to be able to develop a vaccine based on all the testing. However, when they sought to apply their findings at a practical level, the deportations began and they were unable to complete their work.[69]

In the ghetto, bandages that were supposed to ward off lice, which had never been mentioned in the scientific literature, were being sold. Hirszfeld and his team of researchers believed that they had been used by Austrian and Japanese soldiers in previous

67 Boleslaw Rutkowski, "Jakub Penson and His Studies on Acute Renal Failure during Typhus Epidemics in Warsaw Ghetto," *Journal of Nephrology*, 17 (2004), pp. 175–179; Jakub Penson, "Cechy kliniczne epidemii duru plamistego w latach 1940–1941/42 w Warszawie. Badania własne nad przemianą azotową ze szczególnym uwzględnieniem nerek. Metoda wczesnego rozpoznawania," *Polski Tygodnik Lekarski*, 46–47 (1946), pp. 1,399–1,404, 1,478–1,487; Mariola Małecka, "Prof. dr med. Jakub Penson (1899–1971). Życie, działalność i dokonania" (PhD diss., Akademia Medyczna w Gdańsku Zakład Hitorii I Filozofii Nauk Medycznych, 2008), pp. 1,538–1,542, 1,553–1,569. Dr. Milejkowski noted that research on typhus was conducted; see Kermish, *To Live with Honor*, p. 743.

68 Rutkowski, "Jakub Penson," p. 178.

69 Hirszfeld, *The Story of One Life*, p. 208.

wars. They concluded that the bandages were soaked in mercury and emitted toxic vapors. However, in practice, it was difficult to examine their effectiveness against lice, so they decided to grow lice in the laboratory.[70] The staff members who raised the lice applied the bandages to themselves to test their effectiveness. The method proved effective, the cultured lice diminished, and all the lice died within a few days. Thus, new possibilities to fight and to eradicate lice were created. Prof. Hirszfeld and his research team then checked whether the application of mercury could preempt infestation and win the war altogether. Hirszfeld wrote, "There is something pleasant about scientific work, because it is based on hope. Now there are new possibilities in the war on lice and in the ability to produce vaccines." However, everything went down the drain, when the deportations began.[71]

Dr. Stein continued to pursue scientific research in the ghetto, despite the many challenges that he faced as director of Czyste Hospital. His findings on the pathological changes occurring in the brain during a bout of typhus evoked great interest in Berlin. A group of experts in anatomy came from Germany to the ghetto to study his medical discoveries and research.[72]

Research on Starvation in the Ghetto

In February 1942, another group of physicians in the ghetto, headed by Dr. Israel Milejkowski, initiated scientific research on the physiology and pathology of hunger, and pursued its inquiry until July of that year.[73] Marek Edelman, an employee of the children's hospital, wrote that the doctors in the ghetto researched hunger, because the mechanism of death by starvation was not clearly

70 Ibid.

71 Ibid., p. 209, Hirszfeld, *Die Geschicte eines Lebens*, pp. 136–137.

72 Wulman et al., *The Martyrdom of Jewish Physicians in Poland*, p. 64.

73 Moshe Shechter, "Simfoniya Bilti Gmura Shel Rofim Yehudim Mishnat 1942" (An Unfinished Symphony by Jewish Doctors in 1942), *Harefu'a* (Hebrew), 44:9 (1953), pp. 202–205; Rachel Auerbach, *Behutzot Varsha: 1939–1943* (In the Streets of Warsaw: 1939–1943) (Hebrew) (Tel Aviv: Am Oved, 1954), p. 329n4; Ringelblum, *Notes from the Warsaw Ghetto*, p. 294.

understood in medical circles at the time, and it was appropriate to seize the "opportunity" that had come their way. "Never had such an abundance of research material been available to medicine."[74] Myron Winick noted that the purpose of the research was twofold: to make sure that the Germans would never be able to cover up their criminal acts, and to tell the world who were the people who had been murdered.[75]

The decision to undertake such research in the ghetto was evidently prompted by several factors: the high quality of medical personnel in the ghetto; the pervasive hunger and the need to cope with its clinical manifestations, which entailed special study and treatment; and Dr. Milejkowski's instructions. Dr. Milejkowski understood that the phenomenon of hunger in the ghetto was unique—one-time conditions had been created for research on the effects of hunger on physiological systems and for understanding pathological phenomena that were common in the ghetto—which would serve to find cures.[76]

The doctors who took part in the research, themselves suffering from hunger and from the other ravages of ghetto life, investigated the tragic reality with scientific tools and documented it. Despite wretched working conditions—limited medical equipment, a deficient physical structure, and inadequate laboratory resources—after five months of research, they managed to present a professional, high-quality, and unique study that would have taken an entire year to produce under normal conditions.[77] Its goals were to identify the physiological changes and the illnesses caused by starvation that were the most common and those that were relatively uncommon; to differentiate the course of an illness in a state of starvation from that in a normal condition; to determine the extent to which certain illnesses cure themselves in a state of hunger; to detect the causes of symptoms that accompany hunger: edema, exhaustion, tetany, and premature aging; and to identify the

74 Krall, *Shielding the Flame*, pp. 17–20.

75 Myron Winick, "Jewish Medical Resistance in the Warsaw Ghetto," in Grodin, *Jewish Medical Resistance*, pp. 93–105.

76 Shasha, "Harefu'a Bageta'ot," pp. 320–321.

77 Winick, *Hunger Disease*, p. 4.

mechanism by which starvation induces death. Intensive clinical work was conducted—anatomical, pathological, biochemical, and hematological screening, accompanied by the most complex and highly delicate tests on starving patients who had been admitted to the ghetto hospital. Most of the work was scientific. Glucose tolerance, insulin, and adrenaline curves were examined and various tests were performed—EKG and measurements of pH and acidity, blood volume flow, blood circulation velocity, balances of water, nitrogen, and minerals, and so on.[78]

Almost all the doctors who took part in the research did not survive. Some perished during the deportations to Treblinka, and the others were killed when the ghetto was destroyed. They foresaw their demise or guessed that it could happen. In the introduction to the book that he edited on hunger disease, Milejkowski wrote, "We knew subconsciously that the work could be interrupted at any minute."[79] Dr. Milejkowski, who headed the research team, conducted much of the research at the onset of the *Grossaktion*. His remarks in the introduction, written in a building in the cemetery, evoke the enormity of the tragedy that befell the inhabitants and the doctors in the ghetto, on the one hand, and the desire to sustain the human spirit, curiosity, and the possibility of contributing to medical research, on the other. Milejkowski's comments are a kind of testament to the medical world and to humanity as a whole. The following excerpt is indicative:

> I have never felt it as strongly as now when I have to write an introduction to this work. This is an unbelievable moment since the work was originated and pursued under unbelievable conditions. I hold my pen in my hand and death stares into my room....
>
> This work was never finished. It was interrupted on July 22, 1942. This was a crucial day in the history of the Warsaw ghetto—the day when the deportations, the mass murder, began. Yes, deportations, mass murder, synonymous words

78 Shechter, "Simfoniya Bilti Gmura," p. 202.
79 Winick, *Hunger Disease*, p. 4.

in the history of the ghetto. The monstrosity of it will be fully understood only in the future.

Let us be silent—as silent as the empty houses in the empty streets of our ghetto. In this prevailing silence lies the power and the depth of our pain and the moans that one day will shake the world's conscience.

The history of the Warsaw ghetto can be divided into two periods—before July 22, 1942, and the period following. The first period was characterized by general hunger, the second period by massive death. It is not surprising, therefore, that when the second period started, the work on hunger stopped. The hospitals and laboratories were destroyed and, most important, the human element, our workers and the subjects of our work, were gone....It is a history full of content! One detail should not be omitted: the work on the manuscript is being carried out in one of the undestroyed rooms of the cemetery buildings. It is symbolic of the basis and the conditions under which we live and work....In a certain sense, one may define hunger as a phenomenon in Jews' lives. Among non-Jews, you do not find a "hunger" for science, for work, and even for life akin to that of the Jewish people. This, perhaps, is where one should seek the origin of the pathological cause of antisemitism....The topic of our work, however, is prosaic, commonplace hunger, hunger in the physical sense. From this standpoint, we Jews stand outside the fence of the competition, particularly now. We should consider it an honor to roll this general topic into a scientific problem in order to quench our hunger for science and knowledge at the expense of our physical hunger....Our work was interrupted several times but was never liquidated. If it may be discussed in historical terms, it is truly an "unfinished symphony" by Jewish doctors in 1942.[80]

80 Taken from two translated versions: Winick, *Hunger Disease*, pp. 3–4, and Moshe Schechter, "Simfoniya Bilti Gmura," pp. 204–205.

Milejkowski requested that if none of the researchers survived, the manuscripts would be forwarded to Prof. Witold Orlowski for publication. Indeed, it was Orlowski, head of the Faculty of Medicine at the University of Warsaw, who preserved the papers. Another copy was given to a non-Jewish attorney named Galecki.[81] The study in Polish and a translation into French were published in 1946 by the JDC, and there is also a partial translation into Yiddish. In 1979, it was translated into English in its entirety.[82] Many of those who took part in the research and its documentation also taught at the underground medical school. For most of them, it was their last scientific endeavor.[83]

Dr. Milejkowski brought together the finest of the doctors who worked at the ghetto hospital. All were remarkably talented and many were experts in their fields who were well versed in the research literature. Some were scientists who had the background and the credentials to advance the research. This explains their impressive accomplishments.[84] Participating in Milejkowski's inaugural staff meeting were Dr. Emil Apfelbaum, head of the department of cardiology at Czyste Hospital, an acknowledged expert on blood diseases; Dr. Julian Fliederbaum, an expert in internal medicine and a refugee from Vilna, who headed the hospital facility on Stawki St.; Dr. Anna Braude-Heller, an admired and renowned pediatrician in Poland and the director of Bersohn and Bauman Children's Hospital; Dr. Mieszysław Kocen, born in

81 From the introduction to Milejkowski's book on hunger disease, in Winick, *Hunger Disease,* p. vii; Schechter, "Simfoniya Bilti Gmura," p. 202; Dr. Israel Rom (Rotbalsam) testimony, YVA, O.3/2357.

82 See the Introduction to this book, footnotes 9 and 22. The study was referenced as early as the late 1940s and the early 1950s. Dr. Milejkowski redacted its results in manuscript form in Polish. This manuscript, smuggled out of the ghetto and tracked down by Dr. Apfelbaum, one of the researchers, was printed in a limited number of copies. The study made its way to the United States in 1966. In 1979, Myron Winick produced the first English edition of the study and updated it. Martha Osnos, who escaped from Warsaw to the United States at the beginning of the war, translated the study from Polish into English. See Myron Winick, "Jewish Medical Resistance," pp. 52–53.

83 Roland, *Courage under Siege*, p. 114.

84 Winick, *Hunger Disease*, p. xi.

Łódź and an expert in blood diseases; and Dr. Josef Stein, a noted pathologist who held distinguished academic degrees and directed Czyste Hospital in the ghetto, and an apostate Jew.[85]

The meeting ended with a plan to carry out the most comprehensive research on hunger ever conducted to that time. It was resolved that each department would plan and carry out the research in its field of specialization. Under the influence of Dr. Braude-Heller, it was decided that both children and adults would be studied. The researchers wished to make a meaningful contribution to science. The tests that were planned were so sophisticated that special equipment had to be smuggled into the ghetto to perform them.[86]

Several research groups were set up. One of them, headed by Dr. Julian Fliederbaum, performed observations on the clinical aspects of hunger among adults and on the metabolic changes that it induced. Another group, directed by Dr. Anna Braude-Heller, investigated the same aspects among children. A third group, under Dr. Emil Apfelbaum, looked into the pathophysiology of the circulatory system in hunger disease. A fourth group, headed by Dr. Michael Szajnman, examined changes in peripheral blood cells and bone marrow. A fifth group, under Dr. Simon Fajgenblat, researched ophthalmological changes. A sixth group, run by Dr. Josef Stein, used autopsy findings to examine anatomical changes caused by hunger disease.[87]

The research group was composed of twenty-eight physicians who assisted the project in various respects. Almost all perished. Dr. Fliederbaum and Dr. Milejkowski evidently committed suicide; Dr. Kocen and Dr. Stein were murdered in Treblinka; Dr. Braude-Heller was killed in a bunker during the ghetto uprising. Dr. Apfelbaum survived and assisted in the preparation and the publication of the research findings. In 1946, he died of a heart attack on a street in Warsaw at the age of fifty-six.[88] Not all

85 Ibid., pp. vii–viii.

86 Winick, "Jewish Medical Resistance," pp. 103–104.

87 Shasha, "Harefu'a Bageta'ot," p. 321.

88 Winick, *Hunger Disease*, pp. viii. Dr. Israel Rom (Rotbalsam) testified that he was with Dr. Stein in the transport to Treblinka. He reported that Dr. Stein, who

the material that was researched survived. Some findings were not put in writing, because some of the researchers died before they were able to do so. Part of the material was lost in the *Aktionen*. Ultimately, the deportations and the transport of the doctors and patients to Treblinka put to an end to the project.[89]

On July 6, 1942, about two weeks before the beginning of the deportations of the Jews of Warsaw to Treblinka, Dr. Milejkowski met with Dr. Apfelbaum, Dr. Stein, Dr. Fliederbaum, and Dr. Cohen, who reported the results of the scientific research on hunger.[90] The researchers' last meeting appears to have taken place in August 1942, during the *Grossaktion*. Dr. Milejkowski informed those assembled that this would indeed be their final meeting and divulged the place in the cemetery where he was concealing the research findings. Almost a week later, few of the participants in the meeting were still alive.[91] The research activity had to be kept secret from the Germans, because its discovery would have not only terminated the work but would have doomed the researchers to certain death. Thus, the work was conducted underground. Dr. Apfelbaum testified to having seen groups of SS and Gestapo men combing the hospital for research documentation after a ban on scientific work by Jews had been decreed.[92]

The results of the research are unique and cannot be duplicated even in the best and most sophisticated laboratories, because of the lack of requisite "human material." Although some of the findings have been lost, the remnant is the most comprehensive research on hunger ever performed. The doctors described the clinical findings in minute detail and with descriptive clarity that endures to this day.[93] The harsh conditions in the ghetto afforded the possibility of observing the

was injured and bleeding, sat next to him. Under the conditions and the lack of air aboard the train, his condition was terminal. See Dr. Israel Rom (Rotbalsam) testimony, YVA, O.3/2357.

89 Winick, *Hunger Disease*, p. ix.

90 Czerniaków, *The Warsaw Diary*, p. 375.

91 Blady Szwajger, *I Remember Nothing More*, p. 37.

92 Dr. Emil Apfelbaum testimony, YVA, M.49.E/4510.

93 Winick, "Jewish Medical Resistance," p. 104.

progression of hunger disease from an unprecedented research perspective. The patients researched were chosen painstakingly to include only persons suffering from hunger disease, without other complications, such as infectious conditions.[94]

One hundred and forty patients participated in the study: 70 adults and 40 children at the ghetto hospitals, and 30 others. The adults' daily nutrition over a period of months comprised a few calories and small quantities of protein and fats. The official ration of 800 calories per day included 3 grams of fat and 20–30 grams of vegetable protein. Most of the diet was composed of carbohydrates from sources such as dark bread, rye flour, potatoes, and small quantities of butter, lard, cooking oil, sugar, and soup. Vitamins and minerals, particularly the fat-dissolving vitamins A, D, E, and K, were lacking, as were calcium and iron. The protein was of poor quality.[95]

Dr. Julian Fliederbaum, who compiled the findings of the effect of hunger on adults, stressed the uniqueness of the study in the Warsaw ghetto as compared to other scientific research on the same topic conducted elsewhere. Shortly before he perished in the ghetto at the onset of the *Aktionen*, he managed to summarize the findings and added that the study in the ghetto had broadened knowledge on the topic and had applied new methods.

> Hunger is as old as the history of mankind. We know of hunger in China, in Russia, during the Civil War, and in Germany during World War I. Still, the clinical aspects and the biochemistry of continuous hunger, as well as the pathogenesis of the symptoms, are not very well described. Because of the inappropriate conditions for conducting scientific work, the clinical aspects of hunger edema were not carefully investigated during the 1914–1918 war. Using the latest scientific methods, we will try to extend what studies there have been.[96]

94 Winick, *Hunger Disease*, p. ix.
95 Ibid., pp. 13, 37.
96 Ibid., p. 13.

The study in the Warsaw ghetto was conducted for a lengthier time period and addressed more intensive hunger than previous studies had. Most of the patients were dying and the clinical stages of the process were documented. The outcome was the most detailed description of starving to death ever performed in research.[97]

A study on child malnutrition in Africa was undertaken by Cicely Williams in 1934, preceding the Warsaw ghetto research project by about eight years.[98] Williams investigated low-protein and calorie-deficient diets among children, and identified typical phenomena associated with malnutrition: edema, skin diseases, premature hair whitening, stunted growth, and protein insufficiency. She defined this disease as kwashiorkor.[99] Although the findings of the ghetto research closely resemble those of Williams, it is not known whether the researchers in the ghetto were familiar with her work. In addition to corroborating the previous findings and producing similar results, doctors at Bersohn and Bauman Children's Hospital identified additional indicators, especially with regard to the lymph nodes. They reported radicalized enlargement of the nodes, despite the absence of a local allergic reaction or any other sign of inflammation. Finding it difficult to identify the cause, they suggested several hypotheses: heightened activity of the glands, latent infection, or perhaps a relative protuberance due to bodily contraction resulting from weight loss and muscular atrophy.[100]

The hunger researchers in the Warsaw ghetto discovered several important phenomena in human metabolism at a time of hunger. Their conclusions about carbohydrate metabolism

97 Ibid., p. 38.

98 C. D. Williams, "A Nutritional Disease of Childhood Associated with a Maize Diet," *Arch Dis Child*, 8 (1933), pp. 423–433; C. D. Williams, "Kwashiorkor: A Nutritional Disease of Children Associated with a Maize Diet," *Lancet*, 2 (1935), pp. 1,151–1,152.

99 The term originated in an African expression that means "disease of the rejected baby." Indeed, it occurs in children from infancy up to age three who are forcibly weaned—"rejected"—due to the birth of an additional baby in the family. Forced weaning and transition to a low-protein diet induce the condition in the rejected baby.

100 Winick, *Hunger Disease*, pp. 59–61.

in hunger are the most extensive in the medical literature. Their findings on the acid-base balance are also very comprehensive. Although their study on nitrogen and mineral metabolism was not completed, the part that was conducted contributed to subsequent research.[101] The researchers examined the phenomenon of the adaptation of the human organism to hunger, which had never been studied before. They found that the process resembles, but is not identical to, that of hibernation among certain mammals, when they "sleep" through the winter. The adjustment to hunger made the patients very weak and vulnerable, and any minor stress had the potential of causing this process to collapse, bringing on severe outcomes, including death.[102]

Changes in cardiac and circulatory system functioning were examined using conventional techniques. The parameters measured were systemic blood pressure, systolic and diastolic; venous and capillary pressure; and EKGs, both in baseline situations and in response to medications. Levels of biochemical substances in blood, such as sugar, urea, and electrolytes, were measured as well. On the basis of these and other findings, such as from autopsies, the researchers developed hypotheses that attempted to explain the phenomena that they observed among people in protracted states of hunger. Some of these hypotheses remain accepted to this day.[103]

In researching the cardiovascular system, they found that blood volume among persons with hunger disease rises, and the pulse slows and often weakens, accompanied by low blood pressure.[104] When metabolic disorders, such as severe anemia and bone marrow depression, were observed, various treatments were attempted, including the administration of iron, liver extracts, and blood transfusions, but with limited success.

Much of the ophthalmic and field of vision research has been lost. The only surviving document, produced by a large team of experts, describes clinical and pathophysiological diagnoses of the

101 Ibid., p. x.

102 Winick, "Jewish Medical Resistance," p. 104.

103 Winick, *Hunger Disease*, p. x.

104 Winick, "Jewish Medical Resistance," p. 104.

eye that are unique and innovative in medical research. A special test by two ophthalmologists—the first of its kind, in Myron Winick's opinion—proved that intra-ocular pressure declines among persons with hunger disease. It was hypothesized that this is a compensation mechanism to protect the eye from the low blood pressure that was typical among these patients.

The doctors found the standard test for tuberculosis to be unreliable among people with hunger disease. Even highly concentrated injections of tuberculin, which was used at the time to diagnose tuberculosis, did not elicit a typical skin reaction among them. It is now known that the lack of response traces to the poor functioning of the immune system, exactly as the ghetto physicians hypothesized. Among patients suffering from a low-calorie intake from protein sources, the immune system is suppressed.[105]

The study describes autopsy reports, including documentation on microscopic tissue testing. At that time, histological research, which deals with the structure of tissues, was in its infancy. The researchers began to develop research patterns, but they did not have time to include detailed data in their study, due to the deportations. This unique and horrifying documentation points to salient organic changes that occur in states of starvation.[106] The doctors predicted that rehabilitation from hunger disease would have to be slow. Uncontrolled eating by patients with severe hunger disease at the beginning of their recovery would cause a rapid increase in metabolism and, in turn, excessive pressure on the heart, cardiac insufficiency, and death. However, the physician researchers could not test this hypothesis, since they did not have the option of rehabilitating their patients. Had the doctors who accompanied the forces that liberated the concentration camps known about the hunger disease research that had been performed in the Warsaw ghetto, it is almost certain that many who had lived to see the liberators but perished shortly thereafter would have survived.[107]

105 Winick, *Hunger Disease*, pp. x–xi; Winick, "Jewish Medical Resistance," p. 104.
106 Winick, *Hunger Disease*, p. xi.
107 Winick, "Jewish Medical Resistance," p. 104.

In the autopsy rooms, pathologists and students conducted difficult examinations of hundreds of corpses. Dr. Stein and Dr. Fenigstein, the doctors who participated in the research, described some of the difficulties that accompanied the research work, particularly in its final stages, during the *Grossaktion*.

> Unfortunately, the poor nutrition and poor general living conditions in the ghetto created a very difficult climate for scientific work. The lack of libraries, the lack of instruments and reagents, and the low morale associated with the constant fear of losing one's life were ever present for all. Autopsies were abundant. They should have been accompanied by histological studies. Unfortunately, the work on the histopathology of hunger started only a few months before July 22, 1942, when the massive deportations started and the hospital, its institutes, laboratories, autopsy rooms, and library were completely destroyed, making any further work impossible....Organs preserved in formalin were completely destroyed. Therefore, the following studies do not contain the exhaustive anatomical and histological description of hunger disease that was anticipated. Instead, we will present a statistical and macroscopic analysis of autopsy material.[108]

The ghetto physicians confronted illnesses that could have been cured had they had the resources to treat them. They personally contracted the illnesses that they investigated and knew what they were facing.[109]

There is no doubt that Milejkowski viewed research as a form of spiritual response, the "sole response to the murderers." He concluded his introduction to the hunger study by making an appeal to the doctors.

> A last few words to honor you, the Jewish doctors. What can I tell you, my beloved colleagues and companions in misery?

108 Winick, *Hunger Disease*, pp. 209–210.
109 Ibid., p. 43.

> You are a part of all of us. Slavery, hunger, deportation, those death figures in our ghetto were also your legacy. And you by your work could give the henchman the answer "*Non omnis moriar*," I shall not wholly die.[110]

The study of the detailed clinical manifestations of hunger as researched by the Warsaw ghetto doctors,[111] yields a palpable and chilling sense of the torments of hunger, and of the physical and mental decline of all those who suffered from it. Given that almost all the Jews in the ghetto suffered from hunger, although not all reached the condition known as hunger disease, this study offers another way to understand the situation in the Warsaw ghetto.

* * *

This chapter elaborated on the organizational aspects of the Warsaw ghetto medical system. Figure 1 below charts the entities that operated in and influenced health care in the ghetto and provides an understanding of the complex conditions under which the medical system operated. The Nazis introduced a deliberate anti-health policy toward the Jews, which brought on catastrophic conditions and foisted responsibility for dealing with them on the doctors and leaders in the ghetto. Those responsible for this were the heads of the Reich health care system, the director of the German Health Department in the General Government, and the German doctors who had been placed in charge of the health of the Warsaw residents, both on the Aryan side and in the ghetto.

Subordinate to them, the chairman of the Judenrat and his staff, the director of the Judenrat Health Department, and many other officials had to work with subtlety, because of the severely limited maneuvering space allowed them. The TOZ health care

110 Ibid, p. 5. The expression *Non omnis moriar* comes from a poem that the Roman poet Horace (8–65 CE) addressed to the muse Melpomene in which he expresses his confidence that, by virtue of his works, his memory will outlast his death. See Shasha, "Harefu'a Bageta'ot," p. 322.

111 For the gist of the findings, see Offer, "Ma'arach Harefu'a Begeto Varsha," vol. 2, appendix E, pp. 257–269.

organization, which had a long-standing tradition of professional medical service, operated alongside the Judenrat. TOZ had to coordinate its efforts with the Judenrat and with the ghetto's relief entities, foremost the various Jewish Self-Help organizations and CENTOS, the child welfare organization. As long as the United States stayed out of the war, as it did until late 1941, the JDC provided some assistance—under the severely restrictive conditions that the Nazi occupier had laid down—to organizations that had operated under its auspices before the war, mainly TOZ and CENTOS. In addition, several Jewish agencies that operated in neutral countries managed somewhat legally to provide minimal aid within the framework of the relief organizations that operated in Poland during the war.

FIGURE 1

Institutions and Entities Significantly Involved in Health Care in the Ghetto

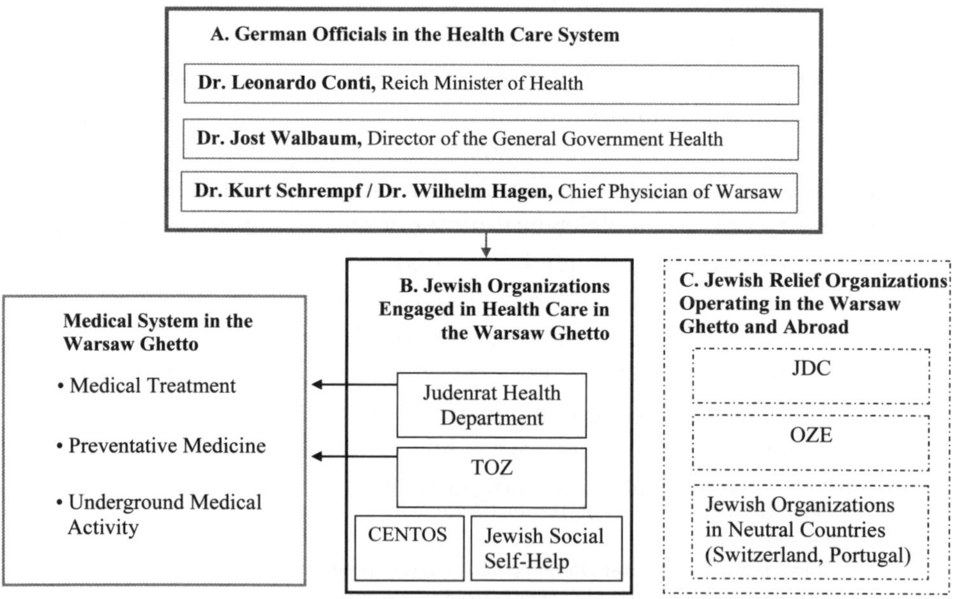

FIGURE 2

Medical System Operating through the Judenrat in the Warsaw Ghetto: Institutions and Their Activities

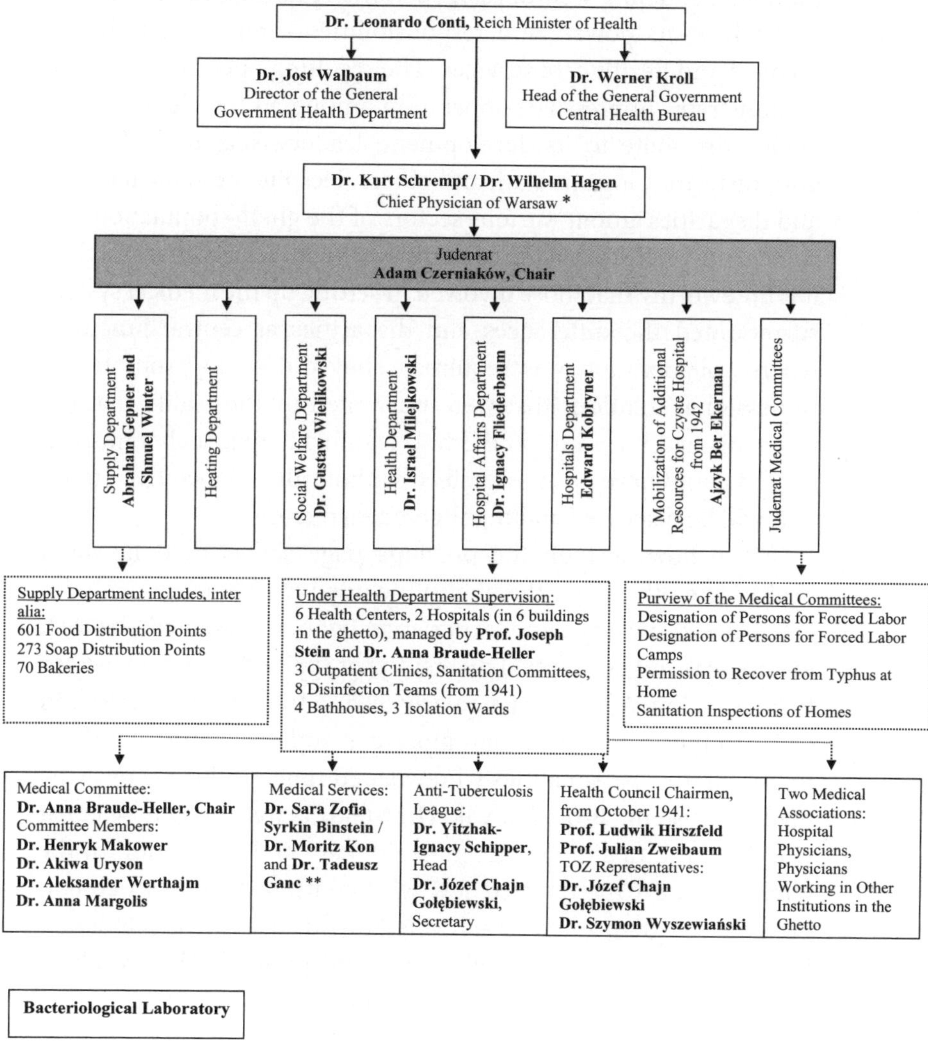

* Dr. Wilhelm Hagen replaced Dr. Kurt Schrempf in 1941. In 1943, Dr. Hagen and Dr. Walbaum were transferred from their positions.

** In 1941, the Department of War on Epidemics of TOZ was transferred to the Judenrat and placed under the management of Dr. Sara Zofia Syrkin Binstein. In 1942, Dr. Hagen appointed Dr. Kon and Dr. Ganc to replace Dr. Syrkin Binstein.

Figure 2 charts the alternative medical system that the Jews in the ghetto established through their own efforts. It indicates the planning of an organizational structure based on a professional rationale, entailing well-developed views regarding the domain of leadership—its powers and responsibilities—and the field of the medical and health care services. The resulting operational system demonstrates impressive cooperation among all the elements that could contribute to its development: leaders, scientists, doctors, administrators, logistic staff, and others. Despite the acute tensions and disparities among various sectors of the ghetto population—as were plainly reflected in the contemporary sources and in research—it is noteworthy that those involved in setting up the medical system surmounted the differences and disparities at central junctures where collaboration was required. They did so to promote the professional solutions that were warranted by the reality that the Germans had forced upon them. It is unlikely that such a medical system could have been assembled without the cooperative efforts that will be discussed and highlighted farther on.

The flowchart on the previous page shows that the main health care officials in the ghetto included men and women with extensive knowledge and experience, who represented the rich ideological and conceptual diversity that typified Jewish society in Poland and in Warsaw, particularly during the interwar period. In order to illustrate this human mosaic, it suffices to mention three representative personalities who wielded much influence over the medical system: Prof. Ludwik Hirszfeld, a well-known scientist who held multiple positions in health care and prevention in the ghetto, was a Christianized Jew who continued to go to church even in the ghetto. Dr. Israel Milejkowski, head of the Judenrat Health Department, was a physician and public leader who held clear Zionist views. The engineer Adam Czerniaków, chairman of the Judenrat, was an assimilated Jew by the standards of the time. The confines of this study do not allow for a deeper and broader discussion of these personalities, which would require recourse to additional sources, such as the biographies of each of them.

Czerniaków, appointed to head the Judenrat by the Germans in October 1939, took systemic steps to organize responses to the many immediate health care needs in the ghetto and participated in bold initiatives. Figure 2 indicates that the Judenrat and those who dealt with the health of the inhabitants of the ghetto adopted the goals of modern public medicine and acted according to its principles. Countries that advocate public health policies consider it their duty to balance the health needs of the individual, the needs of society, and the environmental conditions. Public health officials engage in three main pursuits: (1) fortifying the population's resilience against the environmental dangers by dealing with hygiene, nutrition, vaccinations, medications for contagious diseases, and the like; (2) enhancing environmental health conditions by improving sanitation, ventilation, water, and food, and by eliminating sources of contamination (3) reinforcing the institutional health care system so that it may serve the aforementioned goals by eradicating disease, prioritizing resource allocation, conducting research on preventive and curative care, providing health education, promoting legislation, and troubleshooting.[112]

The medical policy adopted by the Judenrat and the others who dealt with the ghetto population's health, as shown below, resembles that practiced in a modern state. In such a state, the public's health is no less important than curing the individual. The war on epidemics, which requires the legal and police enforcement of sanitation and medical standards, cannot be waged by the individual alone. Medical knowledge ceases to be the individual's concern as the state undertakes functions of medical education, research, and licensing. This is the origin of the concept of "public health," which, like defense, cannot be reduced to the health of the individual constituents of the public.[113] All these methods—in all the domains in which a public health system engages—

112 Richard P. Wenzel, "Control of Communicable Diseases," in Robert B. Wallace, Neal Kohatsu, and John M. Last, eds., *Maxcy-Rosenau-Last Public Health & Preventive Medicine* (New York: McGraw Hill, 2008), p. 57; eBook, http://alraziuni.edu.ye/book1/nursing/Public%20Health%20and%20Preventive%20Medicine,%2015th%20ed%20(2008).pdf.

113 David Heyd, *Etika Verefu'a* (*Ethics and Medicine*) (Hebrew) (Tel Aviv: Broadcast University, Ministry of Defense, 1990), p. 25.

were adopted in the ghetto, despite the deprivation and the harsh conditions.

It is necessary to understand the actions taken by Czerniaków in this context: (1) the establishment of organizational entities to deal with the diverse fields of health: a hospitals department, a health department to deal with the entire range of medical and sanitation problems, a medical committee to eradicate epidemics, an anti-tuberculosis league, and sanitation courses; (2) a policy of allocating a large share of the Judenrat's paltry budget for health care services; (3) support for activities to promote health that clashed with the Germans' orders at personal risk and in collaboration with various officials whom he had appointed; support for the establishment of an underground medical school; support for medical research; submission to the Germans of memoranda, containing claims backed by science that the measures they imposed caused epidemics; organization of professional lectures for ghetto doctors; (4) considerable personal attention to urgent issues concerning the operation of the medical institutions (5) attempts to maneuver the tension between ongoing management on the basis of internal needs and the Germans' dictates—an obvious source of strain, as Figure 1 clearly indicates.

Our description of the professional characteristics of the Judenrat's health policies in the ghetto did not overlook the harsh criticism that was leveled against Czerniaków. Special caution is required in any critical discussion of the Judenrat's activities in the field of health, as in every other area of activity in which the Judenrat engaged in the ghetto. The Judenrat attracted tremendous censure for the obvious reason that it was appointed by the Germans to carry out their orders, while at the same time being responsible for managing all areas of life and meeting the urgent needs of the Jewish population.[114] Many activists in the Jewish Social Self-Help and the underground newspapers

114 On the difference between a Jewish headship and the Jewish leadership in the Holocaust, and the role of headships in the German policy, see Michman, *Holocaust Historiography*, pp. 160–172.

adopted a staunchly, systematically, radically, and sweepingly critical attitude toward the Judenrat's activities—including its handling of medical matters.[115] The reproach, usually from TOZ and the self-help organizations, pertained to matters of policy and implementation regarding issues of health care and morbidity factors. Notably, in my estimation, even though Czerniaków was not innocent of all error in the policies that he promoted, the overall alternative health care system that he was instrumental in establishing—in conjunction with all the others who were involved in medicine and sanitation in the ghetto—overshadows the critics' points of argument.

As for the question of the involvement and participation of all the entities that engaged in health care in the ghetto, as emphasized in the texts and figures above, it is also important to relate to the TOZ health care organization and its position in the overall system. TOZ, which had an impressive professional tradition among the Jews of Warsaw, in particular, and of Poland, in general, continued to make its contribution even under the conditions in the ghetto. The impression created by the various sources mentioned in this study is that TOZ looked out for the weak and the refugees, while the Judenrat dealt only with institutional issues. This impression impairs the balanced and complete view of the ghetto's medical system in its entirety. Our argument is that TOZ did indeed focus on helping the disadvantaged, just as it had before the war, but the distinction between it and the other players in the health care field is erroneous and misleading, even if its own staff members depicted it that way.

Many TOZ operatives cooperated with the head of the Judenrat Health Department, Dr. Israel Milejkowski, who represented the Judenrat's health care policies, and many of them sat on medical committees that had been set up on the Judenrat's initiative. Some worked concurrently at institutions affiliated with both. This collaboration was also manifested in the underground medical activities, such as the establishment of the clandestine medical school and of the medical studies that were set in

115 See Gutman, "Emanuel Ringelblum," pp. 92–93.

motion with the support of the Judenrat and of members of other organizations. Thus, we contend that TOZ contributed its share to the joint effort, which benefited from TOZ's obvious advantages—its professionalism and strong social orientation. Despite the disagreements and criticism that it expressed, TOZ continued to work for the unification of the ranks and consciously chose to play an important part in what we call in this study "the medical system in the Warsaw ghetto."

In the following remarks, Dr. Israel Milejkowski expressed this sense of sharing a common fate, despite all the differences, and the unification of forces for the protection of the health of the Jews and their survival in the ghetto. His responses to a questionnaire from members of the Oneg Shabbat underground archive in the ghetto bring into sharp focus his Zionist ideological outlook, his description of the ideological and social stratifications and differences in the ghetto, and his sense of responsibility for maintaining a vision of the entire population, with all its diversity, as a Jewish concept and a public mission at this unique historical moment for the Jews in the ghetto under German tyranny.

> My ramified and highly intensive work in the area entrusted to me on the health board and in hospitalization for the Jewish community in the Ghetto, takes up all my waking hours and leaves me no free time to meet with various people in different community spheres and hear their views on the present situation.
>
> I head the health service charged with combatting epidemics and am responsible for the hospital department. In addition, I head the Jewish Medical Association here in the Ghetto with a membership of over eight hundred doctors. All these activities leave me very little time and my impressions are therefore gleaned from my daily work and practice and—to the extent possible—I will attempt to state my conclusions in general terms....
>
> Here in the Ghetto we must make every attempt to survive this terrible period of our being. Endurance and survival—

must be our current slogan.... I will borrow two terms from medicine: endogenous and exogenous. Internally we must do everything possible to permit endurance and survival. But externally the oppressor's whip cracks forcing us to perform tasks and deeds beyond the ability of our frail strength. The oppressor's conduct towards us can be expressed in the words of the officers of the children of Israel to Pharaoh, "there is no straw given unto thy servants, and they say to us, make brick..."[116] We are told to perform tasks which we are in no position to execute in Ghetto conditions, precisely because of the difficult conditions themselves.

Therefore, taking this into account, I always try—within the realm of my authority—to act in such a way as to undermine the control exerted by "them," and with my orders and prescriptions temporarily alleviate the whip lashes....

To properly appreciate the picture of Ghetto life, we cannot judge simply by what is seen in the streets. I discern two layers in the Ghetto which can perhaps be illustrated in the following manner: the entire Jewish community in the Ghetto can be said to have been cast into a large cauldron of boiling water atop a high flame—the flame of our tribulations. In this boiling water two layers can be discerned—an upper and a lower. The upper layer seethes and bubbles all over its surface. The bottom layer also seethes, but more quietly, with less fuss.... to appreciate the true face of the Ghetto, we must plunge below the surface....

...in its layer of the Jewish Ghetto population we find modest but highly important phenomena, full of light and vigor...which finds expression in the house committees... organized Jewish life where the true Jewish qualities of mercy and charity find realization.

In addition, quiet, unassuming work also is going on in other fields...public kitchens, medical courses, as well as other studies in order to equip the younger generation to grow up with skills. Intensive medical research is being

116 Exod. 5:16.

carried out on death through starvation and typhus. The entire clinical—and unfortunately plentiful—material is being studied and conclusive medical results of the research are being prepared....

...We simply want later—after the cataclysm—to be able to show the world that even these terrible trials could not break us. At this very moment a small scientific conference is in progress at the hospital, devoted to Ghetto problems which includes scientific papers, addresses and discussion. The result of this work will later be published and will be, I hope, of great interest the world over....

Our prospects after the war appear quite dim to me. If the present war were a war between two avowed ideological camps, between democracy and fascism, one might then imagine that with the final triumph of democracy over Hitlerism, our situation will improve materially, though not in the national sense. Nor will antisemitism slacken; on the contrary, it will get stronger. For the practical lesson Hitlerism is teaching all the nations how Jews can by physically and spiritually stamped out is so enticing, so attractive that the nations liberated from Hitler's regime will not deny themselves the pursuit of Hitler's ways....

But this entire problem has now become even more complicated because of a third factor which is taking on major proportions in the world...bolshevism....It is clear that bolshevism does not solve the Jewish national problem.

For the Jewish intellectual or the one who has no national sentiment of "Jewish identity," bolshevism is a radical way of solving the problem of the suffering and persecuted masses of the Jewish people....

In this entire entanglement I see only one recourse open for our people, and that is [Mandatory] Palestine. After the war, we must, we have to, emigrate to [Mandatory] Palestine.... to establish ourselves as a nation in our permanent home....

...I find wholeness in the religious Jew. He does not suffer from the "heartbreak" and "doubts" which devour the soul of the enlightened Jew....

And now a few words on my attitude towards converts in the Ghetto. My attitude is a direct result of my two positions regarding the problem: firstly, the medical and secondly, the Jewish-ethical. I understand the soul and disposition of the convert who was brutally cast into the Ghetto with us. I can feel how difficult it must be to be a "*Zwangs-Jude*" (a Jew by force), to live and suffer with the masses of Jewry from whom he's always tried to flee, and to make a final break forever.

The convert was led to conversion because of the woeful manner in which he was raised by parents who tried to free their child of the Jewish burden. For the most part he did it himself for material reasons. And suddenly there came to the world the mammoth Hitlerian cataclysm…which unfurled the flag of zoological anti-Semitism not only with respect to first-generation converts from Judaism, but also with respect to half and quarter Jews up to the fourth generation.

How should we receive these dissident brethren of our origin? The Gemara says that even if a Jew sins, he is still a Jew. And here my conscience dictates to adhere firmly to the Jewish-ethical prescription: "Though shalt neither avenge nor bear grudge"—In our ethical development we stand high above petty account-settling with brother-sinners, and particularly in times of trouble. As a doctor I see the converts who live with us in the Ghetto as people with a severe spiritual complex. Therefore from this viewpoint—no, not viewpoint, but feeling—I relate to them without hatred whatsoever, but also without fondness.[117]

117 Kermish, *To Live with Honor*, pp. 741–746.

FIGURE 3

TOZ Activities

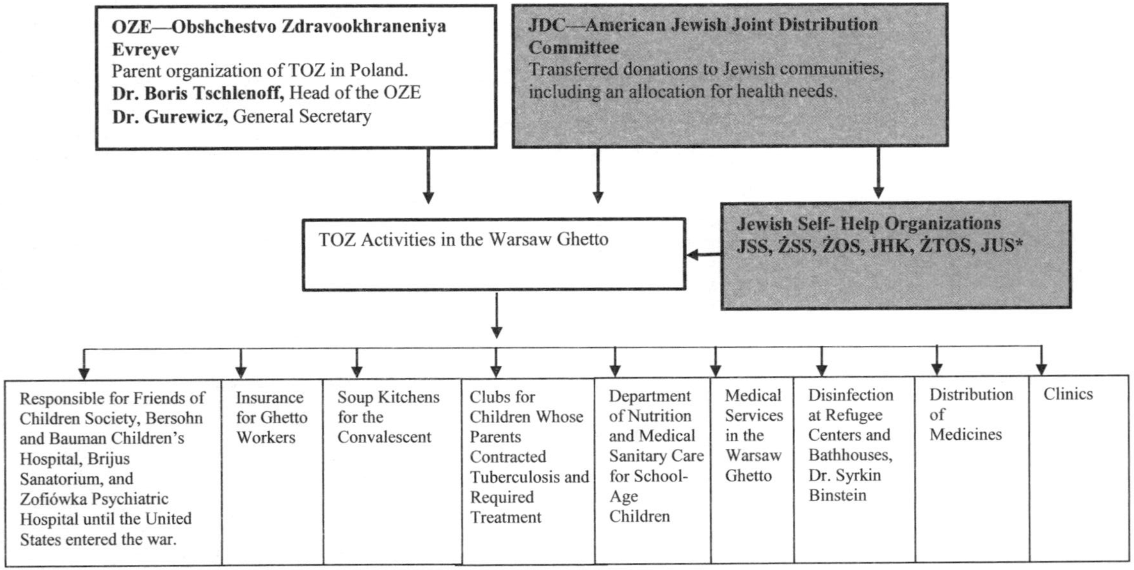

* Jüdische Soziale Selbsthilfe, Żydowska Samopomoc Społeczna, Żydowskie Opieki Społecznej, Jüdisches Hilfskomitee, Żydowskie Towarzystwo Opieki Społecznej, Jewish Relief Office.

FIGURE 4

A "Jewish Medical Network" under Nazi Occupation—TOZ in Warsaw as the Heart of Medical Services for All Jews in the General Government[118]

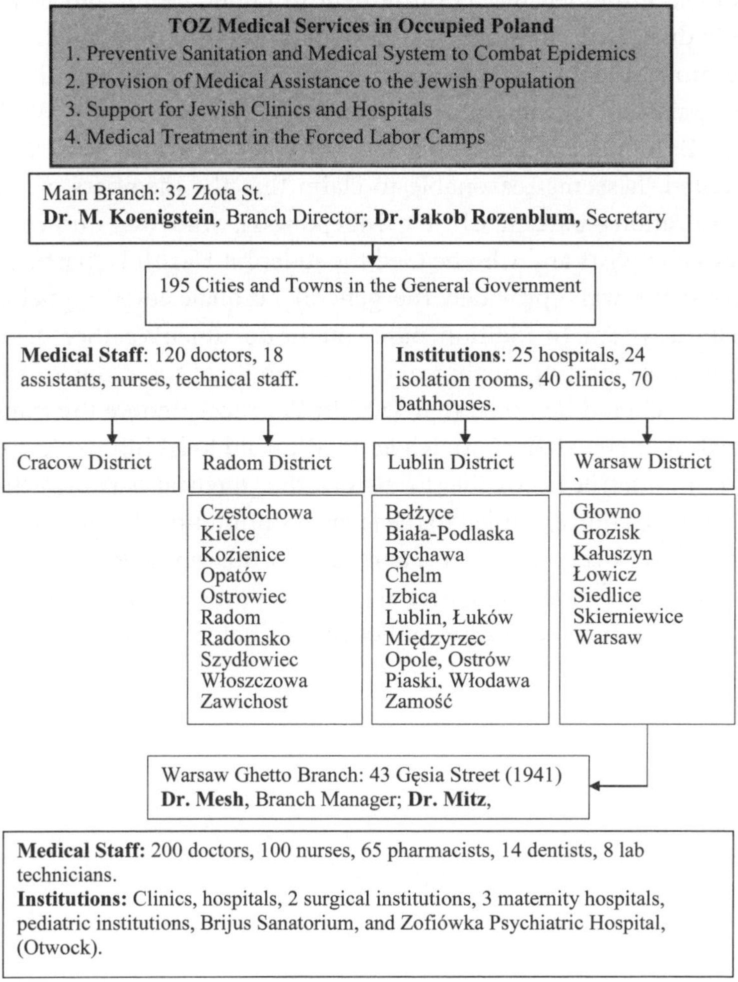

118 Report by Emanuel Patt on welfare activity for the Jews of Poland, March 1941, JDC, AR.33–44, file 814; report by Dr. Wulman on TOZ activity, May 1940, JDC, AR.33–44, file 840. According to the May 1940 report, the Warsaw branch was responsible for 195 cities and towns. The March 1941 report, produced after many ghettos had been established, cited 35 branches in cities.

This study and the figures above demonstrate the highly impressive initiatives that TOZ undertook in an attempt to meet the medical and health care needs amid a protracted state of catastrophe under Nazi occupation. The foundations of the organization's social outlook, grounded in a commitment to public health and to the individual, with an emphasis on helping the disadvantaged, and the professional knowledge and organizational experience that it had amassed during eighteen years of activity preceding World War II found expression in the extensive activities that TOZ initiated. It seems reasonable to claim that the members of this organization—particularly Dr. Milejkowski, who was one of its prewar activists and who headed the Judenrat Health Department during the war—provided the general rationale for the ghetto's medical system. In addition, based on the documents gathered, but without elaborating further due to the limits of the scope of this study, it should be noted that TOZ in Warsaw—despite the tragic situation there—helped to deliver medical aid to additional Jewish communities. It is possible to discern the "medical network" that the organization extended to the Jewish communities in the ghettos throughout occupied Poland and explain this singular activity as a corollary of TOZ's activities as a countrywide organization that had served the great masses of Polish Jews before the war.[119]

119 Offer, "Ma'arach Harefu'a Begeto Varsha," vol. 2, appendix A.18, pp. 70–92.

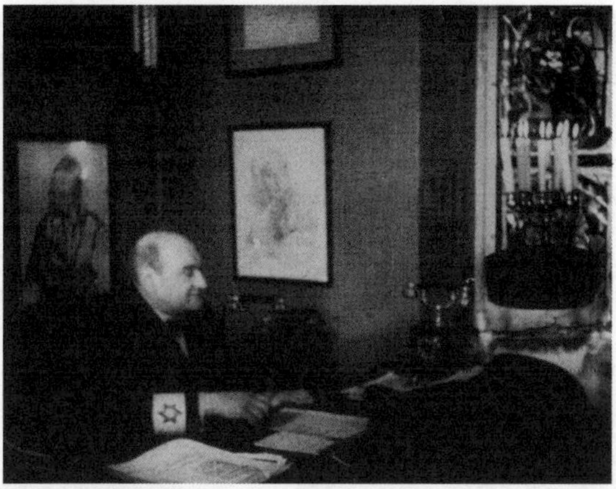

Adam Czerniaków (1880–1942), chair of the Judenrat in the Warsaw ghetto, 1940. Photo Collection, YVA, 46644.

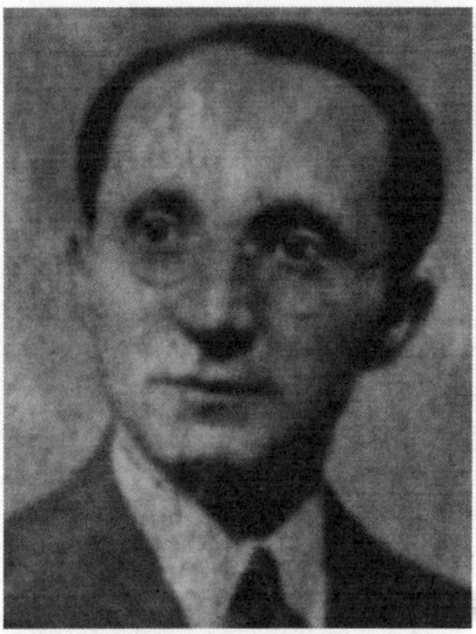

Dr. Israel Milejkowski (1887–1943), director of the Judenrat Health Department in the Warsaw ghetto and the initiator of the hunger study. Photo Archive, GFH, no. 53942.

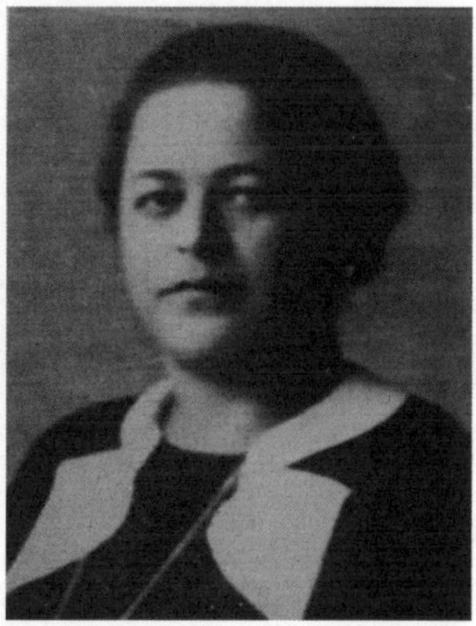

Dr. Sara Zofia Syrkin Binstein (1890–1943), internist, co-director with Dr. Milejkowski of the Health Department in the Warsaw ghetto, and a leader in the war against epidemics. Courtesy of Livia S. Yanowicz.

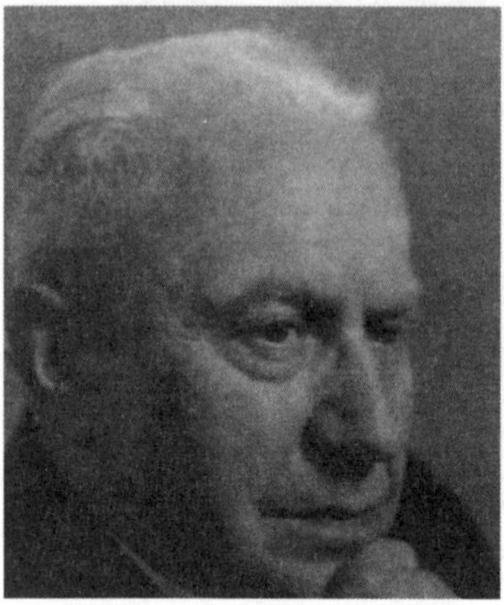

Prof. Ludwik Hirszfeld (1884–1954), world-renowned serologist and microbiologist, and physician in the Warsaw ghetto. Courtesy of Ruti Ben Shahar.

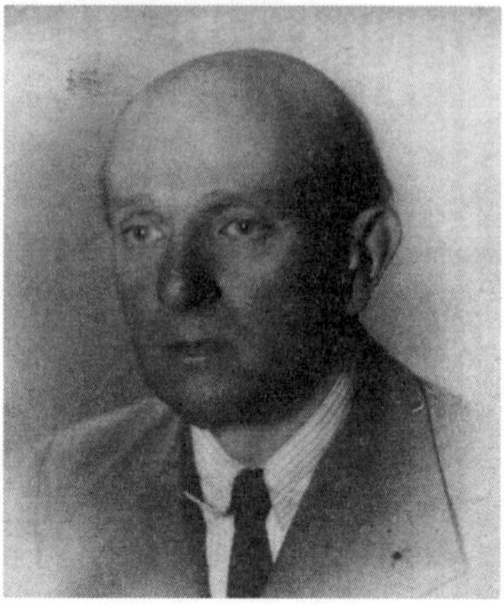

Prof. Juliusz Zweibaum (1887–1959), histologist and embryologist, and one of the founders and the director of the underground medical faculty in the Warsaw ghetto. Courtesy of his granddaughter Zofia Karlowicz Perzyńska.

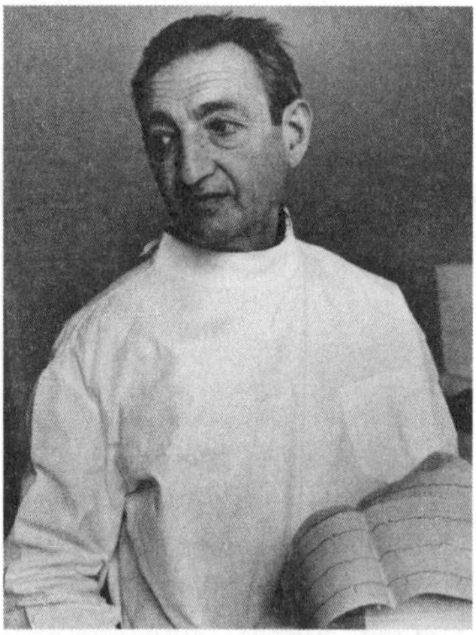

Dr. Marek Edelman (1919 or 1922–2009), a courier for Bersohn and Bauman Children's Hospital and a leader of the Warsaw Ghetto Uprising, who became a cardiologist after the war. Photo Archive, GFH, no. 4613/11.

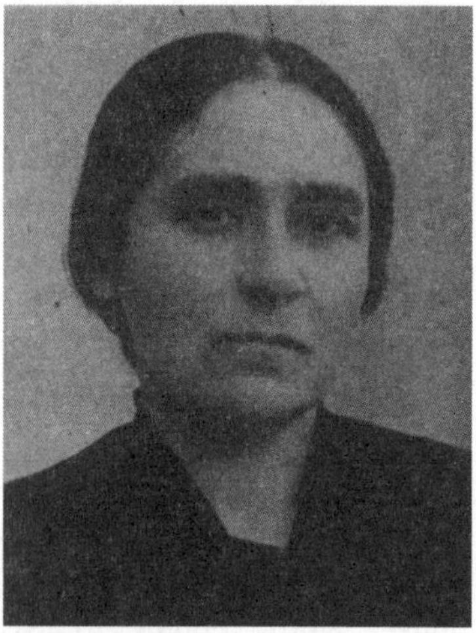

Dr. Anna Braude-Heller (1888–1943), director of Bersohn and Bauman Children's Hospital in Warsaw and in the ghetto. Photo Collection, YVA, 73176.

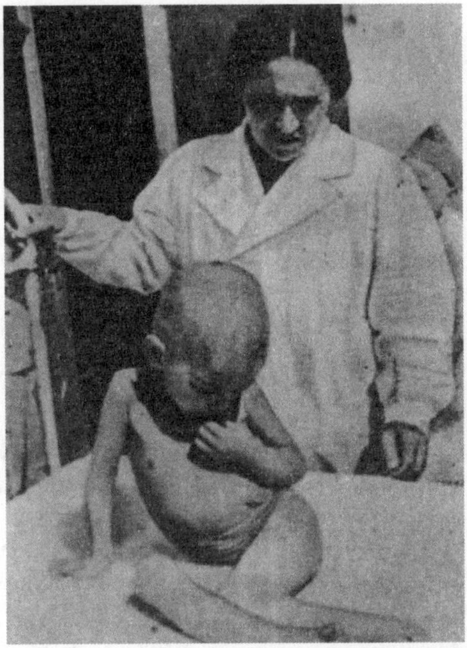

Dr. Anna Braude-Heller treats a child at Bersohn and Bauman Children's Hospital. Photo Archive, GFH, no. 2885.

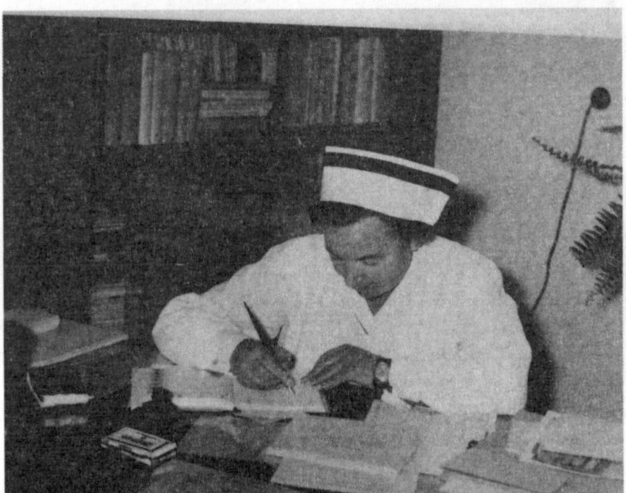

Luba Blum-Bielicka (1906–1973), principal of the nursing school in the Warsaw ghetto. Courtesy of her daughter, Aviva Blum-Vaks.

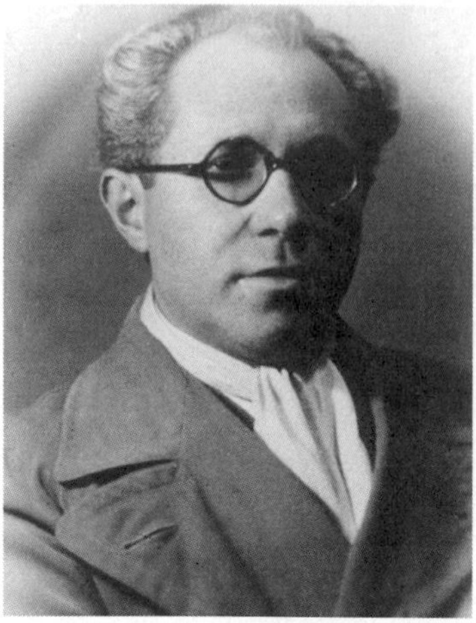

Dr. Emil Apfelbaum (1890–1946), head of the department of cardiology at Czyste Hospital and hunger study researcher in the Warsaw ghetto. Photo Collection, YVA, 3384/14.

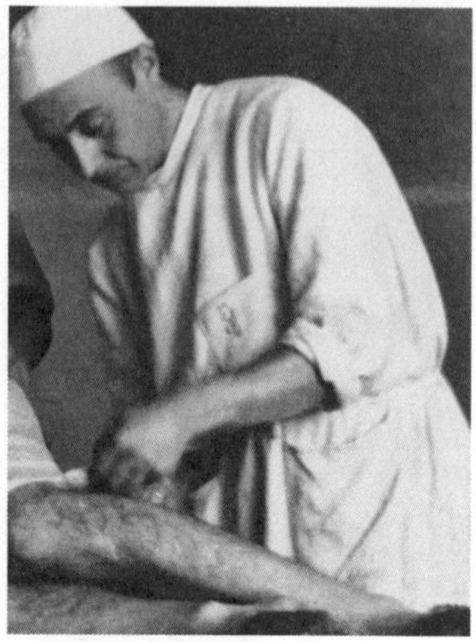

Prof. Ludwik Stabholz (1911–2007), surgeon at Czyste Hospital who taught anatomy in the underground medical faculty in the Warsaw ghetto. Courtesy of the Stabholz family.

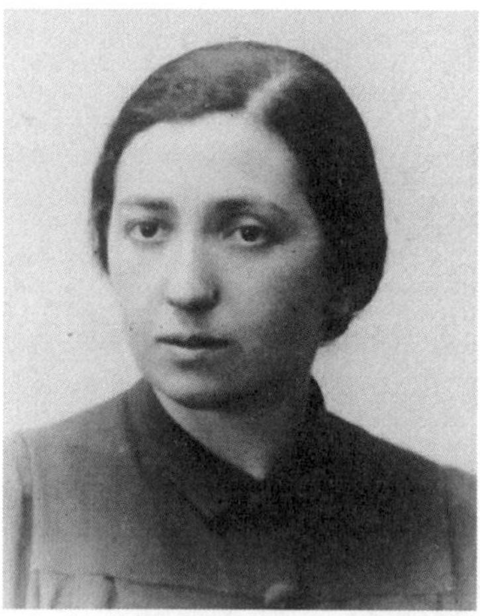

Dr. Natalia Julia Lipsztat-Muszkat (1908–1943), pediatrician at Bersohn and Bauman Children's Hospital. Courtesy of Prof. Mordechai Muszkat.

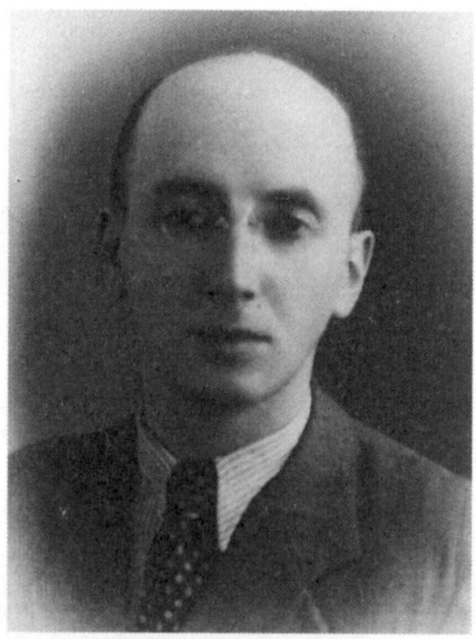

Dr. Abraham Paweł Lipsztat (1903–1943), director of the infectious diseases department at Czyste Hospital and physician at the refugee disinfection unit. Courtesy of Prof. Mordechai Muszkat.

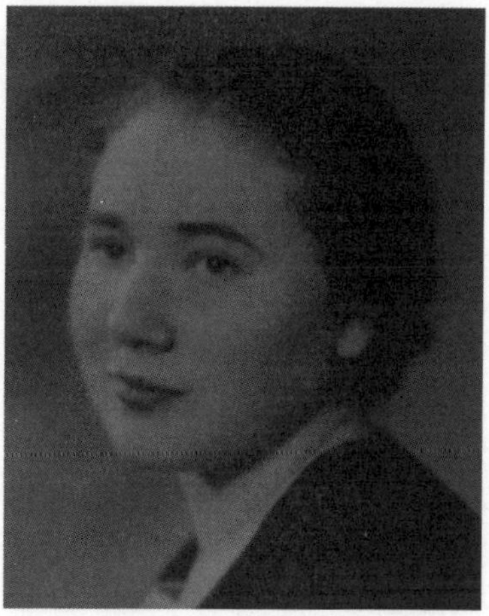

Dr. Adina Blady Szwajger, physician at Bersohn and Bauman Children's Hospital. Photo Archive, GFH, no. 1324.

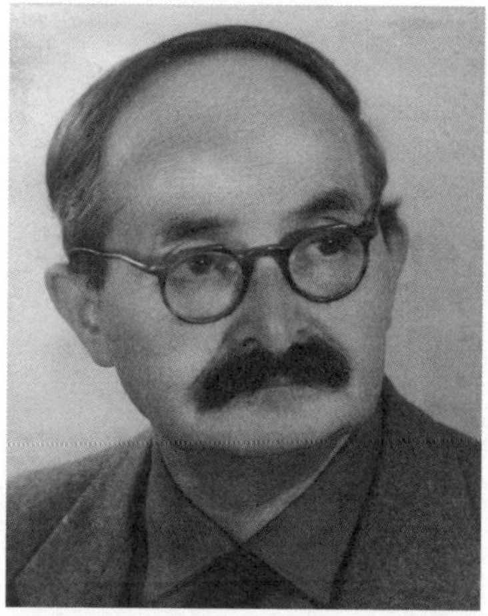

Dr. Mordechai Lensky (1890–1964), physician at Czyste Hospital and at the clinics in the Warsaw ghetto. Courtesy of his son, Prof. Yaacov Lensky.

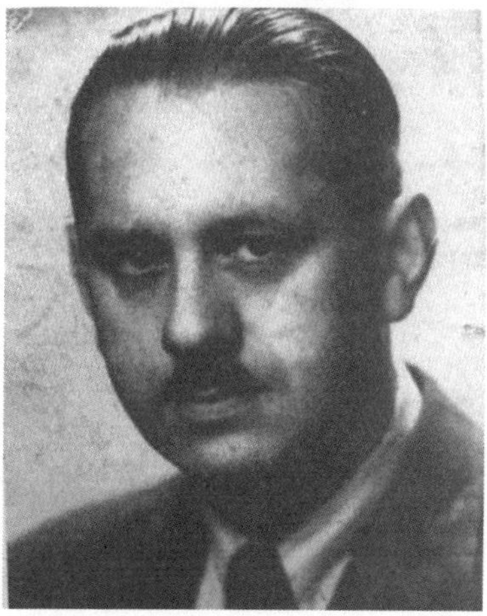

Dr. Maurycy Brandwein (1898–1943), physician in the surgery department at Czyste Hospital. Courtesy of his daughter, Shulamit Tzeder.

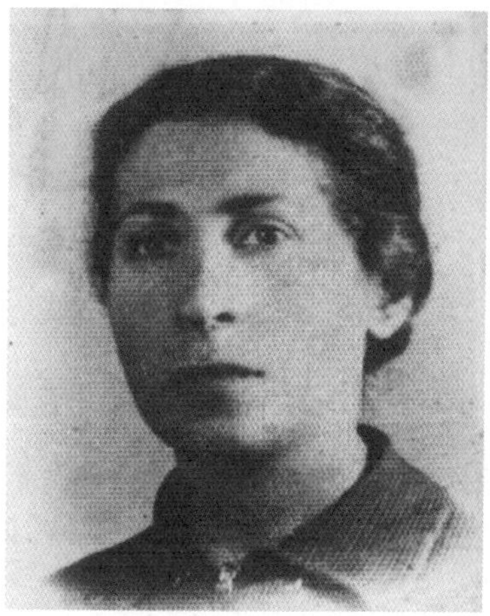

Sabina Gürfinkel-Glocer, nurse at Czyste Hospital. Photo Collection, YVA, 3526/4.

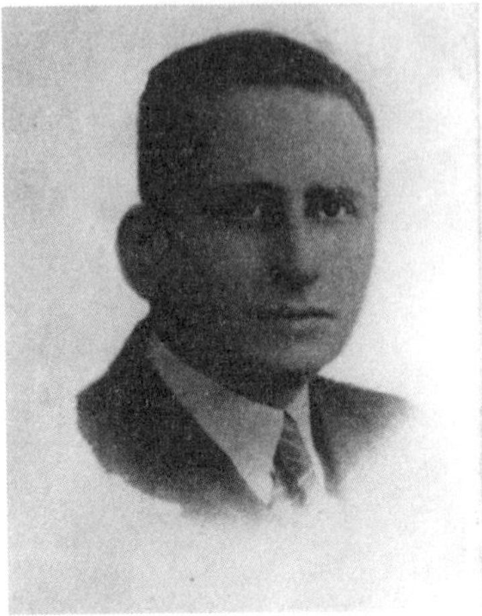

Dr. Jakub Munwes (1894–1943), internist at Czyste Hospital. Photo Collection, YVA, 5027/883.

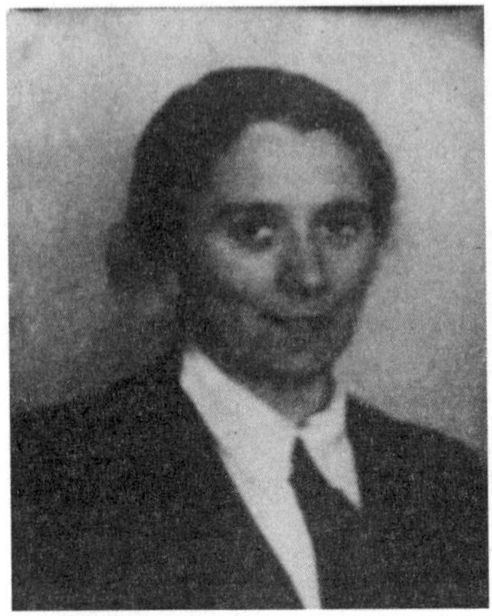

Nurse Ala Gołąb-Grynberg (1904–1943). Photo Archive, GFH, no. 1112.

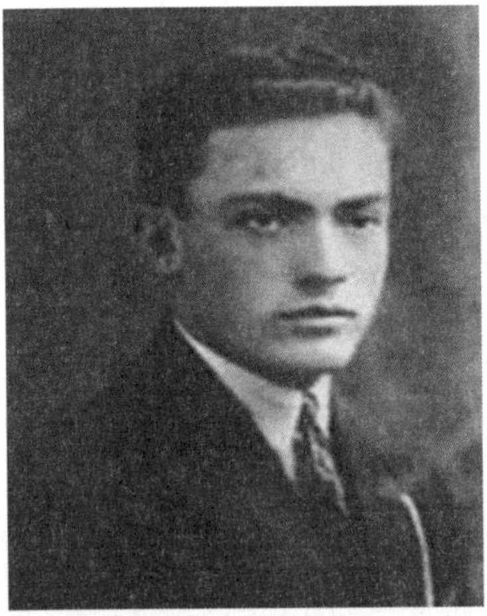

Dr. Simcha Lederman (1909–1942) participated in the hunger study in the Warsaw ghetto. Courtesy of his nephew Prof. Avi Ohry.

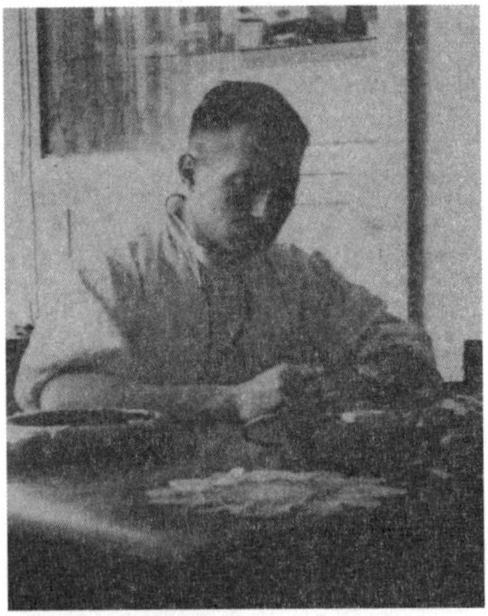

Dr. Marek Balin (1918–2006), a medical student who worked at Czyste Hospital in the ghetto and completed his studies after the war, 1947. Courtesy of his sister Halina Birenbaum.

PART THREE

The Challenges to the Medical Profession

Living Conditions, Diseases, and Ethical Dilemmas

Chapter Six

Factors Affecting Illness and Health

The foregoing clarifies beyond all doubt that the epidemics among the Jews were a direct outcome of the ghastly overcrowding in the apartments, the suffering, the impossibility of making a living. All health regulations will be useless; they will not help to improve the situation. Neither will protection from the scourge be attained by structurally sequestering the population and isolating the Jewish-inhabited parts of the city from the rest of the population. The typhus bacteria will not be stopped by warning signs and barbed-wire fences. The most effective ways to fight them are by providing adequate nutrition and sufficient clothing, rebuilding destroyed structures, and integrating the Jews into the breadwinning population.[1]

When the war broke out on September 1, 1939, German aircraft circled over the homes of Warsaw, sowing death, destruction, and fire. Although the population sought refuge in cellars and public shelters, thousands perished and tens of thousands sustained injuries. In addition to the mounds of debris, the streets filled with human corpses, carcasses of horses, heaps of bricks, and piles of shattered glass.[2] A disinfection team gathered the dead. Horrific sobbing and wailing of those trapped and buried

1 Memoranda by Jewish doctors to the Germans addressing the causes of typhus and proposals to combat it, AŻIH, ARI.85; YVA, M.10.AR.1/85.

2 Dr. Moshe Tursz testimony, YVA, O.3/438; Auerbach, *Tzava'ot Varsha*, p. 47.

alive erupted from the shelters.[3] On September 23, 1939—Yom Kippur—Warsaw was bombarded all night long, especially the Jewish quarter.[4] Hundreds of buildings were set ablaze and thousands of Jews were buried under the ruins. The city was left without electricity, cooking gas, telephone service, or radio, and there were shortages of bread, water, medicine, and bandages. The plight of the wounded was particularly dire. Thousands were homeless and people crowded into every building that still stood. Under the unsanitary conditions that set in, the outbreak of a ghastly epidemic was a foregone conclusion.[5]

Crowding and Hygiene

The war brought on a severe decline in the health of the population, especially that of the Jews. A typhus epidemic broke out at this time among the residents whose homes had been destroyed. So many people were ill that everyone was afraid to allow others to enter their homes for fear of contagion. The disruption of all infrastructure caused morbidity, and mortality escalated.[6] The destruction and devastation in Warsaw remained evident many weeks after the city had surrendered. After capitulating, it had a population of 1,300,000, including 360,000 Jews. About 20,000 people had lost their lives in the fighting and approximately 47,000 had been wounded. Half of the 20,000 residential buildings in the city had sustained damage, including many hospitals. Czyste Hospital was among those damaged.[7]

3 Ringelblum, *Yoman Vereshimot*, p. 5.

4 There is no proof that the Germans deliberately targeted the Jews in their sorties or timed their decrees to coincide with Jewish festivals. See Gutman, "Warsaw: Jews during the Holocaust," in Gutman, *Encyclopedia of the Holocaust*, p. 1,602.

5 Kaplan, *Scroll of Agony*, pp. 36–38; Berg, *The Diary of Mary Berg*, p. 6–7; Czerniaków, *The Warsaw Diary*, p. 76; Turkow, *Hayo Hayta Varsha Yehudit*, pp. 24–26; Gutman, *The Jews of Warsaw*, p. 7; Hirszfeld, *The Story of One Life*, pp. 173–174.

6 Trunk, "Epidemics and Mortality," p. 84.

7 Auerbach, *Tzava'ot Varsha*, p. 54; Cohen, "Harefu'a Besherut Ha'idiologiya," p. 141; Roland, *Courage under Siege*, p. 20; Gutman, *The Jews of Warsaw*, p. 8.

Many residents of the Jewish quarter became "local refugees." The arrival of masses of refugees from surrounding villages in the district inflated their numbers. When the Jewish quarter later became the ghetto, the damage it had sustained made it difficult to live there.[8] The ghastly overcrowding created in the ghetto impaired the ability to maintain basic sanitation and caused the spread of infectious diseases. According to Ringelblum, in October 1940, before ghettoization, 350,000 of the 425,000 Jews in Warsaw were living in the Jewish quarter, which had been marked as an epidemic-infested zone. Even before the ghetto was sealed, the population density in the Jewish quarter was nine times higher than that in the rest of the city.[9] Upon ghettoization, about 140,000 Jews from the affluent quarters of Warsaw had to move into the rundown neighborhood, following the evacuation of the 110,000 Polish inhabitants. The Jews had to find housing and, lacking any means of transport to take their belongings with them, they lost their property.[10] The ensuing overpopulation in the ghetto was such that it was difficult to circulate in the overcrowded streets.[11] Karmelicka St., for example, was so narrow that you could barely walk among the masses of people.[12]

It is difficult to present accurate statistics because the components of population density changed frequently. The size of the population varied, due to the deportations and evictions from other towns to the ghetto, as well as to mortality. The number of housing options decreased as the ghetto boundaries were

8 Roland, *Courage under Siege*, pp. 20–21.

9 Ringelblum, *Notes from the Warsaw Ghetto*, p. 63; report by Emanuel Patt, Welfare Activity for the Jews of Poland, JDC, AR.33–44, file 814. Dr. Patt reported that housing density in the Jewish quarters was 5 persons per room on average. However, it was common to find rooms that accommodated 10, 12, or 15 people.

10 It is difficult to estimate the exact number of Jews who were forced to enter the ghetto and the number of non-Jews who were evicted from it. The sources give similar figures. See, for example, the lecture by Waldemar Schön, head of the Warsaw District Resettlement Department in Arad et al., *Documents on the Holocaust*, pp. 222. Schön referred to the transfer of 138,000 Jews and the eviction of 113,000 non-Jews. See also Ringelblum, *Notes from the Warsaw Ghetto*, pp. 63, 72; Gutman, *The Jews of Warsaw*, p. 60.

11 Dr. Moshe Tursz testimony, O.3/438, pp. 7–8.

12 Turkow, *Hayo Hayta Varsha Yehudit*, pp. 35–36, 41.

constricted. According to various estimates, upon ghettoization, the number of residents in the ghetto ranged from 380,740 to 590,000. Population density was also gauged by occupancy per room. These data vary from period to period and from source to source. Most estimates range from 7 to 12 persons per room.[13] According to Trunk, the density data do not fully reflect the grave reality, because they do not include more than 150,000 refugees, and because statistics do not describe the suffering caused by overcrowding. Many refugees lived in a room measuring about 25 square meters with 25 people.[14]

The ratio of the population to the area of the ghetto is an important parameter for understanding the problem of overcrowding. The ghetto boundaries underwent many changes. The area was reduced from the time that it was demarcated in November 1940 to July 1942, when the transports to Treblinka began. In March 1941, the area of Warsaw measured 141,500 dunams, and the ghetto was allocated 3,400 dunams, which was a scant percentage of the area of the city for about one-third of its population. Only 61,295 of the 284,912 dwelling units in the city, about one-fifth, were in the ghetto. On the Aryan side, the average number of people per dunam was 6.6. In the ghetto, it was 130.8—twenty times greater.[15]

The ghetto area continued to change. In the middle of September 1941, for example, more than ten months after the ghetto had been established, Ludwig Fischer, the Nazi governor of the Warsaw district, initiated a plan that would reduce and ultimately liquidate the small ghetto. The German Sanitation Department in Warsaw, which was under the authority of

13 Many sources remark on this. For various estimates, see Mendelsohn, *The Polish Jews*, p. 10; Gutman, *The Jews of Warsaw*, p. 60; Arad et al., *Documents on the Holocaust*, pp. 226–227; Blumental and Kermish, *Hameri Vehamered Begeto Varsha*, p. 355; Trunk, "Epidemics and Mortality," p. 87; Blatman, *Geto Varsha—Sipur Itona'i*, p. 143.

14 Trunk, "Epidemics and Mortality," p. 88.

15 Ibid., p. 87. The data on this topic vary, evidently due to different reporting dates and changes in the size of the area of the ghetto. See, for example, Blatman, *Geto Varsha—Sipur Itona'i*, p. 142; Gutman, *The Jews of Warsaw*, p. 60; Roland, *Courage under Siege*, p. 27; Offer, *Haluk Lavan Bageto*, appendix B.6, p. 541.

Dr. Hagen, opposed the scheme for fear that it would exacerbate overcrowding, which would cause the epidemics to spread even more. Nevertheless, more than 50,000 Jews were evicted from their homes and transferred to other precincts in the ghetto.[16] Menachem Linder,[17] the ghetto economist and demographer, described the demographic calamity in the ghetto and noted that the Jewish quarter had always been known as being the most congested in town.

> Another 100,000 Jews [refugees] were forcibly crammed into this anthill, and if we add 100,000–120,000 Jews who reached the ghetto from elsewhere in Warsaw, we get an inkling of the teeming, swarming nature of the place and of its sanitation conditions.[18]

As more and more refugees arrived and more housing was required, the Germans reduced the area of the ghetto.[19] The newspaper *Biuletyn* reported in October 1941 that precisely before the winter, as cold weather combined with hunger aggravated the typhus epidemic, the ghetto streets again filled with wagons of refugees.[20]

Basic sanitary conditions in the ghetto were truly wretched. The area set aside for the ghetto was one of the poorest in Warsaw. Most of its buildings were old and lacked basic sanitation. Apartments had neither showers nor toilets. The residents used

16 Ringelblum, *Notes from the Warsaw Ghetto*, pp. 217, 222; Trunk, "Epidemics and Mortality," p. 89.

17 Linder (b. 1911), wrote extensively from the mid–1930s onward on diverse topics related to the Jewish people and the Warsaw community. One of the most prominent researchers at YIVO in Warsaw before the war, he operated in the ghetto in underground circles associated with Zionist pioneering youth movements, was active in culture, and played a leading role in Jewish self-help. Linder was murdered by the Germans on the "Night of Blood," April 18, 1942; Blatman, *Geto Varsha—Sipur Itona'i*, p. 146. For more on Linder, see Ringelblum, *Yoman Vereshimot*, pp. 102–105.

18 Blatman, *Geto Varsha—Sipur Itona'i*, p. 148.

19 Turkow, *Hayo Hayta Varsha Yehudit*, pp. 35–36, 41.

20 Blatman, *Geto Varsha—Sipur Itona'i*, p. 170. See also Berg, *The Diary of Mary Berg*, p. 59; Hirszfeld, *Die Geschichte eines Lebens*, p. 120; Hirszfeld, *The Story of One Life*, p. 190.

a common latrine, situated in the courtyard, and they had to go to public bathhouses to bathe. Streets reeked of human waste. In addition, because there was a lighting problem, some tenants used malodorous candles and coal lamps. The courtyards were small, crowded, and the smell of garbage was revolting.[21] The living conditions were fertile ground for epidemics. The electricity in many buildings had been disconnected or restricted so severely that people spent the entire day in darkness. The residents of the buildings facing the street across from Pawiak Prison were ordered to black out their windows. "I hardly need describe what it means for the occupants' eyes and lungs, their state of mind, this continual dark existence without fresh air, even ghetto air," Lewin wrote.[22]

The soap in use was a sticky paste that disintegrated upon contact with water and did nothing but spread the dirt.[23] In December 1941, the sanitary conditions became worse. Sewage pipes froze and the latrines in many buildings became unusable. Feces were often thrown out with the garbage and waste-removal carts rarely arrived. There was serious fear of an outbreak of cholera.[24] In July 1941, the Jewish police reported on the dire anti-sanitary situation in the ghetto that they had encountered during a patrol. Under the threat of shutting down an entire street for two weeks, due to the state of filth there, disinfection teams were ordered to improve the situation.[25] The *Biuletyn* reported that the cause of the epidemics was not racial origin, as the Nazi propaganda would have it, but poor domestic hygiene in overcrowded housing.[26]

21 Roland, *Courage under Siege*; Szac-Wajnkranc, *Halaf Im Ha'esh*, p. 10; Gutman, *The Jews of Warsaw*, p. 60.

22 Lewin, *A Cup of Tears*, p. 97.

23 Berg, *The Diary of Mary Berg*, p. 60.

24 Ibid., p. 107; Roland, *Courage under Siege*, pp. 42–43; Ringelblum, *Yoman Vereshimot*, pp. 373–374.

25 Czerniaków, *The Warsaw Diary*, pp. 261–262.

26 Blatman, *Geto Varsha—Sipur Itona'i*, p. 143.

Nutrition

In his notes, Ringelblum stated, "The Germans' true goal in establishing the ghetto was to starve the Jewish inhabitants." He added that Auerswald, the Nazi superintendent of the ghetto, spared no effort to implement the Germans' scheme of inducing the Jews' slow death. Only by virtue of smugglers—Jewish and Polish—was the plan not fully realized.[27] The Germans imposed scant food rations distributed by means of food ration coupons, for which they received payments. Already in the beginning of January 1940, food ration coupons to purchase foodstuffs were distributed and purchased at official prices.[28]

The closure of the ghetto allowed the Germans to control all movement in and out of it. In May 1941, they established an institution called the Transferstelle to manage this exchange, granting it sole responsibility for allowing food and other supplies to enter and exit the ghetto. Only foods acquired using the food ration coupons, as well as small amounts of supplies from the Jewish Social Self-Help, were allowed into the ghetto. These meager quantities doomed the ghetto to death—it was just a matter of time. The Germans intended to sever the ghetto from economic and social life, and to exploit its manpower and equipment by providing slightly larger food rations to those serving the war effort.[29] The German administration in the General Government allocated fewer than 200 calories per Jew, less than one-third of the allotment per Pole, and less than one-tenth of the quantity earmarked for each German.[30] An average adult requires 2,000–2,400 per day. Hans Frank, the governor of the General Government, wanted to kill the Jews by restricting their daily diet to 200 calories. Although Dr. Wilhelm Hagen, the Warsaw municipal physician, wanted to raise the allocation to

27 Ringelblum, *Ktavim Aharonim*, pp. 209–210.

28 Gutman, *The Jews of Warsaw*, pp. 26–27, 66–67.

29 Ibid., pp. 143, 151–152, 193–196; Blatman, *Geto Varsha—Sipur Itona'i*, pp. 164–165; Trunk, *Judenrat*, p. 80; Ringelblum, *Ktavim Aharonim*, p. 204.

30 Joseph Kermish, "Nigudim Ma'amadiyim Begeto Varsha," in Gruenbaum et al., *Entziklopediya Shel Galuyot*: *Varsha*, vol. 6, p. 572 n15.

2,000 calories, the ration was not changed. In Roland's opinion, the implementation of the Germans' food rationing policy depended on the local officials.[31]

From the establishment of the ghetto until January 1941, the authorities did not strictly enforce the closure, and women and children were allowed to leave the ghetto through some of its gates and to return with bread.[32] When Heinz Auerswald was appointed ghetto *Kommissar* in May 1941, half a year after ghettoization, he sought to isolate the ghetto population further and to prevent smuggling in order to make the ghetto an independent, closed economic entity, although he could not provide its inhabitants with sources of livelihood.[33] Wishing to increase the ghetto's productive potential, he attempted to reduce mortality and to improve food rations, contrary to Governor Frank's policy.[34]

In May 1941, the Nazi governor of the Warsaw district, Fischer, informed Czerniaków that it was not his goal to starve the Jews and that the rations were likely to be increased, but no changes were made. Czerniaków blamed this on the Transferstelle's policy.[35] In early November 1941, he wrote, "My head spins and my thinking is getting muddled." He continued to say that the food rations were to be increased, but the whole thing turned out to be all talk but no action because nothing at all was achieved.[36] According to Ringelblum, the official ration was less than even one-tenth of normal consumption.[37] All rations were distributed at prices set by the authorities. However, the distribution mechanism was rigid, unwieldy, and ineffective. It was not possible to buy the provisions included in the rationing system on the Aryan side, because the authorities kept these supplies off the open market. Basic commodities were requisitioned for military purposes, and

31 Roland, *Courage under Siege*, pp. 102–103.

32 Ringelblum, *Yoman Vereshimot*, p. 207.

33 Cohen, "Harefu'a Besherut Ha'idiologiya," p. 173; Gutman, *The Jews of Warsaw*, pp. 98–100.

34 Arad et al., *Documents on the Holocaust*, pp. 244–246.

35 Czerniaków, *The Warsaw Diary*, pp. 239, 243, 245. For an example of the rigid policy of the Transferstelle's director, see Czerniaków, *The Warsaw Diary*, p. 192.

36 Ibid., p. 295.

37 Ringelblum, *Polish-Jewish Relations*, pp. 79, 81.

it was impossible to provide the ghetto with essential foods at official prices.[38]

On August 24, 1942, at the height of the deportations from Warsaw, Frank wrote, "It is not necessary to dwell on the fact that we are sentencing 1.2 million Jews to death. That much is clear. And if the Jews do not die of starvation, it will be necessary to step up anti-Jewish measures, and let us hope that too will come to pass."[39] At the beginning of the war and long before the establishment of the ghetto, there was widespread hunger in Warsaw.[40] It was so acute that people hacked meat off the corpses of horses on the sidewalks. Prices of basic goods skyrocketed. Large food warehouses went up in flames. Transport was paralyzed, which impeded the ability to deliver food to the city. Already then, fourteen months before ghettoization, "Man has become an animal, concerned only with brute existence and fear of starvation," Kaplan wrote.[41] After occupying the city, the Germans set up field kitchens to distribute food to the population. The Jews stood with everyone else in the long lines, but they were shoved aside by Polish hooligans. The food rations for Jews were smaller than those for non-Jews, and the number of food rations was not increased in accordance with the number of incoming refugees.[42]

Four months into the occupation, the cost of living in Warsaw was increasing daily. Grain and other basic foods were being transported to the Reich, because of the famine that prevailed there, despite the Wehrmacht's victories.[43] In addition, about eight months before their internment in the ghetto, the Jews were taken away for forced labor under starvation conditions. Over time, the shocking phenomenon of children begging on the streets escalated.

38 Blatman, *Geto Varsha—Sipur Itona'i*, pp. 156, 164–165.

39 Gutman, *The Jews of Warsaw*, p. 64; Trunk, "Epidemics and Mortality," p. 91.

40 Kaplan, *Scroll of Agony*, pp. 27, 30, 34–35; Ringelblum, *Polish–Jewish Relations*, p. 36.

41 Berg, *The Diary of Mary Berg*, pp. 5–6, 14; Czerniaków, *The Warsaw Diary*, pp. 76–77; Ringelblum, *Yoman Vereshimot*, p. 5; Kaplan, *Scroll of Agony*, pp. 27, 35.

42 Turkow, *Hayo Hayta Varsha Yehudit*, p. 14; Kaplan, *Scroll of Agony*, p. 43; Ringelblum, *Notes from the Warsaw Ghetto*, p. 22.

43 Kaplan, *Scroll of Agony*, pp. 97–98.

About two months before ghettoization, during the funeral of some toddlers from a children's home, the children from the institution placed a wreath on their graves with the inscription, "To the Children Who Have Died from Hunger—From the Children Who Are Hungry."[44] In May 1940, soup kitchens were opened for Jews who were so malnourished that this was the only food they ate.[45]

Shortly after ghettoization, poverty and hunger took on the magnitude of a national disaster.[46] In mid-January, manifestations of hunger appeared: *khapers* (snatchers), in the language of the ghetto, who swiped bread from passersby on the streets.[47] Many Jews starved to death. Numerous families were pauperized at once. Next to almost every building, people slumped on the ground, pleading for help.[48] Entire families sprawled on sidewalks, begging for bread, but no one reached out to them.[49] In late February 1941, the official ration allowed only a minuscule portion of bread, while the price of bread on the black market was exorbitant.[50] In April 1941, food supplies did not suffice even for the fortunate few who could earn a little through peddling, clerical work, or trade.[51] Around Passover in April 1941, there were dreadful scenes at the offices of the refugee organizations. Thousands of people, including those considered affluent, waited for matzot and food parcels.[52] Toward the end of the month, people were fainting and

44 Ringelblum, *Notes from the Warsaw Ghetto*, p. 52.

45 Krall, *Shielding the Flame*, pp. 16–17.

46 Blatman, *Geto Varsha—Sipur Itona'i*, p. 140.

47 Ringelblum, *Yoman Vereshimot*, p. 231; Edelman, *The Ghetto Fights*, p. 26; Kaplan, *Scroll of Agony*, p. 244; Turkow, *Hayo Hayta Varsha Yehudit*, p. 42; Blatman, *Geto Varsha—Sipur Itona'i*, p. 144.

48 Kaplan, *Scroll of Agony*, p. 237; Ringelblum, *Yoman Vereshimot*, p. 232; Berg, *The Diary of Mary Berg*, pp. 47–48.

49 Kaplan, *Scroll of Agony*, p. 255.

50 Ten zlotys for half a kilogram of dark bread; 15–17 zlotys for the same quantity of white bread; Berg, *The Diary of Mary Berg*, p. 44.

51 Kaplan, *Megilat Yesurin*, p. 479.

52 Ringelblum, *Notes from the Warsaw Ghetto*, p. 154. On refugee aid in the Warsaw Ghetto, see Lea Prais, "Harefu'a Vehabriyut Begeta'ot Vilna, Kovna, VeShavli, 1941–1944: Bein Hapitaron Hasofi Leproduktivizatziya" (Medicine and Health in the Ghettos of Wilna, Kovna, and Shavli, 1941–1944: Between the Final Solution and Productivity) (Hebrew) (Master's thesis, The Hebrew University of Jerusalem, 1998), pp. 124–172.

dying on the streets. The cost of living, political events, such as the Nazi conquest of Yugoslavia, and the forced labor camps had an impact on the situation in the ghetto. Food prices continued to rise, and bread and potatoes were no longer available.[53]

In addition to the paltry food rations, the quantity of food ration coupons distributed was not commensurate with the actual number of ghetto residents. In May 1941, for example, 420,000 bread coupons were distributed to 460,000 people, creating an acute shortage of bread. Bread deliveries were sporadic and chaotic.[54] Hunger was so onerous that "terrible things," as Czerniaków put it, happened in the hospitals and the refugee points. Children starved to death. Women wound barbed wire around their breadbaskets to prevent *khapers* from seizing their food. In the ghetto workshops, workers fainted from hunger. People began to loot bakeries.[55]

Food parcels that saved many lives reached the ghetto until June 1941, when Germany invaded the Soviet Union. Thereafter, the parcels stopped arriving and the situation worsened.[56] By the end of that year, most of the ghetto population was starving, as attested to by the many deaths in the hospitals and orphanages, and by the clinical findings.[57] Mothers concealed dead children to receive their food rations and even placed corpses in the street after blurring their identities.[58] According to Kaplan, about two months before the beginning of the deportations, 60 percent of the population were literally starving, 30 percent were malnourished, although their situation did not appear to be terrible, and only 10 percent earned an adequate living.[59] Those who remained in the ghetto during the deportations suffered from grievous hunger. The Germans stepped up their watch over the ghetto gates, and Gestapo men replaced regular soldiers, who

53 Ringelblum, *Notes from the Warsaw Ghetto*, p. 154.

54 Ibid., pp. 276, 293.

55 Czerniaków, *The Warsaw Diary*, pp. 232, 235, 243, 247.

56 Turkow, *Hayo Hayta Varsha Yehudit*, p. 45.

57 Kermish, "Nigudim Ma'amadiyim," pp. 565–566.

58 Roland, *Courage under Siege*, p. 100; Czerniaków, *The Warsaw Diary*, p. 300; Ringelblum, *Yoman Vereshimot*, p. 306.

59 Kaplan, *Scroll of Agony*, p. 333.

regularly accepted bribes, thus, reducing smuggling. Dr. Lensky wrote that the Germans could have annihilated the Jews in the ghetto easily, simply by starving them. However, he believed that they wished to conceal the genocide and, therefore, they shipped the Jews to die in the East, where they could torture them as well.[60]

In the general hunger tragedy, starvation among the children was most egregious. Starving and abandoned youngsters appeared on the ghetto streets, their emaciated arms extended toward passersby, pleading for bread. People hurried past, ignoring the small, outstretched hands and shutting out the sobbing.[61] Mortality and deportations to forced labor camps of adults left thousands of children without parents, relatives, or other guardians. The plight of the refugee children was particularly severe.[62] By July 1941, massive numbers of children in rags with obvious physical symptoms of hunger disease sat in the streets.[63]

Coping with hunger was especially problematic for those who observed the Jewish dietary laws. While some upheld these rules scrupulously, many compromised and ate non-kosher food. The Nazis banned ritual slaughter, but this was not a major problem, since there was rarely any meat in the ghetto. Kosher food was available until late 1941, and refugees could receive it in kosher soup kitchens. Rabbis strived to encourage and reinforce the observance of kashrut. However, under the grim ghetto conditions, fewer and fewer people were able to keep kosher.[64]

60 Lensky, *A Physician inside the Warsaw Ghetto*, pp. 140–141.

61 Blatman, *Geto Varsha—Sipur Itona'i*, p. 230.

62 Ringlelblum, *Notes from the Warsaw Ghetto*, pp. 133, 140; Kermish, "Nigudim Ma'amadiyim," pp. 569–570; Blatman, *Geto Varsha—Sipur Itona'i*, p. 231.

63 Berg, *The Diary of Mary Berg*, pp. 76–78; Ringelblum, *Notes from the Warsaw Ghetto*, pp. 133, 241.

64 Roland, *Courage under Siege*, p. 105. On the hardships attending to observing the dietary laws, see Szymon Huberband, *Kiddush Hashem: Ktavim Miymei Hashoah* (Tel Aviv: Zachor, 1969), pp. 100–111. Ritual slaughterers slipped out of the ghetto to villages, and the meat was smuggled into the ghetto after they did their job. The illegal operation was facilitated by bribing both Poles and Germans. The Orthodox did not trust the clandestine operation, because it mistrusted that the religious requirements were stringently observed. Some in the ghetto bought meat that had been smuggled in from Otwock, where kosher slaughtering continued. Live cattle were smuggled into the ghetto and slaughtered there as well.

Morbidity from hunger disease appears to have been very high, although no continuous records have survived, such as those maintained on typhus, for example. Several factors appear to explain the absence of comprehensive, quantitative documentation of this disease: 1) The symptoms of hunger disease, as observed in the ghetto, were unique, and there were not enough precedents for the grave clinical aspects of the illness. This prompted the ghetto physicians to study hunger disease. 2) Hunger disease patients died before doctors could diagnose the disease. 3) Because of the many complications associated with hunger disease, it was difficult to diagnose. Moreover, the disease was not considered a contagion and, therefore, it was not mandatory to report it to the German authorities. In the refugee centers, where records have survived, in contrast, the incidence of hunger disease was very high[65]—up to 70 percent in 1942 in certain centers.[66]

The most appalling phenomenon in the ghetto was cannibalism. Hunger and general misery drove a few individuals to nourish themselves on the flesh of cats, rats, and even on human corpses. *Undzer Hofenung* (Our Hope), the underground newspaper of the General Zionist Party, reported in March 1942 that a woman had consumed part of the body of her eleven-year-old son. Czerniaków noted the incident in his diary and protested to the Germans about the situation that their policies had brought about in the ghetto.[67] Some imputed the state of hunger to the Jews' resigned response to their oppression. In late August 1941, Ringelblum claimed that the Jewish masses were passively dying of hunger with silent sighs and without protest.[68] Dr. Adolf Polisiuk, writing during the deportations, reported that the population showed no sign whatsoever of passive resistance.

65 Blatman, *Geto Varsha—Sipur Itona'i*, p. 212.

66 Trunk, "Epidemics and Mortality," p. 121. Examples of morbidity rates are 50 percent at 9 Stawki St., 62 percent at 3 Dzika St., 63 percent on Grzybowska St., and 73 percent on Żelazna St.

67 Czerniaków, *The Warsaw Diary*, p. 329; Kermish, "Nigudim Ma'amadiyim," p. 569; Blatman, *Geto Varsha—Sipur Itona'i*, pp. 178, 224; Krall, *Shielding the Flame*, p. 17; Turkow, *Hayo Hayta Varsha Yehudit*, p. 76.

68 Ringelblum, *Notes from the Warsaw Ghetto*, p. 206.

Hunger had become so severe that people volunteered to report to the Umschlagplatz in exchange for a kilogram of jam and three loaves of bread.[69]

Most of the deaths in the ghetto were from hunger and its corollaries. In Prof. Hirszfeld's judgment, no medical measures could have helped the population that was starving to death.[70] The Germans' policies and the development of the war had an impact on the hunger that prevailed in the ghetto. The high cost of living made food difficult to obtain on the black market and frustrated the efforts to improve nutrition in both quantity and quality. From the outbreak of the war until the onset of the occupation, anarchy prevailed in Warsaw. Official ration coupons were used to obtain minute portions of necessities of life, food, and clothing. It was also possible to purchase these items on the black market at a steep cost.[71] At the beginning of the occupation, the Germans threatened to execute profiteers, which put an end to commerce in food and created perceptible shortages. Discrimination against Jews in the distribution of food staples was introduced.[72] In May 1940, rations of bread and other basic goods for Jews were slashed[73] to starvation levels.[74] Prices of meat, butter, and vegetables surged that month, and milk and tea could not be acquired.[75]

When the ghetto was sealed, contact and trade between the Jews and the villagers were cut off, and food was transferred to German control. The goods in the shops disappeared immediately, leaving those who had not cached supplies in advance in misery. At this time, Poles came and went undisturbed, bringing groceries to the ghetto at prices many times higher than those in the Polish

69 Dr. Adolf Polisiuk diary, GFH, no. 3182.

70 Hirszfeld, *The Story of One Life*, p. 223.

71 Kaplan, *Scroll of Agony*, p. 44. Kaplan, *Megilat Yisurin*, pp. 32, 44, 235–236.

72 Gutman, *The Jews of Warsaw*, pp. 25–26.

73 Blatman, *Geto Varsha—Sipur Itona'i*, pp. 148–149.

74 Gutman, *The Jews of Warsaw*, pp. 25–26, Ringelblum, *Notes from the Warsaw Ghetto*, p. 41. For a comparison of the bread and sugar allotments of the Jews and the non-Jews in Warsaw in 1940, see Offer, *Haluk Lavan Bageto*, appendix B.8, p. 543.

75 Kaplan, *Megilat Yisurin*, pp. 235–236.

market.[76] In early December 1940, the shopping frenzy that had prevailed during the first days of the ghetto ceased and prices came down, even though many non-Jews often bought goods from the Jews in the ghetto.[77] For the time being, there was no acute shortage of food products in the ghetto and the crackdown on smugglers was yet to come.[78] In mid-March 1941, Poles were denied access to the ghetto, and prices rose toward the end of that month.[79]

The quantities of food that ration coupons could purchase were scant. Poles paid 10 grosz for a monthly food ration per person, whereas Jews paid 1.10 zlotys.[80] April–May 1941 was a particularly difficult period. Food shortages worsened and prices skyrocketed, due to reports about developments in the war and transport difficulties.[81] The stores were emptied and merchandise was hoarded in expectation of selling it at higher prices later on.[82] Food prices soared from October 1940, a month before ghettoization, until June 1941. The sources describe average increases of 300–600 percent.[83] In April 1942, shops in the ghetto were adequately stocked, but only non-Jewish customers who slipped into the ghetto or affluent Jews could afford to shop there.[84] About two months before the *Grossaktion* began, prices rose from one hour to the next.[85] When the deportations began, food prices increased at once. Jews who were working in the forced labor brigades outside the ghetto smuggled food back and sold it at particularly high prices, even to victims who sat starving on the Umschlagplatz, awaiting transport to Treblinka.[86]

76 Ringelblum, *Yoman Vereshimot*, pp. 186–187, 196–197; Ringelblum, *Notes from the Warsaw Ghetto*, pp. 86, 92; Kaplan, *Scroll of Agony*, pp. 225–226, 230.

77 Ringelblum, *Yoman Vereshimot*, p. 200.

78 Ibid., p. 207.

79 Ringelblum, *Notes from the Warsaw Ghetto*, pp. 139, 147.

80 Kaplan, *Megilat Yisurin*, pp. 478–479.

81 Gutman, *The Jews of Warsaw*, pp. 66–67; Blatman, *Geto Varsha—Sipur Itona'i*, p. 144; Ringelblum, *Notes from the Warsaw Ghetto*, pp. 175, 180–181, 272.

82 Ringelblum, *Notes from the Warsaw Ghetto*, p. 147.

83 Trunk, "Epidemics and Mortality," pp. 94–95; Offer, "Ma'arach Harefu'a Begeto Varsha," vol. 2, appendix B.7, p. 167.

84 Blatman, *Geto Varsha—Sipur Itona'i*, p. 167.

85 Kaplan, *Scroll of Agony*, p. 333.

86 Lensky, *A Physician inside the Warsaw Ghetto*, pp. 140–141.

The diet was poor, since only bread usually reached the ghetto. Other basics, such as flour, sugar, jam, meat, eggs, and the like were distributed infrequently and in small quantities. According to a report from the Judenrat supply department, the amounts actually received fell far short of the allotted quotas, which themselves were paltry.[87] The average daily food consumption of a working male before the war—2,380 calories per day--dwindled steadily in the ghetto. Daily allowances plunged to 460 calories in December 1940 and to only 153 in July 1941.[88] The caloric value of the food ration in January–August 1941 was less than one-tenth of the minimum required. There was no allotment for fats at all.[89] In 1942, rations were even smaller and distribution even less frequent.[90] In April of that year, for example, the monthly ration was 2 kilograms of bread—66 grams per day—200 grams of sugar at sporadic intervals—6.6 grams per day—and varying quantities of coffee, salt, jam, soap, and laundry detergent.[91]

No one could survive on the official rationing. According to one memoir, the official monthly rations were insufficient for even three days.[92] In practice, people were able to increase their caloric intake slightly by smuggling food, buying it on the black market, and the like. The sources and studies that discuss the calorie count offer various estimates, due to references to different periods of the existence of the ghetto and to different sources of information, as well as to the lack of clarity regarding the official number of calories and the illegal number, and so on. The average estimates fall in the range of 300–800 calories for the poor, 1,000–1,150 for the middle class, and 1,500–1,700 for the wealthy.[93]

87 Trunk, "Epidemics and Mortality," p. 92; Offer, "Ma'arach Harefu'a Begeto Varsha," vol. 2, appendix B.8, p. 167.

88 Roland, *Courage under Siege*, pp. 101–102.

89 Trunk, "Epidemics and Mortality," p. 93n32.

90 Ibid., p. 92n29.

91 Blatman, *Geto Varsha—Sipur Itona'i*, pp. 156, 164–165.

92 Gutman, *The Jews of Warsaw*, pp. 67–68; Offer, *Haluk Lavan Bageto*, appendix B.9, pp. 544–545.

93 See, for example, Edelman, *The Ghetto Fights*, pp. 25–26; Hirszfeld, *The Story of One Life*, p. 224; Roland, *Courage under Siege*, pp. 103–104; Lensky, *A Physician inside the Warsaw Ghetto*, p. 47. On social disparities in the ghetto, see, for

The quality of the food was wretched. According to the reports of the bacteriology lab that operated as an adjunct of the Judenrat Health Department, more than half of the food inspected in July–December 1941 was unsatisfactory.[94] In February 1942, more than half of the flour samples contained excess water and minerals, such as talcum—up to 20 percent, in some cases—magnesium, and lime, not to mention sundry weeds and mold.[95] In May 1941, spoiled onions and withered carrots were supplied. Small rotten fish were sold in the ghetto, which were sometimes the main sources of nourishment. Higher-quality meat and fish could be obtained, but at such high prices that only the few truly affluent could enjoy them.[96] Glasses of water sweetened with saccharin and razor-thin slices of bread were sold on the ghetto streets. Women sold a jelly made from horse bones and peddled fishcakes that the inhabitants called "stinky."[97] In December 1941, the Germans allocated a large shipment of potatoes to the ghetto. Initially intended for German soldiers, the potatoes had frozen. They could not be cooked, but they could be fried in inedible oil—itself an expensive commodity in the ghetto.[98] The vegetables delivered to the ghetto were contaminated, because they were transported in garbage wagons, due to the shortage of more appropriate means of transport. This triggered a dysentery epidemic in the summer of 1942.[99]

The high cost of living and the daily difficulties in obtaining basic food were compounded by the proscription against options to earn a livelihood. The German decrees toppled the Jews of Warsaw into economic disaster and crippled the community's

example, Kaplan, *Megilat Yisurin*, pp. 478–479; Wein, *Pinkas Hakehillot*, p. 106; Grupińska, "Conversation with Adina Blady Szwajger," pp. 157–158; Kermish, "Nigudim Ma'amadiyim," pp. 557–560, 563–565.

94 Trunk, "Epidemics and Mortality," p. 93. See the report from the Chemical-Bacteriological Institute of the Judenrat, July–December 1941, YVA, M.10. AR.1/191. Offer, "Ma'arach Harefu'a Begeto Varsha," vol. 2, appendix B.10, p. 168.

95 Blatman, *Geto Varsha—Sipur Itona'i*, p. 224.

96 Berg, *The Diary of Mary Berg*, p. 51.

97 Ibid., p. 78.

98 Ibid., p. 110.

99 Lensky, *A Physician inside the Warsaw Ghetto*, p. 68.

functioning.[100] The occupier's anti-Jewish economic policies included expropriating factories, businesses, and all Jewish property; severing economic relations with the local population; and exploiting Jewish labor for the German war effort.[101] During the very first stages of the occupation, most Jews no longer engaged in paid labor and had to fall back on their savings or sell their belongings for food that barely allowed them to subsist.[102] Ghettoization created another economic catastrophe for the Jews—a definitive one that cost them their jobs outside the ghetto and their sources of income.[103]

The Judenrat implemented its economic policy within the ambit of the German restrictions. The only productive activities permitted were those of a few home-based enterprises that adapted themselves to the Germans' needs. Other workshops produced goods that could be smuggled to the black market.[104] Unlike in other ghettos where the slogan "salvation by labor" was coined, the policy of the Warsaw Judenrat was one of non-intervention. However, the sheer size of the Jewish population in Warsaw lured Germans and Poles to do business in the ghetto, exploiting the Jews' wretched status under the Nazi regime.[105] In June 1941, about 40,000 persons in the ghetto were economically active, supporting

100 For an itemization of the various economy-related edicts up to ghettoization, see, for example, Kaplan, *Scroll of Agony*, pp. 42–46, 48–50; Kaplan, *Megilat Yisurin*, pp. 93–94, 125–126, 166, 171–172; Opochinsky, *Reshimot*, pp. 58–59; Gutman, *The Jews of Warsaw*, pp. 18–25; Wein, *Pinkas Hakehillot*, p. 100; Ringelblum, *Notes from the Warsaw Ghetto*, pp. 11, 18, 69; Mendelsohn, *The Polish Jews*, pp. 14–15; Hirszfeld, *The Story of One Life*, pp. 240–241; *The German New Order in Poland*, pp. 227, 558–560; Szac-Wajnkranc, *Halaf Im Ha'esh*, pp. 8, 11; Itamar Levin and Rachel Neiman, *Walls Around: The Plunder of Warsaw Jewry during World War II and Its Aftermath* (Westport: Greenwood Publishing Group, 2004), Chapters 1 and 2.

101 Gutman, *The Jews of Warsaw*, p. 72.

102 Wein, *Pinkas Hakehillot*, p. 99; Szac-Wajnkranc, *Halaf Im Ha'esh*, p. 8.

103 Ringelblum, *Notes from the Warsaw Ghetto*, p.77n2; Szac-Wajnkranc, *Halaf Im Ha'esh*, p. 26.

104 Gutman, *The Jews of Warsaw*, pp. 75–77.

105 On the economic aspects, see ibid., pp. 145–158; Kaplan, *Megilat Yisurin*, pp. 478–479; Wein, *Pinkas Hakehillot*, p. 106; Mendelsohn, *The Polish Jews*, p. 19; Ben-Shalom, *Ha'ezra Ha'atzmit Hayehudit*, pp. 54–55, 60–61.

a population of around 120,000, including dependents.[106] At the end of that month, the ghetto population was 435,700. Therefore, about one-fourth of the inhabitants lived under viable conditions, while the rest were hungry and dependent on public support.[107] Ringelblum wrote admiringly about the adaptability, enterprise, and professionalism that the ghetto inhabitants displayed in coping with the economic problems.[108] Despite his positive assessment, the data show that most people in the ghetto did not earn enough to buy even minimum sustenance and, therefore, they were doomed to starvation, illness, and death.

The Judenrat's main activities included attempts to improve the quantity and quality of the food rations. After ghettoization, the ZZ—Zakład Zaopatrywania (supply department)—was the Jewish entity in charge of supplying all the legal commodities allotted to the ghetto.[109] Its manager, Abraham Gepner, was known as being a Judenrat official who aided the ghetto population. However, the ZZ could not persuade the Germans to increase the food rations and operated strictly in accordance with the rules and permits issued by the Germans.[110] The ZZ was scathingly criticized in the ghetto for allegedly systematically oppressing the population, failing to distribute food in a proper and timely manner, and engaging in fraudulent acts that resulted in the distribution of spoiled food.[111]

Several months before ghettoization, the Judenrat imposed a tax on bread ration coupons, which prompted criticism for ostensibly adhering to the principle of "egalitarianism," rather than

106 Trunk, "Epidemics and Mortality," p. 89n19.

107 Ibid., p. 90n22. See also Offer, "Ma'arach Harefu'a Begeto Varsha," vol. 2, appendix B.11, p. 169. The method used to calculate employment varies from one source to another. See Gutman, *The Jews of Warsaw*, p. 77; Czerniaków, *The Warsaw Diary*, pp. 305, 378; Judenrat Statistics Department Report, no. 29, March 17, 1942, GFH, no. 11250, p. 17; Trunk, "Epidemics and Mortality," p. 90; Blatman, *Geto Varsha—Sipur Itona'i*, p. 154.

108 Ringelblum, *Polish-Jewish Relations*, pp. 61–63.

109 Trunk, *Judenrat*, p. 103.

110 Roland, *Courage under Siege*, pp. 104–105.

111 Kermish, "Nigudim Ma'amadiyim," p. 572.

levying the tax on the wealthy.[112] In mid-July 1940, after intense debates about exempting the poor from the bread tax, the Judenrat did exempt more than 40,000 people from paying this tax. Later that month, it distributed bread ration coupons at no charge for several days.[113] A year later, in July 1941, Czerniaków opposed a motion by members of the Judenrat to raise the price of bread, but he was unable to dissuade them.[114] The Judenrat introduced a tax on every bread ration coupon issued to family members. Those who could not afford the levy received permits from their "courtyard committee" that exempted them.[115] In January 1942, Czerniaków increased the number of exemptions. About 150,000 people—roughly a third of the ghetto population—were exempted. Several heads of house committees, who were expected to help implement the provision exempting the poor, did not comply with the instructions and were even incarcerated by the Jewish police for this.[116]

Judenrat officials rebelled against the high cost of living and sought relief for themselves. In response, Czerniaków was compelled to boost the rations for the Jewish police to match those of the police on the Aryan side, leaving less for the rest of ghetto residents.[117] The Judenrat did help the ghetto's weakest groups. In February 1942, for example, poor children received food supplements, bread was supplied to the schools still operating in the ghetto, special soup kitchens were set up for children, and 63,125 breakfasts were distributed each month—around 2,100 per day. At the same time, Judenrat employees, welfare workers, and those working for German companies received extra food.[118] That month, the Judenrat managed to increase the number of food ration coupons, and its departments drew up plans to provide

112 Ibid., p. 570.

113 Czerniaków, *The Warsaw Diary*, pp. 173, 174, 177.

114 Ibid., p. 254.

115 Kaplan, *Megilat Yisurin*, pp. 278–279.

116 Czerniaków, *The Warsaw Diary*, p. 312.

117 Ibid., p. 251.

118 Judenrat Statistics Department Report, no. 29, March 17, 1942, GFH, no. 11250, pp. 2, 6.

additional food, which would be manufactured in the ghetto, and to operate new workshops.[119]

Czerniaków summoned the Jewish police to carry out surprise inspections of shops that packed their display windows with luxury goods. Food was confiscated and handed out to indigent children on the streets and in shelters.[120] In mid-June 1942, in order to assist street children and to give more food to the poor, Czerniaków attempted to reduce the bread supplements granted to favored groups, but the Germans would not allow it.[121] The Judenrat's efforts to improve nutrition were not spared criticism. For example, Kaplan wrote, "The kehilla [Judenrat] is not even supporting us with enough to satiate a dog. First it imposed heavy taxes on every chew and swallow."[122] The food supplements given to those in high and powerful positions in the ghetto were criticized as well. Stanisław Adler, a member of the Jewish police, found the sight of the portly figures of Józef Andrzej Szeryński, chief of the police force, and his deputy, against the background of the starving ghetto population, tragic.[123] Some Judenrat officials arranged for themselves food ration cards that exceeded the quota.[124]

Welfare organizations and house committees also joined the struggle to procure food for the ghetto. In September 1939, they were already helping to feed the hungry at soup kitchens with the assistance of the JDC, which operated in Poland until early 1942, when the United States entered the war.[125] During the first months of the occupation, about 80,000 meals were served daily

119 Ibid., p. 3.

120 Czerniaków, *The Warsaw Diary*, p. 345.

121 Ibid., pp. 367–369.

122 Kaplan, *Megilat Yisurin*, pp. 478–479.

123 Roland, *Courage under Siege*, p. 101.

124 In March 1942, employees of the Judenrat and its extensions were allowed a bread supplement. A bread supplement of 10 kilograms per person per month was also alloted to 2,200 policemen. About 30,000 workers, 6,000 Judenrat staff, and 8,000 inpatients, as well as persons in aid institutions, received an extra allotment of 4 kilograms of bread that month. The rest of the population received only 2 kilograms. Blatman, *Geto Varsha—Sipur Itona'i*, p. 204; Kermish, "Nigudim Ma'amadiyim," p. 572; Szac-Wajnkranc, *Halaf Im Ha'esh*, pp. 43–44.

125 Kaplan, *Scroll of Agony*, p. 29.

to adults and children in Warsaw in seventy soup kitchens. The number of meals then plummeted, due to financial difficulties at the JDC. In mid–1941, more than half a year after the ghetto had been established, it was reported that half of the 500,000 people in the ghetto were indigent and in need of assistance, but only 120,000 portions of soup per day could be provided.[126] In January 1942, 80,000 soup portions continued to be distributed daily. Relief organization activists noted that the assistance provided by the Jewish Social Self-Help could sustain its recipients only for a short period—which simply prolonged their suffering—because it lacked the enormous sum of money required to be able to save them. Those who frequented the soup kitchens, subsisting on the soup and the rationed morsel of bread, died a slow death.[127]

The house committees also helped to keep tenants fed and made efforts to assist the poorest among them. These committees emerged among the public with the assistance of welfare organizations and the JDC shortly after the occupation began. In cooperation with the Judenrat, almost every house committee set up its own soup kitchen. Its members bought food on the market and their wives prepared the meals on a voluntary basis. After several months of activity and as the situation worsened, this important endeavor came to an end.[128] These soup kitchens served severely watered-down soup to the poor,[129] which benefited only those who had some other source of nutrition but could not sustain those most in need. Entire families went to eat at the soup kitchens, where many died as the staff looked on.[130]

Although the Judenrat, the Jewish Social Self-Help, and the house committees did everything possible, it was not enough to surmount the hunger crisis among the population. They sought to make up for the shortage of basic foods in illegal ways, foremost by smuggling. The German authorities fought this clandestine

126 Roland, *Courage under Siege*, p. 106.

127 Kermish, "Nigudim Ma'amadiyim," p. 565; Ringelblum, *Yoman Vereshimot*, p. 297; Lensky, *A Physician inside the Warsaw Ghetto*, p. 98.

128 Lensky, *A Physician inside the Warsaw Ghetto*, pp. 113–115.

129 Ibid., p. 114.

130 Auerbach, *Tzava'ot Varsha*, p. 82.

enterprise, imposing fines and severe punishments, including execution, on those caught smuggling food.[131] In December 1941, Czerniaków wrote, "We legally received 1,800,000 zlotys' worth of food in the ghetto monthly and, illegally, 70,000,000 to 80,000,000 zlotys' worth." Thanks to smuggling, basic foods were available, but they were very expensive and could not meet the needs of the many inhabitants.[132] The Germans turned a blind eye to smuggling, as long as it squared with their goals, possibly in return for bribes and not by virtue of real permits.[133] In April–May 1941, more and more exit routes from the ghetto were blocked and the smuggling paths were restricted.[134] Those who organized the smuggling of food and those who benefited from the contraband met a tragic and gruesome end. Despite the financial gain reaped by some of the smugglers, their actions must be deemed manifestations of public and private efforts, which should be viewed as a positive achievement in a human and a national sense.[135]

Effect of Cold Weather

Under these conditions of deprivation, it was difficult to survive the horrific cold that afflicted the inhabitants of Warsaw during the first winter under Nazi occupation. No coal was available,[136] since

131 In November 1941, eight people were shot in the Jewish prison for such offenses. Baila Kesselberg, who was caught smuggling and was given a prison sentence, described in her testimony the hanging of Jews as punishment for the transgression of smuggling. See Baila Kesselberg testimony, YVA, M.10. AR.1/470.

132 Czerniaków, *The Warsaw Diary*, p. 305. Many sources address the matter of smuggling. See, for example, Trunk, *Judenrat*, pp. 111–114; Gutman, *The Jews of Warsaw*, pp. 67–88; Szac-Wajnkranc, *Halaf Im Ha'esh*, pp. 10–11, 41–42; Hirszfeld, *The Story of One Life*, p. 191; Turkow, *Hayo Hayta Varsha Yehudit*, pp. 45–47; Auerbach, *Tzava'ot Varsha*, pp. 75–77; Ringelblum, *Polish-Jewish Relations*, pp. 79–82, 85–88; Roland, *Courage under Siege*, pp. 110–112.

133 Szac-Wajnkranc, *Halaf Im Ha'esh*, pp. 10–11.

134 Ringelblum, Notes from the Warsaw Ghetto, p 165.

135 Auerbach, *Tzava'ot Varsha*, pp. 75–77.

136 Czerniaków, *The Warsaw Diary*, pp. 106, 113; Turkow, *Hayo Hayta Varsha Yehudit*, pp. 35–36; Blatman, *Geto Varsha—Sipur Itona'i*, p. 140; Kaplan, *Megilat Yisurin*, pp. 177–178.

the occupation authorities had confiscated the reserves that had been amassed and prepared before the war had begun. The Poles rarely distributed the coal rations for which they charged high prices, and the heating supplies barely reached those in need.[137] There was a shortage of clothing, which was stolen from the shops, most of which were shut down.[138] As their distress mounted, large families would gather in a small room that they heated with their breath, spending the night sleeping on tables and chairs.[139] The cold and exhaustion forced poor families to bundle up in cushions and blankets even during the day and to sleep in their clothes. Under these conditions, filth accumulated and lice multiplied, transmitting lethal typhus from person to person.[140]

Not surprisingly, the number of frostbite victims escalated steeply in the winter of 1939–1940, as well as during the following two winters. Before the war, cold-related injuries were uncommon in Warsaw.[141] From late December 1939 on, people froze to death. Masses of Jewish refugees arrived at the hospital at this time, setting in motion the tragedy of freezing to death as hundreds of people died of cold-induced gangrene of the legs. The homeless, who had been forced to wander the streets, were not the only victims of frostbite—patients in the inadequately heated hospital were also its victims.[142] In the first winter in the ghetto, frozen corpses lay scattered on every corner up and down Leszno St.[143]

During a severe frost in October–November 1941, the apartments lacked the three main resources used for heating: coal, gas, and electricity. Most of the inhabitants could not even get a glass of hot water.[144] After the first snow, the frozen bodies of seventeen children were discovered on some steps and in various recesses among the ruined buildings. As the phenomenon of

137 Kaplan, *Megilat Yisurin*, p. 133; Gutman, *The Jews of Warsaw*, pp. 26, 113.

138 Kaplan, *Scroll of Agony*, p. 98.

139 Ibid., pp. 177–178.

140 Gutman, *The Jews of Warsaw*, p. 113.

141 Roland, *Courage under Siege*, pp. 21–22.

142 Dr. Emil Apfelbaum testimony, YVA, M.49.E/4510.

143 Ringelblum, *Notes from the Warsaw Ghetto*, p. 20; Kaplan, *Scroll of Agony*, p. 237; Berg, *The Diary of Mary Berg*, pp. 36–39.

144 Ringelblum, *Notes from the Warsaw Ghetto*, pp. 233–234.

children freezing to death became widespread, the ghetto police opened a special home to take in children off the streets.[145] In January 1942, refugees in shelters also began to freeze to death.[146] More and more frozen bodies appeared on the streets—lying in the building entrances, spines bent and knees folded—people succumbed as they tried to fight off death.[147]

Ringelblum pointed an accusing finger at the Judenrat's heating department, which was in charge of distributing coal. He charged that they allocated this resource only to Judenrat employees and their cronies. In his opinion, it was possible to deliver coal to at least one apartment in each building, but this never occurred to them and, thus, the poor were doomed to freeze to death.[148] Ringelblum bluntly accused the Judenrat of having done nothing, other than set up a center to gather children taken off the streets on its own initiative. In his opinion, the main reason for the lack of coordination between the Judenrat and ŻTOS, the Jewish self-help organization, was the Judenrat's strong desire to wipe out ŻTOS and weaken its influence. This prompted the Judenrat to oppose the participation of ŻTOS in the winter relief operation,[149] which clearly attests to the tension

145 Ibid. On January 7, 1942, the *Gazeta Żydowska* reported that the home had indeed opened at 35 Twarda St., using the proceeds from a "Month of the Child" fundraising drive. See also Ringelblum, *Notes from the Warsaw Ghetto*, pp. 334–335; Berg, *The Diary of Mary Berg*, p. 109. On the matter of child mortality, see, for example, Blatman, *Geto Varsha—Sipur Itona'i*, pp. 231–232; Deborah Dwork, *Children with a Star: Jewish Youth in Nazi Europe* (New Haven and London: Yale University Press, 1991), pp. 202–204; Janusz Korczak, "Shnei Aronot Metim Birehov Smucha Uvirehov Shliska" (Two Coffins on Smocza St. and Śliska St.), in Shevach Eden, ed., *Iyunim Bemorashto Shel Yanush Korchak* (Studies on the Legacy of Janusz Korczak) (Hebrew), vol. 4, (Haifa: University of Haifa, 1993), pp. 140–141.

146 Ringelblum, *Notes from the Warsaw Ghetto*, p. 251.

147 Berg, *The Diary of Mary Berg*, p. 124.

148 Ringelblum, *Notes from the Warsaw Ghetto*, p. 234.

149 Ibid., pp. 237–238. The winter relief operation was an initiative of the Jewish Social Self-Help in collaboration with the Judenrat to help the ghetto inmates to cope with the hardships of winter. This operation, which took place during the week of Hanukkah, was announced on December 7, 1941, during an evening of lectures held at the theater in the ghetto. The Jewish population was recruited to assist. See Turkow, *Hayo Hayta Varsha Yehudit*, pp. 38–39.

that existed between the self-help organizations and the Judenrat. However, caution should be exercised in making judgments about this matter. Kermish blamed the heating department even more harshly, claiming that it robbed the Jewish population of the little coal that the Germans had allocated to it.[150]

Refugees

One of the main causes of the acceleration of morbidity and mortality in the ghetto was the concentration of tens of thousands of refugees there. When the war began, a great influx of Jewish refugees reached Warsaw,[151] fleeing during the German occupation campaign.[152] In addition to these refugees, there were masses of deportees from northern and western Poland, which had been annexed to the Reich in late 1939 and the winter of 1940.[153] Altogether, of roughly 610,000 Jews who had been deported from the cities and towns in the Łódź and the Warsaw districts, no fewer than 100,000 joined the population of Warsaw.[154] Without being given any time to prepare, they were evacuated violently and hastily, loaded onto wagons, and transported to the General Government, specifically to cities with large concentrations of Jews

150 Kermish, "Nigudim Ma'amadiyim," p. 572.

151 According to the sources, a distinction may be made between refugees who fled, due to the situation, and those who were evicted—the exiles—due to the Germans' policies. However, given that they confronted the same problems upon reaching Warsaw, we refer to both groups as "refugees." For more on the refugee problem in the Warsaw ghetto, see Lea Prais, *Refugees in the Fabric of Jewish Life in Warsaw, September 1939–July 1942* (Jerusalem: Yad Vashem, 2015).

152 Dr. Moshe Tursz testimony, YVA, O.3/438; Roland, *Courage under Siege*, pp. 17–18, Kaplan, *Scroll of Agony*, p. 29.

153 Trunk, "Epidemics and Mortality," p. 115n83.

154 Blatman, *Geto Varsha—Sipur Itona'i*, pp. 147, 155–156, 207; Kaplan, *Scroll of Agony*, pp. 93–94, Ringelblum, *Yoman Vereshimot*, p. 23; Gutman, *The Jews of Warsaw*, pp. 15–16; Ruta Sakowska, "Opieka nad uchodźcami i przesiedleńcami żydowskimi w Warszawie w latach okupacji hitlerowskiej," BŻIH, 65–66 (1968), pp. 73–75.

in the Warsaw area. They became a burden to the Jews of Warsaw and altered the social fabric.[155]

The second large wave of deportations in February–March 1941 brought more than 70,000 refugees from the Warsaw district to what was now the ghetto.[156] They were crowded into more than 100 hovels—refugee centers and shelters—where they suffered the agony of hunger, cold, and deprivation. Many ultimately died on the streets.[157] By March–April 1941, the refugee population in the ghetto numbered almost 150,000, about one-third of the total.[158] Approximately 50,000–60,000 Warsaw Jews left the city during the first months of the war, and around 160,000 refugees arrived, bringing the ghetto population to approximately 476,000 in November 1941. There were 360,000 Jews in Warsaw before the war.[159] In March–April 1942, Jews from Germany began to arrive in the ghetto. Unlike refugees from elsewhere in Poland, they arrived well nourished and armed with cash, but this situation did not last for long. They soon began to die like the others. This group also had to cope with the language barrier and foreignness, and with the many difficulties of finding housing in the ghetto.[160]

Despite their efforts, the community and welfare institutions could not meet the multitudinous needs of the tens of thousands of DPs who inundated the city under occupation conditions.[161] The Judenrat oversaw the process of receiving the refugees, while the JHK—Judisches Hilfskomitee (Jewish Relief Committee)—aided by the JDC, assumed the responsibility and concern for their daily care.[162] When the waves of refugees arrived in

155 Arad et al., *Documents on the Holocaust*, pp. 183–186.

156 Mendelsohn, *The Polish Jews*, p. 25; Blatman, *Geto Varsha—Sipur Itona'i*, pp. 146–153, 207.

157 Blatman, *Geto Varsha—Sipur Itona'i*, pp. 155–156.

158 Trunk, "Epidemics and Mortality," p. 115n83; Kermish, "Nigudim Ma'amadiyim," p. 564.

159 Blatman, *Geto Varsha—Sipur Itona'i*, pp. 146–153, 155–156; Offer, "Ma'arach Harefu'a Begeto Varsha," vol. 2, appendix B.12, p. 169.

160 Hirszfeld, *The Story of One Life*, p. 232; Czerniaków, *The Warsaw Diary*, pp. 339, 342, 347, 376; Roland, *Courage under Siege*, pp. 41–42.

161 Kaplan, *Scroll of Agony*, pp. 93–94.

162 Hirszfeld, *A Story of One Life*, p. 229.

Warsaw, the JDC mobilized to provide emergency aid by setting up refugee relief committees that operated in every domain—providing subsistence, clothing, medical aid, and housing; assisting orphans; transferring funds from kin abroad; searching for relatives; and assisting in rehabilitation, through loans, jobs, and training.[163] Due to the devastation and the destruction of many apartments by the German bombardments, it was very difficult to find housing solutions for the thousands of refugees, and many were put up in public shelters—"overnight centers."[164] The living conditions in these refugee centers made the occupants the most miserable population in the ghetto. TOZ, supported by the JDC, mobilized to provide medical aid and attempted to improve hygiene in the centers.[165] The Jewish Social Self-Help, which administered the vast majority of refugee shelters during the first year in the ghetto, organized house committees to assist refugees as well. [166] In November 1941, the Judenrat established a special department to coordinate the care of the refugees, and responsibility for administering all aid to the refugees, including the 141 refugee shelters, was transferred to this department.[167]

The finance department of the Jewish Social Self-Help collected monthly taxes and raised funds to assist the refugees.[168] Those in charge of the shelters actively collected supplies and money for their residents.[169] House committees also collected daily bowls of soup for refugees from residents who still prepared meals in their own kitchens, thus supplementing the meals provided by the soup kitchens of the Jewish Social-Self Help. Notably, the house committees set up 212 soup kitchens to feed newly arrived refugees.[170] However, many refugees did not survive for

163 Sapir, "Joint," p. 569.

164 Turkow, *Hayo Hayta Varsha Yehudit*, pp. 26–27.

165 Dr. Moshe Tursz testimony, YVA, O.3/438.

166 Berg, *The Diary of Mary Berg*, p. 36.

167 Jewish Social Self-Help, Statistics Department Report, no. 6, November 1941, AŻIH, ARI.32.

168 Ibid., p. 31.

169 Ibid., p. 34; Offer, "Ma'arach Harefu'a Begeto Varsha," vol. 2, appendix B.13, p. 170.

170 Turkow, *Hayo Hayta Varsha Yehudit*, p. 40.

long on the thin soup that these kitchens offered, which was their only food, and they died en masse.[171]

In response to the refugees' grievous plight, the Judenrat attempted to organize further assistance for the shelters. In February 1942, it convened a meeting with the participation of 100 representatives of all population groups. Dozens of volunteers were recruited and each one was assigned to look out for one shelter. The volunteers engaged in fundraising among the population to assist the residents of their shelter and continued their activities to feed the refugees.[172] Despite all these efforts, the tragic plight of most of the refugees could not be reversed.

Notwithstanding the efforts of the Judenrat and the Jewish Social Self-Help, some refugees complained about the indifference of the Jews of Warsaw toward them. Some ghetto residents also directed criticism at themselves concerning this matter. Lensky claimed that the Jews of Warsaw left the care of the refugees to the public institutions.[173] Ringelblum described the Judenrat's attitude toward the refugees as "intolerable" and accused it of transferring the shelters to the worst locations.[174] Yitzhak Gitterman, one of the directors of the JDC, argued that the Jews of Poland, in general, and those of Warsaw, in particular, did not demonstrate a proper understanding of the cause of assisting the refugees. Ringelblum wrote that the "thousands of victims of the typhus epidemic among the wealthy of Warsaw are a revenge of sorts for the tens of thousands of refugees who are dying of hunger and disease without their aloof brethren offering them a hand."[175]

Morbidity and mortality rates among the refugees were particularly high. Upon their arrival in the city, refugees had to

171 Ringelblum, *Ktavim Aharonim*, p. 18; Ringelblum, *Yoman Vereshimot*, pp. 18–19; Jewish Social Self-Help, Statistics Department Report, no. 6, November 1941, AŻIH, ARI.32, p. 16.

172 Judenrat Statistics Department Report, no. 29, March 17, 1942, GFH, no. 11250, p. 13.

173 Lensky, *A Physician inside the Warsaw Ghetto*, pp. 82–84.

174 Ringelblum, *Notes from the Warsaw Ghetto*, p. 207.

175 Ringelblum, *Ktavim Aharonim*, pp. 63, 120. For further criticism, see Blatman, *Geto Varsha—Sipur Itona'i*, pp. 212–213; Lensky, *A Physician inside the Warsaw Ghetto*, pp. 82–84; and Ringelblum, *Yoman Vereshimot*, p. 308.

live in the first vacant public places that they found, which were usually synagogues and schools. Hundreds were concentrated in very crowded overnight centers of this type. Every day, new centers were set up. These locations had no heating materials, and the windows of some had been shattered during the bombardments. The refugees suffered from hunger, unbearable cold, and bloody diarrhea. Due to the shortage of latrines, human waste accumulated in piles.[176] Given no opportunity to bathe, infested with lice, and suffering from malnutrition, the refugees spent entire days sprawled on mattresses, unable to get up. The gripping poverty and hunger in the overnight centers eventually sealed the fate of the refugees.[177] This was the situation of the refugees from their arrival at the beginning of the war until the liquidation of the ghetto.[178]

A Jewish Social Self-Help report indicates a downward trend in the number of refugee shelters and residents between May and November 1941—from 15,140 residents in 165 shelters in May to 9,588 in 126 shelters in November.[179] In February 1942, there were 8,275 refugees in 113 shelters sponsored by the Judenrat.[180] Presumably, it was not possible to house the remaining tens of thousands of refugees in the overcrowded centers, and some sought shelter in stairwells, courtyards, cellars, and demolished buildings.[181]

There were three types of refugee dwellings: apartment blocks, large apartments of five or six rooms that housed several

176 Dr. Moshe Tursz testimony, YVA, O.3/438, pp. 5–6.

177 Edelman, *The Ghetto Fights*, pp. 26–27; Berg, *The Diary of Mary Berg*, pp. 59–60; Trunk, "Epidemics and Mortality," pp. 115–117.

178 Ringelblum, *Yoman Vereshimot*, p. 25; Czerniaków, *The Warsaw Diary*, p. 268; Kaplan, *Scroll of Agony*, pp. 246, 251–252; Blatman, *Geto Varsha—Sipur Itona'i*, p. 209; Offer, "Ma'arach Harefu'a Begeto Varsha," vol. 2, appendix B.17, p. 173.

179 Jewish Social Self-Help, Statistics Department Report, no. 6, November 1941, AŻIH, ARI.32, p. 13; Offer, "Ma'arach Harefu'a Begeto Varsha," vol. 2, appendix B.14, p. 171.

180 Judenrat Statistics Department Report, no. 29, March 17, 1942, GFH, no. 11250, pp. 11–12. Even though the Judenrat centralized the refugees' care in November 1941, it appears that other organizations still ran the shelters. In February, there were 2,604 people living in "refugee towns"—housing sites that the Judenrat did not manage directly—as compared with 5,671 in the shelters run by the Judenrat.

181 Trunk, "Epidemics and Mortality," p. 116. According to Trunk, there were nearly 20,000 refugees in the centers in May 1941.

hundred people, and small apartments that were suitable for a dozen or two dozen people. The situation in the blocks was ghastly. About 1,000 refugees lived there under appalling sanitary conditions. Refugees who lived in larger apartments were less isolated than the rest of the population and could find employment more easily. The worst off were those in small dwellings, most of which were cellars. It was very difficult to attend to the refugees who were housed there, because of the distance between them. Prof. Hirszfeld wrote that he saw scenes of horrific suffering, of total desperation and despair.[182]

Upon their arrival, the refugees were taken to isolation stations for disinfection and bathing. The conditions at these locations were atrocious. The isolation station at 109 Leszno St. was one of the most dreadful in the ghetto—it was overcrowded, filthy, chaotic, and it lacked food.[183] After his first shift there, one of the doctors described the terrifying conditions at the location and the inability to provide proper medical aid.

> There's not enough air. Stench, women and children...When we pass by, they extend their hands toward us. Everyone begs. We're truly afraid of everything that's happening. We can hardly tell one face from another. Everyone asks for food. But we doctors—what can we do? I do what I can, and it's not much.[184]

According to a Jewish Social Self-Help report, the cold and filth in the shelters, which lacked heating materials and cleaning supplies, caused the epidemic of lice infestation to spread in November 1941. More and more starving refugees lay on the

182 Hirszfeld, *Die Geschichte eines Lebens*, pp. 154–155, Hirszfeld, *The Story of One Life*, pp. 229–230.

183 Blatman, *Geto Varsha—Sipur Itona'i*, p. 208; Kaplan, *Scroll of Agony*, p. 255; Ringelblum, *Notes from the Warsaw Ghetto*, p. 130. For more on this isolation center, see the testimony of an anonymous doctor regarding the deportees from Grojec in isolation on Leszno St., AŻIH, ARI.1069.

184 Testimony of an anonymous doctor regarding the deportees from Grojec in isolation on Leszno St., AŻIH, ARI.1069. For reports about the doctors' work among refugees and some of the professional hardships encountered at the refugee centers, see the report on the medical situation at refugee centers, AŻIH, ARI.84.

bunks, swollen from hunger. In a report on one of the shelters, a doctor described the situation, which prevailed in most of the shelters. "Cold, dirt, and hunger are claiming casualties among the tenants. The number of deaths is rising. In the corridors and the rooms, there are puddles of mud, due to water leaking from the roof."[185] The hungry refugees could not concern themselves with maintaining order and cleanliness, which aggravated the filth and the dirt.[186] The adult refugees left the shelters during the day in search of work, leaving behind the children, the ill, and the elderly lying in bed.[187]

Dr. Israel Rom (Rotbalsam), a physician at the Warsaw ghetto children's hospital, noted that while the refugee centers contributed significantly to the spread of disease in the ghetto, many refugees died before becoming ill.[188] In the course of 1940, large numbers of refugees died because of the severe hardships that they had suffered during the deportations.[189] By late December 1940, about a month and a half after ghettoization, masses of refugees were dying every day in the shelters.[190] In May 1941, Czerniaków delivered a lecture before members of the German security police about the catastrophic situation in the refugee centers. In February–May 1941, for example, 69 out of 456 residents died in the center at 69 Smocza St.—15 percent in four months.[191] During this period, the mortality rate doubled.[192] At certain centers, the mortality rate was even higher.[193] In late

185 Jewish Social Self-Help, Statistics Department Report, no. 6, November 1941, AŻIH, ARI.32, pp. 15–16.

186 Ibid.

187 Turkow, *Hayo Hayta Varsha Yehudit*, p. 40; Berg, *The Diary of Mary Berg*, pp. 59–60; reports from children's clubs, GFH, no. 4368.

188 Rom, "Mahalot Hayeladim Begeto Varsha," p. 15.

189 Ringelblum, *Notes from the Warsaw Ghetto*, pp. 8, 25; Czerniaków, *The Warsaw Diary*, p. 129.

190 Ringelblum, *Yoman Vereshimot*, p. 215.

191 Czerniaków, *The Warsaw Diary*, p. 232; Czerniaków, *Yoman Geto Varsha*, p. 180, and note ad loc concerning mortality at the refugee "points."

192 Trunk, "Epidemics and Mortality," p. 116.

193 Czerniaków, *The Warsaw Diary*, p. 232; Czerniakow, *Yoman Geto Varsha*, p. 180, and note ad loc concerning mortality at the refugee "points." See also Ringelblum, *Notes from the Warsaw Ghetto*, p. 199.

May 1941, Ringelblum wrote that the refugees topped the list of the dead.[194]

Reports from doctors at the refugee centers indicate that the main reason for the increase in mortality was hunger. The cause of death was hunger-related edema—not higher morbidity.[195] The September 1941 issue of the underground newspaper *Biuletyn* reported on morbidity and mortality among the refugees, stating that 500 of the 8,500 refugees in 127 centers were ill, and that 5 percent of all refugees died each month. Mortality at these shelters was four times greater than the average in the ghetto. About 40 percent of the inhabitants of the refugee centers were infested with lice.[196]

According to the Jewish Social Self-Help, 3,134 people died in the shelters in January–November 1941. The mortality rate increased during these months[197] and continued to do so in 1942. The Bund and Zukunft underground newspaper *Der Wecker* reported that 715 of the 9,030 refugees in the centers died in January 1942. In the center on Dzika St., 439 refugees out of 2,500 perished.[198] The newspaper published by the Union of Armed Resistance Forces in Warsaw reported, for example, that in one building on Miła St., 250 refugees out of 578 died; 430 out of 794 perished in a shelter on Pawia St.; and all 400 refugees in one of the houses on Krochmalna St. died within a three-month period.[199] The report described the sanitary conditions that prevailed at the height of the death toll among the refugee population, the shortage of coal, and the naked, barefoot, lice-infested residents of the refugee center on 2 Leszno. An anonymous witness commented,

194 Ringelblum, *Notes from the Warsaw Ghetto*, p. 181.

195 Blatman, *Geto Varsha—Sipur Itona'i*, p. 212; Ringelblum, *Notes from the Warsaw Ghetto*, p. 219.

196 Blatman, *Geto Varsha—Sipur Itona'i*, pp. 212–213.

197 Jewish Social Self-Help, Statistics Department Report, no. 6, November 1941, AŻIH, ARI.32, p. 13; Offer, "Ma'arach Harefu'a Begeto Varsha," p. 172.

198 Blatman, *Geto Varsha—Sipur Itona'i*, p. 214. The situation in the refugee centers took a terrible turn for the worse in the winter of 1941–1942; see Ringelblum, *Notes from the Warsaw Ghetto*, p. 251. The center on Dzika St. was the largest in the ghetto; see Engelking and Leociak, *Getto warszawskie*, p. 30.

199 Roland, *Courage under Siege*, pp. 41–42.

> About ten weeks ago, forty people died within a week. Now they are also dying uninterruptedly. From what? No one knows. The doctor does not check the ill. They do not even have thermometers to take their temperature. No diagnosis is made. They say they died from cold and starvation. The doctor is afraid to approach the patients.[200]

The sources offer various reasons for the mortality rates in the refugee centers. The main cause of death was hunger. In June 1941, more than 80 percent of refugee deaths were traced to hunger and the trend steadily grew. The centers housed around 20,000 people in May–June 1941, 4.4 percent of the ghetto population of 450,000. However, the proportion of deaths from hunger among them was 20 percent—five times higher than their share of the population.[201] In contrast, death from typhus among the refugees was relatively low, compared with the general population. It seems that the poor suffered less from typhus than the affluent did, although the death rate from typhus also increased among the refugees, as the weakening effects of hunger wore down their resistance. The situation worsened in 1942: there were 1,763 starving refugees among 9,425 in December 1941, and 2,792 among 8,000 in early March 1942.[202] From May to November 1941, about 70 percent of refugee deaths were from starvation, 2.1 percent were from typhus, and nearly one-fourth were from sundry causes.[203]

200 Sanitary conditions at the time of high mortality among the refugees, AŻIH, ARII.161; Offer, "Ma'arach Harefu'a Begeto Varsha," vol. 2, appendix A.34, pp. 161–162.

201 Mortality in the Warsaw Ghetto Report, June 1941, AŻIH, ARI.223; Trunk, "Epidemics and Mortality," pp. 120–121.

202 Trunk, "Epidemics and Mortality, p. 121n100. The newspaper *Yugent-Ruf* reports that 41.5 percent of the residents of the shelters contracted hunger disease during December 1941–February 1942. See Blatman, *Geto Varsha—Sipur Itona'i*, p. 214.

203 Jewish Social Self-Help, Statistics Department Report, no. 6, November 1941, AZIH, ARI.32, p. 13. The monthly data for May–August pertain to deaths in all the shelters. Those for September–November refer only to shelters sponsored by ŻOS. See Offer, "Ma'arach Harefu'a Begeto Varsha," vol. 2, appendix B.18, p. 173, appendix B.19, p. 174.

The sources allow us to parse mortality in the refugee centers by age groups. The death rate in the children's homes was high. Forty-seven of 470 children died in the largest children's home on Dzielna St. in July–August 1940. Mortality escalated in 1941—among 600 children, 178 perished in May, and 155 died in June.[204] Death rates among children and adolescents in the shelters climbed in the last quarter of 1941.[205] An examination of deaths in the four months between August and November 1941 shows that the mortality rates were highest among those aged 45–60, nearly 20 percent, and those over 60, about 25 percent. In the preceding months, the death rate among the latter group had been the highest; it declined thereafter. The average death rate of those aged 35–45, 12.9 percent, was lower than that of those aged 45 and over. The lowest death rate was observed among those in the 25–35 age bracket—9.8 percent. Mortality among those aged 7–25 was slightly higher—10.7 percent—and, surprisingly, the 0–7 age group, which had an 11.5 death rate, resisted death more effectively than did those aged 35 and over.[206]

204 Trunk, "Epidemics and Mortality," p. 116nn90, 91; Mortality in the Warsaw Ghetto Report, June 1941, AŻIH, ARI.223.

205 Jewish Social Self-Help, Statistics Department Report, no. 6, November 1941, AŻIH, ARI.32, pp. 14–15; Offer, "Ma'arach Harefu'a Begeto Varsha," vol. 2, appendix B.15, p. 171.

206 Ibid. See also Offer, "Ma'arach Harefu'a Begeto Varsha," vol. 2, appendix B.20, p. 175.

Chapter Seven

Diseases and Medical Care

At various times, the health care systems in the Warsaw ghetto treated infectious diseases that threatened to spread. The first plague of typhoid fever was followed by typhus and then by a tuberculosis epidemic that persisted throughout the ghetto period. In the end, hunger disease claimed the lives of its victims, day in and day out. The surgery departments were overcrowded and could not admit everyone who required emergency assistance, particularly during the *Aktionen*, as well as in the intervening periods, when Germans shot passersby indiscriminately. During the siege of Warsaw in September 1939, epidemics of typhoid fever and dysentery battered the inhabitants.[1]

Prof. Hirszfeld described the development of these contagious illnesses as observed in the ghetto. Typhus, he said, which erupted in a closed environment, was typified by a high coefficient of transmission, during which the population gradually acquired immunity and the epidemic receded spontaneously. Tuberculosis, in contrast, spread more than typhus did, and its manifestations were more severe, due to hunger. In Hirszfeld's opinion, pediatric diseases were not common because there was a decline in the birthrate, which was affected by some "unclear" factor. He estimated that the decrease in the incidence

1 Einhorn, "Harofe Begeto Varsha," pp. 10–11; Lensky, *A Physician inside the Warsaw Ghetto*, p. 99; Gutman, *The Jews of Warsaw*, pp. 110–111.

of dysentery was also incidental.[2] The Germans thus liquidated the ghetto directly by exacerbating hunger and epidemics. "By using these methods, they would have been able to obliterate the entire Jewish population with no need for crematoria," Dr. Chaim Einhorn would write years later.[3]

Typhoid Fever

When the fighting ended on October 4, 1939, a typhoid fever epidemic broke out in Warsaw.[4] In the wake of the siege and the bombing of the city, the water filtration plants were damaged, and the population was forced to drink polluted water from the river. Sanitary conditions were appalling, and the Jewish hospital was filled with typhoid fever and dysentery patients. Typhoid fever had erupted sporadically in the autumn in Warsaw, even before the war, but the ravages of the fighting caused a major epidemic. The residential areas in the heavily Jewish northern quarters of the city were especially hard-hit by the bombardments. Due to the resulting damage and the severe overcrowding in that area—where about 60 percent of the local Jews and refugees lived—the scourge spread aggressively among the Jewish population. Hundreds of people suffering from high fever, nearly unconscious, streamed to Czyste Hospital. The conditions at the hospital were ghastly, and it was not possible to provide those who had contracted typhoid fever with the special diet that they required.[5]

The epidemic erupted when Warsaw was still under the control of the German Army, and Prof. Wilhelm Richter, the

2 Hirszfeld, *The Story of One Life*, p. 227.

3 Einhorn, "Harofe Begeto Varsha," pp. 12–13.

4 Typhoid fever is a severe illness of the digestive system caused by the Salmonella typhi bacterium in contaminated food or water. The bacterium infects the liver and the gall bladder, and destroys bone marrow. Fever, diarrhea, abdominal pains, headache, weakness, and muscle pain occur after approximately two weeks of incubation. The typical indicators are an enlarged spleen, prominent clusters of skin rash, and a pulse that is not as rapid as expected when there is fever. Sepsis causes death.

5 Dr. Emil Apfelbaum testimony, YVA, M.49.E/4510.

military physician who headed the medical services, was in charge of waging the war on the epidemic. Richter had the water system repaired, and clean water became available again by December 1939.[6] On his orders, a formation of precinct physicians, Jewish and non-Jewish, was set up. Each doctor was responsible for a given area and was tasked with ensuring cleanliness, identifying and hospitalizing the sick, and locating and disposing bodies that had not yet been evacuated from the area. The health care services took drastic measures. All inhabitants, Polish and Jewish alike, had to be inoculated against typhoid fever. By November 1939, the entire population of the city was vaccinated. The Jewish population cooperated; masses of Jews reported to the vaccination stations. Doctors who worked many long days without pay administered the vaccines by order of the health care services. Dr. Mordechai Lensky personally inoculated about 12,000 people. In buildings inhabited by both Poles and Jews, Jewish physicians inoculated everyone. The epidemic stopped after about half of the population had been vaccinated. Morbidity from typhoid fever gradually receded to a level even lower than it was in peacetime.[7]

Reports from TOZ demonstrate the centrality of this organization and its doctors in immunizing the public and treating the epidemics.[8] In the last quarter of 1939, 2,057 cases of typhoid fever were reported among the Jews of Warsaw—an average of 685 per month. The patient count tapered to 540 in December and plunged to 104 in January 1940, 25 in February, and only 10 in April. As the hygienic living conditions improved, the number of persons infected declined from day to day, and

6 According to Dr. Emanuel Patt, only in November 1940, fourteen months after the war had begun, was the damage from the bombardments repaired. See report by Emanuel Patt, "Welfare Activity for the Jews of Poland," JDC, AR.33–44, file 814.

7 Lensky, *A Physician inside the Warsaw Ghetto*, pp. 99–104; Rom, "Mahalot Hayeladim Begeto Varsha," p. 14; Einhorn, "Harofe Begeto Varsha," pp. 10–11; Cohen, "Harefu'a Besherut Ha'idiologiya," pp. 163–164; Trunk, "Epidemics and Mortality," p. 85; Dr. Henry Fenigstein testimony, "Varshever yid," YVA, O.33/1074, p. 9.

8 See, for example, Dr. Wulman's report on medical activity, February 28, 1941, JDC, AR.33–44, file 840.

the epidemic finally came to a halt. The vaccination campaign undoubtedly had its effect.[9] In Dr. Apfelbaum's opinion, the German authorities had intended to increase mortality among those who had fallen ill, but thanks to the Jewish doctors' curative methods, it decreased.[10]

Typhus

Typhus was the cruelest disease that afflicted the Jews of Warsaw and claimed innumerable victims during the war.[11] After the war had begun and Warsaw was mercilessly shelled, and following the cessation of the typhoid fever epidemic, a typhus epidemic erupted. Many Jews were left homeless, living under grim hygienic and sanitation conditions.[12] Nevertheless, there were relatively few cases of typhus in Warsaw in 1939.[13] In December 1939, three months into the occupation, many Jewish refugees were forced to move or escaped to Warsaw. The Jewish public buildings where they were concentrated became a breeding ground for the typhus epidemic. In February 1940, as the spread of typhus accelerated, Czerniaków saw the need for a new isolation facility.[14] Indeed, within a few days, the Judenrat was required to install a quarantine center for typhus patients and their families, and to establish two hospitals to treat typhus patients.[15]

9 Trunk, "Epidemics and Mortality," p. 85.

10 Dr. Emil Apfelbaum testimony, YVA, M.49.E/4510.

11 Typhus, also known as spotted fever—*Fleckfieber*, in German—is a disease brought on by the Rickettsia bacterium. It is transmitted from person to person by means of, among other things, body lice, which were rife in the ghettos. Its symptoms include high fever, shivering, headache, muscular pain, vomiting, and nose and throat infections. About a week after infection, small, clear, red blotches appear on the skin, chiefly on the face and the feet. As the disease progresses, pulmonary, renal, and cardiac infections develop, ultimately causing death, unless the patient receives antibiotic treatment.

12 Turkow, *Hayo Hayta Varsha Yehudit*, pp. 24–26; Opochinsky, *Reshimot*, p. 58; Dr. Moshe Tursz testimony, YVA, O.3/438, p. 4.

13 Roland, *Courage under Siege*, pp. 132–134.

14 Czerniaków, *The Warsaw Diary*, p. 116.

15 Ringelblum, *Yoman Vereshimot*, pp. 20, 23; Rom, "Mahalot Hayeladim Begeto Varsha," p. 15.

In March 1940, *Untersturmführer* Karl Georg Brandt, who was deputy head of IV B 4—the department in the SIPO and the SD that dealt with Jews—demanded data on mortality from typhus in 1939 and in January–February 1940. According to the figures submitted by the Judenrat statistics department, 944 people died of typhus in December 1939 and 1,004 in January 1940.[16] In the Judenrat's official report, it was stated that the Jewish hospital, the only one that admitted patients with infectious diseases, admitted 861 typhus patients in February–April 1940; 104 of them died. The number of typhus patients and of their deaths escalated from month to month.[17] The epidemic, which was mild at first, intensified in March 1940.[18] Ringelblum reported that it had spread to an alarming extent and was claiming more and more lives. One out of every three patients in the hospital died.[19]

Having learned the lessons of World War I, the Germans took stern measures to fight the spread of epidemics and eradicate them, sealing houses where the ill were located, disinfecting buildings and their surroundings, and waging war on lice. Dr. Wilhelm Hagen, the German chief physician of Warsaw, reported that 1,920 typhus patients had been identified during this outbreak—177 Poles, 1 German, and 1,742 Jews, the main casualties.[20] Hagen appears to have drawn these data from Jewish sources that reported similar figures. In an article in the newspaper *Dror* in May–June 1941, for example, Menachem Linder wrote that 1,772 of the 1,920 typhus patients in all of Warsaw between September 1, 1939, and August 31, 1940, were Jewish—more than 90 percent. "In principle, one may say that the identification of Jews with lice, illustrated so graphically

16 Czerniaków, *The Warsaw Diary*, p. 129.

17 The data appear in Judenrat reports. These figures may not reflect the intensity of the epidemic. The Judenrat presumably had an interest in understating the toll and almost certainly did not know about all the typhus patients. See Gutman, *The Jews of Warsaw*, pp. 26–27.

18 Ringelblum, *Notes from the Warsaw Ghetto*, p. 30.

19 Ringelblum, *Yoman Vereshimot*, p. 98.

20 Cohen, "Harefu'a Besherut Ha'idiologiya," p. 165.

in huge posters in March, was confirmed by the objective statistics." Linder also noted that this situation was the result of the horrific overpopulation in the ghetto, and that the disease was engendered by the poor health situation, due to the dire conditions prevailing there.[21]

The epidemic ended in August 1940. German and Jewish sources differ about the factors that successfully suppressed it. According to Hagen, it was the actions taken by the Polish health care system under his direction as the chief physician of Warsaw. According to Jewish documentation, in contrast, the Judenrat and especially the Jewish health care organization TOZ eradicated the epidemic. TOZ reports from that period indicate that the staff of this organization were intensively active in quashing the epidemic.[22] On October 24, 1940, the Polish-language Jewish newspaper *Gazeta Żydowska,* the only one to appear under the auspices of the German occupier in Poland, published details about the epidemic. "Typhus fever, whose first appearance was recorded in December 1939, reached its peak in April with 407 cases. As of June, the epidemic had begun to decline, and it was contained by August, when only a dozen or so cases were recorded."[23]

The epidemic lasted from January to July 1940. The count of reported cases among the Jews rose from 88 in December 1939 to 191 in January 1940, 214 in February, 398 in March, and 407 in April, which was followed by a decline: 123 cases in June, 68 in July, and only 18 in August. Typhus morbidity decreased significantly from May 1940, and the overall mortality rate dropped as well.[24]

21 Blatman, *Geto Varsha—Sipur Itona'i*, pp. 146–148.

22 Cohen, "Harefu'a Besherut Ha'idiologiya," p. 165. See the reports by Dr. Wulman, February 28, 1941; the reports by Dr. Rozenblum et al. about TOZ's work, between September 1, 1939, and June 8, 1940; the TOZ activity report, January 1940–December 31, 1940; and many additional reports in JDC, AR.33–44, file 840.

23 Gutman, *The Jews of Warsaw*, p. 54.

24 Trunk, "Epidemics and Mortality," p. 85. For data on typhus morbidity at Czyste Hospital, February–April 1940, see Judenrat Statistics Department Bulletin, AŻIH, ARII.133; Offer, "Ma'arach Harefu'a Begeto Varsha," vol. 2, appendix B.21, p. 176.

The Germans claimed that the spread of the epidemic and the associated dangers led to the creation of the ghetto in Warsaw. In fact, however, the wave of epidemics of 1940 had practically abated by the time the ghetto was set up, and experts thought that they could extinguish it altogether by adopting remedial measures. After all, there were only 14 cases in December 1940. Nonetheless, from April 1941 onward, an immense wave of the typhus epidemic surged in the ghetto.[25]

When the ghetto was sealed, about 350,000 people were living in severely overcrowded dwellings under dire sanitary conditions. In addition, the Germans sent refugees, whom they had evicted from nearby towns, as well as Jews from Germany and the occupied countries of Western Europe, to the ghetto. As a result, a second wave of the typhus epidemic broke out in the spring of 1941, infecting approximately 100,000 people, until it subsided in July 1942.[26] It began at Mokotów Prison, a facility that was far from the ghetto and that held no Jewish prisoners. Prof. Heinrich Kudicke, a German doctor posted in the General Government as an expert on typhus, headed the Institute of Hygiene in Warsaw and led the war on typhus. The epidemic at the prison was subdued through classical methods, including meticulous delousing, disinfection of laundry and residences, and isolation of patients and anyone who had been in contact with them.

Dr. Hagen claimed that the living conditions at the prison and the treatment of the disease were indicative of what the ghetto would probably face, since the living conditions in both places were similar and, therefore, the methods of treatment should follow suit. However, he realized that the results attained at the prison could not be duplicated in the ghetto, because the procedures could not be fully implemented in the Jewish quarter and because the Jewish population would resist the coercive treatments, which were intolerable. The Jews attempted to conceal typhus patients to avoid the two or three-week quarantine of their homes, which would prevent them from going to work and buying food. With

25 Gutman, *The Jews of Warsaw*, p. 110.

26 Rom, "Mahalot Hayeladim Begeto Varsha," p. 15.

the arrival of additional refugees in the ghetto, it was clear that it would be impossible to prevent and restrain the spread of lice and of typhus under the overcrowded conditions. Nevertheless, Hagen thought all classical measures against lice and typhus should be taken in the ghetto to mitigate the possibility of infecting the population on the outside.[27]

In January 1941, Dr. Hagen arrived in Warsaw to succeed Dr. Schrempf in his post. Recognizing the first signs of an outbreak of typhus, he opposed relocating refugees from other areas to the ghetto, but his opinion was not accepted. Those in charge of public health in Warsaw had planned to inoculate 500 refugees every day but found themselves treating 1,000 people, if not more, and the system broke down.[28] In early January 1941, typhus patients were found only in the Jewish quarter, which provided Hagen with a justification for the isolation of the Jews to prevent the spread of typhus to the Polish population. He changed his view in June 1941, when it became clear that the number of typhus patients in the ghetto was rising considerably with each passing month. He demanded the disinfection, delousing, and two-week quarantine of the many refugees who were arriving in the ghetto, but there was not enough room in the isolation houses to accommodate all the new arrivals. Until April 1941, squads of Poles and Jews participated in the war on the epidemic. Thereafter, the Judenrat employed about 300 people, including doctors, disinfection workers, and police, to carry out disinfection operations and other actions to fight the typhus epidemic.[29] At the same time, it was necessary to close almost all the internal medicine departments in order to hospitalize typhus patients, and a new department, headed by Dr. Abraham Paweł Lipsztat, was opened to admit the masses of patients.[30]

In the opinion of the scientists in the ghetto, the classical method of eradicating the epidemic—delousing, disinfection,

27 Cohen, "Harefu'a Besherut Ha'idiologiya," pp. 168–170.

28 Roland, *Courage under Siege*, pp. 134–135.

29 Cohen, "Harefu'a Besherut Ha'idiologiya," pp. 169–170.

30 Dr. Henry Fenigstein testimony, "Varshever yid," YVA, O.33/1074, p. 9. The department was set up at 109 Leszno St.

isolation—adopted by the Germans to deal with it in the ghetto was fundamentally wrong. Prof. Hirszfeld, Judenrat Chairman Czerniaków, and Dr. Israel Milejkowski, head of the Judenrat Health Department, sent memoranda to the Germans in which they explained the weaknesses of the German policy in the war on epidemics and proposed ameliorating measures. They claimed that the Germans were relying on scientific literature and attempting to quash the disease by means of disinfection teams that engaged in mass delousing, but that the difficulty lay not in reducing the population of lice, but in wiping it out altogether. The well-known German epidemiologist Paul Martini claimed that the real challenge was to kill more lice than were being bred, which could be accomplished by taking the radical action of allowing all the ghetto residents to change and launder their clothes once a week. This would induce mortality among the lice and cause them to retreat spontaneously. Fighting lice by means of remedies and orders from the police was suitable for institutions or closed groups, but not for civilians and masses of people. Evicted from place to place, the Jews had become wretched refugees who were swarming with lice and were too exhausted to deal with them. Gathered together in the ghetto, those who arrived infested with lice mingled with people from clean locations.

Before the war, the city Jews did not contract typhus, which was mainly a disease of the peasants in the villages. However, when the war broke out and the ghetto was established, the Jews became ill with typhus, owing to the Germans' misguided methods to eradicate the disease. The authorities termed typhus a "Jewish disease," which was totally unfounded. They could just as well have called it a "German disease," because it was linked to the German occupation. While it would be an overstatement to blame the German medical system for the outbreak of typhus in the ghetto, the reason for the epidemic did stem from the Germans' modus operandi.[31] In late November and early December 1940, during

31 Hirszfeld, *The Story of One Life*, p. 211; Szac-Wajnkranc, *Halaf Im Ha'esh*, pp. 35–36. See also a memoranda about methods used to fight the epidemic, which was evidently addressed to the Germans and probably written by Hirszfeld, YVA, M.10.AR.1/85; Offer, *Haluk Lavan Bageto*, appendix A.2, pp. 497–504.

the first month of ghettoization, the Germans conducted a sanitary inspection of all the buildings to ensure that there were no typhus patients there and found no incidence of the disease. However, in the Polish quarter, where Jews no longer lived, cases of typhus surfaced every day.

According to Ringelblum, "The theory that the Jews were carriers of the typhus bacteria was utterly useless."[32] Although typhus had not reached epidemic proportions in the first months after ghettoization, it had triggered much panic.[33] However, the harsh winter of 1940–1941[34] and the new influx of refugees to the ghetto in February–March 1941 contributed to a new and fierce outbreak of the disease. From the spring to the autumn of 1941, the epidemic assumed ghastly dimensions. In 1941, 15,449 cases were recorded compared with 1,758 in 1940. The actual number of cases in 1941 was approximately 38,000.[35] Due to the overcrowding in the ghetto streets, there was a risk of bumping into lice-infested people and spreading lice by mere contact. Solicitors, musicians, singers, jugglers, and beggars congregated at the peddlers' stands, blocking the way. These passageways were breeding grounds for the typhus epidemic, which spread in the ghetto because of the hunger, deprivation, cold, overcrowding, and filth, claiming more and more victims. The dead were gathered in the streets and placed in mass graves, and their clothing was sold, causing the epidemic to spread and escalate even more.[36]

In June 1941, about seven months after ghettoization, the menace of epidemics in various parts of the ghetto intensified. The main cause was the lice that infested clothing, which they could not get rid of under the conditions of the ghetto.[37] Typhus spread aggressively that month, bringing about the quarantine of

32 Ringelblum, *Yoman Vereshimot*, pp. 200–201, 211. Ringelblum claimed that the reason for this was that the Poles ate a great deal of fruit, whereas the Jews had access to very little fruit at the time.

33 Ibid., p. 245.

34 Trunk, "Epidemics and Mortality," pp. 96–97.

35 Kermish, "Nigudim Ma'amadiyim," p. 566.

36 Turkow, *Hayo Hayta Varsha Yehudit*, pp. 41–44.

37 Berg, *The Diary of Mary Berg*, p. 66.

280 residential buildings, as well as many offices. When the Jews had to move out, the epidemic surged again,[38] raging throughout the ghetto in July 1941. The doctors lacked the means to cope with the growing number of deaths. Medicines were in short supply and the hospitals were bursting at the seams. Adding beds brought no relief because the number of patients increased from day to day. A "No Space Available" sign was posted on an office window at Czyste Hospital. Bersohn and Bauman Children's Hospital was also full of young typhus patients of all ages and, lacking space, could not admit more.[39] More and more buildings were marked with yellow signs, warning *Fleckfieber* (typhus). The disease struck the poor, in particular, at the overnight shelters, where masses of refugees were housed. The hospitals were converted into special facilities for infectious diseases. Hundreds died and the cemetery could not accommodate them all. "Typhus swarmed everywhere, threatening from every direction; together with hunger, it became the omnipotent master of the ghetto," Marek Edelman wrote.[40]

Typhus spread with particular ferocity in the vicinity of the streets Gęsia, Nalewki, and Nowolipie. Things were slightly better in the "small ghetto," where people were relatively affluent and could afford private medical care.[41] The disease also took a grave toll on the staff of the Oneg Shabbat Archive, who worked with thousands of refugees and people who returned from the forced labor camps—the main carriers of typhus to the population. None of the employees were vaccinated, because they could not afford the high price, and many died of the disease.[42] Several doctors and medical personnel were infected with typhus.[43] The sanitary conditions of the patients were poor. Nurses often found lice under the bandages of the injured and the ill, and the children's bodies and hair swarmed with lice. When the Jewish police began

38 Ringelblum, *Notes from the Warsaw Ghetto*, p. 191.
39 Berg, *The Diary of Mary Berg*, p. 75.
40 Edelman, *The Ghetto Fights*, p. 27.
41 Berg, *The Diary of Mary Berg*, p. 76.
42 Ringelblum, *Ktavim Aharonim*, pp. 9–10.
43 Lensky, *A Physician inside the Warsaw Ghetto*, p. 81.

to get involved in stanching the spread of the epidemic, they too contracted the illness and many died.[44]

In late July 1941, Mary Berg wrote that crowds of beggars congregated on Grzybowska St., where the largest soup kitchen in the ghetto, which was funded by the Judenrat, was located. People who lived on this street were especially hard-hit by typhus, and there were several patients in every building.[45] Those who recovered from typhus shaved their heads to keep their hair from falling out, and women wearing kerchiefs wrapped like turbans were common sights on the ghetto streets.[46] In August 1941, Ringelblum wrote,

> Next to hunger, typhus is the question that is most generally absorbing for the Jewish populace. It has become the burning question of the hour. The graph line of typhus cases keeps climbing. For example, now, the middle of August, there are some six or seven thousand patients in [private] apartments, and about nine hundred in hospitals.[47]

The official number of cases reported that month was 1,805.[48] At the end of that month, Ringelblum wrote that the count had doubled to 70–80 each day. In total, typhus had struck 900 of the 1,400 buildings in the ghetto.[49] In August 1941, *Neged Hazerem* (Against the Current), the underground newspaper of the Hashomer Hatza'ir youth movement, reported that the epidemic had spread mainly where there were concentrations of refugees, claiming thousands of victims per month. The Judenrat made desperate efforts to isolate and disinfect affected apartments and buildings.[50]

In late August 1941, the prognosis for the winter was that the disease would progress with full force. The doctors estimated

44 Roland, *Courage under Siege*, p. 137.
45 Berg, *The Diary of Mary Berg*, p. 80.
46 Ibid., p. 92.
47 Ringelblum, *Notes from the Warsaw Ghetto*, p. 194.
48 Roland, *Courage under Siege*, p. 137.
49 Ringelblum, *Notes from the Warsaw Ghetto*, pp. 195–196.
50 Blatman, *Geto Varsha—Sipur Itona'i*, p. 152.

that one Jew in five would be infected, and some estimates even cited one in two. There were rumors that the ghetto population would be transferred out of Warsaw to eliminate the peril of typhus.[51] In September 1941, the ghetto residents were overcome with anguish because of the increasing number of typhus patients in every family.[52] Late that month, Berg wrote that the epidemic had ballooned to more than 500 cases per day, adding that while the Judenrat Health Department did what it could to counter the epidemic, the number of deaths grew, due to the shortage of medicines and hospital beds.[53] In mid-October 1941, as typhus continued to spread, Czerniaków wrote that the entire staff of the burial department, including himself and his wife, had contracted the fatal disease.[54]

In October–November 1941, 5,894 cases of typhus were reported as compared with 39 during the same period in 1940.[55] In November 1941, one of the underground newspapers of the left-wing Po'alei Tziyon Party *Awangarda Młodzieży* noted that while the number of new typhus cases was difficult to assess, various estimates cited thousands each week.[56] According to the Bund and Zukunft newspaper *Za Nąsza i Waszą Wolność*, 1,971 people came down with typhus in December 1941—1,502 were hospitalized and 469 were treated at home—and in 515 buildings, half of the total, there were typhus patients among the residents.[57] Dr. Hagen wrote that on July 4, 1941, 578 typhus patients were hospitalized in Czyste Hospital and their numbers grew by 50 each day. At the time, he claimed that there were around 3,000 new cases daily and he believed that only one in five cases was reported to the hospital.[58]

51 Ringelblum, *Notes from the Warsaw Ghetto*, pp. 196, 218.
52 Berg, *The Diary of Mary Berg*, p. 83.
53 Ibid., p. 92.
54 Czerniaków, *The Warsaw Diary*, p. 290. Czerniaków also mentioned a widespread theory that not only infected lice but also their excretions, which were dispersed in the air, transmitted the disease. Indeed, Hirszfeld wrote about this theory in his memoirs.
55 Ibid., p. 310.
56 Blatman, *Geto Varsha—Sipur Itona'i*, p. 155.
57 Ibid., p. 172.
58 Roland, *Courage under Siege*, p. 221.

In September 1941, Ringelblum wrote that the vast majority of the typhus patients had gone into hiding and the number of unknown cases was thought to be 4,000–5,000. German sanitation officials estimated their overall number at 14,000.[59] According to some doctors in the ghetto, the actual count of typhus patients was five times the official figure.[60] Dr. Henry Fenigstein wrote in his memoir that 15 percent of the ghetto population contracted typhus, but only 5 percent was cited in the official report to the Germans. Fearing the disinfection that they would have to undergo as a result, many failed to report it.[61]

According to data on morbidity from a study by Jewish doctors in the Warsaw ghetto, 20,399 cases of typhus were reported from January 1940 to November 1942.[62] Given that these data were drawn from reports that the Judenrat statistics department had submitted to the Germans, they presumably do not reflect the actual total number of ill. Israel Gutman wrote that in the course of 1941, 14,661 cases of typhus were recorded but, presumably, only one-fourth to one-third of the cases were known. The patients and their relatives were afraid to report the contagious disease because of the consequent sanctions that their homes would face. Doctors sometimes collaborated in concealing cases and, in other instances, it was impossible to diagnose the disease, especially when the disease struck people who were severely enfeebled by hunger disease.[63] Even if we accept the low estimate of the number of patients who were concealed and unreported—around 5,000—the ratio is estimated at about eight hidden or unreported cases for every five reported. By implication, if 15,449 cases were reported in 1941, another 22,700 were unreported, which brings the total that year to 38,150. It should be noted that the number of typhus

59 Ringelblum, *Notes from the Warsaw Ghetto*, pp. 218–219.

60 Trunk, "Epidemics and Mortality," p. 96; report by an anonymous doctor on the war on typhus, March 1942, AŻIH, ARI.363; see also Offer, *Haluk Lavan Begeto*, appendix A.1, pp. 492–496.

61 See Dr. Henry Fenigstein testimony, "Varshever yid," YVA, O.33/1074, p. 10.

62 Winick, *Hunger Disease*, p. 35.

63 Gutman, *The Jews of Warsaw*, p. 110.

cases reported in all of Poland before the war was 1,640 in 1930 and 4,149 in 1935.[64]

A March 1942 report by the Judenrat statistics department provided exact figures on morbidity and mortality from typhus in 1940–1941 and early 1942. The data show that the typhus epidemic first appeared in January–May 1940 and began to ebb about five months before ghettoization, evidently disappearing totally in August–December 1940. From January 1940 onward, in the first months of ghettoization, it spread again, peaking in October 1941 and then retreating.[65]

Typhus Morbidity in Warsaw, 1940, 1941, 1942[66]

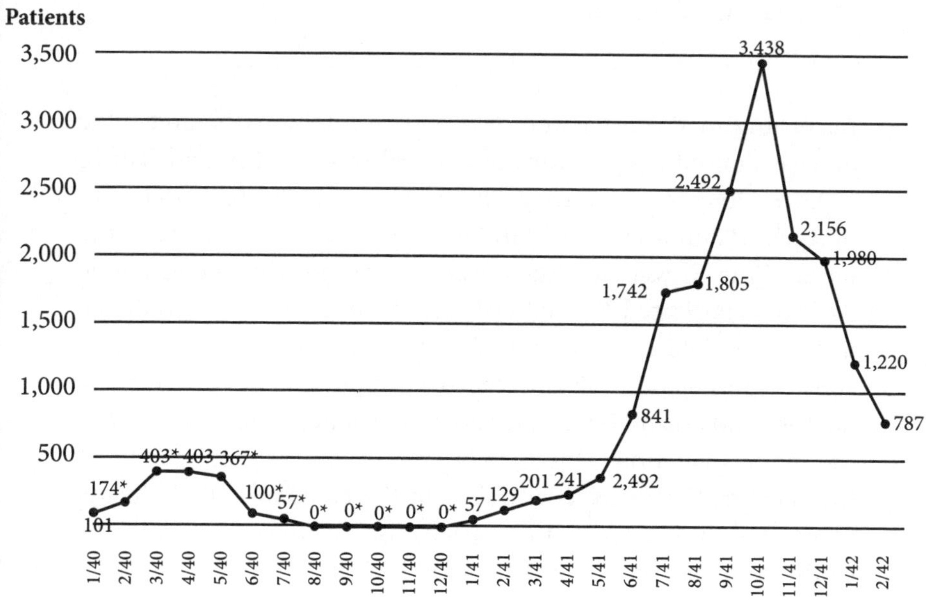

64 Trunk, "Epidemics and Mortality," p. 97.

65 Judenrat Statistics Department Report, no. 29, March 17, 1942, GFH, no. 11250, p. 1.

66 Ibid. The data for 1940 that are marked with an asterisk are approximations based on the original graph.

Morbidity, January–February 1942, as Compared with the 1941 Monthly Average[67]

	Monthly Average 1941	January 1942	February 1942
Hospitalized Patients	2,033	1,707	1,633
Infectious Diseases	1,479	1,188	967
Typhus Patients	1,287	1,220	784
Typhus Patients Treated at Home	512[68]	337	195
Hospital Mortality	410	368	363
Hospital Mortality from Typhus	132	134	96

According to the foregoing data and to additional sources, the disease showed a significant downward trend in the first half of 1942: 1,220 cases in January, 787 in February, 478 in March, 319 in April, 208 in May, and 67 in July.[69] From June 1942, close to the onset of the *Grossaktion*, there were indications that the epidemic had been eradicated.[70] Specifically in the winter, when the epidemic usually escalated, the typhus plague in Jewish Warsaw abated considerably—about 40 percent—as reported by pharmacies, doctors, and hospital staff. This does not stand to reason and defies rational explanation. One possible reason is that most people at the shelters, the main focal points of the epidemics, had already contracted the disease. Some also surmise that the poor wore thick clothing in the winter, which made it difficult for lice to reach their bodies.[71]

67 Ibid., p. 2.
68 Ibid. Registration began only in October 1941.
69 Trunk, "Epidemics and Mortality," p. 97.
70 Gutman, *The Jews of Warsaw*, p. 111.
71 Ringelblum, *Notes from the Warsaw Ghetto*, p. 230.

According to Dr. Tursz, the course of this epidemic followed the progression typical of all epidemics. After cresting, morbidity declined as patients either acquired immunity or were less severely infected.[72] Lensky wrote that the doctors were astonished to see the epidemic cease even though sanitary conditions had not improved. In terms of epidemiology, it seems that there are limits to epidemics, even when they erupt under poor sanitary conditions.[73] Prof. Hirszfeld confirmed that the epidemic began to recede spontaneously for some strange reason, after one-third to one-half of the residents had contracted the disease. The reason for this, in his opinion, is that the workers' quarters and refugee dwellings had high rates of contagion—up to 100 percent—meaning that this entire population, which was at the epicenter of the epidemic, had already been infected and the epidemic receded there. It reemerged in the ghetto and progressed after the *Grossaktion* in late October 1942. Most of the Jews in the ghetto had been deported by then, leaving behind about 500 typhus patients, who were treated in November 1942 at the alternative Jewish hospital that was established after the liquidation of the ghetto.[74] Outside the ghetto, the number of typhus cases in 1940 did not exceed 200, although the population was three times as large as that of the ghetto. The typhus epidemic on the Aryan side began to spread in February 1941, but it was much less severe than it was in the ghetto.[75]

According to Lensky, the mortality rate of typhus was higher than that of any other disease. Although seemingly low—15 percent of those who developed the disease—the large-scale spread of the illness and the Nazis' cruel approach to the disease caused distress and crisis among the Jewish population.[76] Dr. Rom (Rotbalsam) claimed that mortality from typhus was high and that it peaked in

72 Dr. Moshe Tursz testimony, YVA, O.3/438, p. 14.

73 Lensky, *A Physician inside the Warsaw Ghetto*, p. 104.

74 Ringelblum, *Yoman Vereshimot*, p. 404; Lewin, *A Cup of Tears*, p. 198; Blatman, *Geto Varsha—Sipur Itona'i*, p. 431; Roland, *Courage under Siege*, p. 93; Lensky, "Problems of Disease in the Warsaw Ghetto," pp. 282–293.

75 Trunk, "Epidemics and Mortality," p. 97; Berg, *Warsaw Ghetto*, pp. 92–93; Czerniaków, *The Diary of Mary Berg*, p. 193; Offer, "Ma'arach Harefu'a Begeto Varsha," vol. 2, appendix B.22, p. 176.

76 Lensky, *A Physician inside the Warsaw Ghetto*, p. 101.

February 1942 at 20 percent of the cases.[77] There is a connection between physical condition and physical immunity and resilience to bacteria at the point of illness. Therefore, during the first wave in 1940, the death rate from typhus was about 10 percent of the cases; in 1941, it is believed to have been twice as high.[78] In the course of 1941, 4,920 people died in Czyste Hospital; 3,171 of them succumbed to contagious diseases, including 1,580 from typhus. The ensuing death counts in 1942 were 220 in January, 119 in February, 80 in March, and 11 in June. Of 3,130 patients in the second half of 1942, 512 died—16.3 percent. In 1941, the death rate was 11.3 percent. The reason for the upturn in 1942 was the population's weak immune system, as well as the poor diet, a problem that only worsened and claimed the lives of many typhus patients during convalescence.[79]

According to the typhus mortality data that appear in the aforementioned study on hunger by Jewish doctors in the ghetto, from January 1940 to November 1942, 2,724 Jews died of typhus—only 3 percent of all deaths. About one-fourth of all typhus patients died of the disease. Most deaths were due to starvation. Mortality from typhus was much lower.[80] Dr. Hagen estimated that typhus was the cause of 8–10 percent of mortality in the ghetto.[81] According to the Judenrat statistics department report from March 1942, 132 people per month, on average, died from typhus in 1941—roughly one-third of all hospital deaths in the ghetto. In January 1942, 134 of 368 deaths at the hospital were from typhus, slightly over one-third. In February, typhus accounted for 96 out of 363 deaths at the hospital—roughly one in four. Thus, the monthly average was around one-third in early 1942, although the difference between January and February indicates a sizable decrease, evidently due to the waning of the epidemic in 1942.[82]

77 Rom, "Mahalot Hayeladim Begeto Varsha," p. 15.
78 Trunk, "Epidemics and Mortality," p. 97.
79 Ibid.
80 Winick, *Hunger Disease*, p. 35.
81 Browning, "Genocide and Public Health," p. 25.
82 Judenrat Statistics Department Report, no. 29, March 17, 1942, GFH, no. 11250, p. 2. The graph on the following page is based on the data in this source.

Deaths from Typhus among All Hospital Deaths in the Ghetto[83]

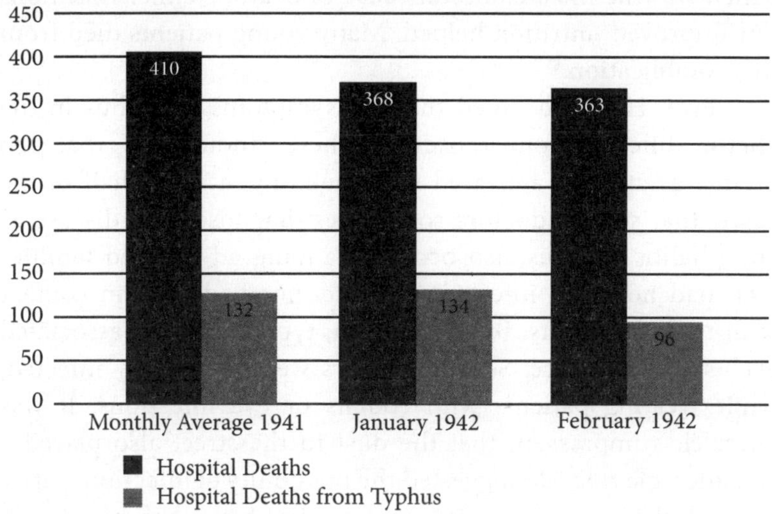

One of the survivors documented her illness: a 40-degree fever, rash, and prostration for two weeks. When she recovered, she had to learn to walk all over again and had lost her will to live. Another survivor's predominant memory of the disease in the ghetto were his bizarre hallucinations, high fever, and total exhaustion. Although only a minority of typhus patients went to the hospital for treatment, Czyste Hospital was always full of these patients. In 1942, during the second eruption of typhus, most hospital wards were crowded with people who had developed infectious diseases.

The symptoms of typhus in the ghetto were unusual. Among patients who suffered hunger disease as well as typhus, the typical symptom of high fever rarely appeared. Some patients reported abdominal pains and the illness was misdiagnosed as appendicitis. The heartbeat of a typhus patient occasionally was difficult to detect, because the disease also affected the myocardium.[84] The nature of the epidemic in the ghetto was particularly harsh. In many cases, during the second week of the disease, the patient's blood pressure suddenly dropped, sometimes resulting in renal

83 Ibid.

84 Roland, *Courage under Siege*, p. 131.

failure (uremia) and shock, concurrently with encephalitis, which was the most common cause of death. Neither injections nor improved nutrition helped. Many young patients died from this complication.[85]

Prof. Hirszfeld noted that the symptoms of typhus in the ghetto differed from those elsewhere. Indications that the brain was affected appeared so frequently, in about half of the cases, that several doctors sometimes diagnosed the disease as encephalitis. Typhus also occurred among advantaged families who had not been infested with lice, nor had been in contact with typhus patients. By implication, typhus was not associated exclusively with lice. Several doctors were apparently infected, while treating patients with coughs or eye infections. It was Hirszfeld's impression that the dust in the street also played a considerable role. He suggested the possibility of infection, partly through the lungs, nose, or eyes, from lice feces that mixed with the dust on the streets.[86]

It is noteworthy that Ringelblum wrote in September 1941 that the course of the disease among the simple masses was relatively mild. Most of those infected actually died in the convalescence stage, when the food that they required was not available. In contrast, those who were in better condition often suffered complications, especially in the brain, which resulted in death in many cases.[87] According to Dr. Einhorn, the mortality rate among people of relatively sturdy body build was higher than among people of ordinary build, but he offered no possible explanation for this.[88] Ringelblum noted that typhus was particularly dangerous for members of the upper social class, who died because they could not fight it off. The phenomenon of high mortality among the intelligentsia had been observed during World War I as well.[89]

85 Lensky, "*A Physician inside the Warsaw Ghetto*," p. 96; Rom, "Mahalot Hayeladim Begeto Varsha," p. 15.

86 Hirszfeld, *A Story of One Life*, p. 226.

87 Ringelblum, *Notes from the Warsaw Ghetto*, pp. 218–219.

88 Einhorn, "Harofe Begeto Varsha," p. 11.

89 Ringelblum, *Notes from the Warsaw Ghetto*, pp. 194–197.

The rates of death from typhus were lower in refugee centers than elsewhere.[90] Czerniaków wrote in early October 1941, "Typhus is raging….Friends and acquaintances are dying all around me—all of them members of the intelligentsia."[91] Rich and poor alike died of typhus, but the death rate among the affluent was higher.[92] A disinfection worker wrote the following remarks in his memoir, after visiting one of the refugee centers:

> Not only the overcrowding, not only the poverty, but also their [the refugees'] poor mental state caused the terrible epidemic to break out. Within a few days, they reached their lowest point. Everyone was hopeless, depressed, and utterly despondent. This is the root of all evil. One group's melancholia passed immediately to others. Three factors contributed to the spread of the epidemic: overcrowding, poverty, and, most importantly, loss of hope. I don't know if anyone is able to describe or write the history of the development of typhus.[93]

Typhus vaccines were smuggled into the ghetto for as long as the ghetto existed. They were not always of good quality and were too expensive for most of the population. Its coffers depleted, the Judenrat could not buy enough vaccines.[94] However, people in prominent positions who had influence were evidently able to obtain them. For example, Czerniaków and his wife were vaccinated several times between December 1939 and February 1942.[95] Mary Berg wrote about a family member who recovered from his illness, due to the injection of a powerful serum into his blood.[96]

90 Trunk, "Epidemics and Mortality," p. 97.

91 Czerniaków, *The Warsaw Diary*, p. 305.

92 Lensky, *A Physician inside the Warsaw Ghetto*, p. 96.

93 Memoir of a member of a disinfection team, AŻIH, ARI.268.

94 Dr. Israel Rom (Rotbalsam) testimony, YVA, O.3/2357; Einhorn, "Harofe Begeto Varsha," p. 11.

95 Czerniaków, *The Warsaw Diary*, pp. 96, 274, 324.

96 Berg, *The Diary of Mary Berg*, p. 108.

In July 1941, when doses of the typhus vaccine arrived from Lwów, which the Germans had occupied the previous month, immunization of the population by means of the "Weigl vaccination" began.[97] Prof. Rudolf Weigl, a world-renowned scientist and the inventor of an important vaccine against typhus, saw to it that it was smuggled into the Warsaw ghetto and thus saved many lives.[98] When the Soviets retreated from Lwów, they left behind tubes of anti-virus serum in a large warehouse, which were smuggled to Warsaw. However, only the wealthy could afford them at thousands of zlotys per dose. Some ghetto residents received mail parcels from Switzerland that contained all sorts of medicines, especially anti-typhus serum. The Swiss medication was better than the Soviet one.[99] The International Committee of the Red Cross also sent a vaccine called Moserschen and officially demanded that it be administered only under the supervision of Prof. Hirszfeld.[100]

The initial price of the vaccine, 400 zlotys, zoomed to 900 zlotys and higher as the epidemic escalated. Hirszfeld believed that two people could be immunized with one dose, as was indeed the practice in the ghetto. However, it turned out that many of

97 Report on war on typhus, March 1942, AŻIH, AR.363.

98 Anolik, "Rofim Polanim Hasidei Umot Ha'olam." In addition to helping to smuggle the anti-typhus compound into the Warsaw ghetto, Prof. Weigl concealed a Jewish family in his home, for which he was awarded the title of Righteous Among the Nations; see Arthur Allen, *The Fantastic Laboratory of Dr. Weigl: How Two Brave Scientists Battled Typhus and Sabotaged the Nazis* (New York: W. W. Norton & Company, Inc., 2014), http://www.amazon.com/dp/039308101X/?tag=slatmaga-20"; see also the excerpt in Allen, "Killing in the Name of Cleanliness: The Shocking Stupidity and Brutality of Nazi Doctors' Response to Typhus," *Slate*, August 5, 2014, http://www.slate.com/articles/health_and_science/science/2014/08/typhus_and_lice_in_jewish_ghettos_nazi_doctors_perverse_groupthink.html.

99 Berg, *The Diary of Mary Berg*, pp. 76–77. There is correspondence detailing how the medicines and vaccines reached their destination from Switzerland. See, for example, JDC, AR.33–44, file 840; GFH, nos. 1933, 4102, 21352. The use of the word "serum" usually refers to "passive immunization," in which antibodies are injected, as opposed to active immunization, in which the pathogen or one of its components is injected to stimulate an immune response. In some sources, there may be a lack of clarity in the use of these terms.

100 Hirszfeld, *The Story of One Life*, p. 209.

the vaccine doses in the ghetto were counterfeit. Before buying a portion, people would hand it over to Dr. Bronisława Fejgin[101] to verify that it contained the Rickettsia bacterium. It was difficult to determine the results obtained by using the vaccine in a smaller than standard quantity. Many people who received the full dose became ill. According to Helena Szereszewska, it was known that the vaccines did not prevent the illness but merely alleviated its progression, and many who were immunized died of the disease. It is important to note that the Germans gave the official in charge of the war on typhus a quantity of Behring, which was used to inoculate members of the disinfection teams and the guard unit of the anti-epidemic committee.[102]

The serum trade infuriated the ghetto inhabitants. Several people were involved in smuggling vaccines. Berg described a young man who looked Aryan—without evidently Jewish features—and who often went to the Aryan side of Warsaw through underground tunnels. Posing as a Pole and holding a counterfeit ID card, he obtained a permit to travel to Lwów, where he bought ampules of the typhus vaccine, paying for them with an advance provided by wealthy individuals for this purpose. His trips were highly dangerous, but immensely profitable.[103] In mid-September 1941, Ringelblum wrote that in addition to the serum that had arrived from Weigl's institute in Lwów, doses stolen from the German hospitals had reached the ghetto. The ghetto inhabitants tried to cope with the typhus problem in various ways, besides vaccination. For example, they walked about with camphor or other chemical substances, so that the acrid smell would drive away the lice. Some spread Lysol and similar disinfectants on their bodies. People stopped allowing the lice-infested beggars

101 Dr. Bronisława Fejgin (1893–1943) was a bacteriologist in Warsaw. During the occupation, she was the director of the Chemical-Bacteriological Institute of the Judenrat. She was killed in January 1943 during the mass murders in the Warsaw ghetto. See Wulman et al., *The Martyrdom of Jewish Physicians in Poland*, p. 339.

102 Report by an anonymous doctor on the war on typhus, March 1942, AŻIH, ARI.363; Ringelblum, *Notes from the Warsaw Ghetto*, pp. 218–219; Szereszewska, *Memoirs*, p. 29. On the war on typhus, see Chapter 9 of this book.

103 Berg, *The Diary of Mary Berg*, pp. 76–77.

to enter their apartments.[104] Prof. Hirszfeld, who had spent many years in Poland administering vaccines against diphtheria, tested the vaccine materials brought into the ghetto and found that they did not provide protection against typhus.[105]

Children's Diseases at Bersohn and Bauman Children's Hospital

Contagious diseases spread, infecting the children in the ghetto as well. Over a five-month period, from the onset of the occupation in September 1939 to early 1940, about 400 youngsters under the age of thirteen who had contracted typhoid fever were hospitalized in Bersohn and Bauman Children's Hospital. Immunization campaigns stanched the epidemic among children, as it did among adults.[106]

Beginning in the spring of 1941, with the surge of the second wave of typhus, the children's hospital treated approximately 1,000 youngsters who had come down with the disease. This made it possible to confirm the well-known fact that the course of typhus was milder among children than among adults. Children's blood pressure usually fell only slightly, if at all; there was almost no uremia; and encephalitis was rare. Mortality was low and many of the children did not require hospitalization. The rash among children mostly was not visible and was mainly on the limbs, and not on the torso, as was typical among adults. Infants rarely developed typhus. However, the cases of those who did were usually very serious, resulting in high infant mortality. Typhus often brought on septicemia or toxicosis, which developed into severe cases of poisoning, now known as septic shock, which usually ended in death.[107]

104 Ringelblum, *Notes from the Warsaw Ghetto*, pp. 218–219.

105 Hirszfeld, *The Story of One Life*, p. 209.

106 Rom, "Mahalot Hayeladim Begeto Varsha," p. 15; Einhorn, "Harofe Begeto Varsha," p. 10; Yehudit Braude testimony, YVA, O.3/2360; Dr. Israel Rom (Rotbalsam) testimony, YVA, O.3/2357.

107 Rom, "Mahalot Hayeladim Begeto Varsha," pp. 15–16.

Dr. Adina Blady Szwajger, who worked in the typhus ward at Bersohn and Bauman Children's Hospital, noted that mortality among children with typhus was not high. However, there was an acute shortage of beds and, consequently, two and sometimes even three children, each with a number pasted on his or her forehead, shared one bed. They suffered from high fever and incessantly asked for water. Since hardly any of them died, they were sent home, very frail, although it was known that they might die of starvation or suffer a slow death caused by hunger edema. The same number of children discharged from the hospital was admitted to the hospital daily. [108]

As stated, the progression of typhus was milder among children than among adults. However, 15–20 percent of young typhus patients showed signs of brain damage, which was practically always fatal. Quite a few patients also died of pneumonia, due to the harsh conditions. Prof. Hirszfeld wrote that other pediatric diseases—diphtheria, scarlet fever, rubella, and so on—were uncommon. In the ghetto's first year, whooping cough was widespread. Interestingly, diphtheria and scarlet fever were most common among children from Germany, while local youngsters tended to be immune and, therefore, they were not inoculated against diphtheria.[109]

Dr. Adina Blady Szwajger recalled that one of the children came down with a strange disease that caused him to lose control of his arms and legs. A neurologist who examined him could not reach a diagnosis. As the boy helplessly screamed in agony, someone had the idea of putting a pencil between the child's constricted fingers and placing a piece of paper in front of him. The boy fell silent and even smiled. He then was given a piece of chalk, and he began to draw images from memory, as well as from his immediate observations. Among other things, he sketched a German soldier handing candy to a child.[110]

108 Blady Szwajger, *I Remember Nothing More*, pp. 33–34.
109 Hirszfeld, *The Story of One Life*, p. 226.
110 Blady Szwajger, *I Remember Nothing More*, p. 35.

Dr. Blady Szwajger also remembered the first case of collective death—babies who had been brought in from a station for abandoned children. Starving, they died of a "posterior infection" in succession within a few weeks. Nutritional care and meticulous maintenance of skin cleanliness were useless.[111] She also described six children, aged four or five, who had lost their ability to speak and whose development had regressed.[112] The illnesses and tragic deaths of children at the ghetto hospital were described in a December 1941 edition of the newspaper *Biuletyn*.

> Fading away in bed, without saying a word, without emitting a sigh, silently dying a hospital death, a creature with a face of an old man—he too is a mere boy. He was distended when he arrived at the hospital. The distention passed and a mask of swollen skin peeled off the skeleton underneath, arms and legs like sticks not properly screwed in, eyes still alive, wide open, in his shriveled face. The distention is gone but the boy is dying. Maybe tomorrow, the day after, or maybe right away, in another moment, he will die, snuffed out like a candle. Indeed, this is how these children die, without the pathos of death—no tears, no kin, no complaint, no sigh. They simply fall asleep and someone, a doctor or a caregiver, steps over to their beds and determines their deaths.[113]

The children of the ghetto suffered from additional diseases, such as tuberculosis, meningitis, rickets, and malnutrition, as described below.

Tuberculosis

Tuberculosis is an infectious disease that spreads under conditions of overcrowding and malnutrition. It was the third epidemic that

111 Ibid., p. 29.
112 Ibid., p. 138.
113 Blatman, *Geto Varsha—Sipur Itona'i*, pp. 235–236.

swept through the ghetto in alarming proportions, affecting adults and children alike. It is difficult to present accurate data, because statistics were not maintained, particularly after the typhus epidemic erupted, when every death was attributed to typhus or starvation.[114] In Winick's estimation, the tuberculosis epidemic would have wiped out the ghetto population had the Nazis not begun the deportations.[115]

When the ghetto was established, there was a widespread tuberculosis epidemic. According to Dr. Einhorn, tuberculosis was found in 15 percent of the population at the very beginning of the ghetto period, including many cases that were in the initial active stage. The incidence of tuberculosis significantly increased, due to the severe hunger that afflicted the ghetto population. TOZ helped to transfer patients to the hospitals or to the sanatorium in Otwock. The rise in the number of pulmonary patients, the shortage of hospital beds, and the refusal of the Nazis to allow the transfer of tuberculosis patients in the ghetto to Otwock made it difficult to halt the epidemic.[116] In a report dated June 28, 1941, the Judenrat Health Department stated,

> The tuberculosis ward received patients in very serious, hopeless condition. They spend a short time with us and die. Most hope that we will save them but we are not able.... Tuberculosis is the most difficult disease under our conditions.[117]

People who were bloated due to hunger or who had recovered from contagious diseases were especially vulnerable to Mycobacterium tuberculosis. The illness struck adults and children alike.[118]

114 Tuberculosis was also widespread in the Łódź ghetto. See, for example, Yitzhak Saar, "Begeto Łódź" (In the Łódź Ghetto), in Dworzecki, *Hama'avak Lakiyum Velabriyut Biymei Hashoah*, p. 46.

115 Winick, "Jewish Medical Resistance," p. 98.

116 Einhorn, "Harofe Begeto Varsha," p. 12; Dr. Chaim Einhorn testimony, YVA, O.3/1836.

117 Health Department report on the fight against tuberculosis, June 28, 1941, AŻIH, ARI.214.

118 Dr. Moshe Tursz testimony, YVA, O.3/438, p. 14.

According to the Judenrat statistics department, the hospitals department began to shut down the typhus ward at Czyste Hospital in March 1942, following the orders of the authorities, and to convert the building into a tuberculosis hospital.[119] Given the acute incidence of TB among children, a special pediatric tuberculosis department had to be opened in 1942, headed by Dr. Anna Margolis.[120]

Dr. Einhorn wrote that the manifestations of tuberculosis encountered were particularly severe: infectious discharges and cavitary tuberculosis, resulting in massive pulmonary damage, which was terminal. Strains of exudative tuberculosis were encountered among children. In certain cases, mainly among those suffering from hunger edema along with overt and severe tuberculosis of the lungs, tuberculin testing yielded negative results.[121] It was possible to detect tuberculosis patients by their glistening eyes and the red blotches on their sunken cheeks, which are caused by high fever. These patients were sent to the X-ray department for imaging and photos. Too weak to stand, they were X-rayed sitting down, propped up on both sides. Many fainted while being examined and regained consciousness only after receiving an injection.[122]

Peretz Opochinsky wrote that a large proportion of children who arrived at the medical facilities already showed overt signs of tuberculosis.[123] Latent tuberculosis, which could only be detected in chest X-rays, was found in 12–15 percent of children and young people who appeared to be healthy. Some were found to have

119 Judenrat Statistics Department Report, no. 29, March 17, 1942, GFH, no. 11250, p. 10.

120 Rom, "Mahalot Hayeladim Begeto Varsha," p. 17. On tuberculosis among immigrants to Israel in the early years of the State of Israel, see Avraham Sternberg, *Behikalet Am* (Tel Aviv: Hakibbutz Hameuchad, 1973), pp. 124–136. Dr. Einhorn wrote that the high incidence of tuberculosis in the ghettos could be inferred indirectly from the results of the testing of the Holocaust survivors. Tuberculosis was found in almost 50 percent of the survivors of ghettos and camps; see Einhorn, "Harofe Begeto Varsha," pp. 11–12.

121 Einhorn, "Harofe Begeto Varsha," p. 12.

122 Lensky, *A Physician inside the Warsaw Ghetto*, p. 23.

123 Opochinsky, *Reshimot*, p. 104.

cavitary tuberculosis.[124] Most of the young tuberculosis patients at Bersohn and Bauman Children's Hospital were between the ages of seven and twelve. Before the war, pulmonary tuberculosis was observed in children of this age in the mildest forms. As hunger overtook the ghetto, the progression of the disease worsened and tuberculosis in advanced stages was diagnosed in these children. Starving children did not even develop high fever, which was usually a very ominous sign. The doctors tried to isolate patients with overt tuberculosis from those in the initial stages of tuberculosis, but soon children with latent tuberculosis reached the wards as well. The youngsters realized that this transition was an indication of looming death. After all, they had seen friends die, sometimes ten or more per day. There was no place to isolate moribund patients.[125]

Children were hospitalized for months on end, away from the brutal realities of the street. Under the existing conditions, there was no chance of recovering from tuberculosis. The patients were not allowed to go out to the garden lest they infect others.[126] Notwithstanding the white beds and the augmented food rations provided by the JDC, the medical profession was powerless against the spreading tide of deadly tuberculosis. When a child began to show signs of convalescence from hunger edema and even began to talk, his or her erythrocyte sedimentation rate (ESR) was checked. If it was found to be high, it was a sure sign that he or she had no more than six to eight days to live.[127] In the statistical records of deaths in the ghetto, exhaustion was usually registered as the cause. Tuberculosis was rarely recorded. Hunger had an enormous effect on the progression and spread of the disease. Those who died of tuberculosis had to be buried in coffins, because it was a contagious illness. Since few inhabitants of the ghetto could afford them, it was necessary to report a different official cause of death. The price of the required death certificate specifying exhaustion as the cause was lower than that of a coffin.

124 Hirszfeld, *The Story of One Life*, p. 225.

125 Ibid.; Rom, "Mahalot Hayeladim Begeto Varsha," p. 17.

126 Blatman, *Geto Varsha—Sipur Itona'i*, p. 236.

127 Blady Szwajger, *I Remember Nothing More*, p. 29.

As early as April 1940, Czerniaków reported cases of tuberculosis.[128] In February 1941, three months after ghettoization, Ringelblum wrote that the spread of tuberculosis posed a great danger to the Jews and that internment in a ghetto would heighten the threat of a widespread epidemic.[129] In November 1941, Czerniaków reported deaths from tuberculosis.[130]According to Trunk, the death toll from tuberculosis had increased tenfold since the beginning of the war: 387 in 1939, 754 in 1940, and 649 in the first two months of 1941. Based on this data, it is possible to estimate that about 3,900 Jews died of tuberculosis in 1941.[131]

The hunger researchers in the ghetto described tuberculosis as accompanying hunger disease. They wrote that a massive increase in cases of tuberculosis occurred during the war, evidently due to a lack of resilience among those suffering from hunger disease, a decline in oxidation, slowed blood circulation, less physical activity, and diminished physical energy. These factors impaired the immune system and, therefore, as noted above, the typical results of tuberculosis detection tests were not observed. Body temperature did not rise and tuberculin tests came out negative, making latent tuberculosis difficult to diagnose.[132]

Exhaustion

Dr. Lensky mentioned a disease unique to the ghetto—exhaustion. He described an acquaintance in the ghetto whose physical appearance changed radically for this reason. "His face grew more haggard from day to day, the hollows of his eyes growing wider and deeper until one day..."[133] Examining him, Lensky found no indications of cardiac, pulmonary, or other organic pathology; he detected only exhaustion. Nutrition was poor, of course, but it was

128 Czerniaków, *The Warsaw Diary*, p. 144.
129 Ringelblum, *Notes from the Warsaw Ghetto*, p. 131.
130 Czerniaków, *The Warsaw Diary*, p. 302.
131 Trunk, "Epidemics and Mortality," p. 121.
132 Winick, *Hunger Disease*, pp. 20–23.
133 Lensky, *A Physician inside the Warsaw Ghetto*, p. 71.

the breakdown of the nervous system, rather than hunger, that had caused both his physical and emotional collapse. Over time, doctors in the ghetto began to specify "exhaustion" on people's death certificates as the cause of death.[134]

Meningitis

Several months before ghettoization, Jews from small towns in the Warsaw area were rounded up and interned in ghettos. In one of these localities, Piaseczno, a meningitis epidemic broke out. Those affected were transferred to Bersohn and Bauman Children's Hospital. It seems that this led to a cerebrospinal meningitis epidemic among the children there, mainly before the ghetto was sealed.[135] The conventional treatment for this illness at the time was to administer a serum by intravenous injection.[136] Dr. Israel Rom (Rotbalsam) wrote that, in these cases, the ghetto physicians at first made use of chemotherapy, administering Daganan and sulphapyridine. Sometimes they administered Daganan in addition to an anti-serum, followed by oral doses of Daganan once every two or three days. The results of tests, conducted by drawing fluid by spinal tap, indicated the latter treatment was better than the combined serum–Daganan course of treatment.[137] Dr. Rom (Rotbalsam) noted that the ghetto physicians obtained these medications for research purposes at no charge from the Spiess pharmaceutical company in Switzerland. They submitted a report on the progression of the disease among fifty patients in the ghetto, which was published in the spring of 1940, omitting the researchers' names, because the Nazis banned the publication of studies by Jews.[138]

134 Ibid. There are reports on exhaustion in other studies on morbidity in the ghettos. See, for example, Dworzecki, "Tofa'ot Patologiyot Begeto Vilna," pp. 11, 34.
135 Rom, "Mahalot Hayeladim Begeto Varsha," p. 15.
136 Blady Szwajger, *I Remember Nothing More*, p. 23.
137 Rom, "Mahalot Hayeladim Begeto Varsha," p. 14.
138 Dr. Israel Rom (Rotbalsam) testimony, YVA, O.3/2357.

Rickets and Malnutrition

In December 1941, the underground newspaper of the left-wing Po'alei Tziyon Party *Awangarda Młodzieży* reported that the Jews of Warsaw were suffering from chronic malnutrition. The condition was more prominent among children, a large proportion of whom suffered from anemia and rickets. The ghetto population was physically enfeebled day by day.[139] Four months later, in April 1942, the Hashomer Hatza'ir newspaper described the Jewish population of Warsaw as chronically undernourished, which was evidenced in particular by the high incidence of rickets, tuberculosis, and anemia among the children. The stamina of both the children and the adults was steadily waning.[140]

Prof. Hirszfeld traced the cause of rickets to the lack of fats containing vitamin D in their diet. The illness was misdiagnosed initially as a neurological or muscular inflammation, and was treated as such. Soon, many people suffered disabling bone fractures. Treatment with edible oils, milk, eggs, and vitamin D supplements had a beneficial effect, but few could afford the cost.[141]

Mental Illness

In February 1940, about five months after the German occupation of Warsaw, Ringelblum reported a substantial rise in the number of cases of mental illness.[142] Shell shock and the distressing conditions in the ghetto appear to have had a detrimental effect on the mentally ill, compounded by the difficulties in obtaining medications for them. Mental illness was triggered among some

139 Blatman, *Geto Varsha—Sipur Itona'i*, p. 160.

140 Ibid., p. 168.

141 Hirszfeld, *Die Geschichte eines Lebens*, p. 147; Hirszfeld, *The Story of One Life*, p. 221. Dr. Yitzhak Saar wrote that rickets had struck most of the population of the Łódź ghetto, irrespective of age and sex. Everyone "goose-stepped," he said, due to vitamin D deficiency. They were unable to solve the problem completely; see Saar, "Begeto Łódź," p. 43.

142 Ringelblum, *Yoman Vereshimot*, pp. 75, 82.

ghetto inhabitants by the beatings inflicted on them by German soldiers. Two months before ghettoization, Ringelblum noted that the climate of war had affected many of the mentally ill, which was manifested in dangerous behavior that reflected their aggressive attitude toward the Germans. Conditions of care in mental institutions were so poor that there was often no choice but to send patients home, because of the lack of resources to provide for them.[143]

The severe mental conditions encountered in the ghetto included acute trauma and schizophrenia, which were treated with electric shock, insulin, and Cardiazol. Nurses injected patients with insulin, monitored hypoglycemia, and administered glucose. The psychiatric department in the ghetto apparently operated under camouflage, due to the fear that the Germans would murder the inpatients.[144]

Gastrointestinal Diseases

Gastrointestinal diseases were widespread in the ghetto. Most were the ordinary, well-known types, but there were also uncommon illnesses as well. In December 1939, a diarrhea epidemic erupted. Agonizingly severe diarrhea accompanied by fever claimed many lives, particularly among the elderly. One doctor tried to diagnose it as intestinal tuberculosis. It spread for no apparent reason and vanished the same way. Two years later, another disease that affected the large intestine spread. Diagnosed as colitis, it clinically presented symptoms similar to those of dysentery: mucus and blood

143 Ringelblum, *Notes from the Warsaw Ghetto*, pp. 35, 50–51, 131.

144 Koren, "Hasiyud Kehelek Misherutei Habriyut," p. 59. Very little has been written on the German policy regarding Jews with mental illness. Koren, "Hasiyud Kehelek Misherutei Habriyut," p. 59; see also R. Strous, "Extermination of the Jewish Mentally-Ill during the Nazi Era—The 'Doubly Cursed,' *The Israel Journal of Psychiatry and Related Sciences*, 45:4 (February 2008), pp. 247–256. On German policy regarding Jews with mental illness in the General Government, see Uzarczyk, "'Schluss mit der Rassenschande!'" On German policy regarding Jews with mental illness in the General Government, see Kamila Uzarczyk, "'Schluss mit der Rassenschande!'"

in the patient's stool, sudden collapse, and high mortality. Blood pressure appeared to plummet dramatically and without warning on the first or second day of the illness. The cause of the outbreak of this disease was also unknown. Some traced it to the contaminated food, which was brought into the ghetto in carts that were usually used to remove feces and garbage. This made sense, because the epidemic peaked in early 1942, when the ghetto sewage system froze over and was not functioning, and the inhabitants piled their trash in courtyards and streets. Since there were not enough carts, the carts used to transport food were used to remove trash as well.

About a month after the German occupation began, Czerniaków wrote that people who died of typhus and dysentery were buried in the cemetery.[145] However, according to Prof. Hirszfeld, gastrointestinal diseases, particularly typhoid fever and dysentery, were relatively uncommon. The immunization of most of the population might explain the low incidence of typhoid fever, but there is no known explanation for the small number of dysentery cases, given the abundance of risk factors.[146] Although the incidence of these diseases did not reach epidemic proportions, as Hirszfeld's testimony implied, people in the ghetto suffered from them. Dr. Korczak reported on the gastrointestinal diseases that children in his orphanage had contracted. Youngsters suffering from dysentery were hospitalized at Bersohn and Bauman Children's Hospital. Pails were placed in the wards during the night for the young patients who could not reach the latrines in time. The buckets were full the next day, which compounded the horrific stench of blood, pus, and feces.[147]

In June 1941, seven months after the ghetto was sealed, Ringelblum noted that despite the need to obtain dysentery vaccines, Czerniaków did not acquire the requisite funds of about 15,000 zlotys.[148] In July–September 1942, amid the *Grossaktion*, a dysentery epidemic broke out, with no remedy at hand. No one in the ghetto, including the members of the Jewish police,

145 Czerniaków, *The Warsaw Diary*, p. 87.
146 Hirszfeld, *A Story of One Life*, p. 226.
147 Roland, *Courage under Siege*, p. 172.
148 Ringelblum, *Notes from the Warsaw Ghetto*, p. 186.

was authorized to approach the former hospital building, which was situated in the Umschlagplatz—where the deportees were forced to wait in appalling conditions, before being packed into the trains.[149]

Other Illnesses

About two months after ghettoization, Ringelblum wrote that scabies had spread in the ghetto because of the shortage of soap.[150] Wilkinson ointment was used to treat the disease. The gray color of the ointment soiled the bedding, which was in limited supply, and could not be laundered and changed as frequently as required.[151] There were also cases of sundry skin diseases in the ghetto, as well as of venereal diseases, such as gonorrhea and syphilis. Some women returned from forced labor with acute infectious diseases. There were also incidences of trench fever, also called Volhynian fever.[152] The patients who were diagnosed with this disease experienced body temperature swings that lasted several months and never subsided altogether. The illness mainly affected the lungs and was often fatal.

Dr. Julian Fliederbaum noted that conditions such as tonsillitis, scarlet fever, measles, rheumatism,[153] and meningitis were very rare in the ghetto, but he did not provide any possible explanation. Asthma and other allergic diseases practically

149 Turkow, *Hayo Hayta Varsha Yehudit*, p. 121; Kermish, "Nigudim Ma'amadiyim," p. 566.

150 Ringelblum, *Notes from the Warsaw Ghetto*, p. 131. There were cases of scabies in other ghettos; see, for example, Dworzecki, "Tofa'ot Patologiyot Begeto Vilna," p. 10.

151 Based on the testimonies of G. Averbuch, Hermann, and Yaffe; see Koren, "Hasiyud Kehelek Misherutei Habriyut," pp. 58–59.

152 Lewin, *A Cup of Tears*, p. 126. Lewin refers to Volhynian fever in his diary by using the Hebrew term *qadahat volinit*. Transmitted by human body lice that carry the Rochalimaea quintana bacterium, it spread among soldiers during World War I; see Jack Edward McCallum, *Military Medicine: From Ancient Times to the 21st Century* (Santa Barbara: ABC-CLIO, 2008), pp. 326–327.

153 It is the opinion of doctors whom I consulted that Fliederbaum probably meant rheumatic fever.

ceased to occur. Many children contracted chicken pox more severely than they would have under ordinary conditions, probably because hunger had weakened their immune system. There were also cases of frostbite, which were treated by rubbing vodka on the affected areas. However, it was difficult to procure this beverage, due to the high demand. There were cases of appendicitis in the ghetto, just as there were elsewhere.[154] There were evidently also cases of malignant tumors. In October 1941, Ringelblum wrote that a friend of his, a former teacher in the ghetto, had died of cancer.[155]

Treatments

As they coped with diseases, the hospitals also attempted to provide various treatments. Mold was used to treat pressure sores. After cleaning and rinsing the bedsores, a special topical ointment was applied. Some were so deep and infected that they defied all remedies and resulted in death.[156] After the *Grossaktion*, many patients lacked any possibility of treating the ulcers that they developed from sitting in hideouts for lengthy periods.[157] A boil, also called a furuncle or furunculosis, was treated by injecting milk into the muscles, as well as with auto-vaccination and Desitin.[158]

People who had bad colds, high fever, or lung infections were treated with cupping and mustard seeds, which were common anti-fever remedies even before ghettoization. When it was still possible to obtain vitamin B12, it was administered to those who suffered from severe malnutrition.[159] Nonconventional methods

154 Roland, *Courage under Siege*, pp. 171–172.

155 Ringelblum, *Ktavim Aharonim*, p. 317. Dr. Yitzhak Saar of the Łódź ghetto wrote that there were no new cases of malignant tumors; see Saar, "Begeto Łodź," pp. 43–44.

156 Based on the testimonies of G. Averbuch, Hermann, Yaffe, and H. Halperin; see Koren, "Hasiyud Kehelek Misherutei Habriyut," p. 58.

157 Lensky, *A Physician inside the Warsaw Ghetto*, pp. 182–183.

158 Koren, "Hasiyud Kehelek Misherutei Habriyut," p. 58.

159 Ibid.

appear to have been used to treat patients at times. For example, syphilis patients were subjected to an artificial malaria shock treatment. This procedure, which was based on the invention of a doctor in Vienna, caused controlled chills. Sulfa, Daganan, digitalis, and strophanthin were administered as well, until the onset of the *Grossaktion* in mid-1942.[160] Pressured by the masses on the streets, the first aid staff were forced to give those dying of starvation injections of camphor that were sometimes mixed with strychnine, which had no medical value.[161] Tonsillectomies were performed in the ghetto.[162] Hernia and hemorrhoid surgeries, caesarean sections, and even colostomies were performed in the hospital as well.[163] Abortions were also common.[164]

Foreskin Restoration

In an attempt to arrange hideouts on the Aryan side, the possibility of performing surgeries to blur evidence of circumcision was discussed. The surgical restoration of the foreskin could mask the Jewishness of men who were hiding under false identities. Prof. Adam Drozdowicz, a microbiologist who worked in the Judenrat's food-inspection laboratory in the ghetto, described how Jewish men in hiding outside the ghetto dealt with the question of camouflaging the mark of circumcision, which the Germans often examined in their efforts to identify Jews in hiding. The doctors in the ghetto had different opinions about the proper method to employ to blur circumcision. The prevailing attitude was that the evidence would be hard to conceal from the prying eyes of an experienced German doctor. The technique that all the physicians preferred was to narrow the head of the penis. This

160 Ibid., p. 59.

161 Ross, "Tahanat Ezra Rishona," pp. 70–71.

162 Turkow, *Hayo Hayta Varsha Yehudit*, p. 361.

163 Based on the H. Halperin testimony, see Koren, "Hasiyud Kehelek Misherutei Habriyut," p. 50.

164 Based on the Kaminski testimony, see Koren, "Hasiyud Kehelek Misherutei Habriyut," p. 50.

technique may have been tested first on cadavers in morgues. Although it yielded good results in certain cases, circumcision could be detected upon careful examination.

In December 1942, after having lost his entire family, Prof. Drozdowicz managed to escape to the Aryan side, where he contacted the gynecologist Tadeusz Gronowski, who had an idea of how to perform such surgery, but had never attempted it. Prof. Drozdowicz was the first to undergo the procedure. It took place in a hideout apartment with only the patient and his doctor in attendance. Thus, Drozdowicz had to assist as the operation proceeded. Conducted under local anesthesia, unlike the method discussed in the ghetto, the surgery was performed on the outer section of the organ. On one side, the surgeon stretched the foreskin to extend it. The technique was effective only in certain cases. When it succeeded, it had excellent results and left only a small scar. Drozdowicz testified that his procedure was an outstanding success.

Many of his friends underwent similar operations. Half of them were successful. Some patients underwent stringent German inspections. A few were even taken to the Gestapo and emerged unscathed. The outcome evidently depended on the flexibility of the tissue. The Gestapo murdered Dr. Gronowski, apparently in a case of mistaken identity that had nothing to do with the clandestine surgeries. Dr. Feliks Zenon Kanabus, known for helping Jews, took over Gronowski's patients. Although accustomed to using the traditional method that was familiar in the ghetto, he adopted Gronowski's technique after Dr. Kanabus' death and arranged safe apartments for convalescence following surgery. Activists in Żegota, the underground Polish Council to Aid Jews, which was established in December 1942, referred young men in need of the operation to Prof. Drozdowicz. Dr. Kanabus considered this an act of social value and the continuation of his prewar activity against antisemitism. He performed thirty to forty operations, many at no charge and some in his home.

Additional physicians engaged in this type of activity. Dr. Andrzej Trojanowski was immensely helpful in fixing "Jewish" noses and assisted people in secret hideouts who required surgery. The doctors who performed these operations considered them humanitarian activities. They assisted those who could not afford surgery—at no charge and at great personal risk. They also conducted several procedures on young children. Irena, Dr. Kanabus' wife and a pediatrician, was very helpful. The pediatric surgeries, which were successful, made it possible to rescue the children in hiding.[165] After the war, Dr. Kanabus and his wife were recognized as Righteous Among the Nations.[166]

165 Microbiologist Prof. Adam Drozdowicz testimony, YVA, O.3/3647. Adam Drozdowicz's real name was Adam (Henryk) Gutgisser. At the onset of the *Aktionen*, he obtained Aryan identity papers under the name of Eduard Drozdowicz. For testimony regarding cosmetic surgery on noses and for camouflaging circumcision, see also Temkin-Berman, *Ir Betoh Ir*, pp. 182–183.

166 Anolik, "Rofim Polanim Hasidei Umot Ha'olam."

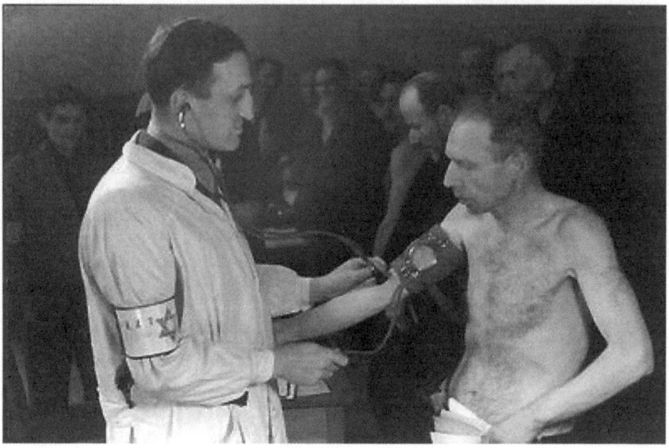

Checking a patient's blood pressure in the Warsaw ghetto, May 1941. Photo Collection, YVA, 24DO8.

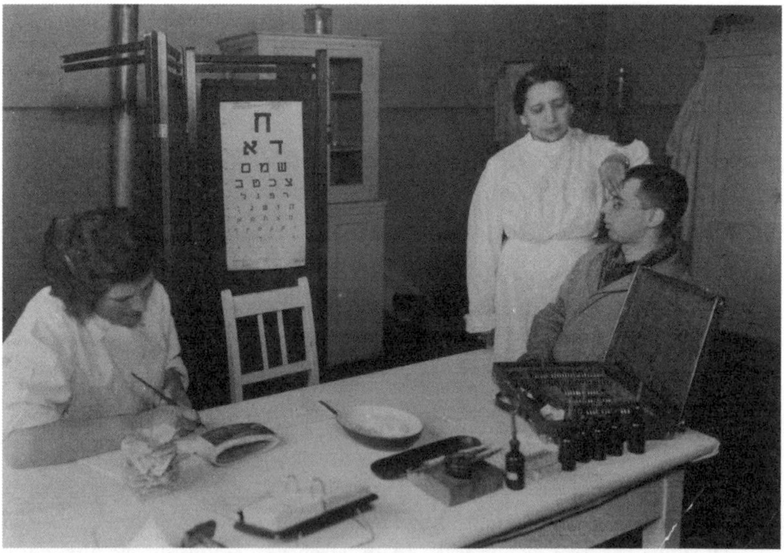

Nurses at work in the ophthalmology department. Photo Collection, YVA, FA35/1980.

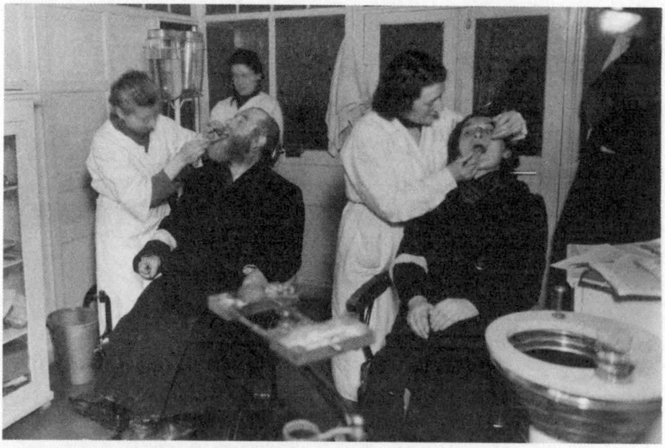

Nurses at work at the TOZ dental clinic. Photo Collection, YVA, 4613/444.

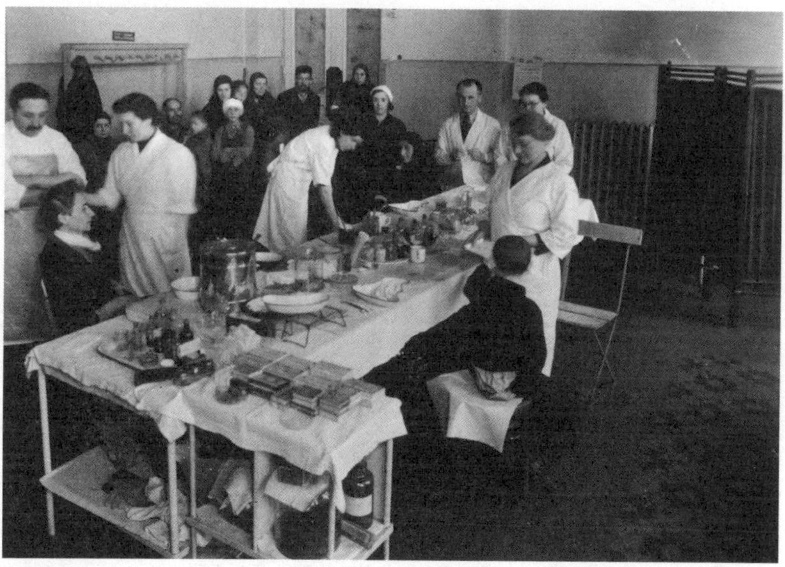

TOZ physicians and nurses at work in the surgery department. Photo Collection, YVA, FA35/1971.

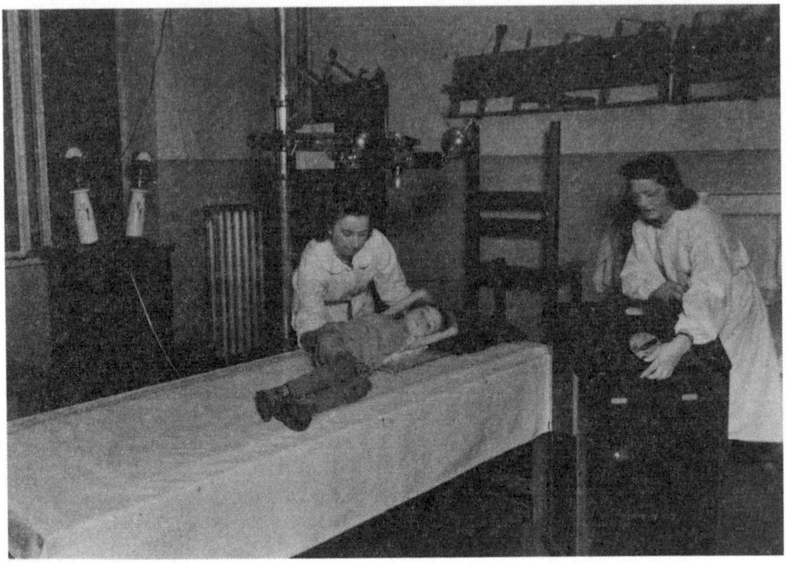

A child undergoes an X-ray. Photo Collection, YVA, FA35/1977.

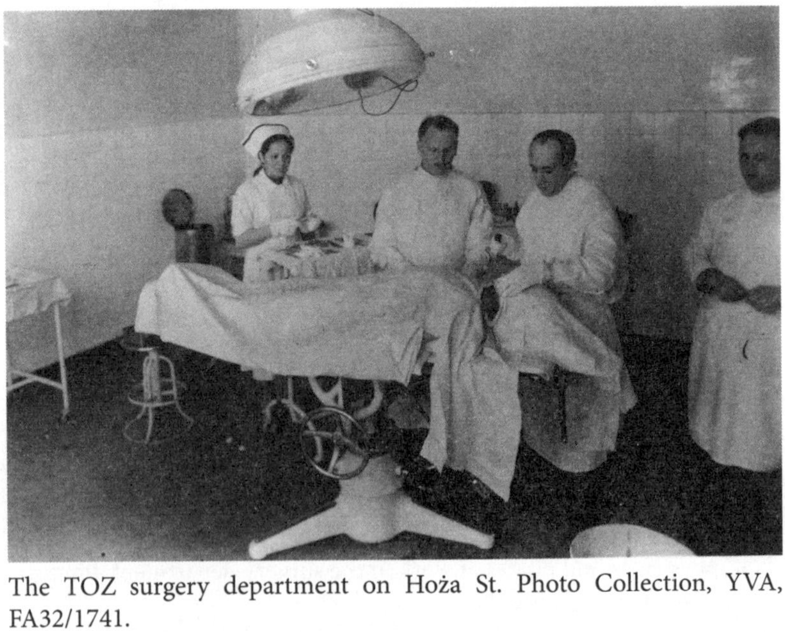

The TOZ surgery department on Hoża St. Photo Collection, YVA, FA32/1741.

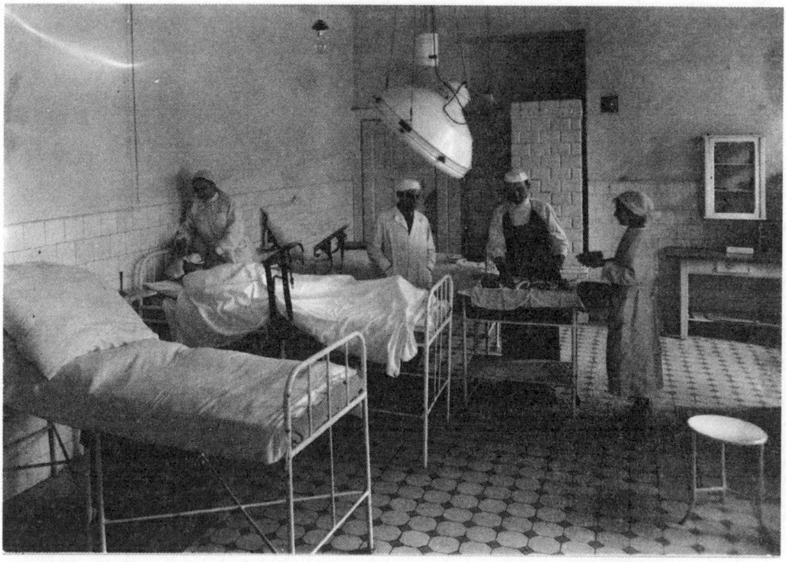

A TOZ maternity ward. Photo Collection, YVA, FA32/1762.

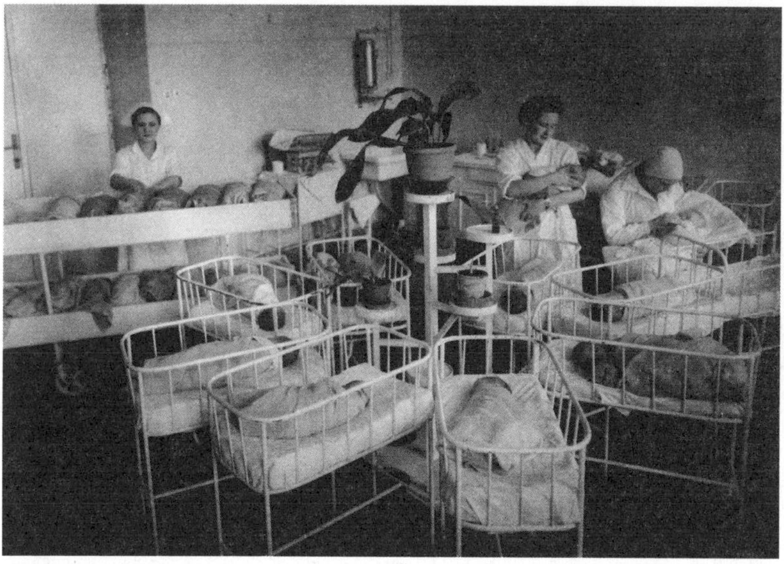

Nursery at the maternity clinic at 35 Twarda St. Photo Collection, YVA, FA32/1277.

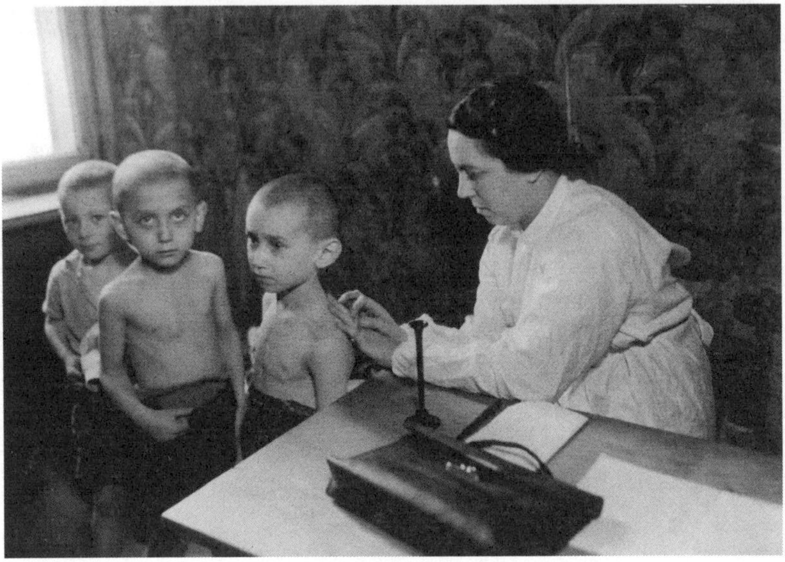

Medical checkups at the children's soup kitchen at 45 Nalewki St. Photo Collection, YVA, FA35/2055.

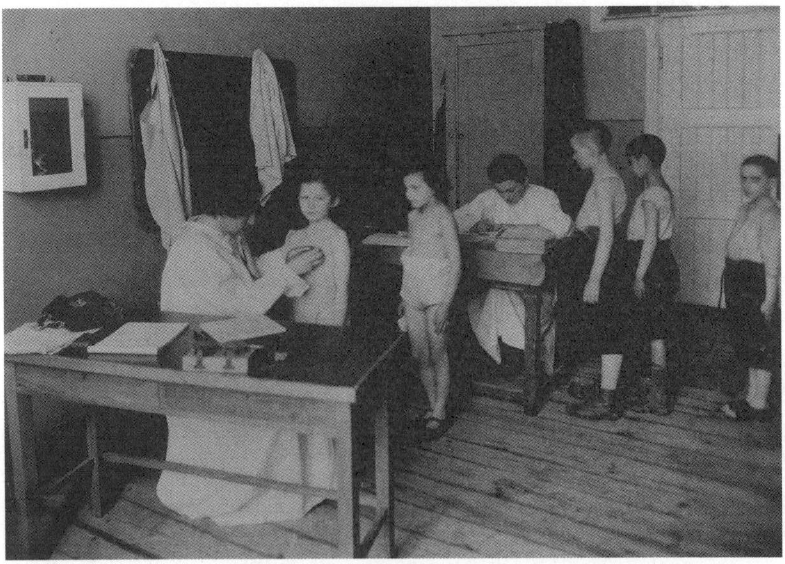

Medical checkups at the children's soup kitchen at 2a Nalewki St. for the distribution of food supplements. Photo Collection, YVA, FA35/2018.

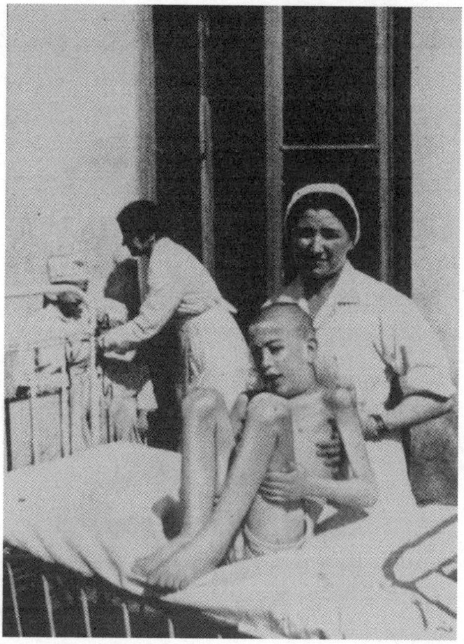

A boy with hunger disease at Bersohn and Bauman Children's Hospital in the Warsaw ghetto, 1942. Photo Collection, YVA, 5493/10.

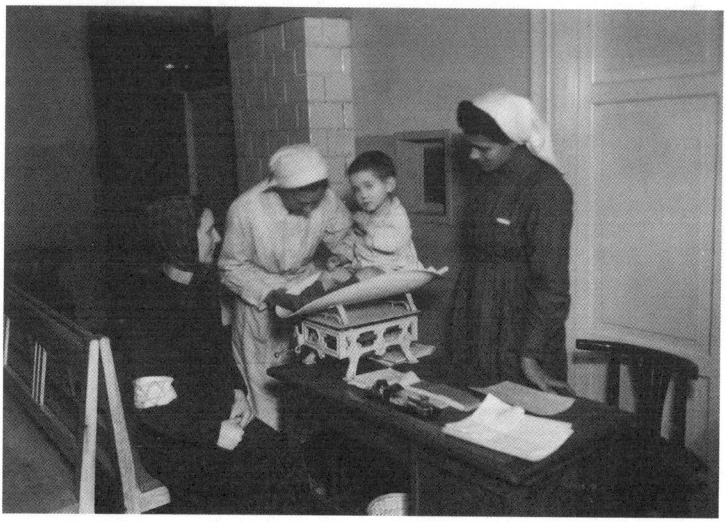

Nurses weigh a toddler at Bersohn and Bauman Children's Hospital in the Warsaw ghetto. Photo Collection, YVA, FA35/2001.

Chapter Eight

Fertility and Mortality

Natural Growth of the Jewish Population of Warsaw

Until the beginning of the twentieth century, the natural growth of the Jewish population in Eastern Europe surpassed that of the non-Jews. The fertility rate was higher and the mortality rate was lower among the Jews.[1] During the years preceding World War I, the fertility rate among the Jews declined and the natural increase of the Jewish population was lower than that of their neighbors due mainly to modernization and secularization processes. During the interwar period, these processes intensified and while the mortality rate among Jews was still lower than that of the general population, the decrease in their fertility rate caused their natural increase to decline relative to the population at large.[2] In the 1930s, the rates of natural increase of the Jews of Warsaw and

1 Jacob Leshchinsky, "Hayishuv Hayehudi Behitpathuto Hakalkalit" (The Jewish Community and Its Economic Development), in Gruenbaum et al., *Entziklopediya Shel Galuyot: Varsha*, vol. 1, pp. 125–126; Mahler, *Yehudei Polin*, p. 19. Mahler explains that the Jewish tradition of reproduction (the commandment of "Go forth and multiply" (Gen.1:22) and adherence to Jewish family purity laws helped to increase fertility, and to prevent sexually transmitted diseases, thus decreasing mortality.

2 Mahler, *Yehudei Polin*, pp. 19–20; Leshchinsky, "Hayishuv Hayehudi," pp. 125–126. See Offer, *Haluk Lavan Bageto*, appendix B.1, p. 534.

of the city's total population were similar.[3] Both populations experienced a demographic decline due to a rise in mortality during World War I, from 1914 to 1918. Since the Jewish fertility rate did not decrease significantly, the downturn in their demographic growth was smaller.

The concentration of refugees in the city, which created harsh hygienic and economic conditions, led to a high mortality rate among the Jews in those years. During World War I, an average of 24.9 per 1,000 Jews died—an increase of more than 77 percent relative to the 1910–1914 period—while the fertility rate of the Jews declined by only 4 percent. Among non-Jews, the mortality rate increased by 58 percent relative to the prewar years, but fertility dropped by 38 percent. According to Leshchinsky, child mortality among the Jews was lower than among non-Jews worldwide.[4] The situation changed drastically during the Nazi occupation of Warsaw.

German Policy on Childbirth, Abortion, and Mortality

A few months after occupying Warsaw and before establishing the ghetto, the Germans displayed an interest in information about mortality, births, and abortions. In late March 1940, Dr. Fritz Arlt, head of the Population and Welfare Department of the General Government Ministry of the Interior, requested information about various aspects of life in the Jewish community, including birth and abortion statistics.[5] In early May 1941, about half a year after ghettoization, Gestapo operatives in Warsaw ordered Adam Czerniaków, chairman of the Warsaw ghetto Judenrat, to provide them with data on births and child mortality. He was also required to present the SIPO in Warsaw with a graph of Jewish mortality in 1939, in 1940, and in the first

3 Leshchinsky, "Hayishuv Hayehudi," pp. 135–136.

4 Ibid., pp. 136, 138; Offer, "Ma'arach Harefu'a Begeto Varsha," vol. 2, appendix B.24 and appendix B.25, pp. 179–180.

5 Czerniaków, *The Warsaw Diary*, p. 133.

few months of 1941. In the middle of May 1941, Czerniaków advised the commander of the SIPO that the scanty food rations in the ghetto had claimed the lives of more than 1,700 Jews in the first half of that month. At the end of May, he again delivered a lecture before the high command of the German police in Warsaw on the state of the Jewish population and its mortality rate. In early October 1941, Czerniaków was ordered to give a lecture on typhus and mortality in the ghetto before Heinz Auerswald, the ghetto *Kommissar*, and many other invitees.[6]

There is no doubt that the Nazi authorities tracked the ghetto's statistics on births and deaths very attentively, and spared no effort to maximize mortality.[7] Along with their keen interest in monitoring changes in mortality and fertility rates, the Germans tried to conceal the death statistics from external bodies. In February 1942, the *Kommissar* arrived in the ghetto with a high-ranking SS officer and a Swiss representative, who questioned the Judenrat about the ghetto and typhus. Before their visit, Auerswald ordered Czerniaków to say nothing about mortality, which stood at 5,123 deaths in January.[8]

Dr. G. Hecht and Dr. Ernst Wetzel, senior officials at the Nazi Party's Office of Racial Policy, determined the Nazis' official approach to the implementation of public medical policy in the General Government. They wrote a memorandum about "the question of treating the populations of the former Polish territories according to racial policy," which was distributed among Nazi leaders on November 25, 1939, and clearly influenced *Reichsführer-SS* Heinrich Himmler.[9] Wetzel and Hecht wrote, "We are indifferent to the hygienic fate of the Jews…their fertility rate must be lowered in every possible way." They proposed reducing the non-Aryan population remaining in the parts of

6 Ibid., pp. 232–233, 235, 242, 286.

7 Kermish, "Nigudim Ma'amadiyim," p. 569.

8 Czerniaków, *The Warsaw Diary*, p. 328.

9 The pamphlet was written at the beginning of the war and, therefore, it is possible to infer that the heads of the Nazi Party's central institutions in Germany had planned the crimes that were committed thereafter. See Dworzecki, *Eropa Lelo Yeladim*, pp. 37–39.

Poland that the Reich had annexed by preventing pregnancy and discontinuing punishment for abortions. They also offered to publicize methods of abortion and contraception, and to recognize homosexuality as a legitimate phenomenon that would not be liable to punishment. The public medical policy toward Poles and Jews aimed to reduce their numbers and to restrict the continuation of their culture.[10]

The conditions in the ghetto made it very difficult to have and to raise children. However, we have no information about a decree against giving birth in the Warsaw ghetto, such as the ban on births in the ghettos in Lithuania.[11] If such an edict had been issued in Warsaw, the sources from that period would surely have mentioned it. On the first anniversary of the Warsaw ghetto, Ringelblum noted in his diary, "In early November 1941, reports arrived from Łódź about a ban on weddings and childbirth among Jews. Pregnant women up to their third month had to abort. In short, the Prussians have renewed Pharaoh's decrees."[12] Ringelblum seems to have been misinformed. No such dictate had been issued in Łódź. It is interesting that as of November 1941, no edict of that nature had been declared in the ghettos of Lithuania, although one was promulgated about three months later, and it is important to note that the Nazi high leadership had been discussing the possibility at the time.

In the course of World War II, the Nazis developed methods to increase the fertility rate in Germany and to improve the German race in order to enhance the biological might of the German people and to aggrandize the German nation. Concurrently, they acted to destroy the biological vigor of undesirable peoples and races. This biological destruction

10 Ibid., pp. 38–39; Browning, "Genocide and Public Health," pp. 21–22.

11 Injunctions against childbirth were first promulgated in the ghettos of Shavli (Šiauliai) and Vilna on February 5, 1942, and in the ghetto of Kovno (Kaunas) on July 24, 1942. On the decree and the elaborate methods used by the Jews to cope with this, see Offer, "Refua Verof'im Begeto Shavli," pp. 52–58, 85–99; Offer, "Medicine in the Shavli Ghetto in Light of the Diary of Dr. Aaron Pik," pp. 164–172; Prais, "Harefu'a Vehabriyut Begeta'ot Vilna, Kovna, VeShavli," pp. 109–129.

12 Ringelblum, *Yoman Vereshimot*, p. 330.

entailed differential planning: all the members of the Jewish people would be annihilated, while the methods to be directed against other peoples would be the murder and abduction of their children, birth control, voluntary and forced contraception, and annihilation by sterilization. In 1940, Hermann Rausching reported that Hitler had asserted in a conversation with him his right to dispose of millions of members of inferior races in some convenient and bloodless manner.

> Why should I not assume the right to do away with millions of racial lowlifes who breed like bugs, and I don't mean to exterminate them but instead will systematically curb their great natural increase…systematically and painlessly, relatively speaking, and in any event without much bloodshed.…It will be one of the most important missions in German politics for all generations to prevent by every means the further growth of the Slavic peoples.…We are fulfilling this very slowly, without bloodshed.[13]

In 1940, about a year before the war between Germany and the Soviet Union broke out, Heinrich Himmler wrote a memorandum, titled "Some Thoughts on the Treatment of the Foreign Peoples in the East," with the aim of lowering these peoples' birth rates. Himmler proposed, among other measures, lowering the level of children's education by teaching arithmetic calculations only up to number 500, abolishing reading instruction, and imposing compulsory obedience to the Germans as a divine law. Administrative measures were taken to reduce births in Poland. On May 27, 1941, an interministerial conference was held at the Reich Ministry of the Interior in Berlin, presided over by Dr. Leonardo Conti, the Reich Minister of Health and director of the Nazi Party's Main Office for Public Health. The minutes of the assembly included a discussion on reducing the fertility rate in Poland. The following steps were proposed: raising the marriage age to twenty-five, officially authorizing abortion, imposing a fine

13 Dworzecki, *Eropa Lelo Yeladim*, p. 37.

for every illegal birth, and decreeing the forced sterilization of any woman who bore an illegal number of children.

In the autumn of 1941, the RSHA, an organ of the SS, drew up a plan to weaken the Slavic peoples based on the assumption that the Germans would achieve great victories in the Soviet Union. According to the scheme, following the German triumph, 50 million Slavs, Poles, Czechs, Ukrainians, and Belarusians would be transferred to Siberia, and the occupied territories would become German colonies. On April 27, 1942, Dr. Wetzel, then director of the Department of Racial Affairs of the Reich Ministry for the Eastern Occupied Territories, submitted a conceptual plan and a position paper for Himmler's general program for the East. The program included anti-pregnancy propaganda, the distribution of contraceptive devices, the opening of special abortion clinics, the training of midwives and nurses for this purpose, propaganda to promote voluntary sterilization and to prevent concerted action to combat infant mortality—a "slow genocide of future generations" or "an absolutely negative demographic policy," as Dworzecki termed it.[14]

In July 1942, the ethnic orders were expanded to include the entire population of the occupied countries in the East. On July 23, 1942, *Reichsleiter* (Reich governor) Martin Bormann, head of the Nazi Party secretariat at Hitler's headquarters, wrote to *Reichsleiter* Alfred Rosenberg, minister for the occupied territories in the East.

> If girls and women in the occupied territories in the East need abortions, we agree…There is great danger that the non-German population in the occupied territories in the East will multiply at a greater rate than before, since the living conditions of the non-German population are becoming much better and safer…must take the necessary measures to prevent non-German populations from reproducing.[15]

14 Ibid., pp. 38–46.
15 Ibid., p. 47.

Various proposals, reports, and ideas were formulated in concrete terms and consolidated in decrees against the Jews. The ban on childbirth in the ghettos of Lithuania and the most stringent implementation of it are concrete examples of the historical process that began with Nazi ideology and culminated in the annihilation of the Jewish people.

A favorable attitude toward sterilization and castration was also part of the idea that crystallized into the scheme of the biological extinction of "racial undesirables," which was broached by the SS Racial and Settlement Main Office. Attempts to put together a program of sterilization by X-ray continued during the war as well. Viktor Brack, a senior officer in the chancellery and one of the heads of the T4 Euthanasia Program, wrote to Himmler on March 28, 1941, that the sterilization by X-ray experiments had been crowned with success. In his memorandum, he also specified the operational methods to implement it.[16] In June 1942, Brack wrote to Himmler,

> According to my impression, there are at least 2–3 million men and women well fit for work among the approx. 10 million European Jews. In consideration of the exceptional difficulties posed for us by the question of labor, I am of the opinion that these 2–3 million should in any case be taken out and kept alive. Of course, this can only be done if they are at the same time rendered incapable of reproduction.[17]

Based on experiments that his subordinates had performed, Brack proposed adopting castration by X-ray, which is "not only relatively cheap but can be carried out on many thousands in a very short time, rather than employing the ordinary sterilization method, which was expensive and time-consuming."[18] Karl Jäger,

16 On the experiments in sterilization and castration by X-ray conducted on the initiative of Himmler and the German doctors, see R. J. Lifton, *The Nazi Doctors: Medical Killing and the Psychology of Genocide* (New York: Basic Books, 1986), pp. 274–276, 278–279; Müller-Hill, *Murderous Science*, pp. 16, 35.

17 Arad et al., *Documents on the Holocaust*, pp. 272–273.

18 Ibid.

the commander of Einsatzgruppe 3, was named commander of the SIPO and of the SD, when civilian rule in Lithuania was installed. In early December 1941, he produced a final report on the Jewish labor force remaining in Lithuania, following the murderous operations there. Jäger wrote, "I am of the opinion that the male working Jews should be sterilized immediately to prevent reproduction. Should any Jewess nevertheless become pregnant, she is to be liquidated."[19]

The formulation of Nazi policy on biological annihilation appears to have found expression in statements by officials in the Nazi ground forces echelons that reverberated among Jewish public figures. By November 1941, Ringelblum reported rumors from the Łódź ghetto about this matter, as previously mentioned. A letter from a junior Nazi official at the SIPO and the SD in Pozńan that was sent to *SS-Ubersturmführer* Hermann Krumey in Łódź in August 1941, concerning "protecting the race as the basis of a biological policy toward populations,"[20] reflected views about the process of biological destruction that should be applied to the occupied peoples. Already then these views were probably widely held in Nazi circles. Reverberations of the missive reached Jewish elements in the Łódź area. Its author presented demands and proposals concerning the biological destruction of the Polish nation and devoted a section to "the extensive sterilization of primitive Polish strata."[21]

> Applying economic pressure on the primitive strata will not prevent [the] possibility of their procreation. Only methods of liquidation can bring this undesired natural increase to an end...The war of peoples is not a political struggle but a biological one.[22]

Therefore, he proposed raising the age of marriage, establishing labor camps for men up to age twenty-five and for women up to

19 Ibid., p. 400.
20 Dworzecki, *Eropa Lelo Yeladim*, p. 43.
21 Ibid.
22 Ibid.

age twenty-one, and imposing taxes on mothers who bore children illegally, among other measures. Rolf Heinz Höppner, another SIPO commander in Poznńan, proposed in July 1942 "the sterilization in the camp of all Jewish women who are able to procreate so that the Jewish problem will be totally solved within a generation."[23]

The ban against childbirth was promulgated in the Lithuanian ghettos in February 1942, after the official decision on the Final Solution was made. Its implementation was deferred by about six months, until August 1942. Since the Jews in the Warsaw ghetto were being deported by then, it was not necessary to publish such an order there. In addition, "natural" mortality in Warsaw, induced by the dire conditions and overpopulation in the large ghetto, made an anti-childbirth order superfluous. In contrast, after the extermination of the many ill and elderly in the ghettos of Lithuania, the healthy and strong Jews who survived were kept there as a forced labor reserve to serve the Reich. Hence, it was necessary to ensure the annihilation of the posterity of the Jews. On February 26, 1942, Ringelblum presented reliable information about "a ban on bringing children into the world" in the ghettos of Vilna and Riga.[24]

Marriage and Conjugal Life

Marriage and sexual relations are two dimensions of the issue of fertility. In December 1941, a year after the establishment of the Warsaw ghetto, there was a rumor that the Nazis intended to ban marriage. After meeting with the *Kommissar*, Czerniaków had the impression that it was likely that some type of decree concerning this matter was imminent.[25] To the best of our knowledge, no such edict was issued in any ghetto in Poland, although it would have been consistent with the German policy described above.

23 Ibid.
24 Ringelblum, *Yoman Vereshimot*, p. 350.
25 Czerniaków, *The Warsaw Diary*, p. 308.

Rabbi Szymon Huberband, a member of the board of the Oneg Shabbat Archive, wrote that no weddings took place during the first three weeks of the war, due to the events and the chaos that prevailed. Those who wished to marry did not even know where their rabbis resided. When migration to the East began, many young people wished to marry before setting out on their journeys. Huberband wrote, "Weddings for young couples who were about to take to the roads became a mass phenomenon." Since the municipal offices were not yet operational, couples who married could not obtain official marriage certificates. To register their marriages, they presented certification from the rabbis who had officiated at their nuptials.

Weddings became frequent during the war. Many marriages that had been postponed due to parental opposition now took place. Nuptials also proliferated, because of the large number of widows and widowers who lost their spouses in the war. Many weddings took place at the time of the move to the ghetto, since it was easier to rent one apartment as a bride and groom rather than one for each person. However, according to Huberband, these wartime weddings were perfunctory events that lacked any hint of joy, and wedding feasts were rare. There were almost no divorce claims during the war. A heightened sense of personal responsibility prevailed during that period. People apparently felt that it was not appropriate to engage in personal conflicts when the nations were embroiled in a bloody war, and that it was better to stay together as a couple than to separate.[26]

In September 1940, roughly a year into the war and the occupation, and approximately two months before ghettoization, Ringelblum wrote that the horrifying reports from the labor camps prompted those summoned for forced labor not to comply. The Nazis responded by abducting dozens of Jews for this service. Since only single men were seized at first, many weddings were held during this period.[27] The onset of the *Grossaktion* in the Warsaw

26 Huberband, *Kidush Hashem*, pp. 92–93.

27 Ringelblum, *Notes from the Warsaw Ghetto*, p. 47; Czerniaków, *The Warsaw Diary*, p. 192. Czerniaków confirmed that married men were not taken to the camps.

ghetto also prompted a wave of bogus marriages. Mothers and sons, and brothers and sisters were married fictitiously in the belief that they could protect their dear ones in this manner. According to Ringelblum, rabbis wrote out ketubot (marriage contracts) without meeting the couples.[28]

The rabbis' attitude toward the issue of marriage in the ghetto is interesting. Rabbi Yehoshua Moshe Aharonson,[29] who briefly served on the Rabbinical Council in Warsaw, wrote that in the presence of important rabbis in that city in 1940, he expressed his opinion under rabbinical law that couples should not marry during that terrible period, because the harsh realities might lead to severe halachic problems. For example, many women might become agunahs—"chained"—unable to remarry in cases when there was no proof of a husband's death. He also believed that single women could hide better on their own, if necessary, and that women sent to labor camps would be more likely to survive, if they were neither married nor pregnant. Aharonson also noted that since promiscuity tended to pervade times of siege and tribulation, it was preferable for women to be unmarried rather than married, in case they were raped or forced to capitulate to demands to have intercourse with a stranger. In addition, the Nazis in Warsaw closed down all the ritual baths and threatened to invoke the death penalty against anyone who violated the closure order. The rabbis continued for some time to attempt to bribe those in charge of the baths to allow them to open, but to no avail.[30]

Until the war began, there were nine privately owned ritual baths in Warsaw and one lavish facility in the Praga quarter that

28 Ringelblum, *Notes from the Warsaw Ghetto*, p. 327; Dr. Chaim Einhorn testimony, YVA, O.3/1836. Dr. Einhorn testified that he and his wife, Helena née Engel, wed at the beginning of the *Aktionen*.

29 Yehoshua Moshe Aharonson (1910–1994) served as Rabbi of Sanok. During the Holocaust, he spent a brief period in Warsaw, returned to his shtetl, and was deported to numerous camps. After the war, he served as a rabbi in the DP camps. After immigrating to Israel, he was named rabbi of Petah Tikva. See Itamar Levine, *Otiyot Shel Esh*: *Eduyot Mitkufat Hashoah Basifrut Hahilhatit* (Letters of Fire: Holocaust Testimonies in Halakhic Literature) (Hebrew) (Tel Aviv: Yedioth Ahronoth and Hemed Books, 2002), pp. 333–334.

30 Ibid., p. 134.

was owned by the Jewish community. All of them were closed when the city was bombarded in September 1939 and were reopened briefly after the ceasefire, until December 1939. Kurt Schrempf, the German chief physician of Warsaw, ruled that these facilities were hotbeds for contagious diseases because, under Jewish law, clean water was piped into them only once every three months. All the ritual baths were shut down under official seal. A notice stamped with a swastika was posted on their gates: "Using or bathing in this bath will invoke the same penalty as for an act of sabotage, ranging from ten years of imprisonment to execution." Warsaw remained without a Jewish ritual bath, and the issue of family purity became a real problem for the daughters of Israel. Religious women, as well as men who immersed themselves regularly, began to travel to towns around Warsaw. Some attempted to immerse in the Vistula (Wisla in Polish) River, but many women contracted lung infections and other illnesses after submerging themselves in the cold water. Through various, clandestine means, they managed to bribe the Polish police and to immerse themselves in one of the ritual baths, and then to operate four other baths, through bribery as well.

When the ghetto was sealed in late November 1940 and its non-Jewish inhabitants had moved out, the baths operated secretly without fear of prying Polish eyes, until early summer 1941. In August 1941, after Dr. Wilhelm Hagen succeeded Dr. Schrempf, the baths were permitted to operate legally for a fee. In early winter 1941, use of the ritual baths declined due to the typhus epidemic and the shortage of heating fuel and, consequently, the fee for using the facility was raised to a level that few could afford. Only two baths out of five in the ghetto continued to operate.[31] Moreover, Rabbi Aharonson ruled that conjugal relations were forbidden during times of war, famine, and religious persecution.

> It is stated explicitly in [*Shulhan Aruch,* section] Orah Hayyim 240:12, that conjugal relations must not be practiced in a year of famine, except among those who are childless. Specifically

31 Huberband, *Kidush Hashem*, pp. 88–92.

> at a time of distress, such as this, a time unprecedented in Jewish history, a time of mass murder, particularly of children and pregnant women, who are among the first to be led to the slaughter, as is known, such relations may be prohibited even to those who have not yet had children...This is how those who feared and trembled [before God] comported themselves at this time of woe.[32]

It seems that conjugal relations in the ghetto were disrupted and diminished, because of the psychological pressures of living under Nazi rule. Most Jews had to share living quarters with others, which made sexual relations difficult, if not almost impossible. The grievous shortage of food also affected sexual desire and impotence—a common phenomenon among prisoners of war. There were also differences in this domain among those who suffered less from hunger and those who were starving, and, of course, there were individual differences.[33]

Sexual activity increased considerably relative to the prewar norms, especially among the young. Teenagers spent much of their time having sex. Many felt that they should experience as much of life as they could before it was too late. Indifference and hedonism were typical of many Jews. Many girls who had not been sexually active before the war engaged in sex in the ghetto.[34] Many women had no fear of getting pregnant, because they had stopped menstruating.[35] Lacking conventional contraceptives, people fashioned condoms out of baby pacifiers.[36] A sense of the fleeting

32 Levine, *Otiyot Shel Esh*, pp. 137–138.

33 Roland, *Courage under Siege*, pp. 48–49.

34 Ibid. It is possible to get an idea about the promiscuity and licentiousness from Rabbi Huberband's writings about the Jewish woman in the war years. See Huberband, *Kidush Hashem*, pp. 116–117.

35 Much has been written about the absence of menstruation among women in the ghettos and the camps. For example, Dworzecki testified that three-fourths of women stopped menstruating. See Dworzecki, "Tofa'ot Patologiyot Begeto Vilna," p. 8. Similar phenomena were reported in Warsaw and Kovno; see Aaron Perzikovitz, "Begeto Kovna" (In the Kovna Ghetto), in Dworzecki, *Hama'avak Lakiyum Velabriyut Biymei Hashoah*, pp. 36–37.

36 Czerniaków, *The Warsaw Diary*, p. 330.

nature of their lives was another factor affecting sexual activity in the ghetto.

The phenomenon of prostitution also emerged at this time. In mid-December 1939, about two months after the occupation began, the Germans, who feared contracting diseases from Jewish women, posted a notice at the public health centers to the effect that Jewish whores who had relations with German guards were committing sabotage. Jewish prostitutes did not receive any medical care at these centers.[37] At the beginning of Nazi rule, the Judenrat was ordered to concentrate the Jewish prostitutes at Czyste Hospital, to examine them, and to make sure they were not ill. In 1940, these women were notified that they had to wear the yellow star, so that German soldiers would not confuse them with Polish whores.

About a month and a half into ghetto life, in late December 1940 and in early January 1941, prostitution began to emerge on the streets. Even highly respected women sank into prostitution. "Distress is causing everything," Ringelblum wrote.[38] Concurrently, a brothel opened for business in the basement of the Britannia Hotel at 18 Nowolipie St. Its owners were members of Group 13, the group that collaborated with the Gestapo.[39] Several brothels operated in the ghetto until the mass deportations began.[40]

37 Ringelblum, *Yoman Vereshimot*, p. 24.

38 Ringelblum, *Notes from the Warsaw Ghetto*, p. 118.

39 Ibid., p. 120. In checkups of women in the DP camps in Germany, Dr. Chanina Lipa Shapira recorded harsh testimonies about the conduct of the Judenrat in the ghetto of Kopyczyńce, where it was required to provide thirty young Jewish women for a brothel in Tarnopol. A similar directive was issued in Łódź, where Rumkowski was ordered to deliver women to an SS officer. Reports also exist about a brothel for Nazi officers in Lublin. An investigation of such cases in the Warsaw ghetto is required. See Chanina Lipa Shapira, *Lo Lishkoah Velo Lisloah: Reshimot Rofe Aliya Bishnat 1949* (Do Not Forgive, Do Not Forget: Writings of an Immigration Doctor in 1949) (Hebrew) (Jerusalem: Kiryat Sefer, 1966), pp. 59, 70–79.

40 Ringelblum, *Yoman Vereshimot*, p. 24.

Births

In October 1941, Ringelblum wrote about several aspects of ghetto life, including that one of the common jokes in the ghetto was about a woman who was having difficulty giving birth and all measures to help were useless. "But the moment her friends left the house, the infant came crawling out of the womb to ask his mother, 'Mama, can I come out now? Have all the *khapers* gone?'"[41] Ghetto humor of this kind reflects women's reluctance to bring children into the world, due to the existential dangers that the newborn would face. In late August 1941, Ringelblum wrote, "[But] there are practically no children under two, simply because there's no milk at all, either for the infants or the nursing mothers. If things continue this way, the 'Jewish question' will soon be resolved very quickly in Warsaw."[42]

Dr. Israel Rom (Rotbalsam), a pediatrician at Bersohn and Bauman Children's Hospital, who took part in the hunger disease research project in the ghetto, wrote that it was no wonder that people did not want children, whose very existence endangered them. He testified that the fertility rate was very low, even before ghettoization, and verged on zero after the ghetto was sealed. By the end of the ghetto era, there were no infants and children under the age of three, because no children were born there. "This natural eradication of the Jewish child as an unnecessary burden is one of the most saddening moments in the whole tragedy that engulfed the Jews of Warsaw in flames."[43] A June 1942 issue of *Yedioth,* the underground newspaper of the Dror Hehalutz movement, reported the conclusion that from the demographic perspective, the ghetto had already destroyed the future viability of the Jews.

> We are witnessing the systematic reduction of the most important group of men in terms of biology and economic

41 Ringelblum, *Notes from the Warsaw Ghetto*, p. 225.

42 Ibid., p. 206.

43 Rom, "Mahalot Hayeladim Begeto Varsha," p. 17.

> activity in the Warsaw ghetto. The number of newborns declined by half compared to that in 1931. The 0–6 age group has declined by 25 percent. These numbers attest to the destruction of Warsaw Jewry.[44]

The Polish statistical abstract for 1947 provides statistics on births and deaths during the first few years of the war.

Births and Deaths among Jews and Non-Jews in Warsaw, Initial War Years[45]

	Jews		Non-Jews	
Year	Births	Deaths	Births	Deaths
1938	6,139	3,680	13,104	10,208
1939*	4,755	8,403	12,958	22,670
January–August	3,179	2,393	9,148	7,167
September–December	1,576	6,015	3,810	15,583
1940	3,676	8,342	12,270	17,976
1941	2,753	43,239	10,404	19,589
1942	428**	39,719***	8,988	19,659

* In the break down of 1939, from January to the outbreak of the war in September and from after the war broke out through December 1939, typos may explain the slight deviation between the figures of deaths of Jews and of non-Jews, which when corrected, 8,408 would appear instead of 8,403 and 15,503, instead of 15,583, respectively.

** First five months of the year.

*** January–July: 24,511; August–December: 15,208.[46]

The number of births dropped sharply—by 31.5 percent among non-Jews between 1938 and 1942, and by more than half

44 Blatman, *Geto Varsha—Sipur Itona'i*, p. 30.

45 Leshchinsky, "Hayishuv Hayehudi," p. 140.

46 Ibid.

among Jews between 1938 and 1941. In the Jewish population, comparison of the first five months of 1941 with the same period in 1942 shows an additional 63 percent decrease. The number of deaths increased more than tenfold among the Jews and nearly doubled among non-Jews between 1938 and 1941. In 1941, the average number of deaths per month among the Jews was 3,603 as compared with the monthly average number of births of 229.4—a ratio of about 1:16. In 1942, there were 3,501 deaths (January–July) and 85.6 births (January–May)—a ratio of 1:41. Mortality escalated drastically, and the fertility rate plummeted.[47]

Despite the grievous situation in the ghetto, not all families forwent procreation. The Jewish fertility rate declined relative to its prewar level, but women continued to give birth, even under ghetto conditions. In 1941, the fertility rate was 45 percent of what it had been before the war in 1938. Even in 1942, as the situation worsened, it continued at 17 percent of its prewar pace.[48] Given the conditions in the ghetto, this should be viewed as a singular phenomenon. There were probably more women who wanted to give birth but were unable to do so, either because they ceased to menstruate, or because of psychological stress.

In order to sustain the monthly average of 230 newborns in 1941 and 86 in 1942, the Judenrat had to arrange appropriate care and assistance for the infants and for their mothers. Dr. Adolf Polisiuk noted in his diary that the maternity ward at the hospital on 1 Leszno St. continued to operate until the *Aktionen* began.[49] There was also a gynecological clinic and maternity facilities in the ghetto. According to TOZ reports sent to the JDC, 200 pregnant women received gynecological counseling in January 1941, and TOZ sent, at its expense, 20 women to give birth at a maternity hospital of sorts at 35 Twarda St.[50] In March 1941, TOZ reported that 202

47 Ibid. See also Havi Ben-Sasson and Lea Prais, "Twilight Days: Missing Pages from Avraham Lewin's Warsaw Ghetto Diary, May–July 1942," *Yad Vashem Studies*, 33 (2005), pp. 7–60.

48 Data on this matter also appear in the underground press. See Blatman, *Geto Varsha—Sipur Itona'i*, pp. 30–31.

49 Dr. Adolf Polisiuk diary, GFH, no. 3182.

50 An overview of TOZ activities, January 1941, JDC, AR.33–44, file 840.

pregnant women had visited the gynecology clinic, 41 births took place at the inpatient maternity home at 11 Elektoralna St., and there were 11 clinical interventions, which may refer to curettages or abortions.[51] A report noted that 1,064 women received care at two mother and child care clinics in April 1941.[52] In May 1941, 120 pregnant women visited the clinics and 45[53] gave birth at the maternity center or at the hospital at 11 Elektoralna St., where 15 surgical treatments were also administered. That month, a report was presented on the number of inpatients in medical institutions and hospitals, including the maternity facility at 35 Twarda St., where 4 mothers gave birth, and at 17 Ceglana St., where 1 had been admitted.[54] According to the TOZ report, births also occurred at refugee centers. For example, there were 3 in May 1941.[55]

In late September 1941, about ten months after the ghetto was established, 1 birth took place in a private hospital. The mother received a bouquet of flowers, as she would have in ordinary days. The baby girl was evidently born healthy, and two nurses devotedly cared for the mother around the clock. Mary Berg described the hospital, which only the wealthy of the ghetto could afford, as luxurious and lavishly equipped.[56] Even the phenomenon of mothers going for a stroll with their infants was discerned in the ghetto. In late July 1941, Czerniaków described mothers heading out with their little ones to a piece of "garden" that had survived behind Święty Duch Hospital, where they sat amid the ruins of the institution, which had been bombarded at the beginning of the war.[57]

51 A monthly overview of TOZ activities in Warsaw, March 1941, JDC, AR.33–44, file 840.

52 TOZ Report, no. 15, May 1941, on the number of people under TOZ medical observation in Warsaw in April 1941, JDC, AR.33–44, file 840.

53 It is possible that there were 75 births, as indicated by the number 30, which was noted in the report in addition to the number 45.

54 A monthly overview of TOZ activities in Warsaw, May 1941, JDC, AR.33–44, file 840.

55 A table presenting medical activities at 130 refugee centers in May 1941, JDC, AR.33–44, file 840.

56 Berg, *The Diary of Mary Berg*, p. 91.

57 Czerniaków, *The Warsaw Diary*, p. 263.

Between May and July 1942, Abraham Lewin commented in his diary on pregnant women in the ghetto, calling those who carried fetuses to full term "national heroes."

> One hardly sees pregnant Jewish women. In the ghetto, people die or are murdered. They are not born…However…there's no rule without an exception. When you circulate in the ghetto and observe passersby carefully, sometimes you can make out a Jewish woman who's pregnant. Today I saw two such women. It left a big impression, I'd say, a tremendous impression. That the Jewish woman today, under the benighted, merciless conditions, can marshal such courage as to bring a new Jewish creature into the world and then raise him—it's heroism and great audacity. If I had the slightest poetic talent to write songs, I'd write a warm paean of praise to the pregnant woman or the young Jewish mother in the ghetto…By virtue of these national heroes, the light of the Jews and of Judaism will not go out altogether, at least symbolically.[58]

There is an abundance of testimonies about the women who gave birth and their newborns, precisely in the context of the *Aktionen*, of all times. The stories about the murder of these mothers and their infants, including those who had managed to go into hiding, left a profound impression on those in the ghetto who documented the harrowing events.[59] According to Chaya Elbaum-Dornbus, the gynecology and maternity clinic at 17 Dzielna St. operated as part of the hospital, until the deportations from the ghetto. During an atrocious *Aktion*, the Germans murdered new mothers, their newborn infants, and the team of nurses.[60]

58 Ben-Sasson and Prais, "Twilight Days," pp. 46–47; Lucy Dawidowicz, *The War against the Jews, 1933–1945* (New York: Holt, Rinehart and Winston, 1975), pp. 297–298.

59 Lewin, *A Cup of Tears*, p. 147; Krall, *Shielding the Flame*, pp. 47, 50; Turkow, *Hayo Hayta Varsha Yehudit*, pp. 166, 167; Blady Szwajger, *I Remember Nothing More*, p. 137.

60 Chaya Elbaum-Dornbus, "Hageto Biymei Hagerush," pp. 607–608.

Even after the ghetto was destroyed, Jews hiding on the Aryan side of Warsaw continued to bring children into the world. A baby, who was born in hiding and was several days old, was one of thirty-six Jews, including Emanuel Ringelblum, who hid in a bunker under the greenhouses of a Polish gardener. On March 7, 1944, the fugitives were discovered and taken to Pawiak Prison. They were shot three days later. The gardener and the Polish midwife who had helped to deliver the baby were imprisoned.[61] Dr. Adina Blady Szwajger also testified about many clandestine births on the Aryan side that took place after the *Aktionen* in Warsaw.[62] In her diary, written when she was an underground activist for Zegota and the Jewish National Committee on the Aryan side, Batya Temkin-Berman wrote the following on November 10, 1944:

> As improbable as it seems, newborn babies were also placed in our care. Under these daunting conditions, there were still [Jews] who gave birth to children. Sometimes the pregnancy was unplanned and there was no way to terminate it. However, there were also cases in which a fully conscious decision was made, despite everything, to give life to new [Jews], believing that these children would be granted better times. Although this always involved innumerable problems, the feat always thrilled us and we tried to help in every possible way, at least materially.[63]

Mortality

Poland's war against Germany and the siege of Warsaw had dire effects on the health of the population, in general, and the Jewish population, in particular. All infrastructure required for basic subsistence was disrupted and mortality escalated.[64] Thousands

61 Auerbach, *Tzava'ot Varsha*, p. 174.

62 Blady Szwajger, *I Remember Nothing More*, pp. 137, 146–148.

63 Temkin-Berman, *Ir Betoh Ir*, pp. 174–179.

64 Kaplan, *Scroll of Agony*, pp. 31, 33, 36; Berg, *The Diary of Mary Berg*, pp. 8–9; Turkow, *Hayo Hayta Varsha Yehudit*, pp. 24–26; Czerniaków, *The Warsaw Diary*, pp. 76–77.

of Jews were killed, and many children were orphaned and were thrown into moldy shelters. The community orphanage was demolished as well.[65] Mortality was very high between September 1939 and May 1940: 1,850 deaths in October; 1,395 in November; and 1,179 in December. In late March 1940, Ringelblum wrote that it had tripled relative to mortality during the corresponding months of the previous year. The bombardments, the severely deteriorating living conditions, and the inflow of refugees and internal DPs from the provinces of western and northern Poland resulted in high mortality rates during these months.[66]

From May 1940, the number of deaths declined considerably. There were 856 in May and in November 1940, the month of ghettoization, there were 445—the lowest number in 1940 and since the outbreak of war.[67] The Nazis decided to lock the Jews in a ghetto on the pretext that the Jews spread diseases precisely after the Judenrat and the Jewish community institutions had overcome the surge in morbidity and had defeated the epidemics by providing the population with medical assistance and vaccinations. In December 1940, the first month of the ghetto, mortality continued to decline. According to Ringelblum, 10 to 12 Jews died every day that month. In the middle of January 1941, about two months after ghettoization, mortality rose significantly to around 90 people each day. In February 1941, deaths became a daily spectacle on the streets. People lay on the sidewalks and in the streets after fainting or dying in the open. These sights became commonplace and no longer made an impression on anyone.[68] The mortality rate increased sharply in April, and the number of deaths rose from 150 to 500 and then to 600, seven times greater than the toll in November 1940.[69]

65 Czerniaków, *The Warsaw Diary*, p. 73; Opochinsky, *Reshimot*, pp. 110, 113.

66 Trunk, "Epidemics and Mortality," p. 84; Ringelblum, *Yoman Vereshimot*, pp. 100–101.

67 Gutman, *The Jews of Warsaw*, p. 64; Offer, "Ma'arach Harefu'a Begeto Varsha," appendix B.26, p. 180.

68 Ringelblum, *Yoman Vereshimot*, pp. 212, 233, 241; Ringelblum, *Notes from the Warsaw Ghetto*, pp. 113, 130.

69 Czerniaków, *The Warsaw Diary*, p. 232; Ringelblum, *Notes from the Warsaw*

The mortality rate in the ghetto reached catastrophic proportions in May 1941[70]— approximately 150 per day.[71] Death roamed all the streets. Children did not fear it. In one of the courtyards, some youngsters were seen tickling a corpse. The streets filled with bodies covered with newspapers and linens. The German governor, Fischer, complained about this and demanded the immediate evacuation of the corpses.[72] On May 8, a record number of ghetto inhabitants died—210. Some Jews may have wished to refrain from eating hametz (leavened food) on Passover, and many practically had to fast during the eight-day festival, because they lacked the appropriate foods, which caused a significant increase in mortality.[73] Menachem Linder refers to May 9, 1941, as "Black Friday."[74] Mortality that month was so high that the house committees had to concern themselves more with the dead than with the living. From the beginning of that month to May 15, 1,700 people died and the death rate continued to climb relentlessly.[75] *Proletarisher Gedank* (Proletarian Thought), an underground newspaper of the Po'alei Tziyon Left, reported in May that there was an appalling rise in mortality, and that death from starvation and exhaustion was escalating at a dizzying pace.[76]

In late July 1941, abandoned corpses were found in homes and on the streets. The Ordnungsdienst reported that the completely decomposed body of a six-year-old lay in front of one building. His mother had abandoned him. Additional bodies were found inside the building.[77] Early in the summer of 1941, Linder wrote that, due to the spreading hunger, "The large number of

Ghetto, p. 165. On the sevenfold increase in mortality among the Jews in the ghetto as compared with the twofold to threefold increase on the Aryan side, see Blatman, *Geto Varsha—Sipur Itona'i*, pp. 143–144.

70 Ringelblum, *Notes from the Warsaw Ghetto*, p. 170.

71 Czerniaków, *Yoman Geto Varsha*, p. 180.

72 Czerniaków, *The Warsaw Diary*, p. 239.

73 Ringelblum, *Notes from the Warsaw Ghetto*, p. 173.

74 Blatman, *Geto Varsha—Sipur Itona'i*, pp. 146–147.

75 Ringelblum, *Notes from the Warsaw Ghetto*, pp. 177–180.

76 Blatman, *Geto Varsha—Sipur Itona'i*, pp. 143–144; Offer, "Ma'arach Harefu'a Begeto Varsha," vol. 2, appendix A.32, p. 151.

77 Czerniaków, *The Warsaw Diary*, p. 261.

dead is turning the Jewish ghetto into a graveyard."[78] In August, ninety-seven deaths on the streets for unknown reasons were recorded. The typhus epidemic was spreading at this time, and thousands of people were dying each month in their homes, the hospitals, the refugee shelters, and on the streets.[79] There were so many bodies on the streets that during the night the burial societies had to gather up the corpses of people who had died there late in the evening.[80] In August 1941, the underground newspaper *Biuletyn* reported that death was rampant in the Warsaw ghetto—5,500 Jews in July, as compared to 898 in January, and about 20,000 in January–July 1941.[81]

In August 1941, the Bund and Zukunft underground newspaper, *Za Naszą i Waszą Wolność*, reported a terrifying increase in mortality from one month to the next. The foremost cause of death was typhus, followed by dysentery—with more than half of the cases ending in death—tuberculosis and heart disease brought on by hunger; malnutrition; and exhaustion. About 70 percent of ghetto inhabitants were starving. Even those who received "soup" at the soup kitchens were doomed to a slow demise. Every mild cold and infectious disease caused death.[82] Ringelblum blamed the alarming rise in mortality on the reduced food supplies and on the typhus epidemic. In July and August, deaths climbed to 5,000–7,000 per month, as compared to slightly more than 1,000 per year before the war, when the Jewish population was smaller.[83]

By late August 1941, the mortality rate was so high among the destitute that entire families perished. The last member of a family lay for several days where he or she had died until the stench of the body reached the neighbors. There were cases in which rats gnawed at the bodies lying in an apartment. Apartments on some streets remained vacant after all their tenants had died. Entire

78 Blatman, *Geto Varsha—Sipur Itona'i*, p. 30.
79 Ibid., p. 152.
80 Ibid., pp. 146–153.
81 Ibid., p. 153.
82 Ibid., p. 154.
83 Ringelblum, *Polish-Jewish Relations*, p. 81.

families often succumbed in one day or within a few days. The orphan population surged because adults, particularly men, died first, followed by the rest of the family.[84] According to the Po'alei Tziyon Left underground newspaper *Awangarda Młodzieży*, mortality climbed from 200 per month before the war to 893 in January 1941, 4,290 in June, 5,550 in July, and 5,560 in August.[85] According to official Judenrat statistics, deaths in July and August 1941 exceeded 5,000 per month.[86]

On March 14, 1942, *Jutrznia* (Dawn), an underground newspaper of the Hashomer Hatza'ir movement, provided details about mortality and its implications. It reported that since the beginning of the war, 260 of the 578 tenants of a building on Miła St. and 450 out of 795 residents of a building on Pawia St. had died—200 in September 1941 alone—45 percent and 60 percent, respectively. Beginning in September 1941, all 400 inhabitants of a building on Krochmalna St. had died. The population of orphans also skyrocketed. There were 11 orphans who had lost both parents and 40 who had lost one in a building of 398 residents on Miła St.[87] In March 1942, 4,951 Jews died in the ghetto, which represents a seventeen-fold increase in the death rate per 1,000 people relative to the prewar rate. In April 1942, about three months before the *Grossaktion* began, 4,432 of the 350,000 Jews in the ghetto had died—twenty times more than the prewar rate. In March and in April, respectively, 290 and 239 died on the streets.[88]

Mortality at the shelters for children reached ghastly proportions. In the largest institution of this type, the one at 127 Leszno St., 47 youngsters among 470 died between July 4 and August 15, 1940. In 1941, the mortality rate was several times higher. Of the 600 children housed there on average, 176 died in

84 Ringelblum, *Notes from the Warsaw Ghetto*, pp. 205–206.

85 Blatman, *Geto Varsha—Sipur Itona'i*, pp. 154–155.

86 Czerniaków, *Yoman Geto Varsha*, p. 180; Offer, "Ma'arach Harefu'a Begeto Varsha," vol. 2, appendix A.32, p. 151.

87 Blatman, *Geto Varsha–Sipur Itona'i*, p. 173.

88 Opochinsky, *Reshimot*, p. 227.

May and 155 died in June.[89] Many children died on the streets.[90] The Jewish ghetto police reported the discovery of 252 corpses on the streets in February 1942, including those of dozens of children.[91] "If an abandoned child dies, it is better for him, but if parents die, even more children are abandoned," Opochinsky wrote in November 1941.[92] By late August 1941, about nine months after ghettoization, indifference to death was strikingly evident. People walked past bodies on the street with equanimity. They seldom visited the hospital to inquire about their relatives' welfare, and they rarely indicated any interest, not even during the last journey of the deceased to the grave or at their funerals.[93] In October 1941, bodies filled the streets and became so much a part of the usual ghetto scene that no one paid any attention to them.[94] Dr. Lensky described how death had become routine.

> Most of them left without much ado, nor the slightest protest…Jews died calmly in their dwellings, and whoever had no comfortable bed at home, like the impoverished refugees for example, would lie down on the sidewalk at night, until his soul departed…At dawn, a Jewish policeman would approach him, cover the body with thick paper and, when that was no longer to be had, use simple newspaper… Passersby who happened to go out early would meet the cadavers…The Jews of Warsaw grew accustomed to such scenes and were no longer that impressed.[95]

After the great wave of deportations, around 35,000 Jews remained in the ghetto. According to *Wiadomości,* the underground newspaper of the Oneg Shabbat Archive, 414 people died in the

89 Czerniaków, *The Warsaw Diary*, p. 237.
90 Opochinsky, *Reshimot*, p. 195.
91 Judenrat Statistics Department Report, no. 29, March 17, 1942, GFH, no. 11250, p. 5.
92 Opochinsky, *Reshimot*, pp. 103–104.
93 Ringelblum, *Notes from the Warsaw Ghetto*, p. 194.
94 Opochinsky, *Reshimot*, p. 149.
95 Lensky, *A Physician inside the Warsaw Ghetto*, pp. 94–95.

ghetto in November 1942—around 1 percent of the remaining Jewish population:[96] 124 were shot by the Nazis; 3 committed suicide; and 287 died of "natural" causes.[97] Writing in December 1942, Opochinsky described the high mortality rate due to work among laborers in the ghetto workshops. For example, the death rate from hunger and grueling labor was no less than 70 percent among those who sewed linens. The composition of a shop's labor force always fluctuated as new victims replaced the dead.[98]

Suicide

According to the sociologist Émile Durkheim, although the phenomenon of suicide runs counter to the religious, social, familial, and political value system, the combination of egoism and the collapse of the social structure tends to lead to a swift rise in suicide rates. When social norms value individual needs over those of the collectivity, indifference to the other may prevail and society may lose its power as a source that contributes to promoting the individual's self-esteem. This creates difficulties in establishing intimate human relations. When an individual lacks minimal concern for the needs and views of others, as well as respect for the values of the group, a sense of loneliness and the absence of social support may result. According to Durkheim, these are factors of suicide.[99]

Lucy Dawidowicz wrote that the suicide rate in the Warsaw ghetto, which was 65 percent of the prewar level among the Jews of Warsaw, was lower than one might have expected.[100] The reason may have been the strong social cohesion prevailing in the ghetto.

96 Blatman, *Geto Varsha—Sipur Itona'i*, p. 431.

97 Roland, *Courage under Siege*, p. 214.

98 Opochinsky, *Reshimot*, p. 187.

99 Lindenthal, "Epidemiological Status," p. 28.

100 Dawidowicz, *The War against the Jews*, p. 292. Dworzecki reported that suicides were very uncommon in the Vilna ghetto as well. See Dworzecki, "Tofa'ot Patologiyot Begeto Vilna," p. 7. On the suicide rate, see also Dworzecki, "The Day-to-Day Stand of the Jews," p. 164.

Durkheim described the power of the group as the most effective means of restraining individual suicides.

> [Individuals], on their part, have no reason to endure life's sufferings patiently. For they cling to life more resolutely when belonging to a group they love, so as not to betray interests they put before their own. The bond that unites them with the common cause attaches them to life and the lofty goal they envisage prevents their feeling personal troubles so deeply. There is, in short, in a cohesive and animated society a constant interchange of ideas and feelings from all to each and each to all, something like a mutual moral support, which instead of throwing the individual on his own resources, leads him to share in the collective energy and supports his own when exhausted.[101]

Dr. Mordechai Lensky, a physician in the Warsaw ghetto, wrote that social and familial partnership warded off an eruption of symptoms of mental illness among individuals.[102] Lindenthal, in contrast, noted that when the odds are stacked against people, for example, during the deportations to extermination camps, social cohesion cannot be reckoned on as a factor to curb suicide. In such a state of affairs, there is increasing social breakdown, and the individual succumbs to suicide.[103]

Suicides occurred already in the very first month of the war. In the middle of September 1939, Kaplan reported that a friend of his, the Yiddish writer Szymon Horonczyk, took his life after his son disappeared in the course of an escape. Disaster had driven him insane. Kaplan wrote sadly and critically,

> Our sages said that a man does not transgress until the spirit of madness enters him. [Horonczyk's] son may not have died

101 Émile Durkheim, "Suicide: A Study in Sociology," in Ian McIntosh, ed., *Classical Sociological Theory: A Reader* (New York: New York University Press, 1997), p. 217.

102 Lensky, "Problems of Disease in the Warsaw Ghetto," pp. 283–293.

103 Lindenthal, "Epidemiological Status," p. 28.

> and may yet come back. And even if he died—one should not sentence oneself to death. But I may be mistaken… Do not judge your fellow until you reach his psychological condition.[104]

In mid-May 1940, information about the Germans' victories plunged the Jewish population into despair and triggered suicides,[105] and suicides among the Jews appear to have increased in October 1940, due to the ghettoization decree.[106]

In Turkow's estimation, suicides were not uncommon in the ghetto, even before the mass deportations began.[107] As early as November, the first month in the ghetto, Czerniaków reported suicides.[108] Ringelblum wrote that there were 7 suicides per week on average before the war, whereas in December 1940, the second month in the ghetto, the average fell to 3 or 4.[109] In May 1941, in contrast, about half a year after ghettoization, suicides increased. Various methods were used, including jumping off high places.[110] On May 20, 1941, for example, 2 refugees took their lives by ingesting strychnine.[111] In mid-September 1941, Czerniaków reported a suicide of a person who leaped to his death.[112] However, suicide was a marginal

104 Kaplan, *Megilat Yisurin*, p. 25.

105 Ringelblum, *Notes from the Warsaw Ghetto*, pp. 40, 70.

106 Czerniaków, *The Warsaw Diary*, p. 205; Ringelblum, *Notes from the Warsaw Ghetto*, p. 79.

107 Turkow, *Hayo Hayta Varsha Yehudit*, p. 148.

108 Czerniaków, *The Warsaw Diary*, pp. 212, 218. There are additional testimonies about suicides at the time of ghettoization. For example, after the German invasion of Hungary on March 19, 1944, a wave of suicides ensued among Jews in Budapest who had been transferred to houses marked with the yellow star. These people could not endure the loss of their homes. On June 21, the people who had made the first suicide attempts by poisoning themselves were brought to the provisional Jewish hospital in Budapest. See Varda Weiskopf, "Beit Haholim Hayehudi BeBudapesht Tahat Hakibush Hanatzi (1944–1945)" (The Jewish Hospital in Budapest under the Nazi Occupation), *Harefu'a* (Hebrew),148:1, pp. 81–84.

109 Ringelblum, *Notes from the Warsaw Ghetto*, p. 113.

110 Ibid., p. 172.

111 Ibid., pp. 180–181.

112 Czerniaków, *The Warsaw Diary*, p. 279.

phenomenon. In September 1941, about ten months after the ghetto was established, Mary Berg wrote,

> It is inconceivable that we have the strength to live through it. The Germans are surprised that the Jews in the ghettos do not commit mass suicide, as was the case in Austria after the *Anschluss*. We, too, are surprised that we have managed to endure all these torments. This is the miracle of the ghetto.[113]

In March 1942, around three months before the beginning of the *Grossaktion*, Kaplan wrote,

> This secret power works wonders in us; as evidence, we don't have cases of suicide...Proud, filled with self-esteem, thousands of German and Austrian Jews put an end to their lives. Not so the...Jews of Poland...this will of ours to live in the midst of terrible calamity is the outward manifestation of a certain hidden power whose quality has not yet been examined. It is a wondrous, superlative power with which only the most established communities among our people have been blessed.[114]

On June 5, 1942, roughly a month and a half before the deportations began, Abraham Lewin noted in his diary that one of the most amazing byproducts of the war was the adherence to life and the nearly total absence of suicide.

> People are dying in vast numbers...but people do not try to escape from life. In fact, just the contrary: people are bound to life body and soul and want to survive the war at any price....The tension of this epoch-making conflict is so great that everybody, young and old, great and small, wants to live to see the outcome of this giant struggle, and the new world order.[115]

113 Berg, *The Diary of Mary Berg*, p. 91. On suicides in the Jewish community and particularly among the Jews of Germany, see Konrad Kwiet, "The Ultimate Refuge: Suicide in the Jewish Community under the Nazis," *Leo Baeck Institute*, 29 (1984), pp. 135–167.

114 Kaplan, *Scroll of Agony*, p. 131.

115 Lewin, *A Cup of Tears*, p. 119.

Jerzy Ross, who worked at the ghetto first aid station, wrote that suicides in the ghetto were few, despite the exceptionally difficult living conditions. From his vast experience in administering first aid in the field, he remembered only a few cases of suicide by hanging, by leaping from multistory buildings, and by poisoning—which constituted the largest share of suicides. He keenly recalled the most dramatic suicide, that of Czerniaków. The staff of the first aid station had been summoned by telephone. Ross and his associates were among the first to arrive and to find Czerniaków, who had committed suicide in his office, sprawled on a sofa next to a desk in the corridor. The first aid doctor carried out the routine tests and established his death. A vial containing a white powder, found on the small desk, revealed that Czerniaków had taken cyanide.[116]

The *Grossaktion* began the next day, triggering a wave of suicides. As the transports headed out one after another, Lewin wrestled with the question of whether or not it would be better for him to put his elderly mother to sleep forever, rather than to hand her over to the murderers. On July 25, 1942, he wrote that there had been many suicides. On August 19, he again noted that masses of Jews were committing suicide.[117] According to a report, dated October 12, 1942, from the governor of the Warsaw district there were 155 suicides in August 1942 and 60 in September.[118] Turkow wrote that the plague of suicides intensified when the transports began. Parents poisoned their young children and children poisoned their elderly parents, each seeking to spare the other horrendous abuse and, ultimately, ghastly death at the hands of the Germans.[119]

116 Ross, "Tahanat Ezra Rishona," p. 72.

117 Lewin, *A Cup of Tears*, pp. 136, 138, 161.

118 Melech Neustadt, ed., *Horban Umered Shel Yehudei Varsha: Sefer Eduyot Ve'azkarot* (Destruction and Uprising of the Jews of Warsaw: Book of Testimonies and Memorials) (Hebrew), 2nd ed. (Tel Aviv: Executive Committee of the General Federation of Labor, 1947), p. 55.

119 Turkow, *Hayo Hayta Varsha Yehudit*, p. 148. On the tragic dilemma of attending to the lethal poisoning of family members, a husband poisoning his wife; a child, his parents; parents, their children; and so on, see Perechodnik, *Hatafkid He'atzuv Shel Hati'ud*, pp. 40–43, 82, 89, 91–92, 138.

The first large wave of deportations ended in December 1942. Ringelblum wrote that during the deportations, when it became clear to some Jewish intellectuals that there was no way out, lacking even 100 zlotys to buy a loaf of bread and constantly under the threat of abduction and of being sent to the Umschlagplatz, several decided to take their fate into their hands and preempt death by means of suicide. The statistics indicate hundreds of suicides, mainly among the intelligentsia. Carrying poison with them became a mass phenomenon among this population.[120] In December 1942, Ringelblum described in his writings the small number of suicides as an astonishing and unique phenomenon under the grim conditions that had been imposed on the Jews. He claimed that the number had reached several hundred, but that this was a minute fraction of the 300,000 Jewish victims who had lost their lives up to that point. In his estimation, the large majority of ghetto inhabitants did not break, but instead carried on physically as long as possible, displaying audacious and effective psychological resistance. From the psychological standpoint, he contended, no people on earth had endured so much for so long as the Jewish people had.[121]

120 Ringelblum, *Ktavim Aharonim*, p. 23.

121 Ibid., p. 24. In Ringelblum's judgment, those who committed suicide during the deportations were heroes. Their numbers would have been greater had they been able to obtain the requisite drugs, but the Jewish pharmacies were locked during the deportations. Most of their staff had been taken to the Umschlagplatz and their entire inventory had been seized and brought to the requisition center. The researcher Konrad Kwiet proposed that suicide be included among the forms of resistance, because it "frustrated" Nazi intentions to persecute the Jews. Dan Michman objected, arguing that if resistance is a form of endurance ("not breaking down"), then suicide cannot possibly be a form of resistance. See Konrad Kwiet, "Problems of Jewish Resistance Historiography," *Leo Baeck Institute*, 26 (1979), pp. 37–57, and Dan Michman, *Holocaust Historiography*, p. 173–174n37, 243. Raul Hilberg mentions suicide as one of many responses of the victims, the few victims who, unlike the majority, did not tolerate the state of aggression and responded in various ways ranging "from suicide to uprising." Raul Hilberg, *Perpetrators, Victims, Bystanders: The Jewish Catastrophe, 1933–1945* (New York: HarperCollins, 1992).

Marek Edelman testified about the doctors who attempted suicide during the *Aktionen*, such as Dr. Irka, who worked at the hospital on Leszno St. When that facility was moved to the Umschlagplatz, she swallowed a phenobarbital pill, put on a nightgown, and lay down in bed. Edelman attempted to save her.[122] In late July 1942, at the height of the *Aktionen*, Dr. Adina Blady Szwajger ingested Luminal the day that the children from the hospital on Leszno St. were taken to the Umschlagplatz. Her friend Dr. Hella Kielson saved her by injecting her with Cardiamin.[123] Dr. Lensky reported that Dr. Izak Lichtenberg committed suicide during the *Aktionen* by taking cyanide.[124] Doctors who escaped from the ghetto to the Aryan side also ended their lives when they sustained injury or could not bear the suffering. For example, in 1944, after Dr. Maurycy Wolf was wounded, evidently in a shelling, he committed suicide by taking cyanide.[125]

Dr. Moshe Tursz testified about the transport of Dr. Jakob Rozenblum, a TOZ executive, Dr. Sara Zofia Syrkin Binstein, an activist in TOZ and the Judenrat Health Department, and Dr. Israel Milejkowski, the director of the Judenrat Health Department, who were loaded onto railroad cars along with thousands of others and taken to their deaths. According to Dr. Tursz, all three probably ingested cyanide on the train.[126] Dr. Polisiuk wrote in his diary that many people who had attempted suicide were found in the hospital wards during the *Aktionen*, including colleagues, such as Dr. Isidor Teichner and Dr. Gershon Lewin of Otwock, both of whom were saved.[127] Mrs. Tenenbaum, the superintendent of nurses at the children's hospital, received a "life number" from the hospital director ahead of a selection. She had a daughter, who did not receive one. After giving the number to her daughter, saying, "Hold this for a

122 Krall, *Shielding the Flame*, p. 108.

123 Blady Szwajger, *I Remember Nothing More*, p. 51.

124 Lensky, *A Physician inside the Warsaw Ghetto*, p. 59.

125 Ibid., p. 23.

126 Dr. Moshe Tursz testimony, YVA, O.3/438, p. 18.

127 Dr. Adolf Polisiuk diary, GFH, no. 3182.

moment, I'll be right back," Mrs. Tenenbaum went upstairs and took phenobarbital.[128]

Funerals and Burial

It is possible to learn about the mortality rate and the death count by examining information about the number of funerals and of exemptions from funeral payments. Presumably, exemptions were granted to the impoverished relatives of loved ones who had died in refugee centers or on the street. According to a report from a house committee on Krochmalna St., 63 bodies were removed from the building in order to avoid funeral expenses.[129] In 1940, there were 8,981 funerals in the ghetto: 2,757 for a fee and 6,224 free of charge. By implication, 70 percent of those who died had been poor.[130] According to the Hashomer Hatza'ir newspaper, *Neged Hazerem*, there were 3,821 burials in the Warsaw cemetery—59 for a fee and 3,762 free of charge. This provides an indication of the poverty rate among the population and, particularly, among those who died.[131]

A comparison of the monthly funeral count throughout the ghetto era with that of the month preceding the war attests to the enormity of the mortality rate in the ghetto.[132] In 1941, the average number of funerals each month constituted nearly 1 percent of the ghetto population—about 10 percent of the total population during the entire year. In January 1942, the rate climbed to 1.35 percent. In February 1942, funerals were held for 1.24 percent of the population. The average size of this population in 1941 numbered 414,772, which contracted by about 8.5 percent to 379,330 by January 1942. The demographic decline continued in February 1942. According to the Judenrat statistics department, 4,618 funerals were conducted in the cemeteries of Warsaw

128 Krall, *Shielding the Flame*, pp. 46–47.
129 Trunk, "Epidemics and Mortality," p. 117.
130 Ibid.
131 Blatman, *Geto Varsha—Sipur Itona'i*, p. 153.
132 Ibid., pp. 150, 172, 178.

that month for 2,147 men, 1,827 women, and 644 children up to thirteen years of age.[133] This source, as well as reports in the aforementioned underground newspaper *Undzer Hofenung*, indicate that mortality was about 8 percent higher among men than among women.

At the beginning of the war, after many were killed in the bombardments, Jews had to contend with the unique issues of burial that were created under the conditions and restrictions of German rule and the hardships of war. A special disinfection team gathered up the dead and took them away in hand-drawn carts, their dislocated limbs dangling.[134] In August 1940, about three months before ghettoization, Kaplan wrote,

> Every great man or leader of his people who passes on in these evil times is carried to his grave alone, with his death and burial unknown to anyone. Since there are no newspapers, there is nowhere to publish death notices... For this reason, in a city as large as Warsaw, no one knows which of his acquaintances are still alive and which are dead...buried in the presence of only half a dozen friends and relatives.[135]

The cemetery remained outside the confines of the ghetto. A permanent guard of German, Polish, and Jewish police was posted at the gate on Gęsia St., facing Okopowa St. The Judenrat was required to give the Germans advance notice of every funeral. The Germans then demanded that a funeral license form, issued by the Judenrat, be filled out.[136] They painstakingly inspected every coffin, having heard that the Jews were using the carts to smuggle food into the ghetto, or people out of the ghetto.[137]

133 Judenrat Statistics Department Report, no. 29, March 17, 1942, GFH, no. 11250, p. 8.
134 Ringelblum, *Yoman Vereshimot*, p. 5.
135 Kaplan, *Scroll of Agony*, p. 176.
136 Turkow, *Hayo Hayta Varsha Yehudit*, p. 34.
137 Ibid.

Numerous funeral agencies that sprouted in the ghetto evacuated the bodies and conducted the funerals. There was an office in almost every other building, a large black sign with white inscriptions indicating the entrance. Each of these businesses had several branches in the ghetto. The largest and best known belonged to Mottl Pinkert, "the king of the dead." The Germans deemed these "undertakers" useful. The workers of these agencies wore special uniforms with white stripes and a black Star of David on their sleeves, and wide-rimmed black hats. Jews paid a great deal of money to acquire such hats and cards that identified them as working for a funeral institution.[138] The employees of these agencies also received crossing permits from the ghetto to the cemetery.[139] Mass burials began to take place in early 1941.[140]

Ghetto inhabitants called the undertakers "black ravens" because they would pounce on the dead, rummage through their pockets, and appropriate whatever they found. They even took their clothing and shoes. They would sell these items to the Poles, who thronged to the Jewish cemetery. Special battalions of Poles dug up the graves of the Jews, exhumed the bodies, and inspected them for gold teeth, which they extracted. The undertakers waged an aggressive war against these "jackals" but to no avail, because they were armed.[141] Lensky remarked critically that Pinkert's business improved from day to day and, therefore, he could sit in a restaurant, eat a sumptuous lunch, and drink beer and wine. When he got up from the table after his meal, he would pat his paunch and throw a few coins to the poor and the beggars on the street.[142] Pinkert's operation provoked great animosity.[143] His funeral wagons traveled through the ghetto for days on end as his employees, their black uniforms decorated with silver medals,

138 Ibid., pp. 43–44; Berg, *The Diary of Mary Berg*, p. 35.

139 Turkow, *Hayo Hayta Varsha Yehudit*, p. 34.

140 Zylberberg, *A Warsaw Diary*, p. 31.

141 Turkow, *Hayo Hayta Varsha Yehudit*, pp. 43–44; Auberbach, *Behutzot Varsha*, p. 30.

142 Lensky, *A Physician inside the Warsaw Ghetto*, p. 93.

143 Szac-Wajnkranc, *Halaf Im Ha'esh*, pp. 31–32.

evoked fear and terror. Until the *Aktionen*, the Germans did not dare to touch them.[144]

The Warsaw Judenrat derived about one-fifth of its total revenue from burial fees.[145] Only the wealthy were interred in the cemetery on Gęsia St. The payment for this service was 500 zlotys, which was, at the time, the equivalent of six or seven dollars. Those who could not afford this payment were buried in the Praga cemetery. The Judenrat was forced to pay the German authorities for the burial plots.[146] In late April 1940, Dr. Schrempf, head of the Sanitation Department at the office of the Warsaw municipal governor, forbade burial in mass graves in the Praga cemetery.[147] In 1941, after ghettoization, the house committees were compelled to assume the considerable expense of burials—up to 30 zlotys per funeral.[148] The committees found it so difficult to cope with the burial problem that one of the committees would not allow new tenants to move in unless they paid a deposit of 20 zlotys—an insurance of sorts in the event of their death.[149]

Every day at 4 A.M. to 5 A.M., undertakers would gather more than ten corpses that random passersby had covered with newspapers, placing a stone on the newspapers so that they would not blow away. Some of the deceased had perished on the streets. Others had died at home, and their families had abandoned their bodies in front of a building, after stripping them in order to sell their clothing, so that the Judenrat would bury them at its expense.[150] The bodies of the poor were loaded onto a simple cart filled with many corpses. Funeral processions in the accepted sense of the term did not take place, because the horse that pulled

144 Ibid., p. 37.

145 Trunk, *Judenrat*, p. 247; Offer, "Ma'arach Harefu'a Begeto Varsha," vol. 2, appendix B.29, p. 184.

146 Lensky, *A Physician inside the Warsaw Ghetto*, p. 53; Berg, *The Diary of Mary Berg*, p. 35; Czerniaków, *The Warsaw Ghetto Diary*, p. 8; Ringelblum, Yoman Vereshimot, pp. 100–101, *Notes from the Warsaw Ghetto*, p. 8. Ringelblum, *Yoman Vereshimot*, pp. 100–101.

147 Czerniaków, *The Warsaw Diary*, p. 142.

148 Opochinsky, *Reshimot*, p. 95.

149 Ringelblum, *Yoman Vereshimot*, p. 330.

150 Edelman, *The Ghetto Fights*, p. 26.

the cart galloped swiftly for sanitation reasons. A regular cart for one person was dispatched only for the affluent. It traveled slowly for 50–100 meters and then proceeded rapidly.[151]

By January 1940, vandalism and looting in the cemetery began to occur.[152] In late March 1940, Ringelblum described the appearance of the cemetery as "shocking." All the trees had been toppled. All the benches and some of the marble tombstones had been looted.[153] In late June 1940, hooligans entered the cemetery and smashed the remaining tombstones with hammers.[154] In September 1941, Ringelblum wrote that horrific depredations were taking place at the cemetery: mass burials in which the indigent dead were grievously dishonored by being tossed into the graves like dogs. In addition, graves were opened at night, gold teeth ripped out, and shrouds stolen. Members of the Jewish police who also engaged in this activity were prosecuted in the ghetto.[155]

German soldiers visited the cemetery by the hundreds, eagerly taking pictures of the dead, the relatives who escorted them to burial, and even the bodies in the ritual cleansing room. Every Sunday, the Nazis visited the Jewish cemetery with their girlfriends. "This [the cemetery], rather than the cinema, was a place of amusement for them. The bereaved regarded them with scorn and loathing, but in the circumstances, silence was the only protest," Michael Zylberberg wrote in his diary.[156] On May 8, 1942, roughly two months before the *Grossaktion*, a large German inscription that prohibited Germans from visiting the Jewish site, ostensibly for sanitary reasons, was displayed in the Jewish cemetery. However, as Ringelblum explained, the German

151 Lensky, *A Physician inside the Warsaw Ghetto*, p. 53; Kaplan, *Scroll of Agony*, p. 255.

152 Czerniaków, *The Warsaw Diary*, p. 105.

153 Ringelblum, *Yoman Vereshimot*, pp. 100–101; Czerniaków, *The Warsaw Diary*, p. 144.

154 Czerniaków, *The Warsaw Diary*, p. 168.

155 Ringelblum, *Yoman Vereshimot*, p. 321; Stanislaw Adler, *In the Warsaw Ghetto, 1940–1943: An Account of a Witness: The Memoirs of Stanislaw Adler* (Jerusalem: Yad Vashem, 1982), p. 167.

156 Zylberberg, *A Warsaw Diary*, p. 31.

masses who frequented the Jewish cemetery to see the heaps of human skeletons in the mass graves began to argue about the Jewish question. Some enjoyed gazing at the victims of Hitler's extermination policy, but others expressed outrage. These visits made a depressing impression on the visitors and, therefore, they were discontinued.[157]

After ghettoization, it was impossible to bury the dead until crossing permits were issued to go to the cemetery on the Aryan side.[158] On May 20, 1941, Ringelblum wrote that the dead were buried in a mass grave from 1 A.M. to 5 A.M. The bodies were interred without the traditional shrouds and, instead, were wrapped in white paper, which was then removed. At first, they were put in graves, side by side. Later, they were buried together in one grave. Land for burial was in short supply by then. Bodies could not be buried deep in the ground, because water seeped in and no soil was available to shore up the walls. Hence, the idea of building a special crematorium for Jews was raised in the German and the Polish Ministries of Health.[159] In late August, the poor were buried in a common grave in front of the cemetery. In the oldest part of the cemetery, piles of sand were heaped over mass graves that emitted a terrible stench on hot summer days.[160] After the January 1943 *Aktion*, the Judenrat issued the order to gather all the victims of the *Aktion* for burial in a mass grave.[161]

* * *

Attempts to determine the death count in the ghetto and to explain the reasons for the deaths have involved a variety of methods,

157 Ringelblum, *Notes from the Warsaw Ghetto*, p. 266.

158 Czerniaków, *The Warsaw Diary*, p. 218.

159 Ringelblum, *Yoman Vereshimot*, p. 181.

160 Ibid., p. 138; Edelman, *The Ghetto Fights*, p. 27.

161 Debora, a girl from the Warsaw ghetto whose mother had been shot by the Germans, described in her diary the difficulties of the burial and her objection to interring her mother in the mass grave. By paying a bribe, she managed to arrange a dignified personal burial for her mother. See Debora's Diary, 1943, United States Holocaust Memorial Museum in Washington (USHMMA), accession no. 2002.74.1.

perspectives, and sources. However, most of the sources yield a similar, woeful picture. At the end of the first year of ghettoization, the underground newspaper *Yugnt Shtime* (Voice of Youth) reported, "Overall, it has been a terrifying year in the ghetto, one of mass dispossession, ghastly poverty and hardship, and funeral agencies at every turn—40,000 dead in the course of one year."[162] According to the many historians who wrote about the mortality rate in the ghetto and as corroborated by data from the hunger disease research conducted there, 6,560 Jews died in Warsaw from the beginning of the war to the end of December 1939, and 8,981 perished in 1940. All told, 15,541 Jews had died before ghettoization. In the course of 1941, 43,000 ghetto inhabitants died—10 percent of the population. From January to June 1942, until the deportations began, another 26,000 perished and it is likely that about 15,000 who were not deported died in August–December 1942. In total, about 85,000 Jews lost their lives from the beginning of the war until June 1942.[163]

Of course, mortality among the Jews of Warsaw before the war was considerably different from that in the ghetto. In 1935–1938, an average of 9.8 Jews died for every 1,000 Jews. In 1941, the numbers soared to somewhere between 96 and 123 per 1,000 in the ghetto.[164] In August 1939, a month before World War II erupted, when 360,000 Jews lived in Warsaw, there were 360 recorded deaths. In August 1941, two years later and more than a year after the ghetto had been established, 5,560 deaths were registered—out of a population of approximately 450,000—the highest mortality rate ever. In August 1939, 0.1 percent of the population died as compared with August 1941, when the death rate rose to 1.2 percent—an increase of 12 times over. Had this

162 Blatman, *Geto Varsha—Sipur Itona'i*, pp. 157–158.

163 Winick, *Hunger Disease*, p. 35; Leshchinsky, "Hayishuv Hayehudi," p. 140; Czerniaków, *Yoman Geto Varsha*, p. 108; Kermish, "Nigudim Ma'amadiyim," pp. 567–569; Blatman, *Geto Varsha—Sipur Itona'i*, p. 153; Ben-Sasson and Prais, "Twilight Days," p. 46; Gutman, *The Jews of Warsaw*, p. 64; Trunk, "Epidemics and Mortality," p. 113.

164 Based on data in Leshchinsky, "Hayishuv Hayehudi," p. 140. Hirszfeld arrived at a similar figure. See Hirszfeld, *The Story of One Life*, p. 223.

trend in the mortality rate persisted, the Jewish population would have been annihilated within five years, without the use of direct mechanisms of killing.

In late 1941 and in the spring of 1942, mortality in the ghetto declined slightly. At that time, there were indications of a steady improvement in the situation. Previously, around the time that the ghetto was established, the Germans' plans had cut short this trend toward relative improvement and stabilization. The ghetto was established to realize the aims of Nazi policy and not in response to local developments. Similarly, the end of the ghetto came about for reasons other than its internal situation. In fact, the ghetto population had managed to weather the worst of its ordeals.[165]

Dr. Hagen reported that 58,000 Jews had died of hunger in Warsaw. According to data collected by the ghetto physicians, only 18,320 of more than 98,000 deaths between September 1939 and December 1942 were attributed to starvation, but the causes of deaths in about 77,000 cases were not identified.[166] While the mortality rate in the ghetto increased, it hardly rose among the Aryan population. The mortality rate in the ghetto was three times higher than that in the non-Jewish side of the city in April 1941 and six times greater in June.[167]

The main reason for the high mortality rate in the Warsaw ghetto was the living conditions in the ghetto itself that caused a deterioration of the hygienic and sanitary conditions of the inhabitants. Shortages of electricity, gas, and heating fuel made it difficult to bathe in warm water, and people seldom bathed at all. In any discussion of the direct causes of death among the Jews of Warsaw, a distinction should be made between 1939–1940 and 1941–1942.

165 Gutman, *The Jews of Warsaw*, p. 65.

166 Roland, *Courage under Siege*, p. 98; Winick, *Hunger Disease*, p. 35.

167 Trunk, "Epidemics and Mortality," p. 118.

Causes of Death, 1939–1942[168]

Year	Months	Total Deaths	Typhus	Rate (%)	Hunger and Exhaustion	Rate (%)	Other	Rate (%)
1939	9–12	6,560	5	0.08	4	0.06	2,056	31.34
1940		8,981	216	2.41	91	1.01	1,032	11.49
1941		43,239	1,991	4.60	10,971	25.37	10,653	24.64
1942	1–6	26,116	512	1.96	7,254	27.78	10,694	40.95
Total		**84,896**	2,724	3.2	18,320	21.58	24,435	28.78

Mortality Rate from Typhus, Starvation, and Other Causes, 1939–1942[169]

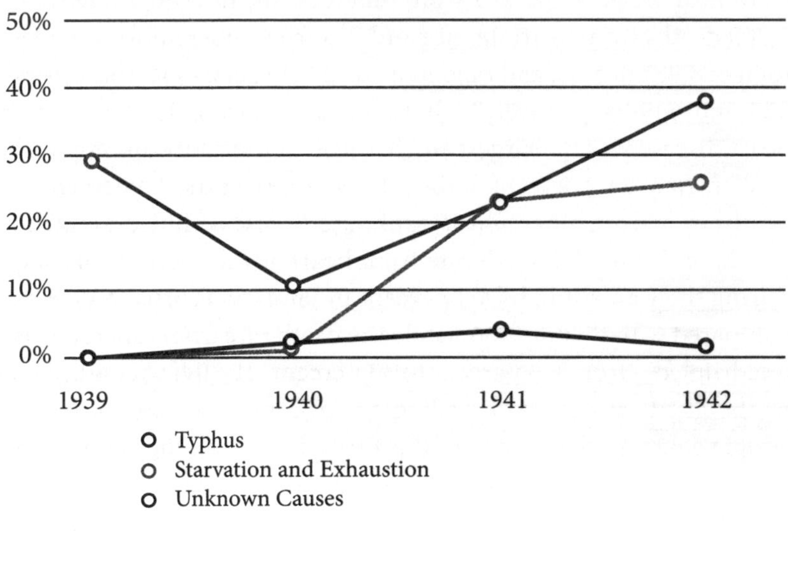

168 Ibid., p. 119. The data in this table was drawn from the hunger disease research in the Warsaw ghetto.

169 Ibid. The graph is based on the data presented by Trunk in "Epidemics and Mortality." See Offer, *Haluk Lavan Bageto*, appendix B.2, pp. 535–537.

In the last months of 1939 and throughout 1940, the death rate from typhus ranged from 0.08–2.41 percent. In 1941 and the first half of 1942, the rate was from 4.6–1.9 percent. Therefore, the number of deaths attributed to typhus was at its highest in 1941.[170] The number of deaths due to hunger and exhaustion rose uninterruptedly, especially in 1941 and the first half of 1942. These two factors explain more than one-fourth of all deaths in 1941 and in 1942. Presumably, the cause of several of the deaths, which had been defined as unknown, was actually starvation and, therefore, the number of deaths due to starvation was higher. According to the data found, 3.2 percent of deaths were due to typhus as compared with 21.58 percent to starvation. We lack data regarding the cause of a large number of the 84,896 deaths cited in the table.

According to Trunk, data exist on other causes of death—heart disease and tuberculosis—that might help us explain some of the numbers that were not accounted for in the table. Of the 6,560 deaths from September to December 1939, there were 1,434 from heart disease and 387 from tuberculosis. In 1940, there were 2,309 deaths from heart disease and 754 from tuberculosis out of a total of 8,981 deaths, and in January and February 1941, there were 523 and 649, respectively.[171] Before the war, from 1931 to 1933, heart disease was the largest single cause of mortality among Jews in Warsaw at 23.9 percent of the total. In those years, 8.3 percent of deaths were from tuberculosis, ranking this disease fifth among the causes of death. The death rate from heart attacks hardly changed during the war, rising by 4.3 percent in January–February 1943 as compared with that in 1936, while the death rate from tuberculosis quadrupled—from 8.3 percent to 33 percent. The living conditions in the ghetto made it a breeding ground for tuberculosis. Many people contracted and died of this disease, because they could not obtain appropriate treatment and proper nutrition.[172]

Based on the research data of the doctors in the ghetto, on Trunk's studies on tuberculosis, and on Roland's tallies, it is

170 Trunk, "Epidemics and Mortality," p. 119.
171 Ibid., p. 120.
172 Ibid., p. 121.

possible to assess the causes of mortality from the beginning of the Nazi occupation to December 1942: 2.8 percent died of typhus and 18.7 percent of starvation and exhaustion. Of the 77,121 deaths that the doctors could not attribute to specific causes, 30.7 percent died of tuberculosis and the remaining 47.8 percent of unknown causes. According to Trunk's data, presumably 28 percent of the deaths whose cause was unknown were due to heart disease. If so, the number of deaths from typhus and tuberculosis increased considerably, while mortality from heart disease increased only slightly. Death from starvation was clearly the result of the state of nutrition in the ghetto.

In the Ringelblum Archive, statistical reports provide data on mortality among the Jews from the time of the establishment of the ghetto in November 1940 to September 1941. The data is broken down according to the following categories: the population at large; children at the central shelter; patients at the two main hospitals, Czyste Hospital and Bersohn and Bauman Children's Hospital; people who died on the streets; and those who perished at the refugee centers administered by TOZ. The main conclusion of the report is that, despite the high morbidity of contagious diseases, the predominant cause of death was starvation.[173]

In 1953, Trunk wrote that 88,568 Jews died in Warsaw between September 1939 and August 1942. In prewar Warsaw, there were 350 deaths per month. Accordingly, there should have been 12,600 deaths in a period of thirty-six months. By implication, 76,000 Jews in Warsaw died of starvation and disease—around 19 percent of the roughly 400,000 Jews living in the ghetto.[174] Lensky claimed that 80,000 died of diseases and other causes, including starvation in 18,000 cases.[175] According to the hunger disease research conducted by the ghetto doctors, the effect of the conditions in the ghetto on mortality was statistically

173 Statistics on mortality among the Jews, 1939–1941, AŻIH, ARI.81; on mortality in the Warsaw ghetto, May 1941, AŻIH, ARI.223; see also "Warsaw Ghetto," documentation on population, mortality, and welfare, 1938–July 1948, YIVO Archives, RG–116–5.3.

174 Trunk, "Epidemics and Mortality," p. 122.

175 Roland, *Courage under Siege*, p. 224; Lensky, "Problems of Disease," p. 293.

significant. The death count among the Jews in Warsaw was 8,981 in 1940; 43,239 in 1941; and 26,116 in 1942, up to the end of June, when the deportations began. Presumably, the mortality rate would have been much higher at the end of that year than it was during the first half of 1942.[176] According to Mendelsohn, mortality among the 370,000 Jews who lived in Warsaw before the war did not exceed 400 per month. In the ghetto, the death count was fifteen to twenty times greater than the prewar figure. Mortality among children was even higher. Seventy percent of the youngsters who were admitted to the children's hospital died.[177]

Turkow wrote that according to official German reports from July 22 to September 12, 1942, 310,332 Jews were "transferred" from the Warsaw ghetto. Taking into account that 60,000 had already been "removed" in the course of various abductions by July 22—according to a report by the Judenrat Labor Office—a total of 370,000 Jews had been expelled from the ghetto. None of these reports included the approximately 90,000 people who died of hunger, epidemics, and other causes. There were 460,000 Jews in the ghetto. In addition to this number, thousands of Jews were tortured and shot. When these figures are added, the death count increases exponentially.[178]

176 Winick, *Hunger Disease*, p. 35.

177 Mendelsohn, *The Polish Jews*, pp. 11–12; Offer, "Ma'arach Harefu'a Begeto Varsha," vol. 2, appendix B.28, p. 184.

178 Turkow, *Hayo Hayta Varsha Yehudit*, pp. 158–159.

Jewish Mortality, Warsaw and the Ghetto, August 1939–June 1942[179]

Month	Deaths	Month	Deaths	Month	Deaths	Month	Deaths
		1/1940	1,178	1/1941	898	1/1942	5,123
		2/1940	1,179	2/1941	1,023	2/1942	4,618
		3/1940	1,014	3/1941	1,608	3/1942	4,951
		4/1940	1,044	4/1941	2,061	4/1942	4,432
		5/1940	856	5/1941	3,821	5/1942	3,636
		6/1940	650	6/1941	4,590	6/1942	3,356
		7/1940	563	7/1941	5,550		
8/1939	360	8/1940	525	8/1941	5,560		
9/1939	1,936	9/1940	489	9/1941	4,545		
10/1939	1,850	10/1940	457	10/1941	4,716		
11/1939	1,595	11/1940	445	11/1941	4,801		
12/1939	1,179	12/1940	581	12/1941	4,366		

179 The data in the graph cover the period from August 1939, the month preceding the war, to July 1942, when the deportations from Warsaw began. The graph is based on the data presented in Winick, ed., *Hunger Disease*, p. 35; Trunk, "Epidemics and Mortality," pp. 119–122; Gutman, *The Jews of Warsaw*, p. 64; Czerniaków, *The Warsaw Diary*; and Blatman, *Geto Varsha—Sipur Itona'i*, pp. 150, 155, 178.

Jewish Mortality, Warsaw, and the Ghetto, August 1939–June 1942

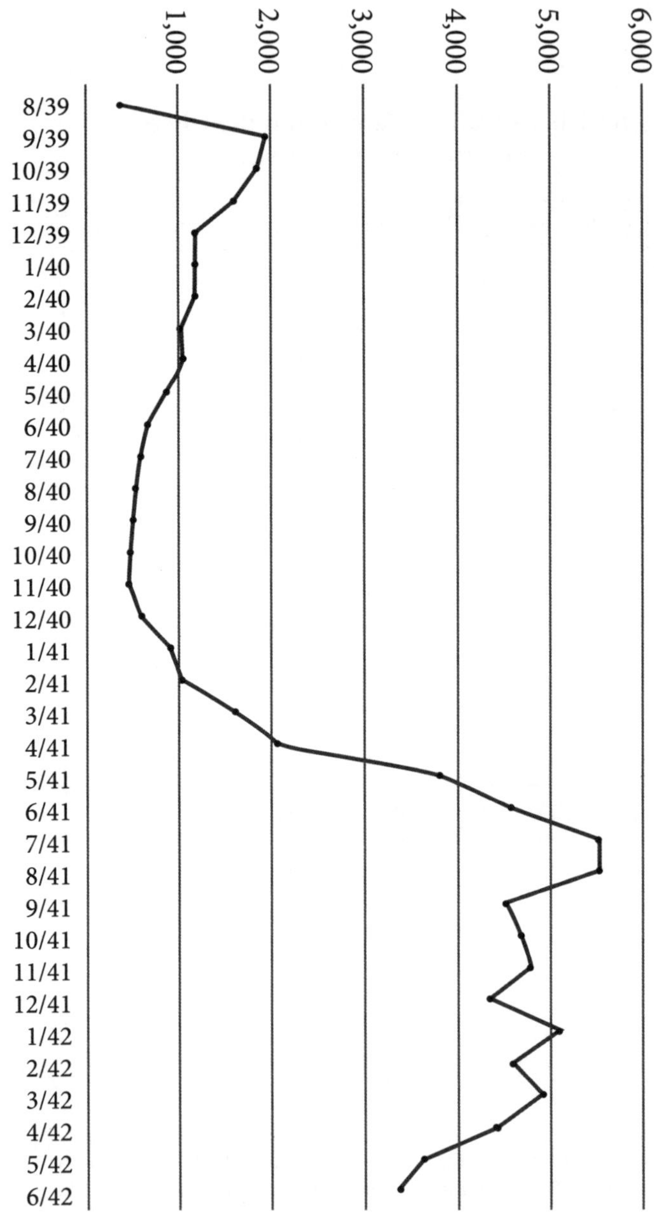

Chapter Nine

The Fight against Epidemics

German Policy on Typhus

It was widely suspected in the ghetto that the Nazis had deliberately spread the typhus bacteria there to test methods of bacteriological warfare intended for use against their enemies. Rumor had it that the Jewish community leaders had no doubt about this, having been informed by world-renowned Jewish bacteriologists whom the Nazis had sent to the ghetto.[1]

The Germans ordered the Judenrat to fight and control the epidemic, and demanded that they organize sanitation squads and operate isolation facilities and public bathhouses.[2] When the typhus epidemic first broke out in Warsaw at the beginning of the occupation and before the establishment of the ghetto, Dr. Kurt Schrempf adopted the "classic" method to eradicate the epidemic: the identification, hospitalization, and isolation of those infected, and a two or three week quarantine of those who had been in contact with them. When the isolation facilities were fully occupied, suspected cases were quarantined in their homes. Many buildings were closed off for two weeks and police were stationed at their entrances. In addition, tenants were deloused and their homes and clothing were disinfected. Schrempf had bathhouses

1 Berg, *The Diary of Mary Berg*, p. 92.

2 Dr. Moshe Tursz testimony, YVA, O.3/438.

and disinfection stations built in various parts of Warsaw but not in the Jewish quarter.[3] He ordered the Judenrat to invest in disinfection facilities, for which the Jews were forced to pay 100,000 zlotys in January 1940.[4] In April 1940, roughly half a year before ghettoization, Ringelblum wrote that the task of disinfection and of taking all the residents of the apartment buildings to the public bathhouse had become a very heavy burden.[5]

In January 1941, about a month after ghettoization, morbidity and mortality from typhus began to escalate. Dr. Wilhelm Hagen, Schrempf's successor, understood that an epidemic had broken out and revised his policy on the treatment of the ghetto population, although he continued to support quarantine, despite being well aware of its dire results. In September 1941, Hagen modified some of the anti-epidemic measures suggested by the Jewish doctors. The two-week quarantine of buildings and the compulsory hospitalization of typhus patients were discontinued, and dwellings were disinfected. The doctors who conducted house inspections twice a week were required to report cases. They also treated patients in their homes.

Hagen also imposed treatment for lice infestation on the entire population, instructing the Judenrat Health Department and the Jewish police to administer the treatment under professional supervision and under the surveillance of German and Polish guards. In 1941, 331,528 people in the Jewish quarter—the majority of the population—were treated for lice, and 78,677 apartments were disinfected. Cold weather, shortages of coal, and resistance by the population impeded the operation.[6] Hagen was frustrated by the response of the Jews who were not eager to comply with the public health measures that he had handed down. In his opinion, only 20–25 percent of typhus cases were reported. Bribery and passive resistance subverted all attempts to enforce the dictates.[7]

3 Cohen, "Harefu'a Besherut Ha'idiologiya," p. 178.

4 Czerniaków, *The Warsaw Diary*, p. 106.

5 Ringelblum, *Yoman Vereshimot*, pp. 95, 98.

6 Cohen, "Harefu'a Besherut Ha'idiologiya," p. 178.

7 Many countries adopt a public health policy to assume control over patients

According to Isaiah Trunk, the public was aware of the Nazi method of combating contagious diseases, which was no less frightening to them than the diseases themselves. Hagen was oblivious to the sense of terror that his medical measures instilled in the ghetto inhabitants for whom two or three weeks in isolation meant starvation, due to the inability to make a living and procure food. Delousing entailed leaving one's home temporarily and exposing it to burglary. Disinfection involved the destruction of clothing and property, and people often had to stand naked and defenseless for a long time in all weathers. Hagen construed the Jews' evasive response to his measures as blind obstinacy that could be subdued only by brutal threats.[8]

In the opinion of the ghetto experts, these measures not only failed to help eradicate disease, but they accelerated its propagation and intensified the suffering. Hirszfeld wrote that it sufficed to find one sick person in an apartment to send all the occupants to the bathhouse. Later, not only did the residents of the dwelling in which the disease was discovered have to undergo treatment, but also those in the adjacent apartments to the right and the left. In addition, the supervising physician was authorized to decree the disinfection of any dirty or neglected dwelling. Prof. Hirszfeld vehemently condemned disinfection as an anti-epidemic measure and accused the Germans of imposing it to heighten mortality. According to Hirszfeld, when cancer was discovered in an organ, healthy tissue was excised as well to make sure that every trace of it was removed. If a few cases of typhus were suddenly detected in a dwelling in a large city where there had not been any typhus patients before, the correct response was to wipe out this locus of

who endanger the public. See, for example, World Health Organization, *Controlling the Spread of Infectious Diseases*, https://www.who.int/healthsystems/topics/health-law/chapter10.pdf (accessed April 14, 2019). One might think erroneously that the Germans' health policies toward the Jews of Warsaw during the occupation were implemented similarly. However, as the ghetto doctors explained, these policies, which created conditions that abetted the spread of disease, and the authorities' powers to stem the spread of the disease for the sake of the public's health, became tools to oppress the Jews.

8 Hirszfeld, *The Story of One Life*, pp. 195, 212–213; Browning, "Genocide and Public Health," p. 25; Trunk, "Epidemics and Mortality," p. 106.

infection thoroughly. Upon discovering many cases of typhus, in contrast, other methods had to be employed and extensive social actions had to be initiated. Even the German epidemiologists advocated this approach.

While Dr. Hagen knew how to combat individual cases of typhus or cholera, he evidently lacked experience in dealing with an epidemic. The members of the disinfection unit sent by the Warsaw municipality to disinfect and to inspect dwellings were young Poles for whom this work was a source of a side income. Many of them pilfered the unattended property as their owners were forcibly led to the bathhouse.[9] People returned from the facility dazed, freezing cold, and hungry after enduring what Peretz Opochinsky called "crafty torments and harassments invented by degenerate, morbid minds to administer torture as would a modern inquisition."[10] Lensky described how the Germans "went berserk as typhus…spread throughout the Warsaw Ghetto."[11] In his opinion, due to their fear that the disease would spread to their own quarter and to their army, they took measures based on hatred and sadistic eagerness to oppress the Jews. According to Lensky, the Germans' sanitary measures appeared to be sound, but they were implemented in a way that aggravated the spread of epidemics and subjected the Jewish population to unspeakable suffering.

There were sixteen bathhouses in the Polish quarter, while the ghetto population, which was about half as large as the Polish one, had access only to four, and the unhygienic conditions and disorder that prevailed made them a breeding ground for disaster.[12] Prof. Hirszfeld accused the German doctors of ignoring the high risk of exposure to infection during hours of waiting at the bathhouses, thereby helping the epidemic to spread.[13] Indeed, the cruel disinfection decree caused typhus to spread at lightning speed. When people heard that someone in their apartment building

9 Hirszfeld, *The Story of One Life*, pp. 190, 212; Gutman, *The Jews of Warsaw*, p. 27; Lensky, *A Physician inside the Warsaw Ghetto*, pp. 101–102.

10 Opochinsky, *Reshimot*, p. 72.

11 Lensky, *A Physician inside the Warsaw Ghetto*, p. 101.

12 Ibid., pp. 101–102; Hirszfeld, *The Story of One Life*, p. 212.

13 Hirszfeld, *The Story of One Life*, p. 190.

was ill, they fled—sometimes carrying pathogen-bearing lice—to other blocks lest their own building be sealed. The Germans' fear of contagion was so great that some Jews managed to frighten away looters and extortionists by threatening them with infection by exposure to the typhus patients supposedly in their homes.[14]

The typhus epidemic created an atmosphere of panic. Rumor had it that the entire ghetto would be evacuated and those responsible for sanitation would be sent to the camps if the epidemic was not quashed. The Germans continued to demand that every case of typhus be reported—on pain of death—and that anyone infected be hospitalized. No one dared to resist these orders, even though it was mortally dangerous to obey them.[15] The German health authorities did nothing to help the ghetto contend with the epidemics and even interfered with the Jews' efforts to combat them. They forbade the importation of anti-typhus serum, forcing the Jews to smuggle it underground. Obviously, the poor could not afford the serum.[16] The German health authorities ordered Czyste Hospital to treat typhus with a preparation called Uliron, which contained toxins and was liable to cause death in certain cases. Every patient who received treatment was filmed and the hospital's medical staff were threatened with punishment if the recommended "cure" was not administered.[17]

Dr. Hagen ordered the Judenrat leaders to summon the doctors to a meeting. Invitations were sent in the winter of 1942, accompanied by a warning that those who failed to attend would be punished. Almost all of the 800 doctors in the ghetto arrived. They were required to register before the meeting began. Hagen, wearing a German uniform, entered the hall accompanied by an SS man who ordered the physicians to rise to their feet. As they remained standing, Dr. Hagen removed his cap, brandished his handgun, laid the weapon on a table in front of him, and launched into a speech.

14 Ringelblum, *Notes from the Warsaw Ghetto*, pp. 194–195.

15 Hirszfeld, *The Story of One Life*, p. 195; Ringelblum, *Notes from the Warsaw Ghetto*, pp. 213, 218–219.

16 Trunk, "Epidemics and Mortality," p. 83.

17 Ibid.

> Jewish doctors, Jewish filth is causing the typhus disease to spread in the Jewish quarter, threatening the Polish population and the German Army as well. Therefore, the Germans' sanitation services will have to restrict the Jewish population's freedom of movement. In cases of disobedience, the most severe punitive measures will be taken. Jewish doctors, you will be personally responsible for implementing the directives that the director of the Polish services will issue to you.[18]

Twirling his handgun, Hagen emphasized that he himself would shoot any Jewish doctor who hid a typhus patient and did not place him or her in isolation in the hospital. He warned explicitly that if typhus was not eradicated, the Jewish population would be evicted from the city. Dr. Milejkowski, head of the Judenrat Health Department, also warned the doctors at this meeting not to treat typhus patients at home but to send them to the hospital.[19]

The city was divided into sanitation precincts under the inspection of Polish doctors and bureaucrats, presided over by a German physician who supervised all health-related matters. Until April 1941, about five months after the ghetto was sealed, the Polish doctors were responsible for sanitation in the Jewish quarter as well.[20] The precinct physicians went from house to house, inspecting cleanliness. These large-scale sanitation inspections terrified the Jews.[21] In several precincts, the Polish doctors engaged in grave acts of corruption. Apart from overtly demanding bribes, they extorted money on the pretext of the lack of cleanliness by threatening to seal houses and shops in places where there were no typhus patients. They also forced people to visit the bathhouse.[22] About a month

18 Dr. Chaim Einhorn testimony, YVA, O.3/1836.

19 Lensky, *A Physician inside the Warsaw Ghetto*, p. 104; Dr. Chaim Einhorn testimony, YVA, O.3/1836; Offer, *Haluk Lavan Bageto*, appendix A.3, pp. 506–507.

20 Lensky, *A Physician inside the Warsaw Ghetto*, pp. 105–106.

21 Opochinsky, *Reshimot*, p. 72.

22 Lensky, *A Physician inside the Warsaw Ghetto*, pp. 104–105; Ringelblum, *Notes from the Warsaw Ghetto*, p. 16.

after the mass "Disinfection *Aktion*" on Krochmalna St., a German engineer named Rinderman complained to Dr. Schrempf about the unethical conduct of the sanitation squad that worked on that street. The inspectors had stolen property, broken down doors and cupboards, and beaten women who refused to tender bribes. The grievance apparently led to a change and, henceforth, the sanitation teams were replaced with Jews under German management.[23]

The quarantine stations, the isolation of dwellings, the disinfection of dwellings and clothing, the bathhouses, and the mass disinfection operations caused the ghetto inhabitants unimaginable suffering, as documentation from the ghetto makes powerfully evident. The quarantine system went into full effect at the centers and stations that served to isolate all inhabitants in any building where a case of typhus had been discovered. These overcrowded and unsanitary locations were themselves detrimental to the residents' health.

> In the course of a month, 1,300 to 1,600 people passed through quarantine. The quarantine represented a veritable hell for the inmates...Fifty to sixty people had to use twenty beds. The isolated persons were to get every day soup twice, coffee and 200 grams of bread, but these rations never reached them...eight to ten persons died of starvation every day... In the daytime, the inmates used to lie on the cots and cry from hunger...Protests were punished by beatings...The staff consisted entirely of Jews and everything was done with the knowledge and participation of the administration.[24]

This system operated from December 1939 to April 1941. In the first year of the occupation, 7,652 people were placed under quarantine. The number of typhus cases at this time was 1,846. For each quarantined patient, four who were not ill were sent as well. As the epidemic spread in the winter of 1941—during

23 Czerniaków, *The Warsaw Diary*, p. 165.
24 Trunk, "Epidemics and Mortality," p. 106.

the ghetto period—the technical difficulties of quarantining so many people mounted. A memorandum dated June 28, 1941, stated that the 1,400 beds in the quarantine center were only half as many as were needed. The health authorities refused to take heed. According to a report to the German authorities, when 5,500 cases of typhus were discovered, 6,000–8,000 people were quarantined.

Two or three weeks of quarantine led to the economic devastation of poor families. The community could not sustain them during isolation and, consequently, the condition and the suffering of the ill deteriorated even more. Hospitalized patients did not receive enough food and their families had to bring some to them. While their families were quarantined, they could not feed the patients, going hungry themselves and leaving the patients to their agonies.[25]

In April 1941, five months after the ghetto was closed off, the isolation method that was implemented at quarantine centers was revised, and they began to isolate and seal the dwellings where typhus patients were found, as well as those adjacent to them. In many cases, thousands of inhabitants were quarantined at the same location and kept under watch by the Jewish administration, until their dwellings could be disinfected. In addition, they were forcibly taken to the bathhouses for disinfection. Initially, all the dwellings in an affected building were disinfected, without exception. Later, beginning on September 26, 1941, doctors from the Health Department were authorized to exempt those found to be clean.[26] People made prodigious efforts, including various kinds of subterfuges, to conceal patients and remove them from their homes in order to avoid isolation and disinfection.[27] Those under quarantine were not allowed even to receive watery soup from the public kitchen. Sometimes a dwelling that was isolated for two weeks was placed under quarantine again, because somebody living there had fallen ill after it had been disinfected. Refugee

25 Ibid.
26 Ibid.; Opochinsky, *Reshimot*, p. 80.
27 Ringelblum, *Notes from the Warsaw Ghetto*, p. 196.

centers remained under quarantine for weeks on end, since new cases of typhus were recorded there every day.[28]

Disinfection units that included preventive sanitation squads disinfected the apartments and removed clothing for disinfection. These groups were notorious for their corrupt practices, which exacerbated the spread of the typhus epidemic in the ghetto.[29] Whenever the disease was discovered in a building, a team from the Jewish police arrived early in the morning and sealed it. Before doing so, the police unofficially advised the house committee of its intention to arrive, and the committee attempted to bribe them in order to take the sting out of the decree. The next to arrive were the Polish and Jewish doctors, Jewish disinfection workers, and German inspectors. Fearing a violent response by the Germans, the house committee did not quibble over the sum of the payment and its chairman discreetly handed over the requested amount. This, of course, caused the process to become more expensive.[30] Against the background of these activities, confrontations sometimes broke out among members of a house committee and between the Jewish police and the committee. On April 5, 1942, for example, an anonymous writer reported that a dispute over the imposition of a quarantine on Nalewki St. had ended with the submission of a grievance by a member of the house committee to the Health Department. The policemen in question were transferred to work elsewhere, but they made sure that the German police beat the committee member.[31]

When the residents of a building were taken by force to the bathhouse, their apartments underwent a "cleanup operation." The doctor issued instructions about the kind of cleaning that each dwelling had to undergo. The ostensible purpose of the disinfection of the apartments was to destroy bacteria, which actually resulted in the destruction of all the property in the dwelling. After the doctor left, the disinfection workers proceeded to dispose of the contents in the apartments, aggressively dragging furniture and appliances into

28 Dr. Moshe Tursz testimony, YVA, O.3/438, pp. 9–10.

29 Ringelblum, *Ktavim Aharonim*, p. 17n37.

30 Hirszfeld, *The Story of One Life*, p. 213.

31 Quarantine on Nalewki St., April 5, 1942, AŻIH, ARI.203.

the courtyard and setting them ablaze. They then began to disinfect the interior, spraying the floors and walls with carbolic acid or Lysol. If they had been paid to exempt the apartment from disinfection, another group of disinfection workers was sent. Instead of spraying the floors with disinfectant, they emptied pails of water onto the surfaces, appropriating the Lysol that could then be sold.[32]

Hundreds of bundles of linens and clothing, dirty and clean, formed mounds in the courtyard, hurled there by the disinfection team. Intended to reach the disinfection furnaces, they lay in the courtyard for a long time. Residents who were allowed to remain in their dwellings slept on sacks of straw and bare mattresses. Those whose apartments had been destroyed had to make do without this bedding, and had to cover themselves with the only coat that they owned. The more thorough and cruel the disinfection, the more profitable it was for the perpetrators.[33] The disinfection team received a minuscule salary, which was paid six months late, so its members compensated themselves by selling pieces of clothing and stealing whatever they could.[34]

The disinfection operation was one of the harshest episodes in the Germans' "war" on the typhus epidemic. It made a mockery of the principles of preventive medicine and exacerbated the scourge.[35] Members of disinfection crews were trained in a twelve-day crash course. At approximately the time of ghettoization, fifty participants had completed the course, which was held at the Institute of Hygiene in Warsaw and was taught by Polish doctors. The head of the military sanitation service in Warsaw, Prof. Wilhelm Richter, administered the examinations.[36]

32 Opochinsky, *Reshimot*, pp. 32–34, 60–72; see also Samuel Kassow, ed., *In Those Nightmarish Days: The Ghetto Reportage of Peretz Opoczynski and Josef Zelkowicz* (New Haven and London: Yale University Press, 2015), pp. 28–30; Kaplan, *Scroll of Agony*, pp. 133–134.

33 Kaplan, *Scroll of Agony*, pp. 133–134.

34 Hirszfeld, *Die Geschichte eines Lebens*, pp. 139–140.

35 Trunk, "Epidemics and Mortality," p. 108.

36 The first course for anti-contagion experts began on November 1, 1940; testimony of one of the participants, June 1942, AŻIH, ARI.221. For the anonymous testimony of a participant in the first training course for Jewish disinfectors, June 1942, see also Offer, "Ma'arach Harefu'a Begeto Varsha," vol. 2, appendix A.1, pp. 7–9.

As the epidemic escalated in the spring of 1941, the number of disinfection squads increased. In September of that year, there were twelve. In early 1942, their numbers fell to eight. At the height of the epidemic, June–August 1941, anyone who volunteered to work in the disinfection brigade was accepted, subject to a recommendation from Dr. Gold, the physician in charge. The Jewish candidates were required to participate in a three-week course that was held at the Judenrat Health Department. The squads were composed of Poles and Jews.

One of the most brutal disinfection actions took place at the end of August 1941.[37] The behavior of the Poles in these squads was so brutal that, pursuant to a meeting in September, attended by Dr. Tadeusz Ganc, superintendent of anti-epidemic operations at the Judenrat Health Department, their work in the disinfection squads was discontinued. German officials supervised the squads and their work.[38]

Only after changes were made and a health reform was introduced did principles of decentralizing and screening begin to be applied in the disinfection process. Now one or two rooms in a dwelling were set aside for disinfection purposes and only places that needed disinfection, in the doctors' judgment, underwent this treatment.[39] However, the process of singling out rooms for disinfection failed to attain its goal. The members of the sanitary units who were mainly concerned with lining their pockets did slipshod work. Wealthy tenants whose dwellings did not require disinfection were subject to extortion by threat of vandalism. Those living in infected apartments paid a ransom to avoid disinfection and, thus, the lice continued to spread. Members of the disinfection teams who engaged in extortion did not bother to seal the windows of rooms that were designated for disinfection by gas. The lice survived, built up immunity, and multiplied.[40]

37 Roland, *Courage under Siege*, p. 138.

38 Trunk, "Epidemics and Mortality," pp. 108–111; report by an anonymous doctor on the war on typhus, March 1942, AŻIH, ARI.363.

39 Trunk, "Epidemics and Mortality," p. 109.

40 Ringelblum, *Notes from the Warsaw Ghetto*, pp. 218–220.

A member of the disinfection teams, known as a *kolumnarz*, described how business was conducted.

> The members of the brigades are primarily interested in their side earnings, which range from 10 to 20 zlotys daily (their regular pay was nominally 6 zlotys a day but actually it came to less). These side earnings come from bribes…In most cases, the house committee…pays for exemptions…The average for an apartment is 10 to 50 zlotys. In dirty apartments, the fee for leaving the contents…depends on the financial means of the owner. In most brigades, the entire income goes into one pool and distribution is by points: 4 points to the physician, 3 points to the head of the brigade, 1.5 to the section leader, 1 point to the ordinary workers—altogether 25 points.[41]

In an anonymous document written in May 1942, about two months before the deportations began, a member of the disinfection squads described episodes that reveal the daily hardships of those who worked in these units, their composition, and his thoughts as he went about his work. He wrote, among other things,

> With blood and tears the ghetto wakes up…hearing the crying of a baby who spent the night under the stars…seeing corpses of people who handed back their ration cards…And we move on apathetically, it doesn't pain us anymore because we have become tough.…You hurry, you run. Hurry to get it done on time, not to be late, [because] if you are late, you lose hope of earning even a shot of liquor…Each time you see more people with the armband of the disinfection squad on their sleeves.

The disinfection worker concluded his writings by expressing the hope that the war would end and his comrades in the disinfection units, whom he considered victims of the catastrophe, would be judged favorably by history.

41 Trunk, "Epidemics and Mortality," p. 111.

> Do not worry, *kolumnarz*, the day will come, perhaps soon, when you'll take off your work uniform and will never have to see it again, and a day will come when you will be a person again. A person with lots of experience. A day will come when you will present a report...and maybe you will appear in it not as a culprit but as an accuser, when the judgment day arrives.[42]

The members of the disinfection units gathered each morning at the offices of the Judenrat Health Department on Leszno St. The composition of the group changed every day; workers did not know whether they would be assigned to work at all, or where. They were stressed about their fate—whether they would earn a slice of bread or not depended on this labor. The supervisor made sure that those not assigned to work would receive food rations. The average worker earned 3.60 zlotys per day. Most members of the disinfection squads were infested with lice.[43]

When doctors identified a typhus patient who was poor, they reported their discovery to the Health Department. When the patient was affluent, they treated him or her for a fee and did not report him to the Health Department, or they authorized a private physician, who also did not report the patient, to provide treatment. When a doctor intended to report someone, he handed the responsibility of actually making the report to the Jewish policeman who accompanied him. The police also benefited from bribes in return for withholding the information. Most of the patients who were hospitalized could not afford to ransom themselves. The wealthy bribed their way out of every stage of the disinfection process.[44] The members of the disinfection units sent the inhabitants of contaminated buildings to the bathhouse. They too first approached the house committee and worked out the payment according to the building's economic situation. Then they set up headquarters in an apartment of the affluent where

42 Thoughts of a member of a disinfection unit, Warsaw, May 23–30, 1942, YVA, M.10.AR.1/31.

43 Ibid.

44 The testimony of an anonymous physician, July 7, 1942, AŻIH, ARI.270.

someone contagious was staying, which made it possible to hide him or her. After the sanitation physician and a member of the house committee jointly determined which apartments had to be disinfected, those apartments and their contents were disinfected. The disinfection materials were defective and insufficient, which rendered the process ineffective.[45] In some apartments, disinfection cells were set up where sulfur candles were lit and the belongings were placed. Since clean belongings were placed with those plagued with lice, they too became infested.

All participants in the disinfection process profited from bribery. It was an open secret. Few workers complained to the Health Department about it. In general, those who did were fired and the system continued to run smoothly. Everyone involved in doing the work, from department and squad managers down to the lowest of the disinfection workers, was tainted with corruption, including conscionable people who tormented themselves for what they did.

> But my conscience, that of a rank-and-file worker...after he handed over his logs was unperturbed...because when you worked in the disinfection squad you had to put your conscience in your coat pocket before getting down to the task...so that it wouldn't get in the way of discharging the simplest duties.[46]

A member of the squad who was in charge of lighting the sulfur in the ovens used to disinfect the clothing described the inefficiency of the disinfection operations, which stemmed from the lack of requisite materials and, in his opinion, from negligence and corruption.

> The company that provided the Health Department with disinfection materials was Chemie on Leszno St. Mr. Golde, the brother of the manager of the disinfection units, and Dr. Goldwasser, the head of the Sanitation Department and

45 Opochinsky, *Reshimot*, pp. 60–84; memoirs of a disinfector, AŻIH, ARI.268.

46 Memoirs of a disinfector, AŻIH, ARI.268.

> the man who managed the distribution of the sulfur are partners in this business…I could not check all the data. If I could, I would have known how great the corruption was…
>
> A disinfection unit had not finished disinfecting a house before the very same house was full of lice. The authorities must have known in advance that the entire endeavor was in vain. I am sure this was a mistake. If the Jews of the ghetto had to take the bitter pill of disinfection, the whole thing should have been done right. In the meantime…everything was limping along…It would take a million miracles for a family that underwent disinfection to remain free of lice.[47]

He then described how the method and the conditions drew him and his comrades into taking bribes.

> Disinfection included four stages: referral of a patient to shower, disinfection in the shower, deposit of clothes in the disinfection cell, and disinfection inside the cell. All four phases were carried out for the sake of appearance, mostly due to apathy and criminal neglect. All it took was for one stage to be done improperly to make the entire job worthless. These cases discouraged anyone who wanted to do the job right. I am a responsible person. At first, I worked as hard as I could. My friends told me that I scattered the sulfur in the cell like a surgeon doing an operation. Sometimes I woke up at night worried about whether I had forgotten to treat some corner. I must compliment myself for having been so dedicated to my work. Nevertheless…I gradually became negligent. I knew that many people were not going to the bathhouse and were infecting others. I also had to make sure the clothing in the cells would not disappear. I did not always succeed…I did not fear inspection. No one came; no one saw.
>
> Everything depended on the disinfection worker's conscience. There was a problem in the way the material was handled—what was high [priority] and what was low

47 Ibid.

> [priority]. No one bothered to obey the instructions that we had been given about this. True, payment for this difficult and dangerous work was low. I never had much money, but I never took a bribe. In March, I found out that twelve disinfection workers had been arrested for taking a bribe. I was furious when all of them were released a few days later. This convinced me that I had nothing to fear, even if I did something that should not be done. That is how my honest character began to change for the worse. One of the tenants once accused me of asking him for money. They did not believe me that this was just slander…Then I thought, like a decent woman whose good name is besmirched for no reason, that if this is how things are, why shouldn't I take a bribe? What's more, my workmates flaunted the money they had received (not all of them) in my face. They said it was the best thing to do, perfectly normal. I stared at them jealously…I worked like a donkey and came home exhausted, without a cent in my pocket. Everything in the ghetto had become very expensive. My comrades helped rid me of my pangs of conscience.
>
> I was not really a criminal, but I stopped being the only saint in Sodom. I did things that I had never done and, even now, I feel disgusted when I remember them. It was tough. It became hard to resist corruption under those conditions of hell and hunger. Laying hands on a little extra money became a vital necessity. In return for a day's work, we received 3 zlotys, net. Clothes and shoes were very expensive, and clothing was ruined and torn quickly when doing disinfection work. A person who wanted to live only on a wretched salary could not continue working in a disinfection unit…and, thus, it happened that we all began to take a little money from the tenants. If only we had been paid a slightly better salary.[48]

Prof. Hirszfeld noted that bribery among the Jews actually helped to keep the Germans' harmful directives from being implemented. It created a new source of income for doctors and

48 Ibid.

disinfection workers—bribes in exchange for non-compliance. Given the high risk involved, large sums were paid. Sometimes people who could not afford to buy off the disinfection workers surreptitiously placed a corpse in the street to evade the disinfection decree on account of the deceased. In other cases, a body was transferred to the home of poor people who, for a fee, were willing to undergo the disinfection and quarantine process. Officially, this tragicomedy was called "the greatest war on an epidemic that history has known."[49]

To avoid suspicion, the doctors, policemen, disinfection workers, doorkeepers, and everyone else who made a living from their fellow Jews' disaster by exempting numerous buildings from disinfection in exchange for bribes had to quarantine buildings to show the authorities that they took the war on filth and disease seriously. Doctors could allow themselves to seal the homes of the poor repeatedly, because the tenants were too wretched to be able to complain.[50] In addition to disinfecting dwellings, quarantining the ill in their apartments, and sending the infected and their family members to the quarantine stations, they imposed a disinfection process by bathing, which was known as the "steaming house" procedure. The operation itself was referred to in Polish as *parówka*.[51] It was a mockery of the elementary principles of preventive medicine and one of the most appalling episodes in the "German war on typhus." The bathhouses were breeding grounds for typhus that caused hundreds, if not thousands, of people to contract the disease.[52]

There were only four bathhouses in the ghetto, including ritual pools, as well as a fifth facility opened by TOZ.[53] Tenants were taken by force to "bathe" in order to disinfect their bodies

49 Hirszfeld, *The Story of One Life*, p. 214.

50 Opochinsky, *Reshimot*, pp. 80–81.

51 Lensky, *A Physician inside the Warsaw Ghetto*, p. 105. According to Lensky, the term was not standard Polish, but was borrowed from the market patois. It was coined probably during the Nazi era for the ad hoc exigency of denoting forced bathing.

52 Kermish, "Nigudim Ma'amadiyim," p. 566.

53 Roland, *Courage under Siege*, p. 144.

and clothes in one of the bathhouses. The four bathhouses had a combined capacity of only 2,000–3,000, which was not enough to treat the tens of thousands of ghetto residents. Hundreds of lice-infested people pressed together for hours, and additional hundreds entered these overcrowded and filthy facilities every few hours. The masses stood crushed together, perspiring and panting with a sense of suffocation. It was fertile ground for contagion.[54]

Polish police hostilely ordered the residents of a building to report to the bathhouse. Those who could afford to bribe the police evaded the decree and stayed home. The gate to the building was closed, leaving no possibility of fleeing to a hideout. The tenants in the courtyard were at the mercy of the police, who beat them with rubber truncheons, and they were forced to join the column of people walking to the bathhouse.[55] On the way, a few attempted to elude the police. They were beaten for doing so. Additionally, the police threatened to shoot marchers who attempted to escape. It was also made clear that those not receiving certification from the bathhouse after their visit would not receive bread coupons.[56] Upon reaching the bathhouse, the marchers endured a series of torments. All were suspected of having lice in their clothing. In order to eradicate them, their clothes had to be disinfected, and the hair of both the women and the men had to be shorn. This process began in the morning and ended in the evening, leaving everyone hungry, tired, and humiliated.[57] While waiting to bathe, people missed the food distribution time and lost their daily meal.[58] They entered the bath in groups of 100 and underwent various treatments for hours. Naked, enfeebled, and starving, they endured the ordeal for almost a full day, until the process was completed.[59]

54 Opochinsky, *In Those Nightmarish Days*, pp. 24–25; Kaplan, *Scroll of Agony*, pp. 133–134.
55 Opochinsky, *In Those Nightmarish Days*, pp. 24–25.
56 Opochinsky, *Reshimot*, pp. 60–72.
57 Kaplan, *Scroll of Agony*, pp. 133–134.
58 Dr. Moshe Tursz testimony, YVA, O.3/438.
59 Kaplan, *Scroll of Agony*, p. 133.

Attendants prodded those entering the bathing facility to move along as quickly as possible, to undress, and to tie their clothing together for disinfection. There was no place to sit down and undress, and people had to sit on top of each other. When they stood up, naked, they had to wait a long time, until their clothing was taken away for treatment. During this time, their hair was shorn. The hall in the bathhouse was unheated and the concrete floor chilled their feet. People short of breath coughed incessantly and the feeble collapsed. Naked bodies cringed in the biting cold. No one believed that he or she would return home healthy after bathing. They passed through four or five rooms and corridors, all unheated, until they finally entered the bathing hall, where shower fixtures had been installed. However, the coal had run out and there was no hot water. Late at night, they received a minuscule piece of soap and took a cold shower. The next day at noon, their clothing was returned. Much of it had been lost or damaged, and everything reeked of the nauseating scent of disinfectant. At the end of the process, the bathhouse staff issued certifications, confirming that the recipients had undergone disinfection and were entitled to bread rations.[60]

Not only buildings were sealed but also entire streets, which included twenty to thirty buildings, whose residents were taken away for bathing and disinfection. Roadblocks were set up on both ends of the street. For a bribe, policemen allowed laborers and traders to set out for work in the morning.[61] Sometimes a street was closed off several times. People who lived on Krochmalna St. under conditions of terrible overpopulation and dire poverty suffered in particular from poor sanitation. In late March 1940, several months before ghettoization, the German Health Office in

60 Opochinsky, *Reshimot*, pp. 72–79. One way in which the Germans tried to ensure that people carry proof of delousing was by enacting a law prohibiting travel by train without such a certificate. To make sure that they would continue to receive further disinfection treatment, the document expired after ten days. Some Jews paid huge sums of money to receive this certification, and the bribes were distributed among the doctors who took part in the disinfection operations. See Roland, *Courage under Siege*, p. 144.

61 Opochinsky, *Reshimot*, p. 81.

occupied Warsaw claimed that this street was a locus of contagious diseases. The officials declared that they would burn it down if they could.[62] In April 1940, the street was closed off along with the thousands of inhabitants. A month later, when the first epidemic broke out, it was sealed again, because thirty new cases of typhus had been found there. Twenty buildings, home to 20,000 people, were quarantined for twenty-three days. It was only thanks to Jews from other areas, who contacted the affected population surreptitiously, that thousands were spared from starving to death.[63]

In March 1941, around four months after ghettoization, Gęsia St. was closed to pedestrian traffic after cases of typhus had been identified there.[64] In late August 1941, during the second typhus epidemic, Krochmalna St. was blocked off for the third time, because sixty unreported cases of illness had been discovered and because the German officials had found the corpse of a boy who had been lying in the street for several days near one of the buildings. When they entered the buildings to determine from where the body had been thrown, they found additional corpses in the courtyard and in the apartments. Consequently, the Judenrat Health Department was forced to inform the German gendarmerie of a new operation to disinfect the street. According to a report from Dr. Hagen, in conjunction with Dr. Milejkowski, Dr. Stein, and Dr. Laski, who was the German head of Warsaw's public health system, he decided to isolate the area again. The inhabitants were taken away for bathing and the buildings were disinfected, while they were away.[65]

About 100 German gendarmes, a similar number of Polish police, and more than 100 Jewish police took part in this cruel operation. Doctors from the Judenrat Health Department, Polish physicians, and officials from Hagen's office also participated.

62 Ringelblum, *Notes from the Warsaw Ghetto*, p. 28; Judenrat report to Dr. Auerswald on the Warsaw Jewish quarter under the *Kommissar*'s rule, May 15, 1941–May 15, 1942, GFH, no. 3909.

63 Czerniaków, *The Warsaw Diary*, pp. 136, 147; Trunk, "Epidemics and Mortality," p. 112.

64 Ringelblum, *Yoman Vereshimot*, p. 253.

65 Roland, *Courage under Siege*, p. 138; testimony about a sanitation *Aktion* on Krochmalna St., March 29, 1942, AŻIH, ARI.93.

The gendarmes were poised to fire their rifles. According to Prof. Hirszfeld, Hagen firmly decided to place Krochmalna St. under quarantine, after an inspection that he had ordered in a number of apartments had turned up several unreported typhus patients, who had taken refuge in attics and in other hideouts. Although the block physician was required to report cases of typhus, this was practically impossible in buildings that housed more than 14,000 impoverished people. Hagen demanded that they bathe and undergo thorough delousing, even though there were not enough showers to accommodate them all. The wretched inhabitants had to lie on the ground in the yard and wait their turn to bathe. The next day, when Hagen came by to check the results of this operation, he found ten to twenty bodies of elderly and ill people, who had not survived the cold winter night under the stars. Hagen responded, as high officials tend to do in such situations, by shifting the blame and dismissing Dr. Sara Zofia Syrkin Binstein from her administrative post at the Health Department.[66]

In documentation from the ghetto archives, an anonymous writer described a disinfection operation in which a friend of his had participated.

> This whole operation…didn't help much…The people were very frightened and hungry. They stood for hours in the street, at night, too…It was useful in only one sense: all the corpses were removed from the area and everyone who had typhus was taken to hospitals.[67]

The underground newspaper *Der Wecker* reported a similar *Aktion* on January 31, 1942, at 93 Dzielna St., where 3,000 people lived.

66 Czerniaków, *The Warsaw Diary*, p. 273; see the testimony of Marek Edelman in Krall, *Shielding the Flame*, p. 19; Blatman, *Geto Varsha—Sipur Itona'i*, pp. 171–172; Ringelblum, *Yoman Vereshimot*, p. 308; Hirszfeld, *The Story of One Life*, pp. 215–216; testimony about a sanitation *Aktion* on Krochmalna St., March 29, 1942, AŻIH, ARI.93.

67 Testimony about a sanitation *Aktion* on Krochmalna St., March 29, 1942, AŻIH, ARI.93.

In its aftermath, dozens contracted colds and pneumonia. The operation took place, not because disease had been discovered, but to punish the tenants for a 700-zloty debt to the Health Department. Members of the disinfection team collected about 2,000 zlotys in bribes from the residents of the building.[68] Such events were in no way unique. In another report about a quarantine at 5 Nalewki St. on April 5, 1942, the anonymous author wrote that the quarantine was imposed in order to collect the money demanded by the Health Department for disinfection.[69]

Anti-Epidemic Measures by the Judenrat

The Judenrat made prodigious efforts and spent huge sums to improve sanitation and health in the ghetto, and to preempt draconian German measures in the event of an epidemic. Nevertheless, its Health Department was unable to improve the health of the inhabitants or even sanitation, mainly due to the German authorities' hostile attitude.[70] The Judenrat set up a special department to combat disease and swiftly trained a group of people dedicated to fighting some of the causes of typhus. The results were negligible, because the ghetto conditions and the lack of resources made vigorous and effective action impossible. Still, from June 1942 on, shortly before the *Grossaktion*, the morbidity curve declined and there were indications that the epidemic had been quashed.[71] The Germans threatened harsher and harsher crackdowns on the pretext of insufficient anti-epidemic action. According to Dr. Tursz, the Judenrat and TOZ disagreed about the measures to take to prevent the spread of epidemics. However, the

68 Blatman, *Geto Varsha—Sipur Itona'i*, p. 223; Trunk, "Epidemics and Mortality," p. 112.

69 Quarantine at 5 Nalewki St., April 5, 1942, AŻIH, ARI.203.

70 Trunk, *Judenrat*, pp. 159–160.

71 Einhorn, "Harofe Begeto Varsha," p. 11; Berg, *The Diary of Mary Berg*, pp. 92–93; Gutman, *The Jews of Warsaw*, pp. 110–111; Lensky, *A Physician inside the Warsaw Ghetto*, pp. 103–104; Zabłotniak, "Epidemia duru plamistego wśród ludności żydowskiej w Warszawie w latach II wojny światowej," pp. 3–21.

Judenrat was forced to obey the Germans' orders and to submit to their supervision.[72]

The Judenrat began to take action on epidemics and hygiene in the first months of the occupation. In February 1940, about half a year after the occupation began, the Germans took Czerniaków hostage, because Jews were not reporting for disinfection as required. By then, isolation houses for typhus patients were already operating and the Judenrat had to cover the costs of disinfection and delousing.[73] In November 1940, several days before ghettoization, Dr. Schrempf summoned Czerniaków to advise him of his dissatisfaction with the results of the Judenrat's actions against the epidemic. Schrempf claimed that this was the second warning that Czerniaków had received and threatened him with arrest the next time. Five days after the transfer to the ghetto, the Judenrat was instructed to install delousing facilities.[74]

With the spread of the epidemic in late June 1941, Czerniaków convened a consultation on the matter and proposed that the house committees, administrators, and doorkeepers be liable for hiding patients and allowing lice to spread. That month, a bathhouse was opened on Prosta St., which received 1,000 people per day. In July 1941, Czerniaków visited the Health Department and the warehouse for disinfection materials. He wrote that he planned to conduct a propaganda campaign to combat typhus in the ghetto. A month later, in mid-August, he submitted a letter about the epidemic to the ghetto *Kommissar*, Heinz Auerswald, and requested a consultation with Dr. Hagen, with the participation of the ghetto physicians and Prof. Hirszfeld. Czerniaków then presented the Germans with memoranda written by Hirszfeld that included a proposal to decentralize the war on the epidemic; scientific criticism of the methods adopted by the Germans in this regard; and evidence of lower morbidity rates from typhus and other communicable diseases among Jews than among their neighbors before the war. Accordingly, Hirszfeld argued that the

72 Dr. Moshe Tursz testimony, YVA, O.3/438, p. 13.

73 Czerniaków, *The Warsaw Diary*, pp. 114–116, 158.

74 Ibid., pp. 215, 218.

current morbidity traced solely to the conditions that the Germans had imposed on the Jews, and presented scientific theories about the proper method to eradicate the epidemic. It required courage on the part of Czerniaków, Dr. Milejkowski, Dr. Bielenki, and Prof. Hirszfeld to submit these documents. The Germans approved the implementation of some of the proposals by the doctors, but the quarantine remained in effect.[75]

Czerniaków persuaded Auerswald to assign an additional aide to Dr. Milejkowski to fight the epidemic and requested 250,000 zlotys in financial assistance to support this struggle. In September 1941, following the disinfection operations on Krochmalna St., an order by Dr. Hagen to hire 200 assistants to implement the anti-typhus measures was promulgated. Czerniaków complained to Auerswald about the disinfection teams' misconduct. At the same time, Dr. Hagen demanded the dismissal of Dr. Syrkin Binstein, the superintendent of the anti-epidemic activities in the ghetto, and of Dr. Milejkowski as well. Czerniaków also ordered the reorganization of the anti-epidemic apparatus and proposed appointing Hirszfeld to coordinate the anti-epidemic activities.[76]

That the Judenrat took action to stem epidemics is beyond doubt, but it did so amid immense objective difficulties. For example, in a March 1942 report by the statistics department, concern was expressed that the melting of frost and the onset of spring would cause a renewed spread of the epidemic, because of the large quantities of garbage that had not been removed, due to a lack of transport vehicles. In addition, the sewage system had suffered damage in many locations in the ghetto, and people had begun to dump sewage in their yards, because they were unable to use their toilets. Steps were taken to haul away the trash in an expeditious manner. The Judenrat asked residents to pitch in and requisitioned all available transport vehicles. Plans were made to evacuate the garbage over a period of six weeks. The German authorities allowed the Judenrat to charge every inhabitant a fee

75 Hirszfeld, *The Story of One Life*, pp. 212–213, 215; Czerniaków, *The Warsaw Diary*, pp. 252–253, 263; memoranda on precipitants of typhus in Warsaw, AŻIH, ARI.185; see Ofer, *Haluk Lavan Bageto*, appendix A.2, pp. 497–504.

76 Czerniaków, *The Warsaw Diary*, pp. 268, 272, 277, 279.

of 50 grosz, payable in two installments. To dispose of the frozen garbage, it first had to be chopped with axes. The house committees helped to mobilize the doorkeepers and the tenants to assume this task and to clean the stairwells. The health centers operating in the ghetto conducted inspections and forwarded reports to the Health Department. In addition, police quarantined buildings where the residents did not cooperate with the measures to remove the garbage. By the end of the month, some progress had been made, but not enough to eliminate the danger.[77] In order to promote garbage removal from the ghetto in the future, a plan to incinerate waste at one of the factories was presented.[78]

The Health Department promoted children's health and hygiene and set aside a bathhouse for the schools' use. In the schools, activities to provide information on hygiene were conducted regularly, including discussions with children, private meetings with parents, and meetings for the staff responsible for hygiene and medical care during which relevant documents were read. Special sanitation inspection committees were set up as well.[79] In February 1942, for example, one such committee inspected refugee shelters, where sanitation was poor due to shortages of water and of heating fuel. These efforts led to some improvement at refugee centers, where maintenance units were charged with maintaining order and cleanliness. However, the work of these groups was fraught with difficulties as the cold and the lack of clothing often made it impossible to send inhabitants to the bathhouses.

The Judenrat also strove to improve conditions at the bathhouses. According to the report, attendance at three active public bathhouses in February 1942 was satisfactory. Each month, the Judenrat disinfected dwellings, oversaw the use of the bathhouses, and inspected thousands of apartments.[80] In late May 1942, about two months before the *Grossaktion*, ghetto *Kommissar* Auerswald rebuked Czerniaków concerning cleanliness.

77 Judenrat Statistics Department Report, no. 29, March 17, 1942, GFH, no. 11250, p. 1.

78 Ibid., pp. 14–15.

79 Ibid., pp. 8–9.

80 Ibid.

Czerniaków personally dealt with the issue for some time by helping the Health Department and the Jewish police. He walked through the ghetto, admonishing custodians of dirty buildings and distributing prizes to those in clean ones. "At such a low cultural level, the ghetto cannot be clean," Czerniaków stated. He blamed the situation on generations of neglect that were now coming home to roost. However, he admitted that the horrific distress and deprivation were making things worse. Only on June 1, 1942, a month and a half before the *Grossaktion* commenced, did the Judenrat assume full responsibility for the removal of waste.[81]

The Health Council that was established by the Judenrat and headed by Prof. Hirszfeld concerned itself mainly with the war on typhus and with reform of this struggle. Hirszfeld tried to tailor his proposals to the needs on the ground. He wrote that it was possible to discern three strata in ghetto society. The poorest inhabitants and refugees, who could not look out for themselves physically, were at the bottom. Hirszfeld examined the homes of the working class and the refugee centers where typhus patients had been found. Most were bedridden, starving, and swarming with lice. The most effective way to treat these wretched people was to isolate them, creating a "ghetto within the ghetto," because they were dangerous. However, such a decision was out of the question and, instead, the conventional method was used to treat these people: bathing and delousing.

The second category consisted of disease-free, working people. Hirszfeld believed that they should be excused from standard disinfection measures and that it would be an error verging on madness to force them to undergo this ordeal. Indeed, it was decided to exempt them from compulsory disinfection. According to Hirszfeld, the third category comprised people who suffered from mild cases of lice infestation. The challenge was to assist them to organize anti-contagion measures themselves, which required supplying them with coal to wash, allowing them to iron their clothing, and assisting them to organize the maintenance of their dwellings. For this purpose, some of the

81 Czerniaków, *The Warsaw Diary*, pp. 360–361.

disinfection teams were converted into auxiliaries to help the inhabitants with the latter. In Hirszfeld's view, by making a good social worker available to such groups, they could accomplish more than the classical disinfection squads could and, therefore, this activity should be promoted and prioritized.

The Health Council convened once a week. Although its discussions yielded practical recommendations, it had no resources with which to implement them. However, it was important that it was assuming responsibility for and committing to efforts to contend with the deteriorating health situation. According to Hirszfeld, its task was the gradual transfer of responsibility for the disinfection activities to the Judenrat in order to change the Nazis' pernicious and brutal methods. [82] Hirszfeld himself felt that the council accomplished little: "our Health Council, vaccinations, and conferences were only for our own mental hygiene."[83] Regulations were published for the public's well-being, which met with resistance. Too many people had an interest in faking disinfection. They went so far as to support the German supervisors of the disinfection units, for whom the old arrangement of bribery was a source of income, and incited resistance against the representatives of the Health Council. The council often had to replace its entire staff, including the doctors.

The Health Council placed advertisements and sponsored gatherings for the public in order to provide information and raise awareness of the causes of typhus and the ways to prevent it. It prepared an exhibition on typhus, which emphasized the suffering and the conditions created by the occupation as the primary cause of the emergence of the disease. Young artists presented artistic proposals.[84] In March 1942, it submitted to the German authorities a request for permission to hold the exhibition on typhus.[85] The liquidation of the ghetto began the

82 Hirszfeld, *Die Geschichte eines Lebens*, pp. 146–147; Hirszfeld, *The Story of One Life*, pp. 217–223.

83 Hirszfeld, *The Story of One Life*, p. 223.

84 Ibid., pp. 217–223; Czerniaków, *The Warsaw Diary*, p. 364.

85 Judenrat Statistics Department Report, no. 29, March 17, 1942, GFH, no. 11250, p. 29.

day before the anticipated date of the opening of the exhibition and all the exhibits were destroyed. Although the Health Council strenuously fought the epidemics, Prof. Hirszfeld did not attribute their decline to the council's intensive activities.

> Strangely, the epidemic began to retreat when we began our activities. Public opinion credited the new direction for this. I do not wish to ascribe this honor to myself and to the sanitation authorities. Our resources were too scanty to eradicate an epidemic on such a scale…The Jewish sanitation authorities do not deserve credit for quashing the epidemic, just as they do not deserve calumny for starting it.[86]

The council also tried to confront the bathhouse and laundering problems. Hirszfeld wrote, "Usually our work was for naught. There weren't enough beds in the hospital. We almost organized a new hospital, but we had to give the building back, when the Jews from Germany came." Engineer Aleksander Szniolis of the Polish Institute of Hygiene was invited to work with the council to redesign the bathhouses. However, Heinrich Kudicke, the German professor who had taken over the institute from Hirszfeld, would not allow Szniolis to assist the Jews. Projects to combat tuberculosis and sexually transmitted diseases were launched. Hygiene in schools and in the labor camps was improved, garbage was removed, and streets were cleaned. A war was waged against scabies, which was spreading rapidly in the ghetto. Food inspections were conducted and the means to cope with contagious diseases were improved, but the problem of hunger defied solution.[87]

In response to the spread of tuberculosis, an organization was established to combat it. Its headquarters were set up in the TOZ building. Dr. Milejkowski, director of the Judenrat Health Department, convened a special meeting with the participation of everyone who could contribute to eradicating the epidemic:

86 Hirszfeld, *Die Geschichte eines Lebens*, pp. 147–148; Hirszfeld, *The Story of One Life*, p. 222.

87 Hirszfeld, *Die Geschichte eines Lebens*, pp. 147-148; Hirszfeld, *The Story of One Life*, chap. 25.

representatives of the Health Department, the Health Council, TOZ, and CENTOS; the directors of the ghetto hospitals, Dr. Braude-Heller, Dr. Stein, Dr. Bielenki, and Dr. Gepner; JDC executives; and social activists in the ghetto. The historian Dr. Yitzhak-Ignacy Schipper was appointed head of the organization and Dr. Józef Chajn Gołębiowski served as its secretary. They decided to establish four tuberculosis clinics and two hospital wards. Efforts were made to arrange larger food rations for tuberculosis patients and high-risk groups, and information and prevention activities were planned, but very little could be implemented. The organization held its last meeting on July 21, 1942, on the eve of the *Grossaktion*. Jewish police burst in on the meeting, demanding that three doctors be surrendered to the prison as hostages of the *Aktion*.[88]

According to Kermish, the suffering of the ghetto inhabitants and the torments of disinfection were also inflicted by the Jews and Poles who did the Germans' bidding: Poles and Jews in the disinfection teams, the Jewish police, and several Jewish doctors who served in the sanitation field under the auspices of the Judenrat Health Department.[89] Some Judenrat sanitation and disinfection unit employees adopted the methods of their Polish counterparts, exempting the wealthy from the dictates in return for money. They became rich on the affliction of the poor Jews and treated everyone involved in the matter cruelly. Officers in the Jewish police—Majors Ganc, Fleischman, and Schmerling—headed these units. Their truncheons always in hand, they issued orders, cursed, and delivered blows to the heads of the "recalcitrant."[90]

The underground newspaper *Jutrznia*, an organ of the Hashomer Hatza'ir youth movement, reported in March

88 Dr. Moshe Tursz testimony, YVA, O.3/438, pp. 14–15; Dr. Józef Chajn Gołębiowski testimony, YVA, O.3/2355; Judenrat report to Dr. Auerswald on the Warsaw Jewish quarter under the *Kommissar*'s rule, May 15, 1941–May 15, 1942, GFH, no. 3909. On sending doctors and other officials to prison on the eve of the deportation, see also Dr. Adolf Polisiuk diary, GFH, no. 3182.

89 Kermish, "Nigudim Ma'amadiyim," p. 567; Trunk, "Epidemics and Mortality," p. 108.

90 Turkow, *Hayo Hayta Varsha Yehudit*, pp. 42–43.

1942 that, while the ghetto had a Health Department that was supposed to fight epidemics, the inhabitants knew that the department's disinfection activities had very little to do with fighting epidemics. Everyone knew that a building was closed off for disinfection only if its tenants failed to reach terms with the department on the amount of the ransom. Disinfection was used to extort the residents. The health centers were derelict in their duties. They did not fight epidemics, even though there was much to do. Instead of looking after people's health, they lined their pockets with the scant means of the defenseless population. "Their activity," the paper concluded, "is another page in the history of the turpitude and corruption of those who rule over us today."[91]

In August 1941, about nine months after the ghetto had been established, Ringelblum issued a caustic critique of the Judenrat Health Department. He described the collapse of the health systems that had fought the epidemics. He accused the department's disinfection units of doing everything to exacerbate the plague of lice. "All the anti-epidemic activities are, in fact, a big scandal perpetrated chiefly by the doctors and the sanitation squads."[92] Disinfection had an effect in only 60 percent of the cases. For a bribe, bathhouses certified that people had used their services. The percent of sulfur used for disinfection purposes was too small and the lice remained alive.[93] Dr. Chai Gorbowicz also criticized the Judenrat's management of the war on epidemics. In his opinion, it was necessary to combat epidemics by addressing the problems that led to them, beginning with the problem of hunger.

> It is impossible to say that the little soup that a few people receive by paying 70 grosz quells hunger. This simply throws sand into hungry people's eyes, as if nothing can be done about it. But action, even a great deal of action, can be taken.

91 Blatman, *Geto Varsha—Sipur Itona'i*, p. 173.
92 Ringelblum, *Notes from the Warsaw Ghetto*, pp. 194–196.
93 Ibid.; Einhorn, "Harofe Begeto Varsha," p. 11.

> The failure is poor organization. Good organization could have saved thousands of people from hunger.[94]

Gorbowicz criticized the disinfection campaigns and the bribery phenomenon, claiming that these disinfection operations were ineffective and that new methods suited to the conditions under occupation had to be sought. In his opinion, it was necessary to treat the epidemic through education and rigorous maintenance of cleanliness at all levels, private and public. He emphasized that people only showered once every three months, because of the shortage of shower facilities. Moreover, the concentration of the homeless in the poorest parts of the ghetto created problems associated with focal points of filth. He concluded that it was necessary to take action against these methods of treatment. "This writer has long since been saying that a special bathroom should be installed in every building." Gorbowicz recommended that people be meticulous about keeping their homes clean and eliminating surplus furniture. He urged them to maintain clean stairwells, yards, garbage cans, and streets, and to ensure the cleanliness of food and baked goods.[95]

Prof. Hirszfeld pointed out the irrationality of the disinfection methods, which were costing the Judenrat treasury about 5,000 zlotys per day. Bribes to forestall disinfection cost 15,000 zlotys per day on average. He reasoned that this money could be used to buy laundry detergent and food for many people. The disinfection process had created a partnership of people who became rich at the expense of the epidemic and the war against it, and who had an interest in preserving the status quo. The tenants, groaning under the burden, were more afraid of disinfection than of typhus. After all, typhus had a 70–80 percent survival rate, while disinfection threatened to destroy everything.[96] Kaplan wrote that the "Health Department" existed for the sole purpose of supervising the state of sanitation, cleanliness, and health. However, even though this

94 Dr. Chai Gorbowicz, "The Struggle against Epidemics," AŻIH, ARI.102.

95 Ibid.

96 Hirszfeld, *The Story of One Life*, p. 214.

activity was undertaken by cultured and highly educated doctors, in practice, they were swayed by financial gain and bribery.[97]

Some sources directed their criticism at the Judenrat and held it responsible for the dire state of hygiene in the ghetto. Kaplan accused the Health Department of negligence, because of its failure to deal properly with the freezing of sewage pipes and, consequently, the breakdown of the sewer system. The underground newspaper *Der Wecker* also blamed the Judenrat for the poor state of sanitation. "The tax is intended for the war on epidemics. Why isn't the kehilla [Judenrat] doing something about this matter?"[98] The communist underground paper *Morgn Frayhayt* (Morning Freedom) blamed the Health Department for the mounds of trash that had piled up in the ghetto. It also claimed that Zamenhof St. had been disinfected, not because typhus had been discovered there, but only because the Health Department clerks needed money. "Will these practices ever end? The Health Department under the Judenrat must rectify the situation!"[99] *Jutrznia,* the underground newspaper of Hashomer Hatza'ir, claimed that the community [Judenrat] unjustly charged all the inhabitants of the ghetto, destitute and affluent alike, the same fee for waste removal. The garbage was not hauled out of the ghetto all winter, because the requisite vehicles were used to transport bricks for the construction of new walls by which "the community lords" profited.[100]

Opochinsky considered disinfection a form of torture, like a concentration camp in a different guise. He claimed that in addition to the Germans and Polish officials who created a climate of antisemitism that influenced the work of disinfection, the Jews who held positions in these activities also behaved cruelly and cynically. Jews brazenly engaged in bribery and in all the wheeling and dealing it entailed. The Jewish police in the ghetto often operated almost independently under the supervision of one Polish policeman, who led the way, creating an atmosphere of violence with the help of his rubber truncheon. However, it

97 Kaplan, *Scroll of Agony*, pp. 342–343.
98 Ibid.; Blatman, *Geto Varsha—Sipur Itona'i*, p. 202.
99 Ibid., p. 201.
100 Ibid., p. 203.

was the Jewish police—the *Shmendriks* (a vulgar form of the word jerk in Yiddish), the "wise guys," and plain old thugs—who finished the job.[101]

The actions taken to prevent and to suppress epidemics sharpen the discussion of the management of the ghetto. The German edicts in this matter raise many questions about the Judenrat's role as the entity responsible for implementing them, on the one hand, and for the ghetto inhabitants' health, on the other. Many questions have been raised about the role of the Health Department as part of the Judenrat and as the agent tasked with meeting the ghetto's health needs; about the involvement of the doctors, police, and doorkeepers; and about the roles of other organizations, such as TOZ and the house committees.

TOZ's Epidemic Prevention Activities

TOZ and a special Department of War on Epidemics set up under the auspices of the Jewish Social Self-Help were partners in the struggle to improve sanitation and eradicate contagious diseases.[102] TOZ worked with refugees and house committees in an attempt to keep epidemics from spreading, while the Judenrat strived to accomplish the same.[103] As soon as the occupation began, TOZ launched a program, with support from the JDC, which included free vaccinations and medicines for the public in general, as well as for bathhouses, disinfection and delousing centers, and refugee shelters. As the first wave of the typhus epidemic intensified, many months before ghettoization, TOZ worked in cooperation with the Jewish population to eradicate it by helping to deliver patients to clinics and hospitals, quarantining families of the ill, bathing those infected, and conducting cleanup operations with the assistance of its sanitation unit.[104]

101 Opochinsky, *Reshimot*, pp. 83–84.

102 Trunk, "Epidemics and Mortality," p. 86.

103 Gutman, *The Jews of Warsaw*, pp. 102–103.

104 TOZ report, September 1939–June 1940, JDC, AR.33–44, file 840; report by Dr. Emanuel Patt on welfare activity for the Jews of Poland, March 1941, JDC, AR.33–44, file 814.

In April 1940, twenty-one refugee centers were shut down due to the severely unsanitary conditions there, and new refugee centers and kitchens were opened and maintained under medical and sanitation supervision. Special action was taken to disinfect the refugees and, in April 1940, roughly seven months before ghettoization, 12,908 people visited nine special bathing facilities for refugees. Six special disinfection squads were set up, which disinfected 198 hostels and laundered 35,000 kilograms of clothing. In addition, a program to provide food to residents of quarantined buildings was organized.[105] TOZ also helped to improve hygiene among thousands of refugees and made slight improvements in the bathing and disinfection methods that the Nazis had imposed. TOZ's Department of War on Epidemics set up a sanitation team and a disinfection unit. On the initiative of Dr. Rozenblum and Dr. Szwalb, TOZ purchased and renovated a bathhouse at 4 Solna St. that served 300 people per day. Its Department of War on Epidemics conducted extensive information and prevention activities for the inhabitants of the ghetto, which may seem strange, given the hopeless situation of the population. Dr. Tursz wrote in his testimony,

> What good are words anymore? How could you speak to people who are swollen with hunger about hygiene and the need to take a bath even though there is no soap...The Warsaw ghetto was characterized by a strange dualism. On the one hand, death was certain and there was no point to any activity. On the other hand, actual work was not considered work, because everything was Sisyphean and hopeless.[106]

With tremendous effort, a "Cleanup Week" that reverberated through the Warsaw ghetto population was organized. Nurses from the Department of War on Epidemics were sent into the field, visiting cellars and attics, talking with residents about keeping clean, and helping people to clean their homes. TOZ

105 Trunk, "Epidemics and Mortality," p. 86.
106 Dr. Moshe Tursz testimony, YVA, O.3/438, pp. 9–12.

also activated a laundry facility that served the overnight centers. Representatives of house committees distributed coupons to the poorest inhabitants to do laundry, free of charge.

The Department of War on Epidemics expanded its social welfare activities with the assistance of Dr. Maurycy Regelman and the social service nurse Ala Gołąb-Grynberg, who were associated with the Jewish Social Self-Help and the network of house committees. Every house committee had a sanitation representative. These representatives formed groups that received instructions from the neighborhood sanitation supervisors. They served as agents of the Department of War on Epidemics, reaching the apartment of every Jew. To the best of their ability, they distributed disinfection materials, including soap, brushes, chlorine, and information sheets with instructions and guidelines. In each neighborhood, doctors gave lectures and mass assemblies were held with the participation of rabbis and well-known social activists.[107]

A Jewish Social Self-Help report from November 1941 indicated that TOZ maintained its "public and social hygiene" activities, whose scope included the inspection of buildings and apartments. However, it did not conduct information campaigns or distribute information sheets. In July 1941, 150 lectures were delivered and 190,000 dwellings were inspected. The quantity of disinfection materials distributed by TOZ peaked at 700 kilograms in July 1941. In November, 6,514 people bathed in the TOZ bathhouses on Gęsia St. and Solna St., 1,664 received haircuts, and 65 bundles of linens and clothing were disinfected. Visits to the bathhouses increased from January to July 1941, numbering 19,250 in July. There was a gradual decline from August to November 1941, with a 45 percent decrease in November relative to August. Haircuts exceeded 3,000 in March and July, but sank to fewer than half as many in October and November 1941.[108]

107 Ibid.; report by Dr. Emanuel Patt on welfare activity for the Jews of Poland, March 1941, JDC, AR.33–44, file 814.

108 Jewish Social Self-Help, Statistics Department Report, no. 6, November 1941, AŻIH, ARI.32, p. 20; Offer, "Ma'arach Harefu'a Begeto Varsha," vol. 2, appendix B.32, p. 187, and appendix B.33, pp. 188–189.

Despite all these efforts, the typhus epidemic spread relentlessly. At least one member of every family contracted the disease. Diseases were particularly common among TOZ staff: doctors, nurses, bathhouse employees, and members of disinfection teams.[109] In February 1942, an urgent meeting was held with the participation of Emanuel Ringelblum, who was one of the most active members of the Jewish Social Self-Help, and TOZ physicians in an attempt to counter the menace of an epidemic by launching a "health month" and extensive activities to improve hygiene. Those in attendance were informed that the situation was grave—the funding required to combat the epidemic was totally lacking, and the existing anti-epidemic measures had lost their effect. In response, they urged TOZ to increase the budget as much as possible. They also resolved to continue offering the public information and lectures.[110]

Even after the *Grossaktion*, which ended on September 12, 1942, when most of the Jews of Warsaw had been murdered in Treblinka and about 60,000 remained in the ghetto, actions were taken to prevent the spread of diseases. The following is an announcement concerning "Cleanup Week":

> Warsaw Judenrat, January 3, 1943
>
> **Attn: Residents of the Jewish Quarter**
>
> Between January 3 and January 9, Operation "Cleanup Week" will take place in the Jewish quarter of Warsaw. Stringent observance of the instructions related to the operation is for your personal benefit. By maintaining cleanliness, you prevent contagious diseases from spreading, and save your lives and those of your families. The Judenrat is confident that you will cooperate in the operation, not only due to fear of punishment for not

109 Dr. Moshe Tursz testimony, YVA, O.3/438.

110 Protocol on "Health Month," February 25, 1942, AŻIH, ARI.43; Offer, "Ma'arach Harefu'a Begeto Varsha," vol. 2, appendix A.26, p. 124.

> cooperating, but mainly because you realize the importance of Operation "Cleanup Week."[111]

On January 18, 1943, two weeks after the announcement appeared, the second deportation from the Warsaw ghetto began, and another 6,000 of the remaining Jews were sent to Treblinka.[112]

Residents' Response to Medical Edicts

Dr. Lensky, a physician at Czyste Hospital in the ghetto, described positive aspects of the way the Jewish population and the Jewish doctors coped with the draconian disinfection and bathing dictates, noting that the populace did everything possible to evade the delousing operations. They preferred to bribe Polish and Jewish doctors and disinfection personnel. Lensky claimed that the population decided to take things into its own hands and to refuse to comply with the appalling decree of disinfection in any way that it could.

> This cruel treatment upset the entire Jewish population. People began to seek ways of defending themselves against the Nazis' violent procedures. As the community leaders' efforts failed, the Jews had no other choice but to take their destiny into their hands.[113]

According to Lensky, the way the Jews handled the edict manifested "great cunning and resourcefulness in those days, and a wonderful vitality." The residents in every building established a committee to liaise with the Judenrat. Forming a "conspiracy of silence," the committees decided not to report typhus cases

111 Notice concerning "Cleanup Week," January 1943, AŻIH, ARI.262; Offer, "Ma'arach Harefu'a Begeto Varsha," vol. 2, appendix A.33, p. 160.

112 Gutman, "Warsaw: Jews during the Holocaust," in Gutman, *Encyclopedia of the Holocaust*, p. 1,621.

113 Lensky, *A Physician inside the Warsaw Ghetto*, p. 102.

and instead to make sure patients would receive medical care at home—a decision that, of course, could not be implemented without the consent and assistance of the Jewish doctors.

The Germans attempted to enforce the disinfection decrees and to track down typhus patients by means of mobile disinfection teams headed by a Nazi or Polish doctor, who conducted surprise inspections in people's homes to flush out the ill. In response, the house committees stringently guarded building entrances and warned tenants of an imminent visit by a disinfection crew. They tried to conceal the patients in their homes in any way possible. However, these preventive measures were difficult to carry out in buildings occupied by the poor. Therefore, buildings in the poorest neighborhoods bore the brunt of the decrees, although they too sometimes devised stratagems to thwart them. Even though many people were treated at home, the epidemic was so broad that most of the poor who fell ill were sent to the hospitals, because the house committees were unable to feed them and ensure effective medical care.[114]

In addition to the severe damage that the disinfection decrees brought about, much of the Jewish population did not trust the Judenrat, which it regarded as representing the Nazi administration, or the Judenrat Health Department and, therefore, it resisted the disinfection procedures that it set forth.[115] The house committees played an important role in the attempt to cope with the disinfection dictates by striving to obtain bread rations and typhus vaccinations during the first epidemic. Each house committee charged a tax of 20 grosz per ration card, assuring itself of a regular if meager income. For each injection, the committee paid only 30 grosz but charged those of means 50 grosz to 1 zloty, bringing in a one-shot income of several hundred zlotys.[116] However, bribery payments emptied the committees' funds, and they were unable to help the residents buy medicines for the ill and bury the dead.[117] In fact, the house

114 Ibid., pp. 103–126.

115 Roland, *Courage under Siege*, pp. 140–141.

116 Opochinsky, *Reshimot*, p. 41.

117 Ibid., pp. 93–94.

committees were tainted with the disgrace of bribery. When it was time for disinfection, they negotiated with the Jewish doctors involved and paid them off to go easy on medical supervision. A committee treasurer sometimes shared the funds collected by the committee with the physician, and the committee members themselves were exempt from the disinfection decree.[118]

* * *

Employing the dual definition of medicine as both medical care and health care, I conclude this chapter by presenting important data on the causes and characteristics of ghetto morbidity, on one hand, and on aspects of health and welfare, on the other. Both sides of the medical coin reflect much of the professional medical challenge that the ghetto inhabitants faced, both as providers of medical services and as the rest of the population, the ill and those concerned with their health who sought to maintain autonomy over their bodies and way of life, even under ghetto conditions.

The deterioration of the health of the Jews of Warsaw resulted from the extreme and adverse changes in all areas of life essential to preserving health due to the ravages of the war and especially to the decrees imposed by the Germans. In fact, the Jews were deprived of the basic conditions for sound health. The main factors that affected illness and health included overpopulation, poor hygienic conditions, starvation rations, loss of livelihood, lack of heating fuel in the bitter cold, and the arrival of thousands of refugees, who could not be properly accommodated. It was for these reasons that epidemics, most conspicuously of typhus, typhoid fever, and tuberculosis, broke out in the ghetto.

The documents on morbidity and health yield important insights on the development of the anti-Jewish policies, on the one hand, and the behavior patterns of their victims, on the other. From the perspective of what may be called the "Jewish medical leadership" in the ghetto—those charged with making crucial decisions on health care policy and its implementation, as discussed

118 Ibid., p. 46.

in the previous chapter—it is evident that professional actions were taken to counter the epidemics that swept the ghetto. These included comprehensive immunization; professional committees to draft anti-epidemic programs; additional professional committees for treating specific illnesses, such as the Anti-Tuberculosis League; studies to illuminate the causes of the epidemics and to propose preventive action; and measures to prevent and eradicate morbidity, to name only a few. These steps improved the population's health in various phases of the occupation. For example, the inoculation and prevention activities conducted in response to the initial wave of typhus and typhoid fever helped to eradicate the epidemics that were brought on by the damage caused by the bombardments during the war and by the overcrowding caused by the arrival of refugees. They were so effective that morbidity waned by the time the Jews entered the ghetto.

The Jewish medical leadership in the ghetto labored to prepare a "scientific medical response" to the Germans' specious claim about morbidity among the Jews. The finest scientists in the ghetto prepared reports, compiling proven data about the history of morbidity among the Jews of Warsaw before the war, and during the war and the ghetto era. It is important to note that they courageously presented these memoranda to the Germans in the hope that they would lead to some change in their health policies toward the Jews. The memoranda indeed demonstrated that the diseases common in the ghetto were caused by the conditions that the Germans had created. Tuberculosis, for example, which had existed among Polish Jews before the war but was considered endemic, attained epidemic magnitudes, because hunger weakened the resistance of the people. Thus, in 1941, about 3,900 Jews died of tuberculosis, ten times as many as had succumbed to this disease in 1939. Before the war, typhus had been uncommon among Jews, and there is no doubt that the ghetto conditions led to its eruption. Accordingly, in 1941, 38,150 people in the ghetto developed this disease, as compared with 200, at most, on the Aryan side.

A comparison of the mortality data in the primary and secondary sources—bearing in mind that they are presented from different angles of observation—yields a similar and dismal picture. From the beginning of the war to June 1942, before the transports commenced, around 85,000 Jews died. The ghetto physicians reported about 98,000 deaths from illness between September 1939 and December 1942. From the beginning of the war to December 1942, typhus accounted for around 3 percent of all deaths in the ghetto and hunger for about 18.7 percent. Of the 77,121 fatalities for which the ghetto physicians did not specify causes, it is presumed that about one-third were from tuberculosis. If so, hunger and tuberculosis together accounted for the majority of all deaths. Thus, contrary to the German misrepresentation of typhus as a "Jewish" disease, both morbidity and mortality were caused mainly by hunger and its complications, which were brought on solely by the ghetto conditions.

The data indicate that the Germans' anti-Jewish policies in Warsaw had no relation to the objective circumstances of morbidity among the Jews. Even if the decisions were in the hands of the local Germans, they did not act according to logical, bureaucratic, or other considerations concerning the condition of the Jews. The Germans based their decisions on the antisemitic, racist, and apocalyptic concepts of the Nazis, as defined by Friedländer.[119] Just as the ghetto was established to implement the Nazis' anti-Jewish policy, and not because of the medical situation, its termination was brought about by the Nazis' extermination policy—not by deterioration in the medical situation there.

The Germans directly murdered about 370,000 Jews during the *Aktionen* and nearly 100,000 died of illnesses due to the devastating living conditions that the Germans imposed on them. In other words, despite the grim conditions, most inhabitants of the ghetto survived, thanks in part to the preventive and curative medical system of the Jews serving the ghetto. As the spring of 1942 approached, morbidity and mortality in the ghetto decreased markedly. Even though this is a typical tendency in epidemics, it is important to note that the epidemics were eradicated shortly before the onset of the deportations. Deportation alone doomed them to collective annihilation.

119 Friedländer, *Nazi Germany and the Jews*, pp. 40, 73–112.

The data on marriages, births, and suicides—areas associated with the fundamentals of human life, health, and welfare—indicate that much of the population yearned to continue clinging to normal life and believed that they would see the end of the Nazi occupation and its horrors. Otherwise, it is hard to explain why they continued to marry and bear children, and why, in view of the tragic reality, the rate of people who despaired to the extent of suicide did not rise.

It is reasonable to assume that the institution of marriage appeared to have gained strength in the ghetto. There are various explanations for this, which require separate study. The new conditions created good reasons for couples to form, in addition to the usual reasons during ordinary times. At the beginning of the war, when migration to the East began, many young Jews chose to marry before heading out. Weddings were also frequent, because there were more widows and widowers. In addition, since only single men were sent to the forced labor camps at first, many weddings took place. Upon ghettoization, there was also a spurt of weddings, because it was easier to rent one apartment as a couple than it was to rent a dwelling as an individual.

As for the question of childbirth in the ghetto, it deserves emphasis that although the birth rate in the ghetto fell short of the prewar level, women continued to bear children, even under ghetto conditions. The birth rate in 1941 was 45 percent of its prewar rate. Childbirth continued amid the worsening conditions of 1942, at 17 percent of the prewar rate. Given the ghetto conditions, this should be seen as a unique phenomenon. From the Nazis' perspective, the policy outlined by Hitler was intended to obliterate "inferior" races by limiting their natural increase.

The policy in the General Government set forth by Dr. Hecht and Dr. Wetzel, senior officials in the Nazi Party's Office of Racial Policy, recommended reducing the Polish population by preventing pregnancies and performing abortions. However, we have no information about an order forbidding childbirth in the Warsaw ghetto. Such a decree was promulgated in the ghettos in Lithuania in February 1942, after the official decision on the Final Solution had been made. Its implementation was postponed to

August 1942, when the deportation of the Jews of Warsaw was in progress, so there was no need to issue such a dictate there. Moreover, the conditions prevailing in the Warsaw ghetto caused "natural" mortality. Following the murder of the ill and the elderly in the ghettos in Lithuania, the healthy Jews who had survived were held as forced laborers for the Reich and, since the Nazis wanted to ensure the destruction of the future of the Jewish people, they prohibited procreation there.

Finally, our research supports the information about the low suicide rates among the Jews of Warsaw during the Nazi occupation. Many of those who documented life in the ghetto noted that suicides were few and explained it as an unusual phenomenon. When the deportations began, in contrast, a wave of suicides ensued, including by many doctors. The sociologist Émile Durkheim believes that people cling to life when they feel they belong to a group. If so, the low suicide rate may suggest that the fundamentals of social cohesion and collective identity held up, even under the test of the ghetto conditions, bolstering the individuals' will to fight for survival. When there was no chance of survival, as many concluded at the time of the deportations, social collapse set in and suicides increased.

Chapter ten

Ethical Dilemmas in the Work of Medical Staff

I approached my associates—coworkers—with this list. It was the most tragic moment in my life. As I read out the list, I announced the death sentence for 600 innocent people, close friends, comrades and workmates, and even my former boss, Dr. H. A. I was forced to read the list to them several times! They could not believe that they were not on the list. They deluded themselves into thinking that they had not heard well or that maybe I had skipped over their names by mistake.... Everyone, including those who were on the list, was gripped with fear and despair, and directed their rage and resentment at those who had produced the list and those included on it. I consoled them with the hope that there would be another list, although I myself did not believe it.[1]

The ghastly reality that had been imposed on the Jews during the Holocaust gave rise to horrific moral dilemmas. To use an expression coined by the American philosopher Thomas Nagel, these dilemmas were classic cases of "bad circumstantial luck"—the misfortune of being in a situation in which any course of action that an individual chooses entails a heavy moral price.[2] This chapter presents the ethical

1 Dr. Adolf Polisiuk diary, GHF, no. 3182.

2 Thomas Nagel, "Moral Luck," in Daniel Statman, ed., *Moral Luck* (Albany: State University of New York Press, 1993), pp. 57–71.

dilemmas entailed in the work of the Jewish medical staff in the Warsaw ghetto during the German occupation.

I propose distinguishing between two types of dilemmas, although the differences between them are not always clear-cut. In one type, medical staff members were required or expected to assist ill or distressed Jews even though such action would expose them to mortal peril. The general question in such dilemmas is: To what extent should doctors or medical personnel in general endanger themselves in order to save lives or to aid those in need? The other kind of dilemma does not involve risk to the medical staff but, instead, conflicting moral values or norms. These are the dilemmas addressed in philosophical discourse. They arise in situations in which a person must discharge two conflicting obligations and cannot fulfill both.[3] There is a debate in philosophical literature about whether such dilemmas exist, namely, whether a situation may arise in which a person is charged with two opposing duties, leaving the individual no way out, and his or her hands inescapably tainted. Here I will not elaborate on this philosophical discussion, but will only say that a study of the acute dilemmas that the Jewish medical staff in the Warsaw ghetto faced casts doubt on the validity of the philosophical position that denies the reality of such dilemmas.

Terrible ethical dilemmas were the daily lot of many officials in the ghetto, particularly those who were affiliated with the Judenrat, but such quandaries seemed to be all the more central and quotidian among medical staff. In addition, medical professionals encountered a dilemma that others did not confront—the question of actively causing people to die. As indicated below, medical staff, like the Judenrat, hesitated to cooperate in the selections. As stated, doctors were forced at times to take actions that led directly to the death of Jews. It is worth adding that a grasp of the ethical problematic of the situations discussed below is not the product of hindsight—the contemporaries were fully cognizant. The medical teams in the ghetto, like others in executive positions in

3 See, for example, Daniel Statman, *Moral Dilemmas* (Amsterdam: Rodopi, 1995), chap. 1.

the ghetto, were often torn between their moral conscience and the professional and human exigencies imposed on them within the framework of their duties. It should also be noted that the commitment of the medical professionals in the Warsaw ghetto to universal moral rules and values was often tested without entailing ethical dilemmas. However, in this chapter, I emphasize issues involving ethical dilemmas that arose in the context of the unique tragedy of the Warsaw ghetto. I begin with dilemmas of the first type, which I call "self-endangerment dilemmas," and continue with moral dilemmas of the second type.

Abandoning Patients to Save Themselves

In September 1939, as the front approached Warsaw, the number of doctors and nurses at Czyste Hospital dwindled. Many were conscripted to the army. Fear of German occupation and concern about how the occupiers would treat the Jews induced some of the other medical professionals to flee. Two days before the Germans entered the Polish capital, many doctors and white-collar staff at the hospital, including the director of the institution, Dr. Henryk Stabholz, escaped. The dilemma arose: Should medical staff serve its patients, even when threatened with danger, or was it permissible for them to look out for themselves and abandon those hospitalized?

This issue beset doctors and nurses at various times in the ghetto. At the beginning of the war and on the eve of the German occupation, many good people tried to save themselves, even at the cost of abandoning their medical work. Admittedly, quite a few returned after finding it difficult to cross over to the Soviet side, but much of the medical staff left immediately before the occupation.

On September 27, the day the Germans occupied Warsaw, the staff at Czyste Hospital chose to remain, despite their fear and dread. Dr. David Amsterdamski and the nurse Sabina Gürfinkel-Glocer were working there at the time. A dialogue that took place between them reflects the fear and the hope nestled in the hearts of the Jews as the Germans moved into the city. "Now hell will open up before us," Sabina said. Dr. Amsterdamski replied,

> Don't despair! Not all the Jews will be killed. Hitler can kill hundreds of thousands of Jews, possibly including us, you and me, but the Jewish people will not be annihilated. We will weather Hitler's era. We must be strong and save whomever we can.[4]

Gürfinkel-Glocer reported that Amsterdamski continued to work indefatigably throughout this time. "It was a question of honor for us to help the doctors and, by pooling our forces, to save those who could still be saved," she wrote.[5]

In the course of their medical and nursing work in the ghetto, the staff repeatedly faced the dilemma of whether to continue their devoted, demanding, and hazardous duties at the hospital, or to seek ways of escaping to the Aryan side of the city in order to save themselves and their families. The quandary was particularly salient on the eve of and during the *Grossaktion*, when the doctors and the medical staff, like everyone else in the ghetto, sought to save themselves. The doctors had formed personal and group relations working together, and they had connections with their colleagues or with their former patients on the Aryan side. This offered them opportunities for survival and rescue, unlike the others in the ghetto who lacked this status, or that of the wielders of authority in the ghetto. During the deportations, many doctors and their families began to cross over to the other side of the city. Those who had Polish acquaintances contacted them and, in many cases, were able to arrange refuge for their entire families or, at least, for their wives and children. Several doctors left the hospital and fled to the Aryan side[6] where, thanks to their relations with the Polish intelligentsia and their fluency in Polish, they easily found shelter and survived.[7]

A large proportion of medical personnel seemed to have found ways and connections to obtain refuge and various services outside the ghetto. According to Dr. Polisiuk, a small number of

4 Gürfinkel-Glocer, "Goralo Shel Beit Haholim Tzhista," p. 588.
5 Ibid., pp. 587–590.
6 Lensky, *A Physician inside the Warsaw Ghetto*, p. 138.
7 Ibid., p. 167.

physicians, including chief physicians, went into hiding on the Aryan side during the very first days of the *Grossaktion*—among those who left the ghetto on September 5, "my manager, Dr. S. That very day, I took over management of the department but only for one day." The *Aktion* in the hospital began the next day.[8] In early 1943, when preparations for the ghetto uprising began, Prof. Stabholz, who was assisting the the ŻOB (Jewish Combat Organization), was urged by Prof. Loth, a Polish physician, to save his family by crossing to the Aryan side. He arranged false papers for Stabholz, including a document attesting to Catholic identity and a new name, Bolesław Dziedzic. Loth even visited the ghetto, placing one of Stabholz's legs in a cast and giving Stabholz a bogus document, signed by an SS officer, certifying that he had been injured while working for the German Reich. A week before the uprising broke out, Stabholz–Dziedzic was transferred to the Aryan side.[9]

Nurse Sabina Gürfinkel-Glocer, who worked in the surgical ward at Czyste Hospital, described her dilemma. "A battle of powerful forces raged in my heart: the duty of a nurse who is commanded to live and die with the patients and the hospital staff, and the sense of motherhood, which ordered me to live at any price in order to save my daughter."[10] After the *Aktion* of January 1943, she decided to send her daughter to the Aryan side. She arranged a hideout for her daughter, said goodbye, and remained in the ghetto.

8 Dr. Adolf Polisiuk diary, GFH, no. 3182.

9 According to Nadav in his article "Limed Anatomiya Begeto Varsha," Stabholz joined his mother and his wife, who had already moved out and had rented a modest apartment not far from the ghetto. A short time later, they returned to the ghetto and witnessed the uprising and destruction of the ghetto. They then moved to Miłosna, a village outside Warsaw, where Stabholz hid in the guise of a disabled person with a cast. In the spring of 1944, he and his wife slipped away, moved toward the Soviet forces that were approaching Lwów, and joined an engineering battalion that was preparing to construct bridges over the River Wisla. With the assistance of a Jewish colonel named Epstein, who was serving with the battalion, they reached Lublin and joined the Polish Army, which had been reconstituted under Soviet patronage.

10 Gürfinkel-Glocer, "Goralo Shel Beit Haholim Tzhista," p. 595.

> Now my heart rebelled against being passive and I decided to save my daughter at all costs, even if it meant separating, although without her my life would not be a life.... The night of the separation arrived. I prayed to God to save my daughter. I escorted her as far as the guard post on Dzieka St., and my husband and the nurse Israelis escorted her from a distance to the guard. Suddenly I heard gunshots from the direction of the guards. I waited for my husband and my friend. She [the latter] arrived first and led me to the hospital. I summoned the last of my strength and went back to work.[11]

Sometime later, Gürfinkel-Glocer decided to flee to the Aryan side to join her daughter. She sadly bid her patients farewell. Although her conscience afflicted her for abandoning her post, she seized the opportunity to save her young daughter and herself. An SS soldier stole the coffee, soap, and syringes that she had hoped to sell in Warsaw to sustain herself and her daughter. One of her former patients helped her to pass through the ghetto gates. Due to housing problems on the Aryan side, she was unable to stay with her daughter, who was murdered some time later.[12]

Nurse Ala Gołąb-Grynberg, who demonstrated exceptional devotion during the deportations from the Warsaw ghetto, turned down an opportunity to survive on the Aryan side, where she had close connections. She firmly believed that her place was with the Jews in the ghetto. She contacted Christian circles on the Aryan side to save Jewish children and to house them temporarily in Polish orphanages and churches. During the ghetto uprising, she was sent to the camp in Poniatowa, near Lublin. Members of the Jewish National Committee's resistance organization, residing on the other side of Warsaw after the uprising, made efforts to extricate her. They repeatedly sent special agents to rescue her, but she adamantly refused. In the camp, she worked at the hospital, set up a children's corner, and took children under her protection. She was resolved not to abandon them. "I must not leave these

11 Ibid., p. 598.

12 Roland, *Courage under Siege*, p. 216.

wretched and helpless lambs," she said, remaining a faithful soldier at her post and bringing joy to these Jewish children until the very end. She perished on November 8, 1943, along with the children and the remaining 15,000 Jews in the Poniatowa camp.[13]

Ringelblum expressed his appreciation for those doctors who chose to remain with their patients to the end and paid for it with their lives.

> We previously mentioned the passive and quiet heroism of the educators, beginning with Dr. Korczak. We recounted how they walked to their deaths willingly, accompanying the children whom they had been nurturing for years. The doctors and nurses at the Jewish Hospital on Stawki [St.]... that bordered this square [the Umschlagplatz]...and where the shouts and cries of the deportees were audible, comported themselves similarly. Everyone knew that the hospital would not be spared from deportation. There were dozens of examples of this in the rural towns, in Lublin, and elsewhere. Therefore, some doctors and nurses left. However, a group of a few dozen doctors and nurses remained and did not abandon the patients until the last moment. When that tragic moment came and more than 1,000 sick people were loaded into the [railroad] cars, a handful of doctors and nurses went with them. Such was the comportment of the people whom the Nazis deemed subhuman.[14]

Dr. Shmuel Stanisław Waller, according to his own testimony, suggested to Dr. Halina Rotsztajn that she leave the Umschlagplatz, whereupon she replied, "My fate is tied to the hospital. I will not leave it." Dr. Rotsztajn treated patients devotedly under gruesome conditions and, along with the hospital staff, was sent with them to Treblinka, where she perished. Her children, who were admitted to a convent, survived.[15] Dr. Polisiuk recorded this story in his diary.

13 Turkow, *Hayo Hayta Varsha Yehudit*, pp. 123–124, 291, 304.

14 Ringelblum, *Ktavim Aharonim*, p. 37.

15 Dr. Shmuel Stanisław Waller testimony, YVA, O.3/2358.

> One of the doctors who had "life numbers" [exemptions from deportation], Dr. Rotsztajn, voluntarily boarded the [railroad] car together with the patients, which she considered her duty to them. Many regarded this act as abnormal. After all, the will to survive was so strong. The heroism of her act was that poignant.[16]

There were other doctors who did not abandon their patients, even when they had a chance to go into hiding on the Aryan side of town. Dr. Waller remembers his last meeting with Dr. Anna Braude-Heller, the director of the children's hospital, in early 1943. When he asked her why she was not using her connections on the Aryan side to save herself, she replied, "I concealed my family there. If I knew that the world would change for the better, that people would be different, I would try to save myself. But I know that people will be just as they are now."[17] Thus, she declined opportunities for rescue in favor of her patients and her medical mission in the ghetto. Toiling unrelentingly, she set up a small pediatric department and ran it in an exemplary manner even after the *Grossaktion*.[18]

Dr. Adina Blady Szwajger described the initial efforts undertaken on the Aryan side to organize the exit and rescue of people from the ghetto. After she left the ghetto, she and her comrades on the Aryan side engaged in procuring papers that would allow individuals to circulate there.

> We took in the people closest to us, our colleagues from the hospital…Then we wrote that letter to the Head Doctor begging her to leave because we had everything ready for her. We got the reply, "Don't worry about me. I've got my own plans." So, for a moment, we believed that, like many other eminent doctors, she had some other way out. But there was only one way for her: together with the hospital.[19]

16 Dr. Adolf Polisiuk diary, GFH, no. 3182.

17 Dr. Shmuel Stanisław Waller testimony, YVA, O.3/2358.

18 Gürfinkel-Glocer, "Goralo Shel Beit Haholim Tzhista," p. 595.

19 Blady Szwajger, *I Remember Nothing More*, p. 65.

The director of the children's hospital did not leave the ghetto. Instead, she repeatedly reorganized the demolished facility. Dr. Adina Blady Szwajger wrote, "And we don't really know how she died. Whether in the flames of the burning hospital, or somewhere in a cellar. Or maybe she was amongst those who were taken away. We don't know."[20]

In early 1943, shelter outside the ghetto was arranged for Dr. Zyf, his wife, and their young daughter. Zyf and his family "looked Aryan," had money, and spoke fluent Polish. However, those among his patients who had been spared from the deportation in January were still in the ghetto and he wished to care for them. He turned down the opportunity to leave the ghetto and the date for his departure was reset to April 20. The uprising and its outcome, the destruction of the ghetto, began on April 19, dooming Dr. Zyf to his death.[21]

After the September 1942 *Aktion*, members of the staff at Czyste Hospital who had moved to the Aryan side transferred their possessions in a car belonging to the government physician who oversaw sanitation in the ghetto. This practitioner visited the hospital several times each week, purchased microscopes and medical instruments from the doctors, and sold them on the other side. His car, large enough to take suitcases as well, set out from the hospital laden with the Jews' belongings. The driver, of course, did this with the government physician's consent. Both were paid well for their services.[22]

Even doctors who had converted to Christianity and who had been forced to enter the ghetto also vacillated about whether to leave and abandon their patients. Prof. Ludwik Hirszfeld reported that senior officials tried to help him emigrate from Poland at the beginning of the war, but to no avail.

> We applied for a pass to Yugoslavia, hoping that this permit would be the easiest to obtain. In Yugoslavia, our

20 Ibid., pp. 38, 65.

21 Roland, *Courage under Siege*, p. 67.

22 Lensky, *A Physician inside the Warsaw Ghetto*, pp. 195–196.

> friends would help us. When they learned about our forced displacement, they reacted in a manner which touched us deeply: at their request, the young king granted me honorary Yugoslavian citizenship, and the Yugoslav government requested our release on the basis that we were indispensable experts. We were informed that our citizenship papers were signed on March 24, 1941. But the war broke out on March 27,[23] and our hope collapsed. Besides, at the same time we received a negative reply from Cracow....My attempts to get in touch with New York were in vain. Indirectly I learned that by that time the Germans were releasing no one to America.

Hirszfeld added that his Polish friends, who had obtained all the necessary documents for him, his wife, and his daughter, had pleaded with them to flee from the ghetto and go into hiding in a village with friends. He faced a difficult dilemma.

> I decided that if I got a chance to go abroad I would. There, I could fight for my people on a larger scale. If, however, this opportunity did not arise, I would stay in the district and would not hide. I did not want future generations and my own conscience to ask me the question: "Fate put you among several hundred thousand unhappy people. What did you do for them? Destiny gave you the key to young hearts. Did you try to open those poor hearts and soothe them?"
>
> So I stayed. I had nothing: no authority, no means, no laboratory. I was a stranger to these people; as a Christian, I was rejected by the masses. I only had a great, boundless compassion. This was my capital and my weapon. I told my wife, "I must stay, but you should leave this hell with our daughter. In the countryside, she may regain her health." I saw how she was torn between a mother's and a wife's instinct, and how the latter won. We told our daughter, "Darling, we

23 On March 27, 1941, the Yugoslavian Army mounted a coup and ousted the regent, Prince Paul, who had signed a pact with Germany and the other Axis countries. Consequently, Germany invaded the Kingdom of Yugoslavia and occupied it on April 6.

> have friends who want to save you. It will be better for us when you are on the other side." But our daughter was made of a noble substance. "Where you are, I shall be too."[24]

In January 1943, following general warnings about an *Aktion*, the small medical staff who had survived at Czyste Hospital decided to hide as many patients as they could. Stabholz, the hospital warehouseman who was devoted to the welfare of the hospital, risked his life during the selections, concealing many people and bolstering the morale of those in hiding.[25]

It is noteworthy that even as the transports to the extermination camps proceeded, there were medical staff members who rescued other Jews by placing them under pseudo-medical guise, exploiting their professional status at personal mortal risk. Various accounts of the drama that took place on the Umschlagplatz indicate that some doctors and nurses chose to endanger themselves in an attempt to rescue as many Jews as possible.

On Leszno St., not far from the hospital, the number of cases of passersby who were accosted and sent to the Umschlagplatz, including doctors and hospital workers, was increasing. Attempts were made to smuggle out the doctors and sometimes other detainees, dressed in white smocks, and to lead them to the hospital for the ostensible purpose of performing surgery. The doctors and nurses involved were liable to forfeit their lives for doing so.[26]

The dilemmas facing medical staff who are required to treat patients at personal risk continue to be debated today. The guidelines of the International Committee of the Red Cross concerning the duties and rights of first aiders in armed conflicts allow medical workers not to endanger their own lives in order to treat the wounded.[27] The Ethics Bureau of the Israel Medical

24 Hirszfeld, *Die Geschichte eines Lebens*, p. 126; Hirszfeld, *The Story of One Life*, pp. 196–197.

25 Gürfinkel-Glocer, "Goralo Shel Beit Haholim Tzhista," pp. 595–597.

26 Edelman, *The Ghetto Fights*, pp. 27, 45–46.

27 See International Committee of the Red Cross, *First Aid in Armed Conflicts and Other Situations of Violence*, https://www.icrc.org/sites/default/files/topic/file_plus_list/first_aid_leaflet.pdf (accessed September 17, 2019).

Association has taken a stand on the question of risk to medical staff, affirming that rights of caregivers, such as to their personal safety, should be taken into account, along with the rights of society and the nation at large. Under the title, "Obligations and Rights of Caregiving Staff Facing Potential Threat," the Israel Medical Association states the following:

> Teams that administer care to casualties in an emergency incur various levels of personal risk in the course of their duty.…As the emergency unfolds, the doctor is duty-bound to assume relevant and immediate personal risk insofar as this will lead to the fulfillment of his/her professional requirement to treat ill and injured patients. However, a medical team that itself sustains injury brings no benefit to the purpose for which it exists.…In the absence of proper advance preparation for the situation it encounters…medical staff will act at their best discretion to help those affected without rendering themselves unable to aid other injured persons.…When a medical team enters the "line of fire," in the event of mortal danger, the doctor together with security officials will weigh the risk of entering the scene of the incident against the need to save lives.[28]

The World Medical Association recognizes the legitimacy of the dilemma regarding the degree of risk that medical staff are required to take in life-threatening situations, but does not take a definitive stance on the best action to take.

Risking Infection from Patients or Withholding Care

Doctors and nurses in the Warsaw ghetto were at risk of contracting grave infectious diseases to which they were not exposed in ordinary times. Indeed, about one-third of the doctors in the

28 Israel Medical Association position paper, May 2008, "Hahebetim Ha'etiyim Be'erua Rav-Nifga'im" (Ethical Aspects of a Mass-Casualty Event) (Hebrew), https://www.ima.org.il/MainSiteNew/EditClinicalInstruction.aspx?ClinicalInstructionId=158 (accessed September 17, 2019).

ghetto contracted typhus and many died from it.[29] Work in refugee centers—focal points of morbidity and mortality—was fraught with daunting dilemmas. The situation in these facilities was tantamount to a "medical disaster" as needs escalated and more patients required the services of doctors and nurses. However, the realistic fear of contracting infectious diseases that were prevalent at these centers, as well as the shortage of medical resources, the hunger, and the living conditions, encumbered the delivery of proper services. Lensky's descriptions shed some light on the dilemmas that doctors in the ghetto faced. When the Health Department through the JDC asked Dr. Lensky to work at the refugee home on Stawki St., Lensky, who was well aware of the dire situation there, gave a noncommittal reply and decided to try to work there for one week.

> Typhus was still rampant. It seemed foolish to put my head in the noose to engage in medical work at a facility where poor hygiene made infection a near certainty, of my own free will, especially when I was under no financial or moral pressure and certainly was not lacking work.[30]

Upon arriving at the shelter to get an impression, Lensky immediately wanted to leave, but his conscience hampered him.

> I was about to turn around and leave but an inner voice kept me there: "If you've already come here, take a look indoors. You might not end up working here, but you owe it to the refugees to witness their living conditions. Going home now would be immoral, running away from the battlefield." This was my conscience speaking.[31]

Dr. Lensky expressed the doctors' moral dilemma: should they be loyal to the ill at any cost, even if it meant contracting life-

29 Hirszfeld, *Die Geschichte eines Lebens*, p. 135; Zylberberg, *A Warsaw Diary*, p. 51.

30 Lensky, *A Physician in the Warsaw Ghetto*, p. 80. The original Hebrew source refers to typhus, unlike in the English version.

31 Lensky, *A Physician in the Warsaw Ghetto*, pp. 80–81.

threatening illnesses, such as typhus, or could it be that, at such times, they must protect their lives, even if it means forsaking the ill. When he came home from his visit to the refugee shelter, Dr. Lensky shared his vacillations with his family. He wished to help these ailing refugees, but his wife tried to dissuade him from accepting the job.

> You are risking your life. Your heart will not stand this. It will fail if you catch fever. We, too, will be at risk, since we have no special room to isolate you when you become ill. Naturally, a doctor may not shirk his duty to heal even if at a risk to his own life. But there are, after all, several candidates for this position. And if you do not apply, some other physician will come along, who has already been ill with typhus and is immune.[32]

Persuaded by his wife's arguments, Lensky intended to tell the JDC that he had decided to pass up the post—but not without suffering pangs of conscience.

> Mixed feelings raged in me, my love for my family was at odds with my conscience. It seemed that thanks to my contacts with the director of supplies at the Joint, I would be able to improve the refugees' economic conditions and thus, indirectly, their sanitary circumstances as well. I thought I could alert the people in charge to the plight of the refugees, and even if not, if none of what I'd witnessed would change for the better, still I was obliged to be with the refugees, to offer them comfort, encourage them, help make them less bitter, rekindle their hopes, relieve their desperation. I couldn't fall asleep that night…tossed and turned, but to no avail.[33]

The issue had immediate practical implications for the health of the medical staff. The nurses who worked at the refugee center informed Dr. Lensky that the people working there—nurses, some

32 Ibid., pp. 85–86.
33 Ibid., p. 86.

of the doctors, administrative staff, and the director—had been infected by those living at the center.

Nurses presumably faced a dilemma similar to that of the doctors and wavered about accepting jobs at refugee centers as well. They worked under appalling conditions: cold, hunger, fear of infection, and a sense of helplessness with respect to their very ability to provide medical care.

> The refugees, too, are suffering from the cold.…They are starving to death. There were 1,200 people here. Now there are less. Every day several persons die of hunger and cold. There have also been many cases of typhus. We send the ill off to the hospital right away. It is right here, opposite our building. The doctors examine the ill here in this very room.…The refugees will starve to death in the course of a few months, all of them.[34]

Dr. Lensky's descriptions of the examinations of the patients and of the medical work undertaken at the refugee center illustrate the dire situation there and the risk entailed in the decision to work at such a facility. Medical personnel exposed themselves to mental hardships and real physical dangers.[35]

Many staff members continued to perform their hazardous duties, despite the severe dilemmas. Dr. Adina Blady Szwajger described contagion from patients and explained the risks involved. A female member of the hospital staff came down with starvation edema. She apparently was expected to quit her job but, in fact, she refused to abandon the ill children whom she was treating. Blady Szwajger herself contracted typhus when she went to a refugee center to administer an injection of glucose to a member of the hospital staff who had fallen ill. At that time, she was working in the hospital's typhus ward. There were three doctors in the department treating 150 ailing children. Because she was now indisposed, she spent two weeks at home, where her

34 Ibid., p. 82.
35 Ibid.

workmates gave her glucose injections to strengthen her heart. After three weeks, she returned to the hospital, rested there for a week or so, and then resumed her duties at the typhus ward.[36]

Prof. Hirszfeld visited the clinics at the refugee centers, where he spoke with doctors and caregivers, and came away impressed with their professional dedication. Many of them developed typhus and quite a few died, thus fulfilling their duties to the very end.[37]

About one-fifth of the staff at the admissions department of Czyste Hospital fell ill with typhus and 8 percent of them died from it. Treatment in this department included shaving and bathing the patients, disinfecting them, and changing their clothing. Therefore, more of the staff were infected in this department than among those who provided inpatient care.[38] Dr. Tursz asserted that many members of the TOZ medical staff also fell ill.[39]

A review of the Israel Medical Association position paper on the limits of the risk that a doctor must assume in the treatment of contagious patients indicates that medical workers today continue to address the ethical issue in this regard. It foists the moral and professional decision onto the shoulders of doctors in the field: "Insofar as the system is unable or unwilling to provide resources… the doctor is not obliged to endanger himself beyond the limits that he sets for himself voluntarily and with his colleagues and experts in the matter."[40] The lines have not been drawn and the dilemma remains unresolved.

Reporting Typhus Patients to the Authorities

Not only did doctors hesitate to work in refugee centers—the focal points for the most severe diseases—but they also faced

36 Blady Szwajger, *I Remember Nothing More*, p. 32.

37 Hirszfeld, *Die Geschichte eines Lebens*, p. 155.

38 Koren, "Hasiyud Kehelek Misherutei Habriyut," p. 77.

39 Dr. Moshe Tursz testimony, YVA, O.3/438.

40 Israel Medical Association position paper, May 2008, "Hahebetim Ha'etiyim," https://www.ima.org.il/MainSiteNew/EditClinicalInstruction.aspx?Clinical InstructionId=158 (accessed April 17, 2019).

a moral dilemma when they examined patients in their homes, which could be anywhere in the ghetto, and diagnosed that they had typhus: whether or not to report them to the authorities. Dr. Lensky's testimony made it clear that many Jewish doctors in the ghetto treated typhus patients in their homes, transgressing the Germans' order to report each case to the sanitation authority on pain of being sent to the camps. He praised the courage and self-sacrifice of the doctors, whose effective assistance largely countered the terror of this decree. Even doctors who did not wish to treat patients in their homes did not report cases to the authority. "The nurses, too, were just as praiseworthy," he noted.[41] The question of reporting was fraught with much indecision, risk, and difficulty. Some doctors accepted bribes for providing home care.

Medical Authority to Determine the Fate of Those Sent to Forced Labor Camps

As mentioned above, one of the harshest dilemmas that officials in the ghetto encountered concerned selections: Should they collaborate in any manner, thus helping the Germans by presenting the lists that they demanded, and, if so, how should they organize these lists? In other words, how should they determine who should live and who should die? The Germans demanded lists not only to send ghetto inhabitants to death camps but also for other transports, such as to labor camps. In any case, the basic moral dilemma was similar.

This discussion begins with the selection committees that screened candidates for forced labor. At the beginning of the occupation in late 1939, the Nazi authorities instructed the Judenrat to fill a large quota of workers for transport to labor camps, placing the choice in the Judenrat's hands. In order to exclude the ill from these transports, it was necessary to establish special committees for medical checkups. A large group of doctors

41 Lensky, *A Physician inside the Warsaw Ghetto*, pp. 12, 103–104.

was charged with examining 150,000 Jewish males aged 14–60. Candidates identified as unfit for labor received a certificate of exemption, as did the staff members of the Judenrat institutions.[42] On February 19, 1940, Ringelblum noted in his diary that a new registration of the Jews of Warsaw for forced labor had begun. A Jewish physician at every enlistment station was tasked with diagnosing illnesses and the Judenrat was responsible for the opinions recorded.[43]

By participating in this operation, the doctors became the Judenrat's partners in implementing the Germans' decree of forced labor. Influenced by the doctors' recommendations, the committee determined who would be sent to which forced labor camp. These decisions were of lethal consequence for individual Jews—for their health, livelihood, and life, as well as their families' lives. Dr. Lensky described the forced labor camps as camps of slow extermination, death camps in disguise.[44]

Doctors were accused of taking bribes in exchange for medical exemptions from forced labor. Their involvement at the labor bureaus subjected them to much criticism. The mass checkup operation left a harsh impression. Stanisław Adler, a member of the Jewish police, described his experience of the situation in the spring of 1941. The medical committee in question performed checkups in offices in a building on Solna St., where people stood in a line several hundred meters long on the street. Ordinarily, an examination would take hours, but a bribe could expedite the process.[45]

Doctors worked hand-in-hand with the Judenrat to exempt people from this ordeal by transferring payments to the committees and to the Judenrat. In early September 1940, Ringelblum wrote that the cost of an official exemption from the labor camps was 10–25 zlotys, which the poor could not afford. The disadvantaged saw this as an income opportunity and agreed to replace the affluent in return for an appropriate payment.

42 Ibid., p. 54.
43 Ringelblum, *Yoman Vereshimot*, p. 80.
44 Lensky, *A Physician inside the Warsaw Ghetto*, p. 55.
45 Adler, *In the Warsaw Ghetto*, pp. 165–166.

However, when rumors about the ghastly conditions in the camps spread, the number of volunteers, even among the most destitute, declined. Against this background, some doctors accepted direct bribes for granting exemptions. The bribery system was so effective that people who had been diagnosed by the doctors as being too ill to make the trip to the camps had to wait a long time for their medical exemptions, because the physicians first awarded them to those who had redeemed themselves, leaving no certifications for those truly entitled to them.

Ringelblum castigated the Jewish doctors for this conduct. "The Jewish doctors are in partnership with the other doctors, who have to sign the medical certificates." He added that there were also brokers in this line of business and that the circle of corruption for exemptions was widening steadily. "With such corruption rife, it is no wonder that the poor have banded together and refused to go to the camps." Ringelblum complained that the labor enlistment was both corrupt and sloppy. Every trifling requirement in the registration process for forced labor entailed awkward bureaucracy that forced individuals to make superhuman exertions. It was necessary to stand in line for two or three days from 5 A.M. onward waiting for a medical checkup. However, it was possible to go through a side entrance for 15 zlotys. "Nothing was anticipated. Complete anarchy and dry rot."[46]

In April 1944, an article in *Biuletyn* reported,

> When the labor camp season begins, it is the same old game, a festival of fleecing: payments for applications, a bribe for a deferral, money passed on to medical committees. Of course, only the wealthy buy their way out of the decree.[47]

In general, forced labor was imposed on young people from the impoverished classes. Only after equipping themselves with documents—the results of urine and blood tests, X-rays, and EKGs—that had to be taken into consideration and thus would

46 Ringelblum, *Notes from the Warsaw Ghetto*, pp. 159–160.
47 Blatman, *Geto Varsha—Sipur Itona'i*, p. 195.

influence the physicians' decisions, did the well-off also report for checkups. These young men could then be integrated in jobs in the community institutions and leave the labor camps behind, while people who were ill sometimes were sent to the camps.[48]

Compulsory Participation in Selections— Determining Who Will Live and Who Will Die

The difficulties in deciding who to send to forced labor camps and who to exempt pale in comparison with the hardships attending selection for transport to death camps, which involved doctors as well. Directors of Jewish hospitals, senior physicians, and medical staff in the ghetto were ordered several times to perform selections among the hundreds of doctors and family members who worked at the various medical institutions. This meant implementing the Nazis' edicts and being directly and personally involved in determining the fate of their colleagues. According to the testimonies, this was a grave dilemma that was tackled in various ways. This marked an escalation in the gravity of the ethical implications that the decision makers had to confront—from making a worker and his or her family more susceptible to the threat of deportation to sealing the worker's fate by including him or her among those being deported to their deaths.

At the beginning of the deportations, members of the medical staff, hospital employees, and their families were entitled to inclusion on a list of hospital workers who enjoyed the benefit of exemption from deportation. As family members gradually were deprived of these rights, they went into hiding in the hospitals.[49] Ultimately, the hospital managers realized that too many people were using their facilities as hideouts,

48 Lensky, *A Physician inside the Warsaw Ghetto*, pp. 54–55. Some doctors were required to work for the Jewish ghetto police; see, for example, Maria Zadziewicz testimony, AŻIH, file 301/2225.

49 Lensky, *A Physician inside the Warsaw Ghetto*, pp. 125, 127–128.

endangering patients and staff. Dr. Stein, the director of Czyste Hospital, wished to avoid responsibility for this situation and ordered doctors who had not been living in the hospital before the *Grossaktion* to move to Pawia St., promising that they would not be harmed there. Carts were allocated to move their belongings. The hospital physicians took up residence at one end of the street and doctors associated with public health institutions lived at the other end, according to the distribution of dwellings performed by a special committee of doctors, which caused bitterness and a feeling of favoritism. The apartments, whose former tenants had been sent to Treblinka, were in appalling condition: broken doors, pipes, and sanitary fixtures, insufficient number of beds, and fleas in the mattresses and on the walls.[50]

Although Stein and the Judenrat had promised those living on this street that they would be protected from deportation, many tenants there were forcibly evicted and sent to Treblinka.[51] Consequently, the hospital management allowed the doctors to send their families back to the hospital, but only during daytime hours. At sunset, the physicians and their families had to leave the hospital and return to their homes. As the *Grossaktion* wound down, the Jewish police, which maintained a permanent presence in the hospital, checked who was there and evicted the family members. No one wanted to leave the hospital. "Until now, it was like an island in a stormy sea. The storm has already lasted for six weeks but has not penetrated the hospital premises thus far, even though Germans and Ukrainians entered the building," Dr. Waller wrote.[52]

In late July 1942, the hospital was ordered to reduce its staff by means of layoffs and to evict those dismissed, as well as their families. With the Jewish population dwindling with each passing day, the SS demanded shorter and shorter lists of hospital staff. Tension in the hospital surged and the composition of the staff

50 Ibid., pp. 125–127; Dr. Shmuel Stanisław Waller testimony, YVA, O.3/2358.

51 Lensky, *A Physician Inside the Warsaw Ghetto*, pp. 125–126.

52 Dr. Shmuel Stanisław Waller testimony, YVA, O.3/2358.

changed each week. As the annihilation *Aktion* continued, the number of staff decreased.[53] This presented the medical authorities with the terrifying task of determining which doctors and nurses were needed and which were not. Dr. Stein, Dr. Aleksander Borkowski, Dr. Szeniszer, and some members of the administrative staff agonizingly carried out this order, striving to retain as many as possible. As usually happened under such circumstances, tragic injustices could not be avoided. Each department reported the number of its patients and staff. The Germans reviewed the lists and informed the hospital that the count would soon have to be reduced by half.[54]

Dr. Waller, who worked at the hospital, claimed that as the ghetto Jews were being deported to death camps, Dr. Stein, who was ordered to fire members of the medical staff, acted according to two criteria: professional distinction and religious affiliation. When those who were dismissed balked at leaving the hospital building, their last refuge, Dr. Stein, assisted by students whom he had hired, mostly Christianized Jews, expelled them en masse. About 500 workers, mostly sanitation and administrative workers, and a few doctors, were left standing with their wives and children in the hospital courtyard. After being forcibly evicted from the hospital grounds, they were surrounded by the Jewish police and taken to the Umschlagplatz. Until the beginning of the *Grossaktion*, the hospital underwent two rounds of layoffs. The institution's doorkeepers were in charge of expelling them and they violently carried out this duty, believing that they would save those who remained by doing so.

The list of workers authorized to continue working was posted on a bulletin board installed at the entrance. In the first round of cutbacks, all the volunteers and some of the nurses were discharged. The nurses had gathered and were sobbing silently. One of the doorkeepers, known for his cruelty, stood guard at the entrance to the wards. Where could they go? There was a tempest outside. Leszno St. was empty and silent. Rickshaws towed by

53 Lensky, *A Physician inside the Warsaw Ghetto*, pp. 127–128.

54 Gürfinkel-Glocer, "Goralo Shel Beit Haholim Tzhista," p. 594.

Jews and carrying Germans or patrols of Ukrainians armed with rifles could appear there at any moment.[55]

When the layoff lists were drafted, with the assistance of Fried, the chief nurse, efforts were made to retain the most senior and professional nurses. However, doctors and nurses were not the only persons expelled from the hospital. At the beginning of the *Grossaktion*, almost all the patients were discharged in anticipation of the many casualties who were expected to arrive at the hospital. Those who could not walk quickly had no chance of survival. When the Germans and Ukrainians checked the rooms and found a patient in bed, they shot him or her at once. The wards were vacated and, within two days, they were filled with victims of German gunfire. Again, there was a shortage of space.[56] Under these circumstances, Dr. Stein's position became extremely difficult, since he had to submit reports about the number of patients and staff from time to time. He struggled to decide how to produce such reports without bringing disaster on the hospital and its workers.[57]

In addition to selecting from among the staff members, the doctors had to do the same from among the patients. Dr. Marek Balin, who worked at the Czyste Hospital facility on Leszno St., described such a selection, which was conducted on August 15, 1942.

> Jews themselves had to surrender their brethren to death and turn over people who were unfit, fragile, unable to walk or whose every move caused then intense pain. To hand over such people to a horrific death….They struggled to keep the secret from the patients, who nevertheless instinctively sensed the encroaching danger. That day, the patients were despondent and there was fear in their eyes. Muffled sobbing was heard from the women's cells. A death sentence was to be issued by their doctors that evening.[58]

55 Dr. Shmuel Stanisław Waller testimony, YVA, O.3/2358.

56 Ibid.

57 Gürfinkel-Glocer, "Goralo Shel Beit Haholim Tzhista," p. 595.

58 Dr. Marek Balin testimony, YVA, O.3/441.

Dr. Marek Balin also described the method that the department directors used to indicate whether or not a patient would be deported.

> They had to place one of two marks next to each name: (+) meant death and (–) indicated remaining in the hospital. The doctors stood at the side of each bed at length, speaking quietly, whispering in Latin, so the patient would not understand the threat of this visit.[59]

Despite the selections and the suspense at the hospital, the hospital grounds were not blockaded until September 6, 1942.[60] At sunrise that day, the Nazi authorities ordered all the Jews to report for inspection, threatening to shoot anyone who failed to comply and who was found outside the inspection grounds.[61] A unit of German soldiers had already appeared in the streets by then. No one knew how many units of this kind were circulating in the ghetto. They turned out to be few but they gave the Germans a psychological edge. Thousands of people could have gone into hiding in the course of this large-scale *Aktion*—hideouts were plentiful—but the Germans had persuaded the Jews to show up.[62]

Panic broke out in the hospital. Everyone realized that this was a death sentence. Dr. Waller wrote that he understood there was no chance of surviving.

> I was not very close to Dr. Stein, I could not rely on our friendship, although I had worked hard at the hospital and there were times when I was the only doctor on duty in the surgical department. I spent entire days in the ward, but I knew that other criteria were considered during the selection. Under the circumstances, I began to look around for a place to hide.…We had long known that a good hideout was worth more than all the Germans' rubber stamps and promises.[63]

59 Ibid. See Offer, *Haluk Lavan Bageto*, appendix, A.6, pp. 521–523.

60 Dr. Adolf Polisiuk diary, GFH, no. 3182.

61 Lensky, *A Physician inside the Warsaw Ghetto*, p. 175.

62 Dr. Shmuel Stanisław Waller testimony, YVA, O.3/2358.

63 Ibid.

There were several hiding places. The hospital building had a well-stocked basement whose entrance was concealed by a cupboard. Only staff members knew about it and Dr. Waller sought refuge there. However, when the others there realized that he was about to move in with a one-year-old child, they vehemently refused to let them hide there. In the meantime, a group of 1,000 people gathered at the hospital entrance in rows of four. Waller, his son, and his wife joined them. Complying with the Germans' order, masses of people clustered on Zamenhofa St. and waited in despair, sobbing, hoping to receive "life numbers," and knowing that they could not count on luck. Implausible as it sounds, even in this hell and under the existing conditions, they had already begun to prepare hideouts in the cellars of the building. Dr. Stein was among those who had compiled the list of recipients of "life numbers." Reaching the courtyard, he immediately was surrounded by hundreds of people. Dr. Waller described the event.

> I grabbed Dr. Stein amid all these people and asked him whether I would receive a number for myself and my family (wife and son), and when he told me that I would not, I was gripped with panic. I seized him by the lapel of his suit so firmly that I tore it and began to remind him, at the top of my lungs, of all the efforts I had made for the hospital. I claimed that he had promised to give me these numbers.[64]

Dr. Stein finally gave Dr. Waller one number, but none for his wife and son. Waller managed to send the two of them to the hospital facility on Niska St. with an ambulance driver. Others were not as fortunate. Waller described meeting Dr. Markusfeld, head of the dermatology ward, and the neurologist Dr. Rotstadt, director of the physical therapy department. They were desperate. Although both were excellent physicians, they had been denied "life numbers" due to their advanced age and were sent to the Umschlagplatz. Dr. Waller reasoned that he had received a number because he was young. He claimed that Dr. Stein thought that, under the circumstances, it was less justified to keep the elderly alive than to

64 Ibid.

sustain the young. Waller testified that he heard the doctors bitterly say, "We spent our whole lives working for Jews, and now they are taking our lives."[65] The mob tried to snatch the "life numbers" from Stein's hands.[66]

They began to remove the holders of "life numbers" from the area, including Dr. Waller. Each person had to present the orange card on his or her way out. Some had managed to acquire bogus cards. At the exit gate, *SS-Untersturmführer* Karl Georg Brandt, the Nazi in charge of destroying the ghetto, stood with several SS men and painstakingly counted each group of four as it left the area. When the tally reached 3,200, he stopped the exodus. If five people in a certain group were found to be holding "life numbers" instead of four, the fifth person was held back even though he or she held a valid number. Those with "life numbers" were allowed to enter the vacated apartments of Jews who had been deported.[67]

Many doctors at the hospital did not receive "life numbers" and were sent to Treblinka, leaving a few department directors and few assistants. The special committee, headed by the director of the hospital, Dr. Stein, and Dr. Milejkowski, director of the Warsaw Judenrat Health Department, drew up the lists, guided by the principle that entire families, not individuals, should be saved. Accordingly, when they decided to award "life numbers" to the department directors, they gave them to their wives and children as well. Although this policy made sense, the administrative workers paid the price, because there were no "life numbers" left for them and most were sent to Treblinka. Assistant physicians also received "life numbers" at the expense of the administrative staff. After the *Aktion*, the hospital began to reorganize at 6–8 Gęsia St. Although the doctors' wives performed physical labor at this time,

65 Ibid.

66 Gürfinkel-Glocer, "Goralo Shel Beit Haholim Tzhista," p. 599.

67 Shmuel Stanisław Waller testimony, YVA, O.3/2358; Dr. Chaim Einhorn testimony, YVA, O.3/1836; Dr. Adolf Polisiuk diary, GFH, no. 3182; Janina Brandwajn-Ziemian, *Młodość w cieniu śmierci* (Łódź: Oficyna Bibliofilów, 1995), published in Hebrew as *Ne'urim Vetushiya Bamilhama: Zihronot Miymei Hashoah* (Youth and Resourcefulness in War: A Holocaust Memoir) (Tel Aviv: Y. Golan, 1994), pp. 78–80. Janina, daughter of Dr. Hieronym Brandwein, grew up in the Warsaw ghetto. Parts of her memoir relate to medical matters.

the remaining staff were sorely embittered by what they considered an enormous injustice to their comrades who had been sent away, including people who had served the hospital for decades.[68]

Dr. Polisiuk's notebooks document in detail the selection that the doctors were forced to carry out among their comrades.[69] Polisiuk wrote that the Jewish population, who still maintained discipline and did not believe the horror stories about Treblinka, obeyed the order almost to the letter.

> We reach the designated place and seized the apartments that had been abandoned at 21 Zamenhofa St. We were all prepared for the events to come and awaited them. In the afternoon hours, we found out that a general selection would be held. The *Gmina*[70] would carry out the selection among its workers on its own, whereas at the workshops and other institutions the selection would be undertaken by...headed by Kraust. Kraust set a quota of...32,900 people for the council. The quota—the general population [to remain] in the area—was set at around 35,000 people.
>
> The *Gmina* board set the quota for its various departments and the directors of each department were instructed to draw up lists of names. For the hospital department, which comprised about 800 people together with the two hospitals and the nearest of kin, a quota of 220 was set. A race for connections and influence ensued.
>
> The public deemed that the *Gmina* should not have taken

68 Lensky, *A Physician inside the Warsaw Ghetto*, pp. 178–179.

69 Dr. Adolf Polisiuk diary, GFH, no. 3182. Dr. Polisiuk was a gynecologist at Czyste Hospital and in the Warsaw ghetto. Two of his notebooks, written in Polish, are kept in the Ghetto Fighters House Archives: "Powiak: Memoir from the Prison," and "Square: Memoir from the Hospital on Leszno St." Dr. Polisiuk remained in the Warsaw ghetto until it was liquidated. He went into hiding in the doctors' bunker during the uprising and, during its final day, he was one of the few who managed to escape to the Aryan side, where he continued to provide medical care to Jews in hiding. He evidently was killed there. See Reuven Ben-Shem, "Batei Holim Yehudiyim BeVarsha," p. 586; Temkin-Berman, *Ir Betoh Ir*, p. 182; Yehudit Braude testimony, YVA, O.3/2360, p. 28; Polisiuk, "Hamatzor Ha'aharon," pp. 310–317; Offer, *Haluk Lavan Bageto*, appendix A.4, pp. 508–515.

70 *Gmina* is the Polish term for community committee, that is, the Judenrat.

on this task. It should not have continued Brandt's deeds, deciding who should remain in the area [the ghetto] and who should be sent to Treblinka. The *Gmina* should not have taken part in this, even if [its non-participation] would have meant more victims among us. It was also known that when the lists were being drawn up, personal influence and connections would outweigh the value of the worker's rights and many years of devoted work—and the majority would surely suffer for these reasons.

....The five-member committee had to decide the fate of 800 people. Those whom they selected should have been those who would be indispensable for the hospital, if one were to be established, and it was they who should have received the temporary right to live in the form of a "number"...the rest would be sentenced to transport to Treblinka.

We were overcome with an uncommon melancholy and disquiet. Many, particularly those from the staff of... threatened not to recognize the list. Outcries were heard, such as "We will turn to the Germans so that they carry out the selection!" or "If left to the Germans, blind fate, not connections, will decide!" They threatened not to allow those holding "numbers" to leave or to tear them up. It turned out later that these "numbers" were ripped up and destroyed at the hospital on Stawki St. There the situation was even more desperate, because the people had no way to leave the area and, therefore, had no opportunity to try to intervene personally. Each of us tried to get our own "number" with the help of personal acquaintances and connections, and amid the tussle for the "number," general confusion reigned. Interpersonal relations turned hostile. Each of us saw everyone else as a rival.

To place as many actual workers as possible on the list, the administration preferred people who were single or childless, but this principle was not maintained with exactitude and there were deviations in favor of some and to the disadvantage of others. Other departments, like Dr. Kon's Health Department, drew up lists of their workers only, leaving family members out. I witnessed a well-known physician, Dr. Stajnsapir, leave the *Gmina* and part from his wife, who walked in a different direction—to the Umschlagplatz....

That concept did not go over in our department. I will not get into the question of which considerations guided our board in selecting specific people. Obviously, such a limited number of people made it impossible to solve this very tragic problem properly and justly, even with the best of intentions and based on the most just premises. Just the same, if Brandt himself had performed the selection, we would have been spared the bitterness and sorrow toward friends and superiors.

All the lists were to be ready by September 7. That day, those chosen to remain were to leave the area and walk home. The public did not know who was on the lists, until almost the last moment. In general, they were required to call out the names on the list. On Monday, September 7, the hospital workers approached me and asked me to present this demand to the director. I thought their position was right so I approached the director, explained the matter to him, and managed to convince him to read out the lists three or four hours before the scheduled time [for the selection]. Since none of the members of the administration wanted to assume the duty of reading out the list, I had to do so with a heavy heart.

Around 250 people were "numbered" on the list, which included thirty doctors, several dozen nurses, and a few maintenance workers. The rest were their wives and children, who were supposed to replace the missing auxiliary staff. As the only doctor in my profession, I was on the list, along with my wife.

I approached my associates—coworkers—with this list. It was the most tragic moment in my life. As I read out the list, I announced the death sentence of 600 innocent people, close friends, comrades and workmates, and even my former boss, Dr. H. A. I was forced to read the list to them several times! They could not believe that they were not on the list. They deluded themselves into thinking that they had not heard well or that maybe I had skipped over their names by mistake.... Everyone, including those who were on the list, was gripped with fear and despair. They directed their rage and resentment at those who had produced the list and those included on it. I consoled them with the hope that there would be another list, although I myself did not believe it.

Just then, realizing that he was not on the list, Dr. Markusfeld committed suicide by leaping from the fourth floor....I bid farewell to the people closest to me, left the area, and turned into the courtyard of the *Gmina*, which was an assembly point, where we were supposed to receive the numbers, those numbers that were supposed to entitle us to remain in the ghetto and to live. Members of the Jewish police already stood at the gate that opened onto the courtyard, preventing "undesirables" from entering. Several people who appeared on the list but were staying at the time in the hospital on Stawki St. were brought to this location in a hospital vehicle. Two leading members of the *Gmina*, Lichtenbaum, Jr. (the director's son), and First, maintained order—without armbands. They had appropriate authorization for this, wearing boots and clutching whips. They beat unauthorized people who tried to infiltrate our ranks (many managed to do so, to the discredit of those in authority), and imposed order even more strictly when Brandt appeared there with the staff of his headquarters. His appearance made us anxious, because we feared an ambush. We were afraid that they would accompany us to the Umschlagplatz, instead of escorting us to our homes.

The first columns left the area at 5 P.M. We were among the last...We headed for the street, which was surrounded by soldiers. The heads of the designated departments escorted us to the residential blocks. We found our apartments looted and plundered. Before the day was out and in the three days following, after (the area) was strictly cordoned off, we escorted those left behind to the Umschlagplatz. A few survived by going into hiding. Many were killed on site and

> many committed suicide (Dr. Rotstadt). The patients from the hospital, together with the rest of the staff, were taken to the railroad cars, including even doctors who held numbers and had stayed behind at the hospital on Stawki St. so that the patients would not be denied medical assistance until the last moment that they were taken away....
>
> Following this selection, a new phase in our lives began—life under the continual threat of being sent to that world from which there is no return, a life without faith in what is human and what is good.[71]

According to Marek Edelman, five "life numbers" were allocated for sixty nurses. The principal of the nursing school, Luba Blum-Bielicka, believed that the best students should receive them. To determine this, she gave her class a one-question exam: "Describe the appropriate nursing care for a patient during the first days following a heart attack." The five who answered best received the "life numbers."[72]

The children's hospital was allotted ten numbers. Its director, Dr. Anna Braude-Heller, initially refused to distribute them, because they sufficed for only a few staff members and doomed everyone else to the Umschlagplatz. All the members of her staff pressed her not to yield the quota of numbers for the children's hospital to other institutions, hoping to save at least some members of their staff. "If you don't do it, none of us will survive. Instead of you, the director of the hospital for adults will step in."

After the selection, Dr. Waller worked with Dr. Braude-Heller at the new hospital on Gęsia St. There she disclosed to him her regret over having treated the technical staff unjustly by preferring to distribute numbers to doctors and their wives and not to

71 Dr. Adolf Polisiuk diary, GFH, no. 3182.

72 Krall, *Shielding the Flame*, pp. 77–78. According to another account, there were twenty "life numbers," which were not enough for all the students remaining at the school. The principal, Blum-Bielicka, had two children, aged four and eleven. They were placed on the list as well. Roland, *Courage under Siege*, pp. 73–74.

veteran workers.[73] Years later, Dr. Adina Blady Szwajger wrote the following:

> Everybody said she had to do it but it was vile, because, after all, none of us would like to decide who is to live and who is to die....Later on, after the war, I asked Arik Heller [Dr. Braude-Heller's son] if he knew why it was us who got "tickets"; that is, people like myself and not the older ones who were a thousand times more valuable. He told me then that his mother had staked her bets on youth, that we might live through it all and still do something with our lives.[74]

Years after the war, Marek Edelman expressed his opinion on this affair in an interview with journalist Hanna Krall. "Is there a standard," he asked, "by which one can determine who has the right to live? No such standard exists," he ruled. But since various delegations approached Dr. Heller and asked her to consent to it, she began to hand out the numbers.[75]

Dr. Lensky criticized the hospital directors and the Health Department for not warning those sentenced to transport to Treblinka about the danger that awaited them, as Dr. Braude-Heller did.[76] However, it should be borne in mind that the staff at the children's hospital was much smaller than that of the doctors at Czyste Hospital, making it difficult, if not impossible, to do the same there.

Whom to Rescue First?

The testimonies describe the dilemma of setting priorities in rescue attempts. Should medical staff be saved first, or should workmates, relatives, and members of the resistance be given

73 Krall, *Shielding the Flame*, p. 46, Dr. Shmuel Stanisław Waller testimony, YVA, O.3/2358.

74 Blady Szwajger, *I Remember Nothing More*, p. 55.

75 Krall, *Shielding the Flame*, p. 46.

76 Lensky, *A Physician inside the Warsaw Ghetto*, pp. 178–179.

priority? Or might it be best to try to aid anyone who comes along and asks for help? The rabbis also faced dilemmas of this nature, when presented with halachic questions.[77] Edelman wrote that people clung to the white smocks of nurses in desperate attempts to survive, pleading to be issued one as well and pounding on the doors of the hospital, where a Jewish policeman stood guard. In one case, Dr. Anna Braude-Heller lifted a boy from his father's arms, after the latter implored her to let her institution save at least his son, and shoved the child into the hospital over the guard's objections.

The testimonies give the impression that there was a preference for workmates, relatives, and members of the resistance. As described by Marek Edelman, "Our people would pick out those who should be saved and I would select them out as sick."[78] Jerzy Ross testified that the first aid staff drove to the Umschlagplatz every day at the time of the transports to help the ill and those who fainted while waiting there.

> We seized these opportunities to rescue relatives and friends, taking them away by car or leading them away dressed in first aid caps, doctors' smocks, and nurses' kerchiefs. This is how I led out and saved my father, who had been captured by the Jewish police, as well as others.[79]

Marek Edelman testified that close associates had priority.

> I was merciless. One woman begged me to pull out her fourteen-year-old daughter, but I was only able to take one more person and I took Zosia, who was our best courier. I

77 See, for example, Irving J. Rosenbaum, *The Holocaust and Halakhah* (New York: Ktav, 1976), pp. 17–46; Esther Farbstein, *Hidden in Thunder: Perspectives on Faith, Halachah, and Leadership during the Holocaust* (Jerusalem: Mossad Harav Kook, 2007), pp. 185–231; Havi Ben-Sasson and Amos Goldberg, *Shnot Ra'inu Ra'a: Prakim Betoldot Hayahadut Hadatit Bitkufat Hashoah* (We Have Seen Evil: Selected Aspects in the History of Religious Jewry during the Holocaust) (Hebrew), vol. 3, (Jerusalem: Yad Vashem, 2008), Introduction, chap. 1.

78 Krall, *Shielding the Flame*, p. 7.

79 Ross, "Tahanat Ezra Rishona," p. 73.

> selected her out four times and each time ended up having to take her out all over again.[80]
>
> I was busy at the Umschlagplatz. With the aid of our people in the ghetto police, I was supposed to select out those whom we needed the most at the time. One day I pulled out a guy and a young woman—he had worked at the printing shop, and she had been an excellent liaison officer. They both died soon afterward—he in the uprising, and she by way of a later trip to the Umschlagplatz—but before that he managed to distribute this paper.[81]

Edelman added in his memoir,

> Helena Szefner, pale and beside herself, brought to the Umschlagplatz after the last blockade, was also taken into the hospital by our comrades and was then, at the first opportunity, taken outside the walls on a doctor's certificate.[82]

The dilemma also arose at Czyste Hospital during the *Aktionen*. Even after all other public and medical institutions in the ghetto were eradicated, the hospital carried on until after the final *Aktion*. The public perceived the hospital as an island of safety at this time, relative to the events in the ghetto during the *Aktionen*. Thus, people sought to save themselves by being hospitalized, placing its management under severe pressure. The administration and the doctors were under the constant threat of death and of the liquidation of the hospital, if the Gestapo physicians, who frequently vetted the lists of patients, were to find healthy and fit people among them. Nevertheless, efforts were made to help individuals find hideouts inside the hospital. Here too, the question of priorities in providing assistance came up. The testimonies reveal that patients were admitted to all the hospital wards on the basis of "pull"—parents of doctors or of

80 Krall, *Shielding the Flame*, p. 7.
81 Ibid., p. 43.
82 Edelman, *The Ghetto Fights*, p. 46.

long-tenured nurses, former staff members who had been fired at the beginning of this or that *Aktion*, or relatives of Judenrat officials. Czyste Hospital was full of fictitious patients, including elderly people who attempted in this manner to elude deportation. Once inside the hospital building, everyone strived in every possible way to stay there. Sometimes surgeons fractured the limbs of family members in order to admit them to the hospital. Czyste Hospital also admitted members of the intelligentsia—writers, artists, and public figures—deemed worthy of rescue at all costs by the medical staff. More than 100 people were admitted as "patients."[83] When the hospital was reopened after the September 1942 *Aktion*, these rescue tactics were employed again.[84]

In a comparison of today's medical dilemmas with those in the ghetto, it is of interest to note the remarks of researchers Priel and Dolev. They examined the ethical considerations that guide activity in a mass-casualty event, which raises dilemmas somewhat reminiscent of the situation in the ghetto in terms of priorities in medical care.

> It is puzzling to discover that the matter of mass-casualty events, which present the medical profession with very sticky, ethical problems, has received scanty attention at the ethical level in the medical literature.... There may be various explanations for this, principally, the repression of a painful and intractable topic.[85]

83 Dr. Adolf Polisiuk diary, GFH, no. 3182; Dr. Shmuel Stanisław Waller testimony, YVA, O.3/2358; Gürfinkel-Glocer, "Goralo Shel Bet Haholim Tzhista," p. 594; Lensky, *A Physician inside the Warsaw Ghetto*, pp. 169–170; Einhorn, "Harofe Begeto Varsha," p. 9.

84 Einhorn, "Harofe Begeto Varsha," pp. 9–10.

85 Yisrael Priel and Eran Dolev, "Shikulim Etiyim Be'et Erua Rav-Nifga'im" (Ethical Considerations in Mass Casualty Situations), *Harefu'a* (Hebrew), 140 (2001), pp. 574–577. The World Medical Association Statement on Medical Ethics in the Event of Disasters states that triage is the instrument to use in contending with a mass-casualty event. The ethical principles that inform medical triage are compassion, independence, causing no harm, and acting justly. The rights of patients, the right of the caregivers to personal safety, and the rights of society and the state are also taken into account. The statement stresses: "It is ethical for a physician not to persist, at all costs, in treating individuals

Euthanasia by Doctors and Nurses during the *Aktionen*

"No words of any human language are strong enough to describe the 'Umschlag' now, when no help from anywhere or anybody can be expected," wrote Marek Edelman in his memoir shortly after the war had ended.

> Nurses search the crowd for their fathers and mothers and, having found them, inject longed-for deathly morphine into their veins, their own eyes gleaming wildly. One doctor compassionately pours a cyanide solution into the feverish mouths of strange, sick children. To offer one's cyanide to somebody else is now the most precious, the most irreplaceable thing. It brings a quiet, peaceful death, it saves from the horror of the cars.[86]

About thirty years after the events, in an interview by the Jewish journalist Hanna Krall, Edelman again described the dramatic ethical decisions that some members of the medical staff made.

> ...the last day of the *Aktion*. On the upper floor, there were a few rooms with children.
>
> As the Germans were entering the ground floor, a woman doctor managed to poison the kids.
>
> You see, Hanna, you don't understand anything. She saved these children from the gas chamber. People thought she was a hero. [Edelman to Krall]
>
> In this hospital, sick people were lying on the floor waiting to be loaded onto the train cars, and the nurses were searching out their parents in the crowd and injecting them with poison. They saved this poison for their closest relatives. And she, this

beyond emergency care.... It is justified when it is intended to save the maximum number of individuals." See https://www.wma.net/policiespost/wma-statement-on-medical-ethics-in-the-event-of-disasters/ (accessed September 17, 2019).

86 Edelman, *The Ghetto Fights*, p. 50.

> doctor had given her own cyanide to kids who were complete strangers![87]

Helena Szereszewska, whose daughter worked as a nurse at the hospital, also described the events there during those difficult hours.

> Some carts drove up to the hospital at seven in the morning. Two Germans came in…and ordered the sick to be carried out onto the carts. She was working in the surgical ward. The doctors and nurses hurriedly poisoned the chronically sick patients by injecting them with large doses of morphine. Some of the patients did not want to go.…When the patients had been driven away, the Germans summoned the staff for a selection…the doctors separately, the orderlies separately, the office staff separately. Both of the Germans were drunk.[88]

On August 24, 1942, Abraham Lewin described in his diary that he wished to spare his mother the suffering and the torments to come.

> The matter of my mother is causing me great anguish. What can be done for her? I have given permission to put her to sleep…rather than give her over to the executioners. But J, who was a doctor, refuses to carry it out. Even the devil could not have conceived of such a situation.[89]

It was evidently Dr. Jakob Tombak, Lewin's brother-in-law, who refused to carry out the mercy killing.

The pediatrician Dr. Adina Blady Szwajger bore indelible memories of the day of the *Aktion* in the hospital.

> All I know is that we went down empty streets…wearing our white gowns…I only remember the hospital gates and

87 Krall, *Shielding the Flame*, p. 9.
88 Szereszewska, *Memoirs*, p. 182.
89 Lewin, *A Cup of Tears*, p. 165.

those stairs strewn with people and that terrible stench of pus and faeces [feces] and that somebody was constantly grabbing at my gown and shouting: "Sister! Sister!"....I know that I kept going up the stairs, trying not to step on people, but there—corpses and living lay all together. I reached...only the infants' ward—no children's wards, just the sick, the wounded and the dying everywhere. But, as I walked around, children began to appear from various nooks and crannies and gathered around me—like birds or puppies....Marysia, who had tuberculosis of the lymphatic glands...said to me, "Doctor, we all know that we haven't got mamas and papas anymore and that we're not going to live through it either. But will you stay with us to the end?" "Yes, Marysia, I'll stay with you to the end," I said. This was only half true, because I did leave but they were already asleep by then and weren't supposed to wake up. Yet sometimes, even now, when I can't sleep, I wonder whether any of them woke up. But it's better not to think about it. But then it never occurred to me. I had no idea that we'd get out. I had a whole day in front of me...

Then Sister Mira came for me...she asked me to go downstairs with her for a moment. When we left the ward, she said—and I can still hear this—"Doctor, please give my mother an injection. I can't do it. I beg you, please. I don't want them to shoot her in bed, and she can't walk." So I asked her what was in the syringe and she told me it was morphine. I knew then what I could do for the children so as to keep my word. Although I didn't know yet that I had been given a "ticket," I did know we'd be separated and I wouldn't be able to help them in that final moment. I asked her if she had a lot of morphine—she said she'd give it to me. Because she knew what I wanted it for....And so that gray-haired lady smiled at me and stretched out her arm. The sister put on the clamp. And I injected the morphine into her vein. And then I saw a few more people who didn't have the strength to move. I asked Mira what we should do and she said, "Help them, surely." So we helped them, too. And by the window there was this woman, swollen from starvation and suffering from circulatory insufficiency, and she kept on looking at us, pleading with her eyes. She was the last one we gave an injection to...

...So when I left the room, I held out my hand and got two large containers of morphine. We didn't say a word to each other, just squeezed each other's hands, I think. I took the morphine upstairs. Dr. Margolis was there and I told her what I wanted to do. So we took a spoon and went to the infants' room. And just as, during those two years of real work in the hospital, I had bent down over the little beds, so now I poured this last medicine into those tiny mouths. Only Dr. Margolis was with me. And downstairs, there was screaming because the Szaulis[90]...and the Germans were already there, taking the sick from the wards to the cattle trucks. After that we went to the older children and told them that this medicine was going to make their pain disappear. They believed us and drank the required amount from the glass. And then I told them to undress, get into bed and sleep. So they lay down and after a few minutes—I don't know how many—but the next time I went into that room, they were asleep. And then I don't know what happened after that. All I know is that I had my "ticket" pinned on me...another four months on Gesia St. where there was a so-called children's ward and two years on the Aryan side. In the morning I helped with pediatrics; in the evening I was a night nurse. Then came the second *Aktion*, followed by the order to shut down this children's home.[91]

More than fifty years after Dr. Adina Blady Szwajger euthanized the infants and the elderly in the midst of the brutal *Aktionen*, she

90 The source of the name Szaulis to refer to Lithuanians is the Lithuanian Riflemen's Union (Lietuvos Šaulių Sąjunga), a Lithuanian paramilitary nationalist organization that joined the German forces together with Ukrainians and Latvians. They were active in exterminating Jews at the time of the Warsaw ghetto uprising.

91 Blady Szwajger, *I Remember Nothing More*, pp. 53–58.

revealed her opinions about euthanasia in ordinary times to the writer Anka Grupińska. According to her worldview, the right to euthanasia exists in one case only, when the person is suffering greatly and has run out of hope. "Life that is no longer life, the life of a person who is effectively already dead—spiritually dead and living with a sense of terrible suffering—should not be prolonged mechanically."[92]

Dr. Adina Blady Szwajger also believed that euthanasia should not be allowed by legislation, because such a statute could be abused. However, individuals do have the right to terminate their lives if they are racked with inhumane suffering and know that all hope is gone. The assessment of hopelessness must be based on medical science rulings in the relevant context. If so, Blady Szwajger believed that individuals are entitled to take their own lives when all is lost.[93]

At the time of the *Aktionen*, Dr. Blady Szwajger attempted suicide by taking sleeping pills with vodka. Failing to end her life, she returned to work at the children's hospital in the Warsaw ghetto. When the Germans broke into the hospital and loaded the patients onto the death transports, she used morphine to euthanize fifteen elderly patients and fifteen toddlers and children. According to Prof. Avraham Steinberg, this is very problematic behavior.

> Any act of homicide, even if committed with humane intentions, is murder, nevertheless. The morphine that was injected caused certain death, and had it not been injected, who knows? Maybe the patients would have managed to go into hiding, maybe the Germans would not have arrived, maybe something would have happened at the last moment.[94]

Prof. Ralph Yodaiken, the Jewish American physician, who researched moral dilemmas among Jewish doctors in the Holocaust, disagreed.

92 Grupińska, "Conversation with Adina Blady Szwajger," pp. 149–150.

93 Ibid.

94 Negev and Koren, "Nisuyim Bivnei Adam," pp. 53–56.

> I believe that Dr. Szwajger, staring into the well of life and death and knowing what was expected, chose the only option for the patients whom she loved and allowed them to die in dignity. Her actions should be seen as a full-fledged act of rebellion. She denied the murderers the pleasure of slaughtering those under her care.[95]

Marek Edelman reported that when the *Aktion* had begun and patients on the ground floor were being evicted, a nineteen-year-old woman on the upper floor of the hospital gave birth, a doctor and a nurse by her side. When the baby was born, the doctor handed him to the nurse. She placed him on a pillow and covered him with another pillow. The newborn bleated for a moment and then fell silent. The doctor neither said a word nor responded in any other way. The mother already knew what she had to do. Edelman told Hanna Krall, "I'm glad that you haven't asked me today, 'And did this woman survive?' the way you asked about the doctor who gave cyanide to the children. Yes, she did survive. She is a very famous pediatrician."[96]

Prof. Hirszfeld described the dilemma that the doctors at the hospital faced during the *Aktionen* and specified the "last social service" that they carried out: euthanizing fifteen elderly people in the hospital.

> The reloading station was a kind of purgatory on the road to hell....Each day, from seven thousand to nine thousand people from the city were brought there....The square was surrounded by a cordon. Whoever got behind the cordon ceased to be a human being and became an animal assigned to work or to death....
>
> ...The dead bodies of orderlies who had been inefficiently performing the role of hangmen were lying next to the railroad cars. Eyewitnesses told me the details of the killings, which made my hair stand on end and which no report can

95 Ibid.

96 Krall, *Shielding the Flame*, p. 47.

> render accurately....The laboratory was not set up, it was not functioning....All my efforts were concentrated on saving persons I knew....Those on the list of community employees at least had some hope of saving their lives. However, hiding one's parents and bringing them some bread was enough of a task to absorb one's entire energy. It was known that the moment would come when most patients would have to be relinquished to their fate. Then what were the physicians to do? Their obligation was to protect their patients. It was impossible to protect all of them from their cruel fate. But a dozen or so patients were the mothers of the physicians. On behalf of professional courtesy, it was decided not to let them be murdered. It was the last service of one colleague to another; those mothers should not die looking at their henchmen; they should fall asleep in peace. When the order arrived that the human contingents from the hospital had to be presented the next day, fifteen elderly mothers of physicians were put to sleep with morphine injections. They had an easy, quiet death. They were buried in a little square in a joint grave. May their deaths lie on the conscience of German physicians.[97]

Killing One to Rescue Many

In her diary, Noemi Szac-Wajnkranc reported that Jews killed babies and children in hiding during the deportations lest they endanger entire groups of sequestered fugitives. Even though the dilemmas related to this scenario do not pertain directly to medical staff and did not manifest themselves in hospitals, medical personnel were sometimes asked to implement such killings.

> We're all sitting in a tiny room. We're thirty people, but others join now and then. Anything to have a roof over their heads, not to lie in the street. Waiting for the inspection.

97 Hirszfeld, *The Story of One Life*, pp. 267–269.

> They've already gone through several buildings.... They don't let children and elderly pass at all.... They kill them on the spot.... They let only 10 percent of all the people go. Everyone who's "freed" gets a number for "life." When you present the number, you can exit the maelstrom. Workers at the "shops" come. Masses, tens of thousands of people, and a group of a few hundred emerges.
>
> ...Children who spent the day playing, oblivious to the horror of the situation, now shut up and sit silently, pressed to their parents. A young woman with a baby on her lap sits right next to the window. I observe her.... The child is a few months old. All day he played and babbled; now he's sleeping.... The woman crouched at his side...I have twelve tablets of Luminal; will they be enough for him?" "I've got ten," I say. "Will you give them to me?" the woman pleads. That night, three children in our room are given the means to go to sleep forever, and a doctor, the father of a three-year-old girl, injects her with a medication that works right away. I hold a toddler in my arms, and in my arms he grows cold and falls asleep.
>
> A sleepless night is followed by an overcast morning. In the world, it brings life, work, delight. What does it bring us? A new torment, new dying. The boy is still suffering, breathing heavily, foam oozing from his mouth. Not enough Luminal...A young woman with graying hair cries..."I can't poison my son, I can't," she wails.[98]

Those who managed to escape to the Aryan side and hide from the German authorities and Polish denouncers faced the same ethical problem. Dr. Adina Blady Szwajger, who had crossed to the other side of town after the January 1943 *Aktion*, described such situations.

> Children are always being born. Even in hiding places and in cellars. But they often die, and it is not always possible to save them. You have only your own hands, but you also need

98 Szac-Wajnkranc, *Halaf Im Ha'esh*, pp. 71–73.

> medicines, and mother's milk, which in this case did not flow at all. The landlady was afraid to bring home more milk than she usually bought. And you also need air, of which there wasn't any in the cellar, and which you can't bring in your hands. And they mustn't cry. The landlords were afraid. Those living with her were afraid. The harassed, terrified mother covered the child's face with a pillow. Because someone had come into the house. So it was no wonder that I had to carry the body of the newborn baby from the house in a cardboard box. A different mother's child, an older baby, a few months old, I carried out in my arms in its swaddling clothes. But I don't wish to remember how I had to drink vodka with the undertakers before they would bury the body somewhere under the wall.[99]

In another case, a mentally ill woman had to be killed, because her behavior endangered the inhabitants of the house and the hideout.

> I don't know, perhaps I should have refused. After all, it wasn't a job for a doctor. Except that no one understood this. There was no other doctor among us at that time. And so I didn't have anyone to talk to, to tell that I would rather die than do this. It would have been easier to die myself than to carry out euthanasia on someone who was mentally ill. She used to run out into the street and shout in Yiddish. She posed a mortal threat for the landlords and for the half a dozen or so young people hiding in the house, among them her own daughter. But I couldn't do it! But I did it. At the request of her daughter.[100]

As stated in the introduction to this chapter, all the dilemmas described were recognized as such at the time.

However, it may also be of interest to mention a dilemma that was not, to the best of my knowledge, acknowledged as such by contemporaries, but is disturbing from today's point of view: medical research by doctors at that tragic time. Without detracting

99 Blady Szwajger, *I Remember Nothing More*, p. 137.
100 Ibid., p. 150.

from the ghetto physicians' medical entrepreneurship, one may wonder whether these studies would meet today's accepted standards for medical experimentation on human subjects. I content myself with pointing out the ostensibly obvious—the studies in the ghetto were not undertaken coercively, they neither exacerbated their subjects' suffering nor worsened their medical condition, and they were undertaken with sensitivity to the patients and to their plight.

* * *

Summing up the topic of this chapter, I note that this study addressed the prominent ethical issues described by the medical staff in the Warsaw ghetto from the beginning of the war to the liquidation of the ghetto. It is possible to sort the dilemmas that the medical workers faced in the Warsaw ghetto into various types.

The first set of issues is characteristic of questions of coping with the commitment to basic and universal moral rules, principles, and values, which in ordinary times underlie personal and public behavioral norms, and create no moral conflict. The ghetto conditions put the inhabitants, individually and collectively, to the special test of upholding these fundamental values in daily life. In view of the health catastrophe caused by the Germans' edicts, the population developed a massive, aberrant dependency on those who staffed the medical and sanitation services, thrusting medical workers into a unique, ethical ordeal every day.[101] For example, the payment of sub-subsistence wages led to the phenomena of bribery and exploitation of the public by medical and sanitation staff. Those who participated in this

101 The use of the term "medical ethics" to refer to the totality of ethical questions relating to medicine attests to an attempt to expose the professionals and their behavioral norms to social criticism from the standpoint of general moral tenets. The assumption is that there is something unique about a doctor's duties to his or her patients. See Heyd, *Etika Verefu'a*, pp. 10–11. Under the ghetto conditions, the public's dependency on its medical service providers, which was already very high to begin with, increased considerably, putting the normative principles of medical service to a unique test.

misconduct harmed others by transgressing basic moral values in a manner that they would surely not have wanted others to inflict on them. Their involvement in bribery extorted the inhabitants of what remained of their money, impaired their health, and even caused the death of entire families. The inhabitants regarded these actions as flagrant violations of the rules of medical ethics and personal morals. Most of the doctors appear to have passed this ethical test honorably, but it is impossible to ignore the fact that the sources identify bribery as a widespread phenomenon.

The second group of moral problems may be characterized as issues of moral conflict, that is, situations in which medical staff members had to decide which duty to fulfill when faced with two worthy but irreconcilable alternatives.[102] An important juncture in this regard concerns the inner dilemma that doctors faced between their professional undertakings and their personal ones. An example of the issues involved is the question of whether medical staff were obligated to treat patients under any conditions, including at personal risk, even to the point of risking one's life in the most extreme case, or whether they were permitted to look out for themselves and abandon the ill. This conflict manifested itself from the very beginning of the war but did so with particular ferocity on the eve of, and during, the deportations, when doctors and staff, like everyone else in the ghetto, wanted to try to save themselves. Some chose to look out for their own lives, while others resolved to remain with their patients until the bitter end.

Additional issues of moral conflict were raised when the medical staff members encountered and were ordered to carry out certain actions under the circumstances imposed on them by the Nazi authorities, which in ordinary times had nothing to do with their duties. The Germans, for example, threatened to put doctors to death for failing to report cases of infectious diseases. Doctors were faced with the dilemma of whether to report the ill, thereby subjecting them and their families to grievous suffering,

102 To understand the concept of "moral dilemma" and its meaning in philosophy, see Statman, *Moral Dilemmas*, chap. 1.

or to help conceal the ill, despite the personal risk entailed. Many doctors treated the contagious patients in their homes, defying the Germans' directives.

Medical staff had to deal with other conflicts during the *Aktionen*. The harsh reality created on the Umschlagplatz and in the hospital confronted them in an extreme manner with the question of prioritizing rescue attempts. There seems to have been a preference for people with close ties. Czyste Hospital took in members of the intelligentsia who, in the judgment of medical staff, had to be saved, in addition to the doctors' families. According to some philosophers, in exceptional dilemmas in which two considerations appear to be in equilibrium, the choice between the rationales has no practical moral significance. The right action is to choose one or the other, never mind which.

This is also true of the dilemmas faced by the doctors in the ghetto who had to tackle the question of preferences in saving lives. However, even in dilemmas involving the saving of lives, the options are not always symmetrical. Although we affirm the value of equality among people, there may sometimes be better reasons to save one person rather than another. This observation is inconsistent with the Hippocratic Oath. Indeed, some believe the oath should be amended in order to provide moral support to medical staff operating in mass-casualty events, when they are required to act according to other criteria, such as the principle of saving as many lives as possible.[103]

In normal times as well, medical staff occasionally are confronted with some of the types of dilemmas described above. However, under the circumstances that were created in the ghetto, these dilemmas became a much more central and extreme part of the routine medical work described above, but under the

103 Ibid., chap. 5; Dolev and Priel, "Hagibuy Ha'eti Lerofe Be'erua Rav-Nifga'im" (Ethical Backing for the Doctor in a Mass-Casualty Event), *Harefu'a* (Hebrew), 130 (1996), pp. 424–426. Only in 1996 did the World Medical Association propose, for the first time, criteria for professional medical treatment to cope with mass-casualty events that address the main problem in such situations—triage and setting priorities for care—in which the principle of doing the best for the maximum number of casualties determines the priorities.

circumstances created in the ghetto, they became a much more central and extreme part of their routine medical work.

The third group of moral problems, in contrast to and unlike those described above, include tragic moral dilemmas that may have been unique to the conditions of medical work in the Warsaw ghetto. A tragic moral dilemma is a special type of conflict in which all the alternatives are dire, and even if it is possible to determine that one is more correct compared to the others, it also severely violates moral values. In the absence of clear moral considerations that serve to identify one course of action as preferable to another, people caught in such a situation feel helpless and cannot decide on the action to take. Under conditions that introduce an element of uncertainty to all the implications of the various alternatives, the dilemma becomes particularly acute. When people are forced to harm others, as well as themselves, which totally contradicts one of the basic values of their worldview, a particularly tragic dilemma is created to the point of undermining a person's life. Even "lesser of all evils" decisions, in which the individual chooses the right course of action under the tragic circumstances, are accompanied by anguish and torment, when they are made and thereafter.[104]

This cluster of ethical problems involves different degrees of blatant evil, which the ghetto doctors and medical teams were forced to confront in the course of their activities. They were required to screen men for forced labor in camps, where many died, and to conduct selections among their colleagues and patients that determined who would be sent to their deaths in Treblinka. The tragic moral dilemmas in this group also include euthanasia, which some medical staff members carried out by terminating the lives of patients without their knowledge and consent, in order to spare them death by brutal torture at the hands of the Germans in the hospital during the *Aktionen*. Some doctors who were asked by patients' relatives to perform euthanasia refused to do so. The sources made it clear that such

104 Statman, *Moral Dilemmas*, pp. 132–136.

decisions were accompanied by grave personal torment. This does not indicate that the doctors made immoral decisions, but only that the outcome of their actions caused them great anguish.[105] Some of those involved noted in hindsight that the dilemma they had faced had a more appropriate answer than the one they had chosen.

Since the medical staff and their families were mainly healthy, selection among them was based on priorities that for the most part were determined according to value judgments rather than medical standards. Many Jews who played a role in this tragic selection believed that the Judenrat and the medical personnel should not have accepted the task of determining who should live and who should die, and instead should have left it to the Germans, even if the tally of victims would have been higher on this account. In their opinion, had they done so, bitterness toward friends and the officials would have been avoided. In any case, after all, too few were entitled to remain to allow for a just solution to the tragic problem.

According to the outlook of the aforementioned philosopher Thomas Nagel, people sometimes have "bad circumstantial luck" in certain situations and in the moral dilemmas that such situations raise. Some people pass these moral tests, while others fail. This applies to the cases presented here. Among the Jewish doctors and nurses in Warsaw, some passed these difficult tests admirably, acting tirelessly and at personal risk to help their suffering brethren. Others engaged in corruption, shirking their professional and human obligations. Many others were somewhere in between. Quite a few studies depict the doctors, nurses, and other medical personnel in the ghetto, almost without exception, as moral saints who were willing to risk their lives and work indefatigably for their ill and needy brethren.[106] Obviously, such a description embellishes a reality that—like any human reality—was much more complex.

105 Ibid.

106 This is the general impression drawn, for example, from Roland's comprehensive study, *Courage under Siege*; Wulman et al., *The Martyrdom of Jewish Physicians in Poland*; and from many other studies.

As we have seen, at least one of the sources presents a tableau of shame, according to which "a large portion" of the doctors failed the moral test placed before them. Other sources, particularly Dr. Lensky's memoir, paint a different scene, in which most of the doctors actually passed the test during that very difficult period. Given the current state of the documentation, we cannot resolve the matter clearly and unequivocally, but even if we could, would it be appropriate and is it necessary to do so? Undoubtedly, the moral portrait of the doctors was complex, as was that of the rabbis and the other leaders in the ghetto, and, a fortiori, that of ordinary people. The conduct of the doctors as individuals was probably not significantly different from that of many of the other individuals in meaningful positions in the ghetto. All were subjected to impossible moral ordeals.

Indeed, the ethical question was omnipresent among the ghetto's health care officials, and the issue of moral challenge was probably one of the dominant aspects of their unique work under the conditions that prevailed. Needless to say, the fate of these individuals was no better than that of the rest of the Jews in the ghetto. After their lengthy, exhausting, and dangerous work in community service, most were sent to the death camps.

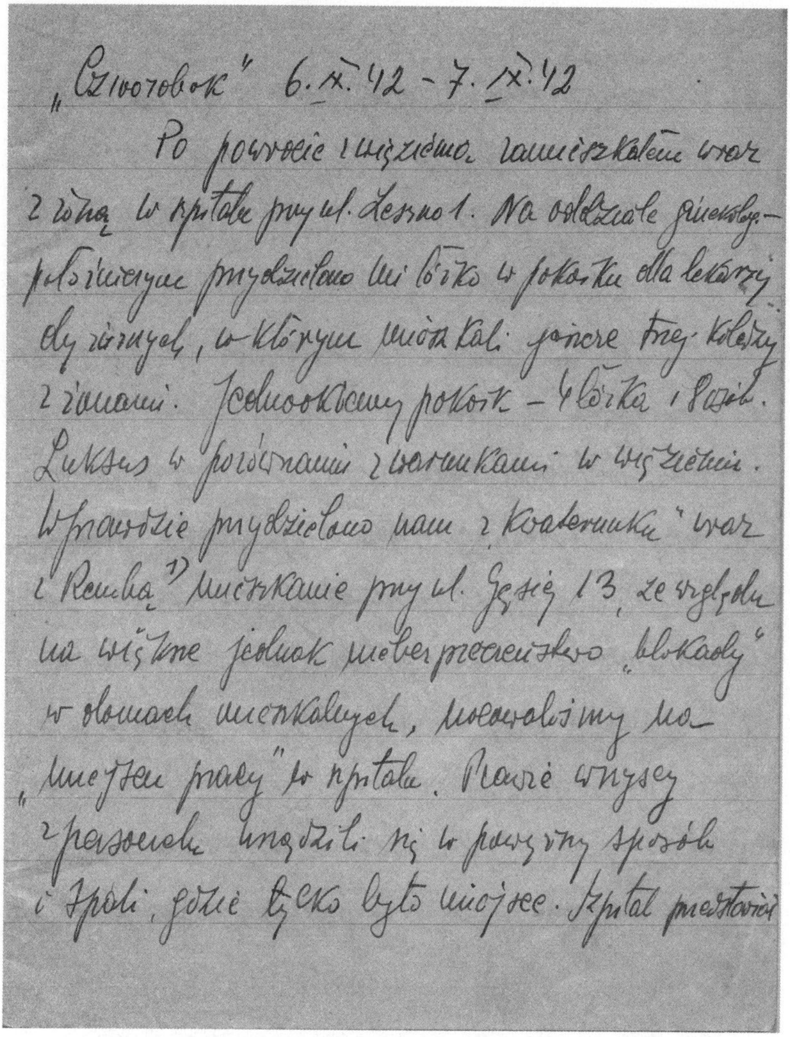

„Czworobok" 6.IX.42 – 7.IX.42

Po powrocie z więzienia zamieszkałem wraz z żoną w szpitalu przy ul. Leszno 1. Na oddziale ginekologiczno-położniczym przydzielono mi łóżko w pokoiku dla lekarzy dyżurnych, w którym mieszkali jeszcze trzej koledzy z żonami. Jednookienny pokoik – 4 łóżka i 8 osób. Luksus w porównaniu z warunkami w więzieniu. Wprawdzie przydzielono nam z Koaterunką" wraz z Rembą 1) mieszkanie przy ul. Gęsiej 13, ze względu na większe jednak niebezpieczeństwo „blokady" w domach mieszkalnych, woleliśmy „na miejscu pracy" w szpitalu. Prawie wszyscy z personelu urządzili się w podobny sposób i spali, gdzie tylko było miejsce. Szpital przedstawiał

The first page of the diary of Dr. Polisiuk, gynecologist at Czyste Hospital, which includes his memoirs of the *Aktion* at the hospital at 1 Leszno St. in the Warsaw ghetto, September 6–7, 1942. GFH, no. 3182.

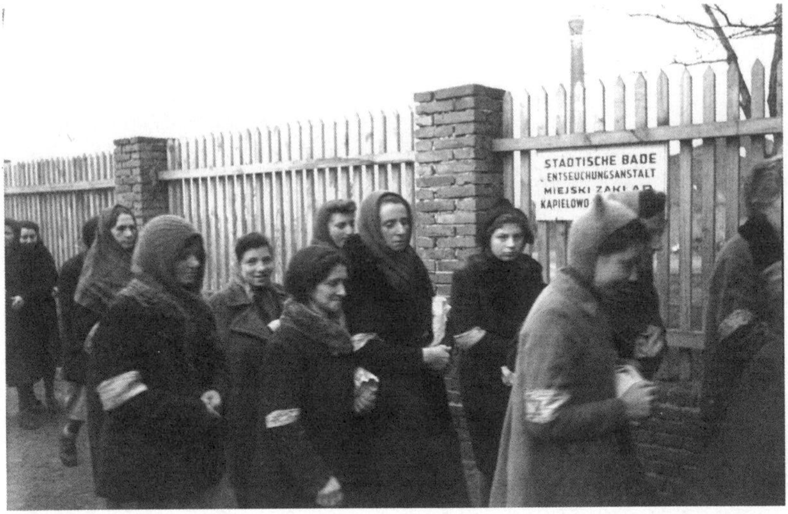

Jewish women wait in line outside the bathhouse in the Warsaw ghetto, May 1941. Photo Collection, YVA, 3955/421.

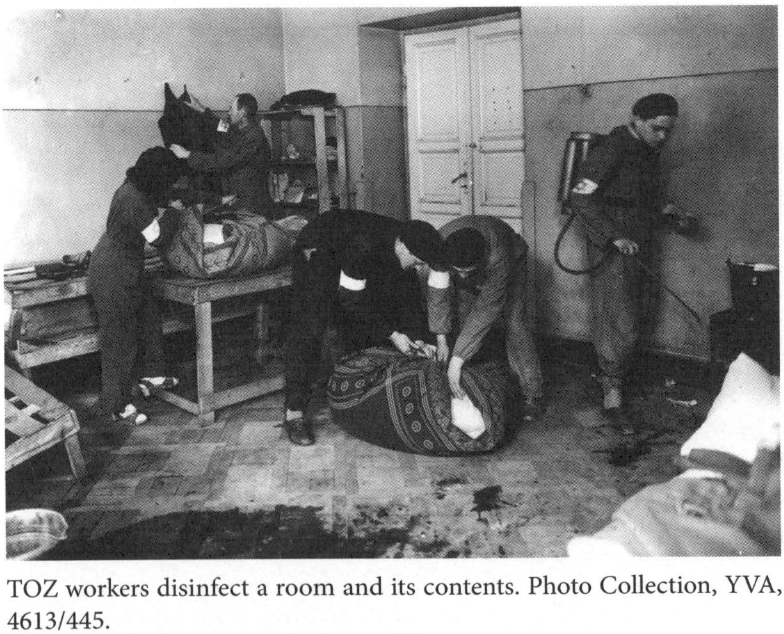

TOZ workers disinfect a room and its contents. Photo Collection, YVA, 4613/445.

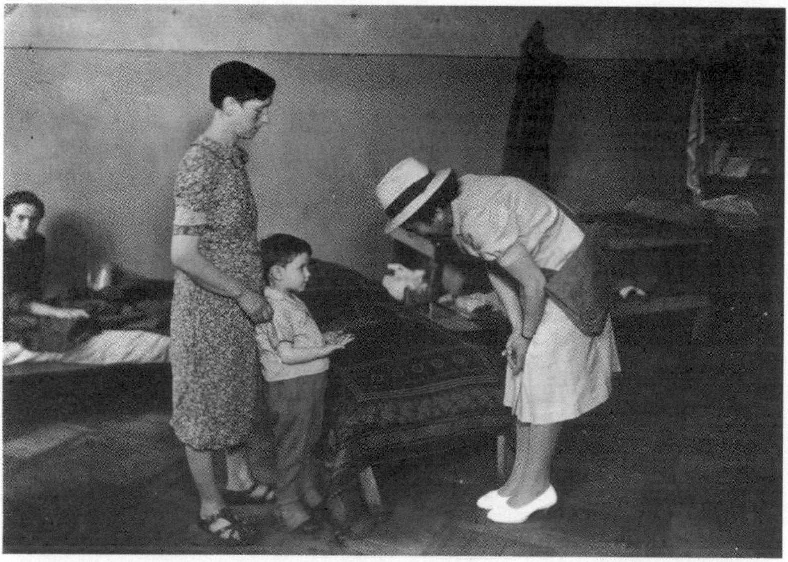

A house call by a specialist from the TOZ Department of War on Epidemics. Photo Collection, YVA, FA35/1986.

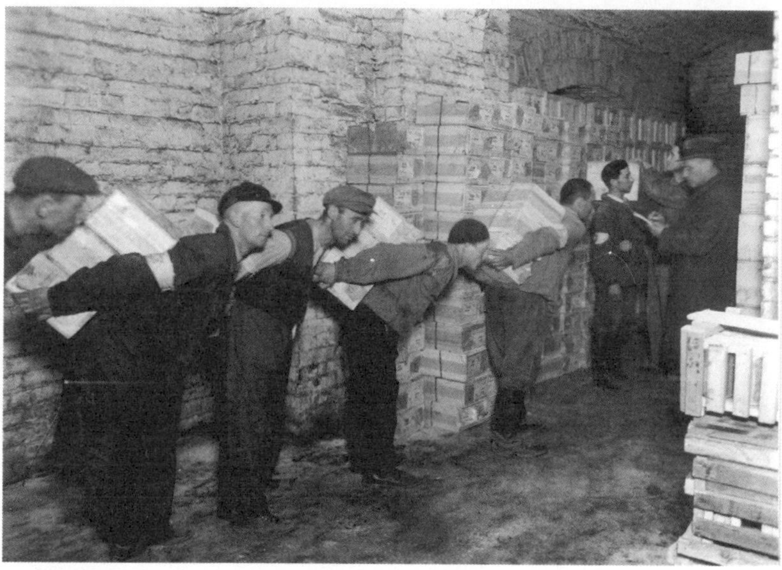

Men carry packages of food in the ghetto. Photo Collection, YVA, FA33/1844.

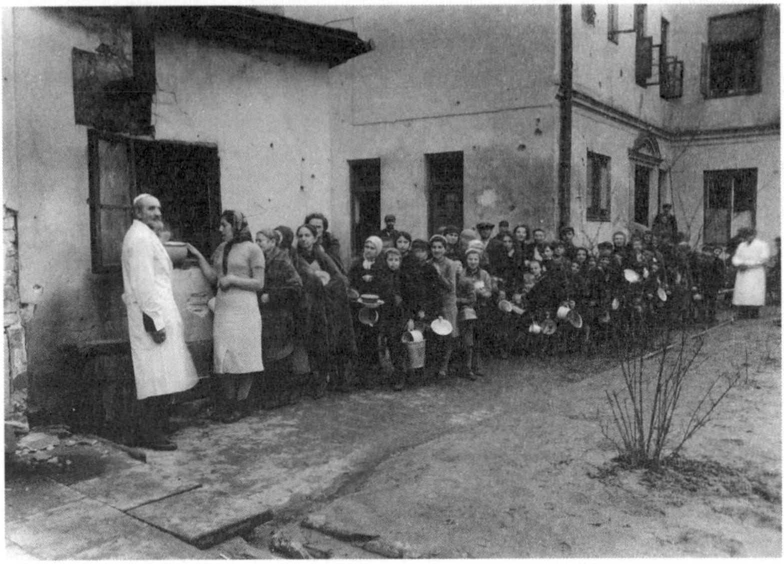

A line of refugees from Lipno and Kalisz in front of the soup kitchen at 7 Dzielna St. Photo Collection, YVA, FA33/1867.

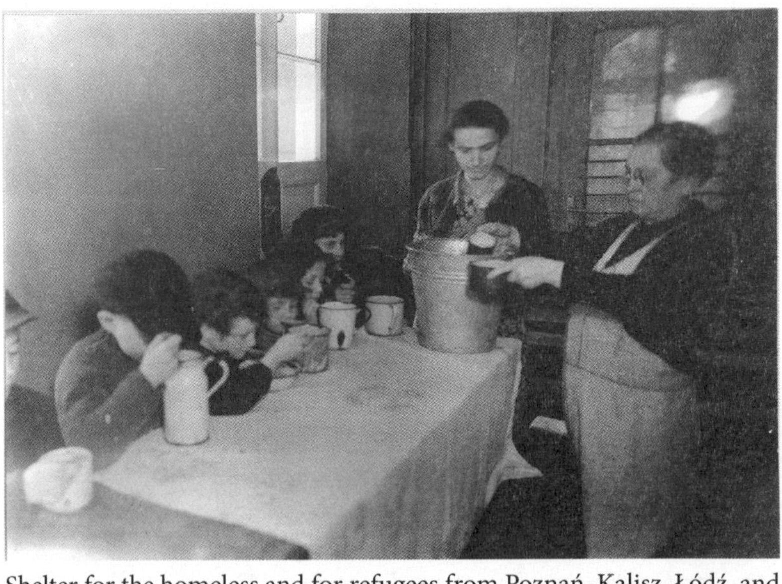

Shelter for the homeless and for refugees from Poznań, Kalisz, Łódź, and Aleksandrów at the former synagogue at 27 Gęsia St. Photo Collection, YVA, FA33/1787.

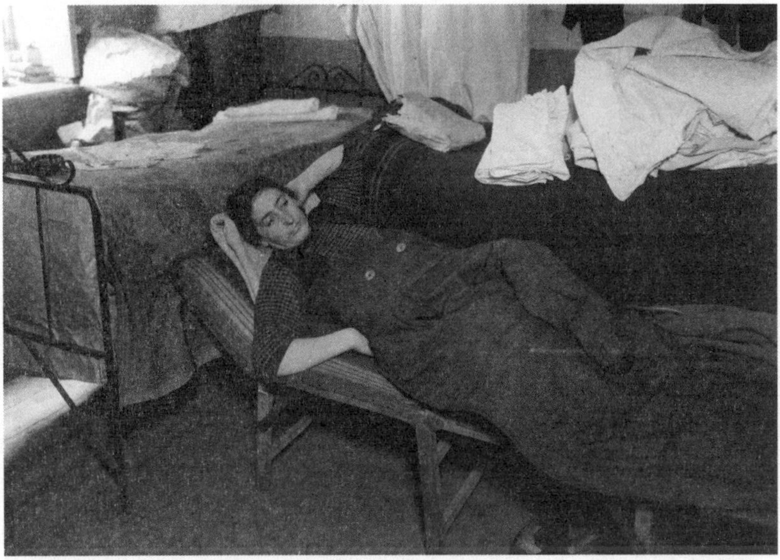

Shelter for refugees from Aleksandrów and Raciaz at the former synagogue at 41 Nalewki St. Photo Collection, YVA, FA33/1779.

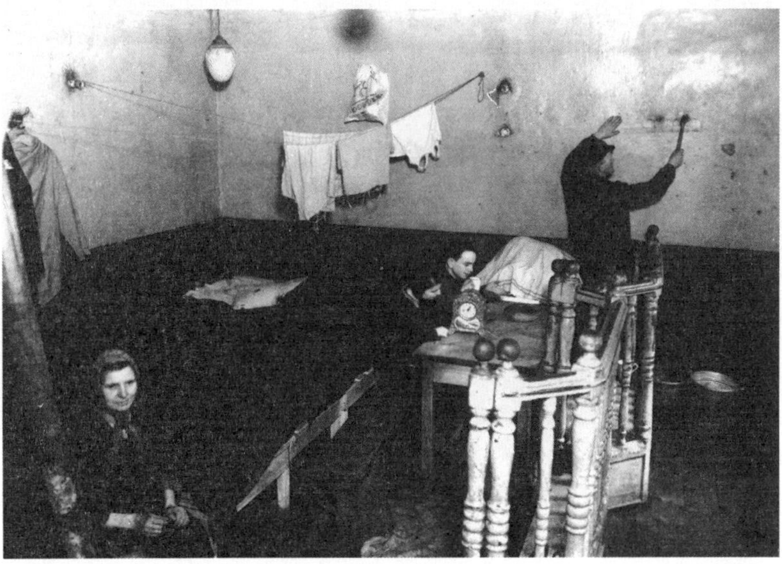

Shelter for refugees from Kalisz, Sierpc, and Łódź at the former synagogue at 47 Żelazna St. Photo Collection, YVA, FA33/1812.

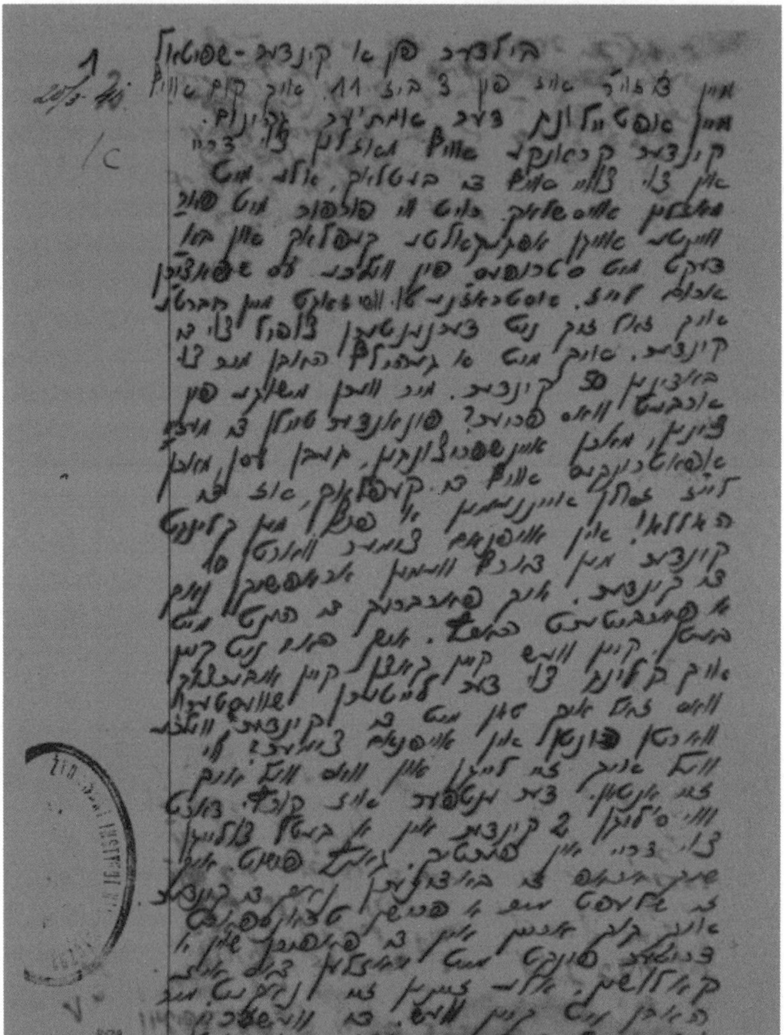

Anonymous testimony regarding the Bersohn and Bauman Children's Hospital. AŻIH, ARI.989.

Conclusion

Holocaust research, first evidenced during the Holocaust itself but truly launched shortly after the end of World War II, has greatly expanded in the past three decades, as is well known. An accepted research method consists of comprehensively differentiating the study of the perpetrators, of the victims, and of the bystanders in the spirit of Raul Hilberg's studies, which I have applied in this book. Although this trichotomy in the context of the Holocaust is problematic in many senses—because there are transitions among the groups and additional categories could be proposed—it largely reflects the approaches of Holocaust scholars over the years. Most of those who study the perpetrators skirt the Jewish aspect. Nearly all researchers of bystanders focus on the comportment of governments, populations, and organizations, and their attitude toward the Jews and their fate. The majority of those who concern themselves with the Jewish victims, mostly Jewish researchers, including prominent Israeli scholars, are mindful of the general framework of perpetration, but wish to view events within a Jewish historical frame. In other words, each research sector heads in its own direction, although there are some exceptions.[1]

1 See Dan Michman, *Holocaust Historiography*; David Bankier and Dan Michman, eds., *Holocaust Historiography in Context: Emergence, Challenges, Polemics and Achievements* (Jerusalem: Yad Vashem, 2008). On the place of the historiography of Jewish medicine during the Holocaust, see Dan Michman, "Resituating the Place of Medicine in the Grand Picture of the Holocaust: Critical Reflections on Mainstream Holocaust Historiography" (lecture delivered at the Second International Conference on Medicine in the Holocaust and Beyond, Western Galilee, Israel, May 7–11, 2017).

The field of medicine in the Holocaust has also fallen into this paradigm. There has even been a remarkable research awakening in the study of Nazi medicine in the past two decades.[2] This area of study focuses on the metamorphoses of eugenic theories and their conceptual integration into the racial doctrine, and addresses the implementation of these ideas during the era of Nazi rule in special research institutes and via the well-developed public health systems in Germany as a modern country. Research in this context emphasizes the ideological exclusion of the Jews from the German race and even from the racial hierarchy, which led to the "justification" for their annihilation.[3] It also stresses the medical experiments performed chiefly in the camps on inmates, who were considered "unfit to live" but fit to serve as guinea pigs in medical research. The material gathered for the trials of Nazi doctors in Nuremburg in 1946–1947 had a significant impact on this kind of inquiry.

On the other hand, Jewish medicine during the Holocaust has also been researched. Doctors who were not professional historians wrote many studies in this context.[4] Interest in this domain, which was keen in the first two decades after 1945—when physician and historian Mark Dworzecki was a central researcher—has enjoyed a rebirth in the past twenty years. Historians who dealt with the matter focused largely on medical systems in several large ghettos in Poland and in Lithuania, in Theresienstadt, in Germany, and in other countries. Generally speaking, they discussed the medical and sanitation systems as manifestations of Jewish steadfastness. Many even wrote admiringly about the achievements attained, justifiably so. This research approach resembles that taken toward the Jewish individual in the Holocaust, as described by Amos Goldberg:

2 On trends in the development of Nazi medicine research and a comparison of these trends with those in the study of Jewish medicine during the Holocaust, see Offer, "Ma'arach Harefu'a Begeto Varsha," vol. 1, pp. 25–30.

3 In this context, note the impact of Zygmunt Bauman's study, *Modernity and the Holocaust* (Ithaca: Cornell University Press, 1991), particularly chap. 3.

4 See an important collection of articles of this kind in Spenser, *Harefu'a Vehashoah*; see also Grodin, *Jewish Medical Resistance in the Holocaust*.

"This image of the victim with his or her interiority intact and with the ability to maintain inner freedom under all circumstances dominates the historical and public discourse of the Holocaust."[5] Studies of this kind deal with these particular issues, as well as others, such as types of illnesses in a specific ghetto, at most. The vast majority do not present the broad historical context.[6] In this book, I sought to provide the broadest and most comprehensive picture possible of the infrastructure of the medical system in the *Zwangsgemeinschaft* (coerced community, in this case, Jewish) in the largest ghetto under Nazi rule—the Warsaw ghetto.

* * *

Raphael Lemkin, the Jewish American jurist of Polish origin, coined the term "genocide" in 1944 in the context of the Holocaust. The term was accepted promptly, and the United Nations adopted the Convention on the Prevention and Punishment of the Crime of Genocide in 1948.[7] Nevertheless, research on genocide was very limited, until it was accelerated in the second half of the 1980s, which has had two main implications for Holocaust research. First, it became a growing trend to view the Holocaust within the

5 Amos Goldberg, "*Holocaust Diaries as 'Life Stories',*" *Search and Research, Lectures and Papers*, 5 (Jerusalem: Yad Vashem, 2004), p. 11.

6 Sporadic studies did attempt to address both sides of the research coin: the perpetrators and the victims. An example of this integration at the early stage of research is the Jewish Polish Holocaust survivor Joseph Wulf and, later, Nava Cohen, in her PhD dissertation in 2003. See Wulf, *Das Dritte Reich*; Cohen, "Harefu'a Besherut Ha'idiologiya."

7 There is much literature about this. See, for example, Ben Meiches and Jeff Benvenuto, eds., *Genocide Studies and Prevention: An International Journal, Revisiting the Life and Work of Raphael Lemkin*, 13:1 (2019); Berel Lang, *Genocide: The Act as Idea* (Philadelphia: University of Pennsylvania Press, 2017); Douglas Irvin-Erickson, *Raphael Lemkin and the Concept of Genocide* (Philadelphia: University of Pennsylvania Press, 2017); John Cooper, *Raphael Lemkin and the Struggle for the Genocide Convention* (Basingstoke and New York: Palgrave Macmillan, 2015); Dominik J. Schaller and Jürgen Zimmerer, eds., *The Origins of Genocide: Raphael Lemkin as a Historian of Mass Violence* (London and New York: Routledge, 2103); Yair Auron, *Genocide: Reflections on the Inconceivable, Theoretical Aspects in Genocide Studies* (Tel Aviv: Contento De Semerik and the Open University, 2015), pp. 14–45.

context of genocide.[8] Second, a debate about the uniqueness of the Holocaust in view of the phenomenon of genocide was sparked.[9] Even if the remarks here are not intended to focus on an overall discussion of the latter issue, I wish to present an insight about the discussion itself based on my study.

In the course of my review of the research literature on both medicine and genocide, an examination of the main books[10] and journals[11] on the topic, which largely mirror the trends in this area of research, revealed that the topic of the medical systems of the victims is nearly absent in genocide studies, with the sole exception of Holocaust research. A cursory review of the research literature

8 On the initiative of Yehuda Bauer, the journal *Holocaust and Genocide Studies* has been published since 1986, initially in Jerusalem and, thereafter, under the auspices of the United States Holocaust Memorial Museum in Washington, DC. In addition, since the 1990s, many university chairs have been established around the world, particularly in the United States, with titles that include the terms "Holocaust and Genocide Studies."

9 For a concise summary of basic issues in this debate, see, for example, Yehuda Bauer, *Rethinking the Holocaust*, pp. 39–68.

10 In the first two decades of the millennium, the literature on the various types of genocide is so comprehensive that detailed reference to it is beyond the scope of this book. See, for example, Donald Bloxham and A. Dirk Moses, *The Oxford Handbook of Genocide Studies* (Oxford: Oxford University Press, 2010); Ben Kiernan, *Blood and Soil: A World History of Genocide and Extermination from Sparta to Darfur* (New Haven: Yale University Press, 2007); Israel W. Charny, ed., *Encyclopedia of Genocide* (Santa Barbara, Denver, and Oxford: ABC-Clio Publishers, 1999 and 2000). In the last year alone, 2018, a search produced more than fifty-three books on the subject of genocide. See, for example, Jutta Lindert and Armen T. Marsoobian, *Multidisciplinary Perspectives on Genocide and Memory* (Cham: Springer International Publishing, 2018); Michèle Valerie Cloonan, *The Monumental Challenge of Preservation: The Past in a Volatile World* (Cambridge: The MIT Press, 2018); Katharine McGregor, Jess Melvin, and Annie Pohlman, eds., *The Indonesian Genocide of 1956: Causes, Dynamics, and Legacies* (Cham: Springer International Publishing/Palgrave Macmillan, 2018); Geoffrey B. Robinson, *The Killing Season: A History of the Indonesian Massacres, 1965–1966* (Princeton: Princeton University Press, 2018).

11 See *Holocaust and Genocide Studies*; *Genocide Studies and Prevention: An International Journal*; *Zeitschrift für Genozidforschung*; *Journal of Genocide Studies*; *Journal of Genocide Research*; *The New England Journal of Medicine*; *Journal of American Medical Association—JAMA; The Lancet Journal*; and the World Health Organization (WHO) publications.

found a lack of data, discussions, and insights about the question of how the victims coped in general, and how they coped medically—an aspect that is so central to genocide events in particular. This is a common thread in a large majority of genocide studies. In contrast, the study of the Holocaust is distinguished by accelerated activity in research on Jewish medical organization. This research began during and immediately after the Holocaust, expanding steadily in the first decade of the twenty-first century through the efforts of doctors and historians alike. There are no indications of a parallel phenomenon regarding any other genocide.[12]

An overview of Holocaust and medical research, in general, and a study of the medical system established by the Jews in the Warsaw ghetto, in particular—compared to research on genocide and medicine—confirms the uniqueness of research on Jewish medicine in the Holocaust.[13] Studies on Jewish medicine in the Holocaust illuminate the phenomenon of the establishment by the persecuted Jewish victims of independent medical systems endowed with modern professional characteristics. I have not found a comparable phenomenon among descriptions of other genocides. It may be assumed that the absence of writings about internal medical self-organization in other cases of genocide is probably not coincidental. No such self-organization appears to have taken place in other cases. It may be assumed that the rapid execution of the genocide in many cases is one of the reasons. Had there been any evidence of such activity, the international media in the age of communication presumably would have covered it. If so,

12 For an initial broad overview that exemplifies the void in research on medical systems of groups of victims in both medical journals and in genocide journals in 1980–2010, see Offer, "Ma'arach Harefu'a Begeto Varsha," vol. 1, pp. 345–349. Articles and books on various aspects of medicine and the genocide are included in the bibliography.

13 For a general overview of research on medicine in the Holocaust, see Miriam Offer, "The Study of Jewish Medicine during the Holocaust: Its Creation and Preliminary Steps," *Korot*, 22 (2013–2014), pp. 129–154; Miriam Offer, "The Study of Jewish Medicine during the Holocaust: Trends and Characteristics of Development," *Korot*, 23 (2015–2016), pp. 111–147. See also the introduction to this book and Offer, "Ma'arach Harefu'a Begeto Varsha," vol. 2, appendix C.1, pp. 191–238, and appendix C.2, pp. 239–247.

research on Jewish medicine in the Holocaust is unique, because the phenomenon, as it occurred during the Holocaust itself, is unique. The characteristics of this uniqueness are discussed below.

The story of Jewish medical organization under Nazi rule during the Holocaust years yields an important insight. The Jews in the ghetto were a segregated and persecuted society, even before the period of annihilation began in 1941, and certainly thereafter. The harsh living conditions to which they were subjected aggravated the poor sanitation and caused diseases in a manner similar to that of other groups who faced genocide and ethnic cleansing. In many cases of persecution and genocide, we generally witnessed a collapse of the medical system of the persecuted and the replacement of its services, if at all, mainly by international organizations. The case that we investigated is much different. Under the dire conditions in Warsaw and in other ghettos,[14] as well as elsewhere in Europe, a hierarchical and rather disciplined health care and medical system was set up to tackle public health challenges, according to modern concepts—concern for sanitation, vaccinations, isolation of infected persons, control of food and water quality, and so on.[15] Other examples include the Jewish hospital in Berlin,[16] the medical system in the Westerbork camp in the Netherlands,[17] the Jewish hospital

14 Almost every large Jewish center had a health care system. The existence of a Health Department in many Judenräte attests to this. See Trunk, *Judenrat*, chaps. 4 and 7.

15 For elaboration on these tasks, see R. Detels et al., eds., *Oxford Textbook of Public Health*, 6th ed., (Oxford: Oxford University Press, 2015), p. 20. For a broader look at the role of public and social medicine in the interwar years and its manifestations in European countries, see Iris Borowy and Anne Hardly, eds., *Of Medicine and Men: Biographies and Ideas in European Social Medicine between the World Wars* (Frankfurt am Main: Peter Lang, 2008).

16 See Rivka Elkin, "Beit Haholim Hayehudi BeBerlin—Sarid Aharon Leyehudei Germaniya Bitkufat Haraih Hashlishi" (The Jewish Hospital in Berlin—A Last Vestige of German Jewry in the Third Reich Era,) *Yalkut Moreshet* (Hebrew), 53 (1993), pp. 53–91. Rebecca Schwoch, ed., *Berliner Jüdische Kassenärzte und ihr Schicksal im Nationalsozialismus* (Berlin: Hentrich & Hentrich Teetz, 2009).

17 Ellen Ben-Sefer, "Gemilat Chesed and Moral Behaviour at Westerbork: Lessons from the Past to Remember for the Future," in Maxwell Elisabeth and Roth John, eds., *Remembering for the Future: The Holocaust in an Age of Genocide* (Basingstoke: Palgrave, 2001), pp. 35–53; Van den Ende, *Vergeet niet dat je arts*

in Hungary,[18] and the health care system in the Theresienstadt ghetto.[19]

The medical system was not limited to providing emergency care and treating the ill. Even during that very difficult period, it continued the "routine" activities that are typical of medical systems: teaching, in-service activities, and research. **The Jews themselves, that is, the persecuted society**, and not the Germans or any outside party, established the system. Modern approaches were applied to confront the problems, despite the many constraints. As previously stated, this phenomenon seems to be unparalleled in any other case of genocide. Namely, it is unique and demands historical explanation.

* * *

The medical and health care system in the Warsaw ghetto clearly has two important components: its systematic organization, including medical training, which relied on organized institutions and health services, and a medical policy that focused on public health, including initiatives for disease prevention, supportive medical research, and other features. These elements did not sprout ex nihilo but were the result of developments, which centered in Europe, from the late eighteenth century onward.

For the purposes of our discussion, two main processes in the formation of modern states since the eighteenth century are important. The first is the consolidation of the centralized state,

bent; Doetz and Kopke, "*und dürfen das Krankenhaus nicht meher betreten*"; Judith Korek Amorosa et al., "Tragedy in the Radiology Department of the Jewish Hospital, Budapest, Hungary," *Radiographics*, 16 (1996), pp. 503–508.

18 Weiskopf, "Beit Haholim Hayehudi BeBudapesht," pp. 81–94. According to the Jewish Hungarian historian and journalist Jenő Lévai, about twenty-one provisional hospitals operated in the Budapest ghetto and in areas outside the walls that had been annexed to it. They were established on the initiative of the persecuted Jews as branches of the provisional hospital that had been set up in a school, after SS soldiers had taken over the Jewish community's buildings, including the hospital, on March 19, 1944.

19 Anna Hájková, "Medicine in Theresienstadt," *Social History of Medicine*, hky066 (2018), https://doi.org/10.1093/shm/hky066 (accessed September 17, 2019); Nadav, *Medicine and Nazism*, pp. 53–64.

with its dominant governing core that shaped organized settings in various areas of life. The second is the transition to the concept of national sovereignty, which drew its first sustenance from the principles of the Enlightenment of the seventeenth and eighteenth centuries, but crossed a watershed with the ascendancy of the concept of the modern nation. National sovereignty in its modern version is no longer construed as that of a group of individuals who enter into a social covenant but as the sovereignty of a "national body." That is, of an entire collective composed of members of the nation who share a deeper partnership than mere citizenship—one that is cultural, historical, or even spiritual and biological, as in its Romantic version.[20]

Since the late eighteenth century and against this backdrop, modern states have developed the belief that it is the duty of their governing institutions to attend to public health[21] by deploying treatment systems that address the public and even dictate its behavior, expanding systems of training and study in medicine and nursing care, and performing experimental medical research to treat or cure diseases, especially epidemics.[22] One of the quintessential manifestations of this was the introduction in various countries of universal vaccinations, sometimes by law, after the development of the smallpox vaccine in the late eighteenth century. Since the goal of promoting public health became a national aim supported by the state, medical research was also encouraged by the state. Germany was one of the leading countries in this field and in medicine in general, particularly after its unification in 1870. Its important medical research institutes include the Kaiser Wilhelm Society.[23] Against this background,

20 The literature about this is extensive. For an important presentation of theory on the topic, see Eric Hobsbawm, *Nations and Nationalism since 1780: Programme, Myth, Reality* (Cambridge: Cambridge University Press, 1992).

21 *Volksgesundheit, santé publique*, public health.

22 David Thomson, *Europe Since Napoleon* (London: Penguin, 1970), pp. 113, 355.

23 The research literature relating to these institutes is vast. See, for example, articles on the official Nobel Prize website, https://www.nobelprize.org/prizes/uncategorized/a-history-of-the-kaiser-wilhelm-institute-for-medical-research-1929-1939 (accessed September 17, 2019). For a comprehensive study on their history during the National Socialist era, see Susanne Heim, Carola

one may say that the extent of development of a given society's public health system is an indicator of the extent of the society's progress in general.

The medical system that was set up in the Warsaw ghetto and its modus operandi eminently reflected these modern public health concepts. Since the establishment of the ghetto—and even before, from the founding of the Judenrat in October 1939—clinics, laboratories, hospitals, and pharmacies operated there; public health measures were taken in consultation with physicians; training facilities for medical and nursing personnel were established; and medical research to cope with common diseases was performed. The ghetto doctors' study on hunger was published in this context, and research on typhus was carried out, addressing two key medical problems in ghetto life. Despite all the restraints and hardships, the medical and health care system in the Warsaw ghetto is clearly indicative of the pronouncedly modern nature of the society, made possible by the processes that took place among the Jews of Poland in the interwar years.

* * *

The rapid organization of the Jewish medical system in Warsaw—initially after the city was occupied in late September 1939 and then about a year later, when most Jews there were forced to move to the ghetto—as well as its scope, diversity, and relatively high level did not arise ex nihilo. It was founded on the infrastructure of Jewish medicine that had developed earlier, especially between the world wars. The uniqueness of Polish Jewry in the field of medicine and health care in interwar independent Poland lies in the development of an autonomous and separate set of professional medical institutions and facilities. Intended to serve primarily the country's large Jewish population, this ethnic–national system required Jewish professionals in all the medical professions. Thus, even if the prominence of Jews as doctors—surpassing their share in the population—was a

Sachse, and Mark Walker, eds., *The Kaiser Wilhelm Society under National Socialism* (New York: Cambridge University Press, 2009).

lengthy tradition of two thousand years,[24] it acquired the additional feature of an independent national infrastructure in Poland during this period. This came about for several reasons.

First, the secularization and modernization of Polish Jewry, which had begun in the second half of the nineteenth century in both the Austro–Hungarian Empire (Galicia) and in Tsarist Russia (Congress Poland), accelerated at this time. This was manifested in many ways, foremost in the growth of political parties. The development of a secular Jewish education system according to modern standards, coupled with the strong flow of young Jews to non-Jewish schools and later to universities, was of paramount importance.[25] The aspiration for professional, social, and economic advancement amplified, among other things, the attraction to the medical profession, which, as stated, was rooted in Jewish tradition. In 1931, there were 4,488 self-employed Jewish doctors in Poland, more than half of all self-employed doctors countrywide, and 2,256 Jewish pharmacists and laboratory workers, roughly one-fourth of all such practitioners in Poland.[26] As we have seen, when the Germans invaded, there were about 800 Jewish doctors living in Warsaw, a considerable number, even if one bears in mind that the population of the Warsaw ghetto exceeded 400,000 at its peak.

Furthermore, in Central and Western Europe, secularization and modernization led to the integration and assimilation of the Jews. The Jewish intelligentsia and white-collar professionals spearheaded these processes. However, this was not the case in Poland. According to Ezra Mendelsohn, in independent Poland, with its highly complex internal and external problems, only nationalism and the Church served as unifying factors, and both Polish nationalism and Polish Catholicism were by nature exclusivist, anti-pluralistic, and antisemitic. Due to the paucity of liberalism in independent Poland, extreme intolerance toward minorities was the rule and the Jews suffered in particular. For

24 For elaboration, see *Encyclopedia Judaica* (Jerusalem and New York: Encyclopedia Judaica, 1971–1972), vol. 11, s.v. "Medicine," pp. 1,178–1,211.

25 Ezra Mendelsohn, *The Jews of East Central Europe between the World Wars* (Bloomington: Indiana University Press, 1983), p. 82.

26 Ibid., p. 27; Mahler, *Yehudei Polin*, p. 159.

this reason, a separate and independent Jewish culture and consciousness evolved in Poland, despite the profusion of disputes, conflicts, and confrontations among the Jews themselves.[27] The Polish state even grounded the status of the Jewish minority in powers that it granted to the communities, particularly in accordance with an order issued by the president of the republic on October 14, 1927. The edict allowed communities to engage in charitable activity and to establish charitable institutions, which became a major factor in the development of hospitals and health care organizations.[28] Some of them also received the support and the involvement of American Jews of Polish origin and, to an important extent, from the JDC. The Jews of Poland kept abreast of professional innovations from abroad through these channels.

In addition to all this, the process described above was accelerated by antisemitism, which worsened over the years. As antisemitism permeated the country's institutions of higher learning, many Jews who wished to study medicine went abroad, mainly to Germany and Austria. They returned with the latest approaches in medicine and nursing, and implemented them in Jewish medical institutions. Thus, Jewish doctors and Jewish medical institutions in Poland, particularly in Warsaw, because of the size of the Jewish community there, were at the forefront of modern medicine.

Indeed, this advanced infrastructure made it possible to cope with the grim medical situation in the Warsaw ghetto during the war. The case study in this book is an example of a medical challenge under extreme conditions, not only in terms of the resources available to those administering treatment but also, and mainly, in view of the diseases and medical problems that they had to confront. It is no coincidence that the research

27 Mendelsohn, *The Jews of East Central Europe between the World Wars*, p. 82.

28 Gershon Bacon, "Hatzlaha Helkit, Hesegim Gdolim: Al Ha'otonomiya Hayehudit BePolin Beyn Shtei Milhamot Ha'olam" (Partial Success, Great Achievements: On Jewish Autonomy in Poland between the Two World Wars), in Israel Bartal, ed., *Kehal Yisra'el: Hashilton Ha'atzmi Hayehudi Ledorotav* (Kehal Yisrael: Jewish Self-Rule through the Ages) (Hebrew), vol. 3, (Jerusalem: Yad Izhak Ben-Zvi, 2004), pp. 351–371, particularly pp. 359, 361.

conducted in the ghetto, which attracted broad professional interest in the post-Holocaust years, focused on hunger and typhus—medical problems that were not characteristic of daily life in an advanced society but were definitely typical of cases of genocide. The knowledge available at the time to contend with these problems was limited and insufficient and, therefore, the emphasis in research was placed on the aberrant. However, the other diseases mentioned in this study, which were not studied systematically, also occurred with extraordinary frequency and, therefore, were documented by the medical teams, who collected information that would be of medical assistance. Even though decades have passed since the Holocaust, and medicine has made amazing strides, it is possible to learn from the measures employed at that time to shed light on case studies of other genocides, at least in terms of the methodology of medical history.

It is important to emphasize that our very ability to present such a detailed description of the medical and health affairs in the Warsaw ghetto is possible because of the copious documentation that remains. This exceptional documentation stems from two sources: the development and high standards of Jewish medicine, as described above, and the powerful motivation of the Jews in the ghetto to document the Germans' lethal onslaught against them that threatened their existence. This impulse has been noted and researched mainly with respect to the establishment of secret archives[29] and the writing of diaries[30] during the Holocaust itself.

* * *

29 Israel Gutman, *Migniza Letziyonei Dereh Historiyim* (From Hidden Treasures to Historical Landmarks: Jewish Archives from the Holocaust Period) (Hebrew) (Jerusalem: Yad Vashem, 1997). David Engel also traces this urge to the perception of historical documentation and the strengthening of the connection between historical writings and public needs as matters of supreme importance, which gained traction in Jewish culture in Poland long before the Holocaust. See David Engel, "Ktivat Hahistoriya Keshlihut Le'umit: Yehudei Polin Umasoroteihem Hahistoriyografiyot" (Historical Writing as a National Mission: Polish Jewry and Their Historiographic Tradition) in Gutman, *Ringelblum: Ha'adam Vehahistorion*, pp. 117–140.

30 Amos Goldberg, *Holocaust Diaries*, pp. 17–23; Goldberg, *Trauma in First Person: Diary Writing during the Holocaust* (Bloomington: Indiana University Press, 2017).

As I have pointed out in this work, an examination of the system deployed by the Jews in the Warsaw ghetto entails several perspectives. First, the picture I offer reveals a great paradox in the rationale that led to the Holocaust from the perpetrators' standpoint. The Nazis' anti-Jewish policy was based on a racist antisemitic ideology that did not recognize Jews as human beings, creatures, or "lives," who have value or the "right to live"; and considered them "subhuman" or "parasites."[31] Ostensibly, this point of departure should have led the Nazis to conclude that concentrating masses of Jews in a closed space would bring on a rapid collapse and unleash uncontrollable diseases. Indeed, in response to Hermann Göring's remark at the well-known meeting of the high-ranking Nazi leadership that followed the *Kristallnacht* pogrom on November 9–10, 1938, "You will not be able to avoid this [occurring] on a massive scale in the ghettos in the cities," Reinhard Heydrich stated,

> From a police point of view, I think that a ghetto, in the form of a completely segregated district with only Jews, is not possible...It would be a permanent hideout for criminals and first of all [a source] of epidemics and the like...The control of the Jews by the watchful eyes of the whole population is better than putting thousands upon thousands of Jews together in a single district of a city where uniformed officials will be unable to check on their daily activities.[32]

However, in practice, the invasion of Poland was followed by the establishment of ghettos, where masses of Jews were concentrated. The Warsaw ghetto was the largest in Poland and in all of Europe. As Browning demonstrated, this was not the outcome of a planned and systematic process. Undoubtedly, the ghettos were considered a short-term, transitional measure. However, as the phenomenon

31 Walter Zwi Bacharach, *Tfisat Ha'adam Ba'idiologiya Hanatzit* (The Perception of Man in Nazi Ideology) (Hebrew) (Tel Aviv: Broadcast University, 1996), particularly chap. 10; Michael Burleigh and Wolfgang Wippermann, *The Racial State: Germany 1933–1945* (Cambridge: Cambridge University Press, 1991).

32 Arad et al., *Documents on the Holocaust*, pp. 111–112.

dragged on beyond expectations, the question of how to deal with it arose. In terms of values and pseudoscience, the German doctors in the General Government toed the racist antisemitic line. That is, they viewed the Jews as carriers and diffusers of epidemics and favored their isolation. Most of them believed that the Jews could be shot or doomed to death by starvation in the ghetto.

In 1940, doctors in Warsaw recommended locking the Jews in the ghetto for health reasons,[33] ostensibly, to prevent the spread of epidemics, just as the epidemic among the Jews had ended. The German doctors knew that ghettoization would not solve the epidemic problem and that the living conditions in the enclosed quarters would have the opposite effect. There was an additional aspect of this, the practical, organizational one. It is worth noting that the director of the General Government Health Department acted to establish a health care system for Poles to protect Germans from the infection. However, nothing of the sort was done for the Jewish population. The Jews had to establish a separate, autonomous administration to deal with their health needs under difficult conditions and without the requisite resources. Dr. Kurt Schrempf, the first German chief physician in Warsaw, adopted this policy.

In January 1941, Schrempf was succeeded by Dr. Wilhelm Hagen, who considered himself then and in retrospect an "enlightened" person. As such, he behaved as though responsible for the health of the Germans and the Poles, and even endangered himself—in contravention of the German health policy—to save Poles who had developed tuberculosis. However, his "responsibility" for the Jews in the ghetto was limited to preventing the spread of communicable diseases from the ghetto to the rest of the city. The fate of the Jews in the ghetto did not interest him. Although he was not a National Socialist, his policy was influenced by antisemitic views. Documents attest that he favored a total closure of the ghetto, upheld the killing of Jews who attempted to escape from it, and applied methods in the war

33 Browning, *The Origins of the Final Solution* (Lincoln and Jerusalem: University of Nebraska Press and Yad Vashem, 2004), pp. 113, 137.

on typhus that were not only cruel but that caused the epidemic to spread.

Nevertheless, the very fact that the German authorities allowed the Jewish medical and health care system in the Warsaw ghetto to develop as it did suggests that the Germans, who were direly afraid of epidemics, implicitly assumed that the Jews would be able to cope with medical problems by providing medical means. Evidence of this, for example, is the Jewish nursing school established in the interwar period that continued to operate legally in the ghetto, because of the Germans' fear of epidemics. It operated according to professional standards from January 1940 to the *Aktion* on January 18, 1943, under the direction of Luba Blum-Bielecka. That this medical institution was allowed to continue indicates that alongside their contemptuous and apprehensive ideological attitude toward the Jews, in terms of dangers to the health of the Aryan population, the Germans realistically assumed that the Jews could cope with the health and sanitation problems in a reasonable way, because there were plenty of doctors and nurses among them. Their assessment was based on their recognition of the reality of the Jews. In practice, the Germans recognized the Jews as human beings—and some even as talented. In light of this, it is important to note that the examination of the Jewish medical system in the Warsaw ghetto reinforces Dan Michman's contention that the conduct of the Jews under Nazi rule should be treated as playing an active role, not only as a form of response to persecution but also in the context of the development of Jewish history in the modern era.[34]

It is also important to point out the transitory nature of the phenomenon described in this book and the reasons for it. The German authorities allowed the Jews to organize a medical system and even relied on it heavily until 1942, as long as the Final Solution had not been decided. As we know, contemporary research has abandoned the intentionalist approach, which had been dominant at the outset of Holocaust research. According to intentionalism, the Nazis' anti-Jewish policy evolved in a linear and deliberate

34 Michman, *Holocaust Historiography*, p. 78.

manner that culminated in the Final Solution. In this context, the Nazis considered the ghettos a preparatory phase for the Final Solution. Although the Final Solution had not yet been decided when the ghettos were established,[35] it is clear today that they were a temporary measure.

The ghettos were provisional settings, where Jews could be kept until a solution could be found "elsewhere." Therefore, the ghettos had to have medical services, even from the Germans' standpoint, although the Germans did nothing to assist the Jews to establish and maintain them. As the ghettos continued to endure, arguments erupted among the Germans in charge of them as to how they should be handled: as productive enterprises or as mechanisms of lethal starvation? However, these questions were debated only in the field. The high authorities in Berlin did not hand down any decisions.[36] After the Final Solution took shape and its implementation began—as happened in Warsaw from July 1942 onward—there was no longer any room for maneuver and the medical system promptly collapsed, its life expectancy reduced to zero.

This last point reinforces the claim that the Jews perceived the living conditions that the Germans had created in the ghettos, which induced death from starvation and disease, as the exacerbation of the persecution of the Jews by the Germans. Today, we know that ghettoization was not part of the Final Solution scheme. However, in the eyes of the Jewish leaders, doctors, underground journalists, and others, it was perceived as the outcome of the view that the Jews could be obliterated by creating conditions that would deplete them in "natural" ways, namely, by reducing infertility and expediting mortality. The educator Chaim Kaplan tellingly expressed this perception in his diary as early as March 10, 1940.

> The gigantic catastrophe, which has descended on Polish Jewry, has no parallel, even in the darkest periods of Jewish history....

35 Ibid., pp. 91–126.

36 Browning, *The Origins of the Final Solution*, pp. 111–169.

> But the founders of Nazism, and the party leaders, created a scientific ideology on deeper foundations [than previous antisemitism in the past]. They have a complete doctrine, which analyzes the Jewish spirit inside and out. Judaism and Nazism are two world outlooks, neither of which is compatible with the other and, for this reason, they cannot live together....The new world, which Nazism will fashion, is directed toward primitive idolatry with all of its attitudes. It is therefore ready to fight Judaism to the finish.[37]

Some forces in Jewish society attempted to resist. Kaplan continued,

> It is our good fortune that the conquerors have failed to consider the nature and strength of Polish Jewry, and this has kept us alive. Logically we should be dead. According to the laws of nature, we ought to have been completely annihilated. How can an entire community feed itself when it has no place in life? There is no occupation, no activity, which is not limited, circumscribed for us.
>
> But here again we do not conform to the laws of nature. A certain invisible power is embedded in us, and it is this secret, which keeps us alive and preserves us in spite of all the laws of nature: if it is impossible to live by what is permitted, we live from what is forbidden....
>
> ...the beaten-down, shamed, broken Jews of Poland. They love life, and they do not wish to disappear from the earth before their time....
>
> Say what you wish, this will of ours to live in the midst of terrible calamity is the outward manifestation of a certain hidden power whose quality has not yet been examined. It is a wondrous, superlative power with which only the most established communities among our people have been blessed.
>
> We are left naked, but as long as this secret power is still within us, we do not give up hope. And the strength of this

37 Kaplan, *Scroll of Agony*, pp. 129–130.

> power lies in the indigenous nature of Polish Jewry, which is rooted in our eternal tradition that commands us to live.[38]

It is necessary to investigate the Jewish medical enterprise in the Warsaw ghetto and, without a doubt, in many other locations, from this angle. After all, why did the ghetto medical staff invest such a massive share of their efforts and resources, which were so limited, to treat patients who were doomed to die no matter what? This question is amplified in light of the detailed analysis of the prodigious and diverse medical activity in the ghetto presented in the first sections of this book. What was the point of sustaining all of the institutions, activities, and studies, if everyone in the ghetto was destined to die? The answer is that, until the deportations began in July 1942, the ghetto inhabitants apparently did not expect the Germans to embark on an active, systematic murder operation; they foresaw only gradual annihilation. They hoped that despite the high mortality, the diseases, and the hunger, many would survive, nevertheless, if only they received proper treatment. Thus, continuing to maintain an active medical system seems to have been rational from the Jews' perspective.

Admittedly, this answer does not address all the questions, because some did express doubts about the rationality of helping the ill, even before the mass deportations. Dr. Chaim Einhorn expressed such doubts in his memoirs.

> As one may gather from our foregoing account, we often asked ourselves whether it was worth continuing to give medical care under such conditions. Despite it all, however, the doctors stayed at their posts until the last moment of the ghetto. And many of them continued their medical work, of this I am sure, to the last moment of their lives, some in the bunkers, some in concentration camps, and some in the ghetto uprising.[39]

38 Ibid., pp. 130–131.

39 Einhorn, "Harofe Begeto Varsha," p. 13.

Furthermore, there is no doubt that the cruel realities of ghetto life presented the medical staff with dire dilemmas, immeasurably graver than the decisions that medical personnel usually face in ordinary times, including taking direct, personal action by order of the Germans that would determine who would live and who would die. Moreover, such dilemmas were many times more frequent under ghetto conditions than they would be in ordinary situations. Thus, amid heroic and courageous feats by medical personnel, there were also instances of morally unacceptable behavior, such as withholding treatment, taking bribes, and the like. Undoubtedly, like many other officials in the ghetto, they were put to impossible moral tests.

How did the medical staff nevertheless manage to continue working under the conditions described? The answer probably has to do with the basic survival instinct that most people possess—the wish to continue functioning until their final breath. Furthermore, the opportunity to alleviate the suffering of people does not lose its value merely because those receiving care might suffer more or even die in the long term. Were this the case, there would be no reason to treat the elderly who, after all, are fated to die soon. Based on events in other cases of genocide, it seems that the aspect of Jewish tradition that so strongly emphasizes the imperative of life and of saving life as a supreme value was preponderant, as Kaplan noted. Prof. Hirszfeld wrote the following in retrospect:

> In the light of subsequent events, however, our scientific achievements appear to me to be a bad historical joke. What does it matter now how the murdered ones intended to combat tuberculosis or venereal diseases? Yet, perhaps, there will be a few who will be touched by knowing how those condemned to death tried to live in dignity and to reassemble the norms of life.[40]

Relating to the sense of duty to perform medical work in the ghetto, Dr. Adina Blady Szwajger wrote,

40 Hirszfeld, *The Story of One Life*, p. 221.

> We weren't there to look at the horror, only to treat the sick or help with a quiet death. But, above all, to save lives because, even though times were bad, as bad as could be, we still wouldn't accept that it was of no use and thought that if we pulled through, we'd save those children and they would survive to the end. So we tried to save them with those scraps of food, medicines and injection, and some of them got better. And when they began to get better, when, from those terrible, swollen lumps, skeletons began to emerge, we'd sometimes even see something resembling a smile. Except that this was the kind of smile that made your hair stand on end and your flesh crawl.[41]

Nurse Sabina Gürfinkel-Glocer, who served in an operating room, noted the pervasive sense of meaning and mission, despite the shortages of everything.

> We had many patients, Jews who needed our help...Jews who had been wounded by the Germans, because they were Jews. It was a question of honor for us to help the patients and, by pooling our forces, save those who could yet be saved.[42]

41 Blady Szwajger, *I Remember Nothing More*, p. 42.

42 Gürfinkel-Glocer, "Goralo Shel Beit Haholim Tzhista," p. 589.

Bibliography

Archive Sources

Yad Vashem Archives (YVA)

M.10.AR.1/31 – Thoughts of a Member of a Disinfection Unit, May 23–30, 1942 (Polish).

M.10.AR.1/85 – Memoranda by Jewish doctors to the Germans addressing the causes of typhus and proposals to combat it (German).

M.10.AR.1/191 – Report from Chemical-Bacteriological Institute of the Judenrat, July–December 1941 (Polish).

M.10.AR.1/204 – Plan for educational work at food distribution centers (Yiddish).

M.10.AR.1/291 – Sanitation operation at 29 Krochmalna St. (Polish).

M.10.AR.1/315 – Anonymous public appeal from doctors and public figures concerning the state of the hospital, June 1941.

M.10.AR.1/470 – Baila Kesselberg testimony, a nurse who posed as a patient at the hospital in Warsaw (Polish).

M.10.AR.1/1099 – Testimony of an anonymous nurse at Bersohn and Bauman Children's Hospital (Yiddish).

M.1.E/934 – Prof. Tadeusz Stabholz testimony (Yiddish).

M.49.E/5883 – Sabina Sanderman testimony, a nurse in Warsaw (Polish).

M.49.E/4510 – Dr. Emil Apfelbaum testimony, history of Czyste Hospital (Polish).

M.49.E/4264 – Luba Bielicka-Blum testimony.

M.49.E/5865 – Luba Bielicka-Blum testimony.

O.33/6403 – Luba Bielicka-Blum autobiography.

O.3/392 – Esther Braude-Grodzinski testimony about her sister, Dr. Braude-Heller (Polish).

O.3/398 – Władysław-Wolf Glocer testimony, husband of the nurse Sabina Gürfinkel-Glocer (Polish).

O.3/438 – Dr. Moshe Tursz testimony about TOZ activity in Warsaw (Polish).

O.3/441 – Dr. Marek Balin testimony (Polish).

O.3/1836 – Dr. Chaim Einhorn testimony (Polish).

O.3/2355 – Dr. Józef Chajn Gołębiowski testimony, member of TOZ board of directors and secretary of the Anti-Tuberculosis League (Polish).

O.3/2357 – Dr. Israel Rom (Rotbalsam) testimony, physician at Bersohn and Bauman Children's Hospital (Polish).

O.3/2358 – Dr. Shmuel Stanisław Waller testimony, physician at Czyste Hospital (Polish).

O.3/2360 – Yehudit Braude testimony about her sister, Dr. Anna Braude-Heller, director of Berson-Bauman Children's Hospital (Polish).

O.3/3647 – Prof. Adam Drozdowicz testimony; he was a bacteriologist who worked in the ghetto laboratory, the Food and Medicines Inspection Institute, under Prof. Mieczysław Centnerszwer (Polish).

O.33/648 – Prof. Tadeusz Stabholz testimony about the medical school (Polish).

O.33/1074 – Dr. Henry Fenigstein, Varshever yid. Shpital betn nazi-rezhim, aroysgegebn durkh farlag Ibergang bey der federatsiye fun poylishe yidn in deytshland, amerikaner zane, 1948, https://digitalarchive.mcmaster.ca/islandora/object/macrepo%3A81178#page/1/mode/2up (Yiddish).

O.33/1558 – Dr. Emil Apfelbaum testimony, history of Czyste Hospital (English translation from Polish).

P.10/38 – Letter from Dr. Dworzecki to the Medical Association about the establishment of the research institute on medicine and the Holocaust. (Hebrew).

M.21/1–17 – Paula Zofia Sanek testimony about Dr. Hagen's criminal actions (Polish).

O.4/515 – The Wulf-Hagen affair: Dr. Hagen versus Jewish historian Josef Wulf, extensive correspondence among Yad Vashem, Wulf, and various elements in an attempt to gather evidence against Hagen; media pieces, and legal documents (Polish, German, Yiddish, Hebrew).

M.49.E./5061 – Dr. Adolf Polisiuk testimony.

Ghetto Fighters' House Museum Archive (GFH)

1145 – Weichert report, including medical aspects of the JUS (German).

1160 – Letter from Michael Weichert to SS and police leader regarding medicines for prisoners (German).

1186 – Letters from Weichert to the Committee for Aid to Jewish War Casualties in Geneva concerning provision to Jewish war casualties (German).

1194 – Report by Dr. Tschlenoff on OSE and TOZ activities regarding shipments of medicines to Poland.

1349 – Dr. Peter-Heinz Seraphim, "On the Economic Role of the Jews in Poland," Ost-Europa Markt, December 1938.

1933 – Correspondence from Dr. Michael Weichert to Dr. Sternbuch of Bikur Holim Society, Switzerland, regarding shipments of medicines to the General Government, 1941–1944 (German).

3182 – Diaries of Dr. Polisiuk: 1. Pawiak—prison memoir; 2. "Square"—memoir from the hospital on Leszno St. (Polish).

3909 – Judenrat report to Dr. Auerswald on the Warsaw Jewish quarter under the *Kommissar's* rule, May 15, 1941–May 15, 1942.

4102 – Correspondence between Dr. Weichert and Bikur Holim Society, Switzerland; letters from Dr. Weichert to SS and police officials in General Government (German).

4368 – Report from counselors at children's clubs, December 1941 (Polish).

5214 – Dr. Einhorn testimony against Dr. Hagen; directive from Hagen concerning punishment by flogging for those leaving the ghetto.

5223 – Envelope containing a list of about 500 doctors who reactivated TOZ in Poland after the war.

6141 – Call for assistance from doctors and intellectuals in Trawniki (Polish).

7783 – Letter from Max Sollman, SS officer and police and SS commander in Warsaw, to Wilhelm Krieger, supreme police and SS commander in the General Government, concerning the tuberculosis plague in the General Government, which he blamed on Hagen; bill for the stay of a certain Jew in the Jewish psychiatric hospital from the Kommissar for Jewish Affairs to chairman of Judenrat in Warsaw (German).

9574 – Confirmation of the delivery of doses of vaccines from the Red Cross and from Dr. Weichert (German).

11250 – Judenrat Statistics Department report, February 1942 (Polish).

19852 – Criticism of Dr. Weichert by representatives of the Jewish National Committee in a letter sent from Warsaw to London (German).

19765 – A physician's testimony about doctors like himself who did not accept any payment for their medical work.

21338 – Letters from Jacob Rosenheim, president of Agudath Israel World Organization in New York, to Elias Sternbuch, Switzerland (German).

21339 – Letters from Prof. Mooser at the Institute of Hygiene of the University of Zurich to Elias Sternbuch, St. Gallen, Switzerland (German).

21342 – Letter from Bikur Holim, Switzerland, to the Jewish Social Self-Help, Warsaw (Polish).

21344 – Correspondence between JUS, Cracow, and Bikur Holim, Switzerland (German).

21351 – Correspondence between the International Red Cross Rescue Committee, Geneva, and Elias Sternbuch, Bikur Holim, Switzerland (German).

21352 – Correspondence between the International Red Cross, Geneva, and Bikur Holim Society, St. Gallen (German).

21356 – Letter from Bikur Holim Society, St. Gallen, to the Jewish Social Self-Help, Cracow (German).

21368 – Letter from the president of Bikur Holim to Lisbon concerning shipment of food and vitamins (German).

Zydowski Instytut Historyczny (Jewish Historical Institute) (AŻIH)

301/2225 – Maria Zadziewicz testimony.

301/2947 – Anonymous testimony about Dr. Anna Braude-Heller, Berson-Bauman Children's Hospital (Yiddish).

370 – Toporol, Ltd. Report, July 1940–December 1941.

4368 – Reports from children's clubs.

ARI.7 – Letter from Dr. Jakub Munwes to the Czyste Hospital Administration Committee (Polish).

ARI.32 – Bulletin of the the Jewish Social Self-Help Statistics Department, November 1941 (Polish).

ARI.81 – Statistical report on the Jewish population of Warsaw, 1939–1941 (Polish).

ARI.84 – Report on the medical situation at refugee centers (Polish).

ARI.85 – Memoranda by Jewish doctors to the Germans addressing the causes of typhus and proposals to combat it (German).

ARI.93 – Testimony about a sanitation Aktion on Krochmalna St., March 29, 1942.

ARI.102 – Dr. Chai Gorbowicz, a doctor in Warsaw, "The Struggle against Epidemics" (Yiddish).

ARI.191 – Report from Chemical-Bacteriological Institute of the Judenrat, July–December 1941 (Polish).

ARI.195 – Regina Wajłowna memoir, nurse at Czyste Hospital, 1939–1941, February 1941 (Polish).

ARI.196 – Nurse Regina Wajłowna testimony, "History of One Case, 1941," (Polish).

ARI.203 – Quarantine on Nalewki St., April 5, 1942 (Polish).

ARI.214 – Health Department report on the fight against tuberculosis, June 28, 1941 (Polish).

ARI.221 – First course for Jewish disinfectors, November 1, 1940 (Polish).

ARI.223 – Mortality in the Warsaw ghetto, 1941 (Polish).

ARI.260 – Health Office Weekly, no. 1, to all Health Office workers, March 8, 1942 (Polish).

ARI.268 – Memoirs of a disinfector (Polish).

ARI.270 – The testimony of an anonymous physician concerning typhus, July 1942 (Polish).

ARI.295 – A document relating to social insurance in Warsaw, 1942 (Polish).

ARI.363 – Report by an anonymous doctor on the war on typhus, March 1942 (Polish).

ARI.428 – Report on various aspects of life in the ghetto (Polish).

ARI.989 – Photos of Berson-Bauman Children's Hospital (Yiddish).

ARI.1069 – Testimony of an anonymous doctor regarding the deportees from Grojec in isolation on Leszno St, 1941 (Polish).

ARI.1099 – Testimony of an anonymous nurse at Bersohn and Bauman Children's Hospital (Yiddish).

ARII.17 – Jewish Social Self-Help report on the doctors' activities in the war on the typhus epidemic in Warsaw, July–August 1940 (Polish).

ARII.43 – Protocol on "Health Month," February 25, 1942 (Polish and Yiddish).

ARII.92 – Jewish Social Self-Help report on TOZ activity, March 1942 (Polish).

ARII.133 – Judenrat Statistics Department Bulletin, May 1940 (Polish).

ARII.161 – Sanitary conditions at the time of high mortality among refugees (Yiddish).

ARII.262 – Notice concerning "Cleanup Week," January 1943 (Polish).

ARII.280 – Report from the hospital and the postal service after the Aktion in 1942 (Polish).

Archives of the American Jewish Joint Distribution Committee (JDC), New York

AR.33–44, file 814 – Report from Dr. Emanuel Patt on welfare activity for the Jews of Poland, March 1941, JDC, based on Judenrat reports to the Germans and data on the TOZ healthcare system during the war.

AR.33–44, file 815 – "The Jewish Situation in Poland during October, November, and December 1937," AJDC bulletin, no. 10, 1938.

AR.33–44, file 821 – TOZ Budget Report, April 1, 1936–March 31, 1937.

AR.33–44, file 822 – CENTOS in Poland report, August 1938.

AR.33–44, file 840 – TOZ reports and correspondence concerning aid for Jews of Warsaw, 1937–1941; correspondence among various players in JDC and elsewhere concerning medical situation in Poland, in general, and in Warsaw, in particular, and concerning budget for feeding and purchase of medicines and inoculations, 1940–1941; report from Mendelsohn, September 1941, on state of health in the Warsaw ghetto; anonymous letter about the epidemic in Warsaw; letters from Elias Sternbuch to president of Agudath Israel concerning inoculations; letter from Dr. Rozenblum and Dr. Koenigstein to the International Red Cross regarding medicines, May 1940; letter from Dr. Rozenblum and Dr. Koenigstein to Wulman about urgent assistance in food and medicines; letter from TOZ Warsaw to Metz, secretary of TOZ Vilna, October 1939; TOZ activity report, May 1940; JDC correspondence with the president of Agudath Israel concerning medicines for Poland, December 1941.

AR.33-44, file 841 – Letter from Henrietta K. Buchman, JDC Poland, to Mr. M. J. Kellner, JDC New York, about TOZ activities in Warsaw at the beginning of the war, November 9, 1939.

YIVO Archives, New York

Poland Collection

RG–116–3.1 – Ludvig Korn, "Hunger-krankhayt kolektive arbet fun yidishe doktoyrim in varshever geto," (Yiddish).

RG–116–5.3 – Spreading of epidemics in Warsaw, December 1939; Warsaw Ghetto: Population, Mortality, and Welfare, 1938–July 1941.

National Library of Israel

002127713 – Lensky, Mordechai, *Der Doktor: Tzvei Vokhen Blat For Popolerer Meditzin un Higyene* (Yiddish).

United States Holocaust Memorial Museum (USHMM)

2002.74.1 – Debora's Diary, 1943.

Archive of the Vilna Gaon Jewish State Museum, Vilnius, Lithuania

Aaron Pik, Shavli Ghetto Diary, manuscript, (Yiddish) (copy in the author's possession).

Private Collections and Interviews

Aviva Blum, survivor of the Warsaw Ghetto, daughter of Luba Blum-Bielicka, director of the nursing school in the Warsaw Ghetto, interview by author, Jerusalem, Israel, November 18, 2007.

Prof. Yaacov Lensky, survivor of the Warsaw ghetto, son of Dr. Mordechai Lensky, a physician who survived the Warsaw ghetto, interviews by author and correspondence with Prof. Yaacov Lensky, and his wife, Dr. Miri Lensky, Rehovot, Israel, May 2011–June 2012.

Shulamit Tzeder testimony, survivor of the Warsaw Ghetto, daughter of Dr. Maurycy Brandwajn, a physician at Czyste Hospital before the war and in the Warsaw ghetto, interview by author, Kibbutz Meggido, Israel, 2007 and 2009.

Printed Sources

Adler, Stanislaw, *In the Warsaw Ghetto, 1940–1943: An Account of a Witness* (Jerusalem: Yad Vashem, 1982).

Apfelbaum, Emil, ed., *Choroba głodowa, Badania kliniczne nad głodem wykonane w getcie warszawskim z roku* (*1942*) (Warsaw: American Joint Distribution Committee, 1946).

______, ed., *Maladie de Famine: Recherches Cliniques sur La Famine Exécutées dans Le Ghetto de Varsovie en 1942* (Warsaw: American Joint Distribution Committee, 1946).

Arad, Yitzhak, Israel Gutman, and Abraham Margaliot, eds., *Documents on the Holocaust, Selected Sources on the Destruction of the Jews of Germany and Austria, Poland, and the Soviet Union* (Jerusalem: Yad Vashem, 1981).

Auerbach, Rachel, *Behutzot Varsha: 1939–1943* (Hebrew) (Tel Aviv: Am Oved, 1954).

Ben-Sefer, Ellen, and Linda Shields, "Courage under Adversity: Luba Bielicka-Blum (1906–1973) and the Nursing School of the Warsaw Ghetto," *Health and History: Medicine in the Shadow of the Holocaust: Australian Reflections*, 18:2 (January 2016), pp. 27–39.

Berg, Mary, *The Diary of Mary Berg: Growing Up in the Warsaw Ghetto*, edited by Susan Lee Pentlin (London: One World, 2006).

Blady Szwajger, Adina, *I Remember Nothing More: The Warsaw Children's Hospital and the Jewish Resistance* (New York: Pantheon, 1990).

Blatman, Daniel, *Geto Varsha—Sipur Itona'i: Mivhar Me'itonut Hamahteret, 1940–1943* (Hebrew) (Jerusalem: Yad Vashem, 2002).

Blum-Bielicka, Luba, "Vegn di 'aktsye' in varshever yidishn shpitol dem 18 Yanuar 1943," *Bleter far geshikhte* (Yiddish), 1:3–4 (August–December, 1948), pp. 211–221.

Blumental, Nachman, and Joseph Kermish, eds., *Hameri Vehamered Begeto Varsha* (Hebrew) – (Jerusalem: Yad Vashem, 1965).

Czerniaków, Adam, *The Warsaw Diary of Adam Czerniaków: Prelude to Doom*, edited by Raul Hilberg, Stanislaw Staron, and Josef Kermish, (New York: Stein and Day, 1979).

______, *Yoman Geto Varsha: 9/6/1939–7/23/1942* (Hebrew) (Jerusalem: Yad Vashem, 1970).

Edelman, Marek, *The Ghetto Fights: Warsaw 1939–1945* (London: Bookmarks, 2013).

Huberband, Szymon, *Kiddush Hashem: Ktavim Miymei Hashoah* (Hebrew) (Tel Aviv: Zachor, 1969).

Kaplan, Chaim Aron, *Megilat Yisurin: Yoman Geto Varsha Chaim Aron Kaplan* (Hebrew) (Tel Aviv and Jerusalem: Am Oved and Yad Vashem, 1966).

______, *Scroll of Agony: Warsaw Ghetto Diary,* edited and translated by Abraham I. Katsh (Bloomington: Indiana University Press, 1999).

Kassow, Samuel, ed., *In Those Nightmarish Days: The Ghetto Reportage of Peretz Opoczynski and Josef Zelkowicz* (New Haven and London: Yale University Press, 2015).

Kermish, Joseph, ed., *To Live with Honor and Die with Honor! Selected Documents from the Warsaw Ghetto Underground Archives "O.S."* (Oneg Shabbat) (Jerusalem:Yad Vashem, 1986).

Korczak, Janusz, "Shnei Aronot Metim Birehov Smucha Uvirehov Shliska," in Shevach Eden, Israel Gutman, Adir Cohen, and Yaacov, Rotem, eds., *Iyunim Bemorashto Shel Yanush Korchak: Meḳorot Hadashim Mehageto* (Hebrew), vol. 4, pp. 140–142.

Lewin, Abraham, *A Cup of Tears: A Diary of the Warsaw Ghetto* (London: Fontana, 1988).

Neustadt, Melech, ed., *Hurban Umered Shel Yehudei Varsha: Sefer Eduyot Ve'azkarot* (Hebrew), 2nd ed. (Tel Aviv: Executive Committee of the General Federation of Labor, 1947).

Opochinsky, Peretz, *Reshimot Migeto Varsha* (Hebrew) (Tel Aviv: Hakkibutz Hameuchad, 1970).

Perechodnik, Calel, *Am I a Murderer? Testament of a Jewish Ghetto Policeman* (Boulder: Westview Press, 1996).

______, *Hatafkid He'atzuv Shel Hati'ud: Yoman Mahbo* (Hebrew) (Jerusalem: Keter, 1993).

Pik, Aaron "*Reshimot Migai Hahariga*": *Zihronot Ktuvim Bageto HaShavla'i (Lita) Bishnot 1942, 1943, 1944* (Hebrew) (Tel Aviv: Igud Yotzei Lita, 1998).

Piotrowski, Stanislaw, *Hans Frank's Diary* (Warsaw: Państwowe Wydawnictwo Naukowe, 1961).

Polish Government-in-Exile, Ministry of Information, *The German New Order in Poland* (London: Hutchinson and Co., 1942).

Polisiuk, Adolf, "Hamatzor Ha'aharon" in Nachman Blumental and Joseph Kermish, *Hameri Vehamered Begeto Varsha* (Jerusalem: Yad Vashem, 1965), pp. 310–317.

Ringelblum, Emanuel, *Ktavim Aharonim: Yahasei Polanim–Yehudim, Yanuar 1943–April 1944* (Hebrew) (Jerusalem: Yad Vashem, 1994).

______, *Notes from the Warsaw Ghetto* (New York: Ibook, 2006).

______, *Polish–Jewish Relations during the Second World War*, editedby Joseph Kermish and Shmuel Krakowski (Jerusalem: Yad Vashem, 1974).

______, *Yoman Vereshimot Mitkufat Hamilhama: Geto Varsha September 1939 Detzember 1942* (Hebrew) (Jerusalem: Yad Vashem, 1993).

Rosen, N., "The Problem of Work in the Jewish Quarter, July 1942," in Joseph Kermish, *To Live with Honor and Die with Honor! Selected Documents from the Warsaw Ghetto Underground Archives "O.S."* (Oneg Shabbath) (Jerusalem: Yad Vashem, 1986), pp. 251–262.

Schatz-Weinkranz, Naomi, *Halaf Im Ha'esh: Reshimot Al Geto Varsha Shenihtevu Bamahvo* (Hebrew) (Jerusalem: Yad Vashem, 2003).

Temkin-Berman, Batya, *Ir Betoh Ir* (Hebrew) (Jerusalem and Tel Aviv: Yad Vashem and Am Oved, 2008).

Turkow, Jonas, *Hayo Hayta Varsha Yehudit* (Hebrew) (Tel Aviv: Tarbut V'chinuch, 1969).

Zylberberg, Michael, *A Warsaw Diary 1939–1945* (London: Vallentine Mitchell, 1969).

Films, Plays, and Newspaper Articles

Braude, Chaim, "Hihrihu Oti Lihyot Malah Hamavet," *Yediot Aharonot* (Hebrew), Special issue for Holocaust Martyrs' and Heroes' Remembrance Day, May 2, 2000, p. 9.

Meredith, Anne, *Out of the Ashes*, film directed by Joseph Sargent (Buckinghamshire: Ardent Productions, 2003).

Milch-Sheriff, Ella, *Baruch's Schweigen* (Braunschweig, 2010), https://www.ellamilchsheriff.com/baruchs-schweigen.

Milner, Iris, "Shfanei Nisayon Shel Atsmam," *Ha'aretz* (Hebrew), April 28, 2000, p. 9.

Nadav, Daniel, "Limed Anatomiya Begeto Varsha, Nitzel Kshehithaze Lekatoli Nehe," *Ha'aretz* (Hebrew), April 16, 2004, p. 10.

Negev, Ayelet, and Yehuda Koren, "Nisuyim Bivnei Adam," *Yediot Aharonot* (Hebrew), Weekend Supplement, April 25, 2003, pp. 53–56.

Nelson, Tim Blake, *The Gray Zone*, film directed by Tim Blake Nelson (Santa Monica, CA: Lionsgate, 2001).

Nesher, Avi, *Past Life* (Tel Aviv: Metro Communications in co-production with Poland's Opus Film, 2016), https://www.jpost.com/Magazine/Past-and-present-with-director-Avi-Nesher-467239.

Offer, Miriam, "Rofim Yehudim Ne'eltzu Laharog Bageto Tinokot Yehudim," *Ma'ariv* (Hebrew), Weekend Supplement, Special Edition for Holocaust Martyrs' and Heroes' Remembrance Day, April 8, 1994, pp. 16–19.

Rappaport, Meron, "Hamahpehan MiNes Tziona," *Ha'aretz* (Hebrew), Supplement, February 11, 2005, pp. 44–46.

Sobol, Joshua, *Ghetto* (London: Nick Hern Books, 1989).

______, *Bamartef* (Hebrew) (Tel Aviv: Or Am, 1990).

Trauban, Tamara, "Im Kvar Anahnu Bageto, Lefahot Nahkor Et Hara'av, *Ha'aretz* (Hebrew), March 11, 2005, p. 10b.

Weiss, Arik, "Mered Intelektuali: Hamehkar Hamahtarti Shel Rofim Yehudim Begeto Varsha," Israeli Television, Channel 13, May 4, 2019, https://13newsco.il/item/news/abroad/europe/ghetto-research-235861/.

Research Literature—Books and Articles

Aaronson, Shlomo, "Heydrich Reinhard," in Gutman, Israel, ed., *Encyclopedia of the Holocaust* (New York: Macmillan, 1990).

Aldor, Leah, "Aspektim Shel Moderna Bashtetl Hapolani: Hatatzlumim Benosei Harefu'a Vehasport Besifrei Hazikaron" (Hebrew) (Master's thesis, The Hebrew University of Jerusalem, 1995).

Aleksiun, Natalia, "Ammunition in the Struggle for National Rights: Jewish Historians in Poland between the Two World Wars," (PhD diss., New York University, 2010).

Allen, Arthur, *The Fantastic Laboratory of Dr. Weigl: How Two Brave Scientists Battled Typhus and Sabotaged the Nazis* (New York: W. W. Norton & Company, Inc., 2014).

______, "Killing in the Name of Cleanliness: The Shocking Stupidity and

Brutality of Nazi Doctors' Response to Typhus," *Slate*, August 5, 2014, http://www.slate.com/articles/health_and_science/science/2014/08/typhus_and_lice_in_jewish_ghettos_nazi_doctors_perverse_groupthink.html.

Aly, Götz, "*Final Solution*": *Nazi Population Policy and the Murder of European Jews* (London: Arnold, 1999).

Amorosa, Judith Korek, Dina Gabaeff, Julia Nagy Fülöp, Marta Fekete Schwartz, and Judith Gönczi, "Tragedy in the Radiology Department of the Jewish Hospital, Budapest, Hungary," *Radiographics*, 16 (1996), pp. 503–508.

Annas, George J., "Military Medical Ethics: Physician First, Last, Always," *The New England Journal of Medicine*, 359:11 (2008), pp. 1,087–1,090.

Anolik, Benjamin, "Rofim Polanim Hasidei Umot Ha'olam" (Hebrew) (paper presented at the Eighth Nahariya Conference on Morbidity and Medicine in the Holocaust, Western Galilee Hospital, Nahariya, May 20, 2007).

Arad, Yitzhak, *Vilna Hayehudit Bema'avak Uvekhilyon* (Hebrew) (Tel Aviv and Jerusalem: Sifriat Poalim and Yad Vashem, 1976).

Aran, Lydia, *Genocide: Critical Essays and Eyewitness Accounts* (New York: Routledge, 2004).

Arbus, Isak, "Memoirs of Heroic Deeds by Jewish Medical Personnel in the Camps," in Michael A. Grodin, ed., *Jewish Medical Resistance in the Holocaust* (New York and Oxford: Berghahn, 2014), pp. 219–226.

Aricha, Ahuva, "Hasherut Hameditzini Bethum Briyut Hatzibor Bere'i Hahistoriya Haklalit Vehayehudit Ufo'alo Begeto Varsha, Kehelek Mipe'ilut Ma'arehet Habriyut Al Irguneha Umosdoteha Hashonim" (Hebrew) (Master's thesis, The Hebrew University of Jerusalem, 2002).

Auerbach, Rachel, *Tzava'ot Varsha: Mifgashim, Ma'asim, Goralot, 1933–1943* (Hebrew) (Tel Aviv: Moreshet, 1985).

Auron, Yair, *Genocide: Reflections on the Inconceivable, Theoretical Aspects in Genocide Studies* (Tel Aviv: Contento De Semerik and the Open University, 2015).

______, *The Pain of Knowledge: Holocaust and Genocide Issues in Education* (London: Routledge, 2018).

Avineri, Shlomo, *Reshut Harabim: Sihot Al Mahshava Medinit* (Hebrew) (Merhavia: Sifriat Poalim, 1966).

Bacharach, Walter Zwi, *Gizanut Besherut Hapolitika: Min Hamonizm El Hanatzizm* (Hebrew) (Jerusalem: Magnes, 1984).

______, *Tfisat Ha'adam Ba'idiologiya Hanatzit* (Hebrew) (Tel Aviv: Broadcast University, 1996).

Bacon, Gershon, "Hatzlaha Helkit, Hesegim Gdolim: Al Ha'otonomiya Hayehudit BePolin Beyn Shtei Milhamot Ha'olam," in Israel Bartal, ed., *Kehal Yisra'el: Hashilton Ha'atzmi Hayehudi Ledorotav* (Hebrew), vol. 3, (Hebrew) (Jerusalem: Yad Izhak Ben-Zvi, 2004).

Bankier, David, and Dan Michman, eds., *Holocaust Historiography in Context: Emergence, Challenges Polemics, and Achievements* (Jerusalem: Yad Vashem, 2008).

Bańkowska, Aleksandra, "Jewish Social Welfare Institutions and Facilities in the General Government from 1939 to 1944: A Preliminary Study," *Studia z Dziejow Rosji i Europy Środkowo-Wschodniej*, 53 (2018), pp. 129–167.

Baron, Shalom, "Kavim Lekoroteihem Shel Yehudei Eropa Bein Shtei Milhamot Ha'olam: Edut Bemishpat Eichmann," in Israel Gutman and Livia Rothkirchen, *Shoat Yehudei Eropa: Reka, Korot, Mashma'ut* (Hebrew) (Jerusalem: Yad Vashem, 1973).

Bartal, Israel, and Israel Gutman, eds., *Kiyum Veshever: Yehudei Polin Ledoroteihem* (Hebrew), 2 vols. (Jerusalem: Zalman Shazar Center, 1997 and 2001).

Batawia, Stanislaw, "Zagłada chorych psychicznie," *Biuletyn Głównej Komisji Badania Zbrodni Hitlerowskich v Polsce*, 3 (1947), pp. 91–106.

Bauer, Yehuda, *American Jewry and the Holocaust: The American Jewish Joint Distribution Committee, 1939–1945* (Detroit: Wayne State University Press, 1981).

______, *My Brother's Keeper: A History of the American Jewish Joint Distribution Committee 1929–1939* (Philadelphia: Jewish Publication Society of America, 1974).

______, *Rethinking the Holocaust* (New Haven: Yale University Press, 2002), pp. 116–117.

Bauman, Zygmunt, *Modernity and the Holocaust* (Ithaca: Cornell University Press, 2000).

Baumslag, Naomi, *Murderous Medicine: Nazi Doctors, Human Experimentation, and Typhus* (Westport: Praeger Publishers, 2005).

______, and Barry Shmookler, "Typhus Epidemic Containment as Resistance to Nazi Genocide," in Michael A. Grodin, ed., *Jewish Medical Resistance in the Holocaust* (New York, Oxford: Berghahn, 2014), pp. 39–48.

Beddies, Thomas, Susanne Doetz, and Christoph Kopke, eds., *Jüdische Ärztinnen und Ärzte im Nationalsozialismus: Entrechtung, Vertreibung, Ermordung* (Munich: De Gruyter Oldenbourg, 2014).

Beinfeld, Solon, "Health Care in the Vilna Ghetto," *Holocaust and Genocide Studies*, 12 (1998), pp. 66–98.

Ben-Sasson, Havi, "Christians in the Ghetto: All Saints' Church, Birth of the Holy Virgin Mary Church, and the Jews of the Warsaw Ghetto," *Yad Vashem Studies*, 31 (2003), pp. 153–173.

______, and Amos Goldberg, *Shnot Ra'inu Ra'a: Prakim Betoldot Hayahadut Hadatit Bitkufat Hashoah* (Hebrew), vol. 3, (Jerusalem: Yad Vashem, 2006).

______, and Lea Prais, "Twilight Days: Missing Pages from Avraham Lewin's Warsaw Ghetto Diary, May–July 1942," *Yad Vashem Studies*, 33 (2005), pp. 7–60.

Ben-Sefer, Ellen, "Gemilat Chesed and Moral Behavior at Westerbork: Lessons from the Past to Remember for the Future," in Elisabeth Maxwell and John Roth, eds., *Remembering for the Future: The Holocaust in an Age of Genocide* (Basingstoke: Palgrave, 2001), pp. 35–53.

Ben-Shalom, David, *Ha'ezra Ha'atzmit Hayehudit Kemisgeret Lepe'ilut Va'adei Habatim Begeto Varsha* (Hebrew) (Master's thesis, The Hebrew University of Jerusalem, 1995), pp. 29, 35.

Ben-Shem, Reuven, "Batei Holim Yehudiyim BeVarsha," in Itzhak Gruenbaum, *Entziklopediya Shel Galuyot: Varsha* (Hebrew), vol. 1, (Jerusalem and Tel Aviv: Encyclopedia of the Jewish Diaspora Co., 1953), pp. 579–585.

______, "Mosdot Ezra Vesa'ad," in Itzhak Gruenbaum, *Entziklopediya Shel Galuyot: Varsha* (Hebrew), vol. 1, (Jerusalem and Tel Aviv: Encyclopedia of the Jewish Diaspora Co., 1953), pp. 587–595.

Berg, Nicolas, "The Invention of 'Functionalism': Josef Wulf, Martin Broszat, and the Institute for Contemporary History (Munich) in the 1960s," *Search and Research: Lectures and Papers*, 4 (2003), pp. 7–38.

Berman, Adolf Avraham, *Bamakom Asher Ya'ad Li Hagoral: Im Yehudei Varsha, 1939–1942* (Hebrew) (Tel Aviv: Hakibbutz Hameuchad and Ghetto Fighters' House, 1977).

Beyrer, Chris, Julian Carlos Villar, Voravit Suwanvanichkij, Sonal Singh, Stefan D. Baral, and Edward J. Mills, "Neglected Diseases, Civil Conflicts, and the Right to Health," *The Lancet*, 370:9587 (2007), pp. 619–627.

Bialostocki, Israel, "Shikum Hayishuv Hayehudi BePolin Aharei Hashoah, 1944–1950," (Hebrew) (PhD diss., The Hebrew University of Jerusalem, 1990).

Blatman, Daniel, "Idiologiya Vehayei Yom-Yom Be'itonut Hamahteret Begeto Varsha," in Israel Gutman, ed., *Migniza Letziyunei Dereh Historiyim: Hartza'ot Mitoh Hakinus: Ringelblum Ve'arhiyon Oneg Shabbat, Arhiyonim Yehudiyim Mitkufat Hamilhama Vehashoah* (Hebrew) (Jerusalem: Yad Vashem, 1997), pp. 90–91.

Bloxham, Donald, and A. Dirk Moses, *The Oxford Handbook of Genocide Studies* (Oxford: Oxford University Press, 2010).

Blum, Alexander, "The Nursing School in the Warsaw Ghetto," in Michael A. Grodin, ed., *Jewish Medical Resistance in the Holocaust* (New York, Oxford: Berghahn, 2014), pp. 173–177.

Blum-Bielicka, Luba, "Szkoła Pielęgniarstwa przy Szpitalu Starozakonnych w Warszawie (1923–1943)," *BŻIH*, 40 (1961), pp. 66–77.

Blumental, Nachman, "Batei Hasefer Bageto," in Itzhak Gruenbaum, *Entziklopediya Shel Galuyot: Varsha* (Hebrew), vol. 6, part 2, (Jerusalem and Tel Aviv: Encyclopedia of the Jewish Diaspora Co., 1959), p. 546.

Borowy, Iris, and Anne Hardly, eds., *Of Medicine and Men: Biographies and Ideas in European Social Medicine between the World Wars* (Frankfurt am Main: Peter Lang, 2008).

Brandwajn-Ziemian, Janina, *Młodość w cieniu śmierci* (Łódź: Oficyna Bibliofilów, 1995),

______, – *Ne'urim Vetushiya Bamilhama: Zihronot Miymei Hashoah* (Hebrew) (Tel Aviv: Y. Golan, 1994).

Bridges, D., "Ma'amad Ha'ahayot Besherutei Habriyut BePolin," *Ahot BeYisrael* (Hebrew), 5 (1959), pp. 35–40.

Brodinger, Regina, *Yomana Shel Ahot Bamilhama Neged Hanatzim, 1941–1945* (Hebrew) (Tel Aviv: Afikim, 1982).

Brouns, Jack, "Medicine in the Kovno Ghetto," in Michael A. Grodin, ed., *Jewish Medical Resistance in the Holocaust* (New York, Oxford: Berghahn, 2014), pp. 155–163.

Browning, Christopher Robert, "Genocide and Public Health: German Doctors and Polish Jews, 1939–1941," *Holocaust and Genocide Studies*, 3 (1988), pp. 21–36.

______, "Nazi Ghettoization Policy in Poland: 1939–1941," *Central European History*, 19 (1986), pp. 343–368.

______, "Nazi Resettlement Policy and the Search for a Solution to the Jewish Question, 1939–1941," in Christopher Robert Browning, *The Path to Genocide: Essays on Launching the Final Solution* (Cambridge: Cambridge University Press, 1992), pp. 3–27.

______, *The Origins of the Final Solution: The Evolution of Nazi Jewish Policy, September 1939–March 1942* (Lincoln and Jerusalem: University of Nebraska Press and Yad Vashem, 2004).

Brunstein Klomekb, Anat, and Itzhak Levava, "A Review of Epidemiologic Studies on Suicide before, during, and after the Holocaust," *Psychiatry Research*, 261 (2018), pp. 35–39.

Burleigh, Michael, *The Third Reich: A New History* (New York: Hill and Wang, 2000).

______, and Wolfgang Wippermann, *The Racial State: Germany 1933–1945* (Cambridge: Cambridge University Press, 1991).

Charny, Israel W., ed., *Encyclopedia of Genocide* (Santa Barbara, Denver, and Oxford: ABC-CLIO, 1999 and 2000).

Chelouche, Tessa, and Geoffrey Brahmer, *Casebook on Bioethics and the Holocaust* (Haifa: UNESCO Chair in Bioethics, Israel National Commission for UNESCO, and the Ministry of Education, 2013).

Ciesielska, Maria, *Lekarza Getta Warszawskiego* (Warsaw: Wydawnictwo Dwa Światy, 2017).

Cloonan, Michèle Valerie, *The Monumental Challenge of Preservation: The Past in a Volatile World* (Cambridge: The MIT Press, 2018).

Cohen, Boaz, *Israeli Holocaust Research: Birth and Evolution* (London: Routledge, 2013).

Cohen, Nava, "Harefu'a Besherut Ha'idiologiya Baraih Hashlishi Vehelka

Bamediniyut Ha'anti Yehudit Bageta'ot Uvemahanot Harikuz" (Hebrew) (PhD diss., The Hebrew University of Jerusalem, 2003).

Cohen, Raya, *Bein Sham Lekan: Sipurim Shel Edim Lahorban, Shvaitz 1939–1942* (Hebrew) (Tel Aviv: Am Oved, 1999).

Cohen-Almagor, Rafael, *Dilemot Be'etika Refu'it* (Hebrew) (Tel Aviv and Jerusalem: Hakibbutz Hameuchad and Van Leer Jerusalem Institute, 2002).

Cooper, John, *Raphael Lemkin and the Struggle for the Genocide Convention* (Basingstoke and New York: Palgrave Macmillan, 2015).

Czerniak, A., "Harofe Hayehudi Baye'arot," in Mark Meir Dworzecki, ed., *Hama'avak Lakiyum Velabriyut Biymei HaShoah: Sidrat Hartza'ot Al Be'ayot Habriyut Bageta'ot, Bemahanot Harikuz Uvaye'arot* (Hebrew) (Jerusalem: Israel Directorate of the World Jewish Congress and the Association of Holocaust Survivor Physicians—Ghettos, Camps, Forests, 1958), pp. 27–32.

Davies, Norman, *Heart of Europe: A Short History of Poland* (Oxford: Oxford University Press, 1984).

Dawidowicz, Lucy, *The War against the Jews, 1933–1945* (New York: Holt, Rinehart, and Winston, 1975).

Doetz, Susanne, and Christoph Kopke, "*Und dürfen das Krankenhaus nicht mehr betreten*": *Der Ausschluss jüdischer und politisch unerwünschter Ärzte und Ärztinnen aus dem Berliner städtischen Gesundheitswesen, 1933–1945* (Berlin: Hentrich & Hentrich, 2015).

Dolev, Eran, and Yisrael Priel, "Hagibuy Ha'eti Larofe Be'erua Rav-Nifga'im," *Harefu'a* (Hebrew), 130 (1996), pp. 424–426.

Dreifuss (Ben-Sasson), Havi, *Geto Varsha—Hasof: April 1942–Yuni 1943* (Hebrew) (Jerusalem: Yad Vashem, 2017).

Durkheim, Émile, *Suicide: A Study in Sociology* (New York: The Free Press, 1951).

______, "Suicide: A Study in Sociology," in Ian McIntosh, ed., *Classical Sociological Theory: A Reader Washington Square* (New York: New York University Press, 1997), pp. 212–231.

Dvir, Batya, "Adam Czerniaków: *Yoshev Rosh HaYudenrat Shel Yehudei Varsha, 1939–1942*" (Hebrew) (Master's thesis, The Hebrew University of Jerusalem, 1993).

Dwork, Deborah, *Children with a Star: Jewish Youth in Nazi Europe* (New Haven and London: Yale University Press, 1991).

Dworzecki, Meir Mark, "Adjustment of Detainees to Camp and Ghetto Life and Their Subsequent Readjustment to Normal Society," *Yad Vashem Studies*, 5, (Jerusalem: Weiss Press, 1963).

______, *Al Mishmar Habriyut Begeto Vilna* (Hebrew) (Tel Aviv: Israel Labor Party, 1952).

______, "Asthenia Hronit Progresivit Vehizdaknut Mukdemet Etzel Nitzolei Shoah," Rofeh Hamishpaha (Hebrew), 1 (1970), pp. 3–7.

______, "Be'ayot Demographiyot Uviyologiyot Shel Aliyat Nitzolei Artzot Hashoah," *Niv Harofe* (Hebrew), 3–4 (1957), pp. 3–14.

______, "Be'ayot Psiho-sotziologiyot Shel Yeladim Yehudim Shehuhbe'u Etzel Lo Yehudim – Bitkufat Hashoah, *Dapim Refu'iyim* (Hebrew), 1–6 (1966), pp. 244–250.

______, *Beyn Habetarim* (Hebrew) (Jerusalem: Kiryat Sefer, 1956).

______, "The Day-to-Day Stand of the Jews," in Israel Gutman and Livia Rothkirchen, eds., *The Catastrophe of European Jewry: Antecedents, History, Reflections: Selected Papers* (Jerusalem: Yad Vashem, 1976), pp. 386–399.

______, *Eropa Lelo Yeladim: Tohnit Hanatzim Leheres Biyologi* (Hebrew) (Jerusalem: Yad Vashem, 1958).

______, "Hakongres Habeinle'umi Leheker Mahalot Tkufat HaShoah," *Yad Vashem Bulletin* (Hebrew), 3 (December 1954), pp. 4–7.

______, "Hamada Harefu'i Vehamatzpun Harefu'i," *Dapim Refu'iyim* (Hebrew), 12 (1953), pp. 303–313.

______, ed. "Hama'vak Al Hakiyum Vehabriyut Bageta'ot Biymei Hakibush Hanazi," *Dapim Refu'iyim* (Hebrew), 6 (1946).

______, ed., *Hama'vak Lakiyum Velabriyut Biymei Hashoah: Sidrat Hartza'ot Al Be'ayot Habriyut Bageta'ot, Bemahanot Harikuz Uvaye'arot* (Hebrew) (Jerusalem: Israel Directorate of the World Jewish Congress and the Association of Holocaust Survivor Physicians—Ghettos, Camps, Forests, 1958).

______, "Hameri Harefu'i Hayehudi Bitkufat Hashoah," *Yediyot Beit Lohamei Hageta'ot* (Hebrew), April 1955, pp. 20–22.

______, "Hameri Harefu'i Hayehudi Vaharefu'a Haposha'at Hanatzit Bitkufat Hashoah," *Niv Harofe* (Hebrew), 9–10 (1953), pp. 3–15.

______, "Hapatologiya Shel Halev Bageta'ot Uvemahanot Harikuz," *Dapim Refu'iyim* (Hebrew), 17 (1958), pp. 3–14.

______, "Hapatologiya Shel Tkufat Hashoah Vehasha'eret Hapatologit

Etzel Nitzolei Hashoah" *Dapim Refu'iyim* (Hebrew), 15 (1956), pp. 3–11.

______, "Hara'av Hametuhnan: Hashita Hametukhnenet Hanatzit Shel Hoser Tzuna Vera'av Be'artzot Hakibush, Bageta'ot Uvemahanot Harikuz—Ehad Hagormim Laheres Habiyologi Shel Ha'amim Hakovshim," *Niv Harofe* (Hebrew), 7–8 (1958), pp. 3–35.

______, "Hasterilizatziya Vehakastratziya Haplilit Bekarnei Harentgen," *Dapim Refu'iyim* (Hebrew), 13 (1954), pp. 3–20.

______, "Heker Mahalot Tkufat HaShoah," *Niv Harofe* (Hebrew), 3–4 (1955), pp. 3–9.

______, "The International Red Cross and Its Attitude toward the Jews in the Nazi-Occupied Countries," in Israel Gutman and Efraim Zuroff, eds., *Rescue Attempts during the Holocaust: Proceedings of the Second Yad Vashem International Historical Conference, Jerusalem, 1977* (Jerusalem: Yad Vashem, 1977), pp. 71–110.

______, "Mahalot Ha'or Bageta'ot Uvemahanot Harikuz," *Niv Harofe* (Hebrew), 14 (1955), pp. 3–12.

______, *Mahanot Hayehudim Be'Estonia, 1942–1944: Hatmurot Beshitat Hahovalot Uveshitat Hamahanot, Amidat Ha'asirim, Hamahteret, Habrihot Laye'arot* (Hebrew) (Jerusalem: Yad Vashem, 1970).

______, "Prof. Klauberg, Miyozmei Hasterilizatziya Hahamonit," *Niv Harofe* (Hebrew), 1–2 (1956), pp. 3–20.

______, "She'erit Haplita Beyisra'el, "Mehkar Be'ayot Demografiyot Uviologiyot," *Gesher* (Hebrew), 1 (1956), pp. 83–113.

______, "Tofa'ot Patolologiyiot Begeto Vilna Uvemahanot Harikuz: Ma Hayta Hadmut Hasanitarit Shel Geto Vilna Vehahayim Bo," in Meir Mark Dworzecki, ed., *Hama'avak Lakiyum Velabriyut Biymei Hashoah: Sidrat Hartza'ot Al Be'ayot Habriyut Bageta'ot, Bemahanot Harikuz Uvaye'arot* (Hebrew) (Jerusalem: World Jewish Congress and Physicians Association and Holocaust Survivors, 1958), pp. 33–36.

______, *Yerushalayim DeLita Bameri Uvashoah* (Tel Aviv: Mifleget Po'alei Eretz Israel, 1951), pp. 286–308.

______, "Yisra'el—Eretz Hanitzolim," *Niv Harofe* (Hebrew), 1–2 (1955), pp. 3–6.

Eckart, Wolfgang U., *Medizin in der NS-Diktatur: Ideologie, Praxis, Folgen* (Köln: Böhlau, 2012).

Eckstein, Benjamin, "Tipul Refu'i Bayehudim Bemahanot Mauthausen," *Yalkut Moreshet* (Hebrew), 30 (1981), pp. 107–114.

Efron, John Maurice, *Medicine and the German Jews: A History* (New Haven: Yale University Press, 2001).

Eighteenth Israel Medical Association World Fellowship International Conference: "Advanced Technologies and Medicine," Programs and Abstracts, 95th Year Anniversary, Jerusalem, April 11–15, 2007.

Einhorn, Chaim, "Harofe Begeto Varsha," in Mark Meir Dworzecki, ed., *Hama'avak Lakiyum Velabriyut Biymei Hashoah* (Hebrew) (Jerusalem: Israel Administration of the World Jewish Congress and Association of Holocaust Survivor Physicians—Ghettos, Camps, Forests, 1958), pp. 9–11.

Elbaum-Dornbus, Chaya, "Hageto Biymei Hagerush," in Itzhak Gruenbaum, *Entziklopediya Shel Galuyot: Varsha* (Hebrew), vol. 6, part 2, (Jerusalem and Tel Aviv: Encyclopedia of the Jewish Diaspora Co., 1959), p. 618.

Elkin, Rivka, "Beit Haholim Hayehudi BeBerlin—Sarid Aharon Leyehudei Germaniya Bitkufat Haraih Hashlishi, *Yalkut Moreshet* (Hebrew), 53 (1993), pp. 53–91.

______, *Halmut Halev: Hemshekhiyut Utmura Bepe'ulot Hasa'ad Veharevaha Shel Yehudei Germaniya Tahat Hashilton Hanatzi, 1933–1945* (Hebrew) (Jerusalem: Yad Vashem and Leo Baeck Institute, 2004).

Engel, David, "Ktivat Hahistoriya Keshlihut Le'umit: Yehudei Polin Umasoroteihem Hahistoriyografiyot, in Israel Gutman, ed., *Ringelblum: Ha'adam Vehahistorion* (Hebrew) (Jerusalem: Yad Vashem, 2010), pp. 109–130.

______, "'Masoret Nega'im?' He'arot Al Hamegamot Hapolitiyot Vehatarbut Hapolitit Shel Yehudei Polin, in Israel Bartal and Israel Gutman, eds., *Kiyum Veshever: Yehudei Polin Ledoroteihem* (Hebrew), vol. 2, (Jerusalem: Zalman Shazar Center, 2001), pp. 649–665.

______, "Remove the Evil from the Midst of Thee: On the Concept of Collaboration in the Trials of Michael Weichert," in Shmuel Almog, Israel Gutman, Yehuda Bauer et al., *The Holocaust: History and Memory Essays Presented in Honor of Israel Gutman* (Jerusalem: Yad Vashem, Avraham Harman Institute of Contemporary Jewry, The Hebrew University, 2001), pp. 1–24.

______, "*Who Is a Collaborator? The Trials of Michael Weichert*," in Slawomir Kapralski, *The Jews in Poland*, vol. 2, (Craców: Judaica Foundation and the Center for Jewish Culture, 1999), pp. 339–370.

Engelking, Barbara, "Moral Issues in Emanuel Ringelblum's Writing from World War II," in Israel Gutman, ed., *Emanuel Ringelblum: The Man and the Historian* (Jerusalem: Yad Vashem, 2006), pp. 34–54.

______, and Jacek Leociak, *The Warsaw Ghetto: A Guide to the Perished City* (New Haven: Yale University Press, 2009).

Even, Leah, Orit Hershlag-Elkayan, and Shaul Menashe Shasha, eds., "Habituyim Hakliniyim Shel Mahalat Hara'av Beyeladim Bageta'ot," *Harefu'a* (Hebrew), 142 (2003), pp. 345–349.

Faigenbaum, Moshe Yosef, ed., *Sefer Biała Podlaska* (Yiddish and Hebrew) (Tel Aviv: Kupat Gmilut Hesed al shem Kehilat Biala-Podlaska, 1961), https://www.jewishgen.org/yizkor/Biala_Podlaska/ (accessed July 2, 2019).

Farbstein, Esther, *Hidden in Thunder: Perspectives on Faith, Halachah, and Leadership during the Holocaust* (Jerusalem: Mossad Harav Kook, 2007).

Farfel, Zvi, "Harelevantiyut Shel Harefua Begermaniya Hanatzit Lesugiyot Refu'iyot Beyameinu: Tafkida Hamahriya Betahalih Hahashmada," *Yalkut Moreshet* (Hebrew), 71 (2001), pp. 43–56.

Fernandes, Ashley, "Nazi Medicine and the Holocaust: Implications for Bioethics Education and Professionalism," in John J. Michalczyk, ed., *Nazi Law: From Nuremberg to Nuremberg, London and New York* (New York: Bloomsbury Academic, 2018), pp. 139–153.

Fishkin, Guy, "Ani Megiya Lamahlaka Vehagehenom Amiti," *Ma'ariv* (Hebrew), April 8, 2013, p. 5.

Fleck, Arye, "Al Refu'a Bitkufat Hashoah," *Harefu'a* (Hebrew), 82:3 (1972), p. 136.

______, "Refu'a Umada Bitkufat Hakibush Hanatzi," *Harefu'a* (Hebrew), 32:2 (1997), pp. 91–92.

Friedländer, Saul, *Nazi Germany and the Jews: The Years of Persecution, 1933–1939* (New York: HarperCollins, 1997).

Friedman, David Aryeh ed., *Sefer Hakongres Ha'olami Harishon Shel Rof'im Yehudim* (Hebrew) (Tel Aviv: Harefu'a, 1936).

Friedman, Philip, "Holocaust Historical Research and Its Problems," in Israel Gutman and Livia Rothkirchen, eds., *The European Holocaust:*

Background, History, Significance Jerusalem: Yad Vashem, 1973), pp. 437–448.

Fund, Naama, Avi Porath, Nachman Ash, Varda Shalev, and Gideon Koren, "Comorbidity Rates between Holocaust Survivors and Individuals in the General Population in Israel," *JAMA Netw Open*, 2:1:e186643 (2019), doi:10.1001/jamanetworkopen.2018.6643.

Galilee Declaration: http://english.wgalil.ac.il/category/Declaration http://www.medicineaftertheholocaust.org/galilee-declaration/ http://mededirect.org/mimeh/galilee.cfm

Gardemann, J., "Primary Health Care in Complex Humanitarian Emergencies: Rwanda and Kosovo Experiences and Their Implications for Public Health Training," *Croatian Medical Journal*, 43:2 (2002), pp. 55–148.

Garrard, Eve, and Geoffrey Scarre, eds., *Moral Philosophy and the Holocaust* (London: Ashgate Press, 2003).

Garrison, F. H., *An Introduction to the History of Medicine*, 4th ed. (Philadelphia and London, 1929).

Gelber, Nathan Michael, "Letoldot Harof 'im Hayehudim BePolin Beme'a Hashmone Esre, in Joseph Tirosh, ed., *Shai LeYeshayahu: Sefer Yovel Le R. Yeshayahu Volfsberg* (Hebrew) (Tel Aviv: Hapo'el Hamizrachi Cultural Center, 1955), pp. 347–371.

Gelber, Yoav, "Ha'itonut Ha'ivrit Be'eretz Yisra'el Al Hashmadat Yehudei Eropa, 1941–1942," *Dapim Leheker Hashoah Vehamered* (Hebrew), 1 (1970), pp. 30–58.

Gerlach, Christian, "Extremely Violent Societies: An Alternative to the Concept of Genocide," *Journal of Genocide Research*, 8:4 (2006), pp. 455-471.

Goldberg, Amos, *Holocaust Diaries as "Life Stories"* (Jerusalem: Yad Vashem, 2004).

______, *Trauma in First Person: Diary Writing during the Holocaust* (Bloomington: Indiana University Press, 2017).

Goldbort, Yuval, and Avraham Ohry, "Ludvig Flek: Hoker, Rofe Ufilosof " (Hebrew) (lecture delivered at the Second Nahariya Conference on Medicine and the Holocaust, Nahariya, May 8, 2002).

Golden, Juliet D., "'Show that you are really alive,' Sara-Zofia Syrkin Binsztejnowa's Emergency Medical Relief and Public Health Work in

Early Interwar Poland and the Warsaw Ghetto," *Medizinhistorisches Journal*, 53:2 (2018), pp. 125–162.

Goldenberg, Myrna, "Review of *Murderous Medicine: Nazi Doctors, Human Experimentation, and Typhus*, by Naomi Baumslag," *Genocide Studies and Prevention*, 1:3 (2006), pp. 375–376.

González-López, Esteban, and Rosa Ríos-Cortés, "Medical Student's Opinions on Some Bioethical Issues before and after a Holocaust and Medicine Course," *IMAJ*, 18:5 (May 2016), pp. 257-260.

Grajek, Stefan-Shalom, *Shlosha Yemei Krav* (Hebrew) (Tel Aviv: Ma'arachot, 1972).

Grodin, Michael A., ed., *Jewish Medical Resistance in the Holocaust* (New York, Oxford: Berghahn, 2014).

Gross, Jan Tomasz, *Polish Society under German Occupation: The Generalgouvernement, 1939–1944* (Princeton: Princeton University Press, 1979).

Grupińska, Anka, "Kah Be'emet: Bishnat 1942 Yatzati Min Habayit Ule'olam Lo Shavti Elav: Siha Im Adina Bladi-Shvaiger" in Anka Grupińska, *Sehor Sehor: Sihot Im Lohamim Migeto Varsha* (Hebrew) (Tel Aviv: Hakibbutz Hameuchad, 2002).

Grynberg, Michal, ed., *Words to Outlive Us: Eyewitness Accounts from the Warsaw Ghetto* (New York: Metropolitan Books, 2002).

Gumpert, Martin, "The Physicians of Warsaw," *The American Scholar*, 18 (1948), pp. 285–290.

Gürfinkel-Glocer, Sabina, "Goralo Shel Beit Haholim Tzhista" in Itzhak Gruenbaum, *Entziklopediya Shel Galuyot: Varsha* (Hebrew), vol. 6, part 2, (Jerusalem and Tel Aviv: Encyclopedia of the Jewish Diaspora Co., 1959), pp. 587–590.

Gutman, Israel, "Emanuel Ringelblum: Historion Vezmano," in Israel Gutman, *Emmanuel Ringelblum: Ha'adam Vehahistorion* (Hebrew) (Jerusalem: Yad Vashem, 2006), pp. 78–108.

______, *Encyclopedia of the Holocaust* (New York: Macmillan, 1990).

______, "Jews during the Holocaust," in Israel Gutman, ed., *Encyclopedia of the Holocaust*, vol. 4, pp. 1,602–1,603.

______, *The Jews of Warsaw, 1939–1943: Ghetto, Underground, Revolt* (Bloomington: Indiana University Press, 1989).

______, *Migniza Letziyonei Dereh Historiyim: Hartza'ot Mitoh Hakinus*

"Ringelblum Ve'arhiyon Oneg Shabbat, Arhiyonim Yehudim Mitkufat Hamilhama Vehashoah" (Hebrew) (Jerusalem: Yad Vashem, 1997).

______, ed., *Sugiyot Beheker Hashoah: Bikoret Vetruma* (Hebrew) (Jerusalem: The Zalman Shazar Center, Yad Vashem, 2008).

______, "Yehudim–Polanim–Antishemiyut," in Israel Bartal and Israel Gutman, eds., *Kiyum Veshever: Yehudei Polin Ledoroteihem* (Jerusalem: Zalman Shazar Center, 2001), vol. 2, pp. 605–639.

______, Avraham Wein, Shlomo Netzer, and Gideon Greif, eds., *Toldot Yehudei Varsha Mireshitam Ve'ad Yameinu* (Hebrew) (Jerusalem: Keter and Association of Warsaw Jewry in Israel, 1991).

______, and Michael Berenbaum, *Anatomy of the Auschwitz Death Camp* (Bloomington: Indiana University Press, 1998).

Gutterman, Alexander, "Hatza'oteihem Shel Yehudei Polin Letikunim Bema'amadam Hahuki Hakalkali Hahevrati Vehatarbuti Bitkufat Haseym Hagadol" (Hebrew) (Master's thesis, The Hebrew University of Jerusalem, 1975).

Hájková, Anna, "Medicine in Theresienstadt," Social History of Medicine, hky066 (2018), https://doi.org/10.1093/shm/hky066 (accessed September 17, 2019).

Halecki, Oscar, *A History of Poland* (London: Kegan Paul, 1983).

Halpin, Ross, *The Essence of Survival: How Jewish Doctors Survived Auschwitz* (Sydney: Sydney Jewish Museum, 2014).

______, *Jewish Doctors and the Holocaust: The Anatomy of Survival* (Berlin and Jerusalem: De Gruyter Publishing and Magnes Press, 2019).

Heim, Susanne, Carola Sachse, and Mark Walker, eds., *The Kaiser Wilhelm Society under National Socialism* (New York: Cambridge University Press, 2009).

Herzog, Rachel, "Hitarutam Shel Rofim Nitzolei Shoah Bahevra Hayisra'elit Uvema'arekhet Habriyut Beyisra'el, 1945–1957" (Hebrew) (PhD diss., Ben-Gurion University of the Negev, 2015).

Heyd, David, *Etika Verefu'a* (Hebrew) (Tel Aviv: Broadcast University, Ministry of Defense, 1990).

Hilberg, Raul, *The Destruction of the European Jews* (Chicago: Quadrangle, 1967).

______, *Perpetrators, Victims, Bystanders: The Jewish Catastrophe 1933–1945* (New York: HarperCollins Publishers, 1992).

———, and Stanislaw Staron, "Mi Haya Adam Czerniaków?" *Yalkut Moreshet* (Hebrew), 27 (1979), pp. 107–111.

Hinton, Alex, "Genocide and Mass Violence: A Conceptual Turn? *Journal of Genocide Research*, 9:1 (2007), pp. 13–14.

Hirszfeld, Ludwik, *Die Geschichte eines Lebens* (1950).

———, *Historia jednego życia* (Warsaw: Czytelnik, 1950).

———, *The Story of One Life* (New York: University of Rochester Press, 2010).

Hlamides, Nikolaos, "The Greek Relief Committee: America's Response to the Greek Genocide," *Genocide Studies and Prevention*, 3:3 (2008), pp. 375–383.

Hobsbawm, Eric, *Nations and Nationalism since 1780: Programme, Myth, Reality* (Cambridge: Cambridge University Press, 1992).

Höffken, Bernd, *Schicksale jüdischer Ärzte aus Nürnberg nach 1933* (Metropol Verlag: Berlin, 2014).

Hohendorf, Gerrit, "The Sewering Affair," in Volker Roelcke, Sascha Topp, and Etienne Lepicard, eds., *Silence, Scapegoats, Self-reflection: The Shadow of Medical Crimes on Medicine and Bioethics* (V&R Unipress: Göttingen, 2015), pp. 131–147.

Holland, Walter Werner, Roger Detels, and George Knox, eds., *Oxford Textbook of Public Health* (Oxford: Oxford University Press, 1984).

Horton, Richard, "Offline: Medicine and the Holocaust—It's Time to Teach," *The Lancet*, 394:10193 (2019), https://www.thelancet.com/journals/lancet/ article/ PIIS0140-6736(19)31608-3/fulltext.

International Committee of the Red Cross, *First Aid in Armed Conflicts and Other Situations of Violence*, https://www.icrc.org/sites/default/files/topic/file_plus_list/first_aid_leaflet.pdf.

Irvin-Erickson, Douglas, *Raphael Lemkin and the Concept of Genocide* (Pennsylvania: University of Pennsylvania Press, 2017).

Israel Medical Association, "Hahebetim Ha'etiyim Be'erua Rav-Nifga'im" (Hebrew), position paper, May 2008, https://www.ima.org.il/MainSiteNew/EditClinicalInstruction.aspx?ClinicalInstructionId=158 (accessed September 17, 2019).

Jakobovits, Immanuel, *Jewish Medical Ethics—A Comparative and Historical Study of the Jewish Religious Attitude to Medicine and Its Practice* (New York: Bloch Pub, 1975).

Jenss, H., and P. Reinicke, *Der Arzt Hermann Strauß, 1868–1944:*

Autobiographische Notizen und Aufzeichnungen aus dem Ghetto Theresienstadt (Berlin: Hentrich & Hentrich, 2014).

Jütte, Robert, "Die Vertreibung jüdischer und staatsfeindlicher Ärztinnen und Ärzte," in Robert Jütte, ed., *Medizin und Nationalsozialismus. Bilanz und Perspektiven der Forschung* (Göttingen: Wallstein, 2011), pp. 83–93.

Kagan, Solomon Robert, *Jewish Medicine* (Boston: Medico-Historical Press, 1952).

Kaiser Wilhelm Institute for Medical Research, https://www.nobelprize.org/prizes/uncategorized/a-history-of-the-kaiser-wilhelm-institute-for-medicalresearch-1929-1939 (accessed February11, 2020).

Kassow, Samuel D., *Who Will Write Our History? Emanuel Ringelblum and the Oyneg Shabes Archive* (Bloomington: Indiana University Press, 2007).

______, ed., *In Those Nightmarish Days: The Ghetto Reportage of Peretz Opoczynski and Josef Zelkowicz* (New Haven and London: Yale University Press, 2015).

Kater, Michael Hans., *Doctors under Hitler* (Chapel Hill: University of North Carolina Press, 1989).

Kermish, Joseph, "Nigudim Ma'amadiyim Begeto Varsha," in Itzhak Gruenbaum, *Entziklopediya Shel Galuyot: Varsha* (Hebrew), vol. 6, part 2, (Jerusalem and Tel Aviv: Encyclopaedia of the Jewish Diaspora Co., 1959), pp. 557–579.

Keys, Ancel, Josef Brozek, Austin Henschel, Olaf Mickelsen, and Henry Longstreet Taylor, *The Biology of Human Starvation* (Minneapolis: University of Minnesota Press, 1950).

Kiernan, Ben, *Blood and Soil: A World History of Genocide and Extermination from Sparta to Darfur* (New Haven: Yale University Press, 2007).

Klaus-Peter, Friedrich, "Rassistische Seuchenprävention als Voraussetzung national-sozialistischer Vernichtungspolitik: Vom Warschauer 'Seuchensperrgebiet' zu den 'Getto'—Mauern (1939–1940)," *Zeitschrift für Geschichtswissenschaft*, 7 (2005), pp. 609–636.

Klee, Ernst, *Euthanasie im NS-Staat: Die Vernichtung lebensunwerten Lebens* (Frankfurt: S. Fischer, 1983).

Kochavi, Yehoyakim, "Hermann Göring," in Gutman, Israel, ed., *Encyclopedia of the Holocaust* (New York: Macmillan, 1990).

______, and Asher Cohen, eds., "Hayei Yomyom Betkufat Hashoah," *Dapim Leheker Tkufat, Hashoah* (Hebrew), 10 (1993).

Koren, Leah, "Hasiyud Kehelek Misherutei Habriyut Begeta'ot Varsha, Vilna, Kovna, 1939–1945" (Hebrew) (Master's thesis, Tel Aviv University, 1987).

Kossoy, Edward, and Abraham Ohry, *The Feldshers: Medical, Sociological, and Historical Aspects of Practitioners of Medicine with Below University Level Education* (Jerusalem: Magnes Press, 1992).

Kottek, Shmuel, ed., "Ma'amarim Refui'yim Al 'Hamatat Hesed' Le'umit Sotzialistit," *Korot* (Hebrew), 19 (2009), pp. 3–117.

Kozłowska, Magdalena, "In Sunshine and Joy? The Story of Medem Sanatorium in Miedzeszyn," *East European Politics & Societies*, July 2013, doi: 10.1177/0888325413494772 and http://www.yivoencyclopedia.org/article.aspx/Medem_Sanatorium.

Krall, Hanna, *Shielding the Flame: An Intimate Conversation with Dr. Marek Edelman, the Last Surviving Leader of the Warsaw Ghetto Uprising* (New York: Holt, 1986).

Kranich, Kai, *Anpassung im Nationalsozialismus: die Universität Breslau und die Aberkennung von Doktortiteln* (Wrocław: Oficyna Wydawn, 2012).

Krischel, Matthis, *Urologie und Nationalsozialismus: Eine Studie zu Medizin und Politik als Ressourcen füreinander* (Stuttgart: Franz Steiner Verlag, 2014).

Kümmel, Werner, "Die Ausschaltung rassisch und politisch mißliebiger Ärzte," in Kudlien Fridolf, ed., *Ärzte im Nationalsozialismus* (Köln: Kiepenheuer & Witsch, 1985), pp. 56–81.

Kunz, Dieter, ed., *Deadly Medicine: Creating the Master Race* (Washington, DC: United States Holocaust Memorial Museum, 2004).

Kwiet, Konrad, "Problems of Jewish Resistance Historiography," *Leo Baeck Institute*, 26 (1979), pp. 37–57.

______, "The Ultimate Refuge: Suicide in the Jewish Community under the Nazis," *Leo Baeck Institute Yearbook*, 29 (1984), pp. 135–167.

Lang, Berel, *Genocide: The Act As Idea* (Philadelphia: University of Pennsylvania Press, 2017).

Leaning, Jennifer, "Diagnosing Genocide: The Case of Darfur," *New England Journal of Medicine*, 351:8 (2004), pp. 735–738.

Legros, Dominique, Christophe Paquet, Fabienne Dorlencourt, and Elizabeth Le Saoult, "Risk Factors for Death in Hospitalized Dysentery Patients in Rwanda," *Tropical Medicine & International Health*, 4:6 (1999), pp. 428–432.

Lensky, Mordechai, *A Physician inside the Warsaw Ghetto* (New York and Jerusalem: Yad Vashem and The Holocaust Survivors Memoirs Project, 2009).

______, "Beit Haholim Hayehudi Tzhista," *Dapim Leheker Hashoah Vehamered* (Hebrew), 1 (1951), pp. 102–107.

______, "Problems of Disease in the Warsaw Ghetto," in Shaul Esh, ed., *Yad Vashem Studies on the European Jewish Catastrophe and Resistance*, vol. 3, (Jerusalem: Yad Vashem, 1959), pp. 83–293.

______, "Rof'im Yehudim Mefursamim," in Itzhak Gruenbaum, *Entziklopediya Shel Galuyot: Varsha* (Hebrew), vol. 6, part 2, (Jerusalem and Tel Aviv: Encyclopedia of the Jewish Diaspora Co., 1959), p. 307.

Leshchinsky, Jacob, "Hayishuv Hayehudi Behitpathuto Hakalkalit," in Itzhak Gruenbaum, *Entziklopediya Shel Galuyot: Varsha* (Hebrew), vol. 1, (Jerusalem and Tel Aviv: Encyclopedia of the Jewish Diaspora Co., 1953–1956), pp. 125–219.

Levin, Itamar, *Otiyot Shel Esh: Eduyot Mitkufat Hashoah Basifrut Hahilhatit* (Hebrew) (Tel Aviv: Yedioth Ahronoth and Hemed Books, 2002).

______, *Walls Around: The Plunder of Warsaw Jewry during World War II and Its Aftermath* (Westport: Praeger, 2004).

Lifton, Robert Jay, *The Nazi Doctors: Medical Killing and the Psychology of Genocide* (New York: Basic Books, 1986).

Lindenthal, Jacob Jay, "Abi Gezunt: Health and the Eastern European Immigrant," *American Jewish History*, 70 (1981), pp. 420–441.

______, "The Epidemiological Status and Health Care Administration of the Jews before and during the Holocaust," in Michael A. Grodin, ed., *Jewish Medical Resistance in the Holocaust* (New York, Oxford: Berghahn, 2014), pp. 16–17.

Linder-Ganz, Ronny, and Rotem Starkman, "Yesh Mashehu She'anahnu

Lo Yod'im Al Hashoah? Hamered Harefu'i Begeto Varsha," *TheMarker* (Hebrew), April 17, 2015, pp. 8–10.

Lindert, Jutta, and Armen T. Marsoobian, *Multidisciplinary Perspectives on Genocide and Memory* (Cham: Springer International Publishing, 2018).

Livshitz, Anatol, Avraham Ohry, and Shaul Shasha, "Tahlua Meuheret Bekerev Nitzolei Shoah," *Harefu'a* (Hebrew), 148:4 (May 2009), pp. 224–228.

Lowy, Ilana, *The Polish School of Philosophy of Medicine: From Tytus Chalubinski (1820–1889) to Ludwik Fleck (1896–1961)* (Dordrecht: Kluwer, 1990).

Lutkiewicz, Stefan, "Hirszfeld Ludwik," *Encyclopedia Judaica*, vol. 8, (Jerusalem: Keter, 1971), p. 530.

Mahler, Raphael, *Toldot Hayehudim BePolin Ad Hame'a Ha-19: Kalkala, Hevra, Hamatzav Hamishpati* (Hebrew), vol. 4, (Merhavia: Hakibbutz Hameuchad, 1946), pp. 98–105.

———, *Yehudei Polin Bein Shtei Milhamont Ha'olam: Historia Kalkalit–Sotzialit Be'or Hastatistika* (Hebrew) (Tel Aviv: Dvir, 1969).

Małecka, M., *Prof. dr med. Jakub Penson (1899–1971): życie, działalność i dokonania* (Gdansk: Akademia Medyczna w Gdansku Zakład Historii Filozofii Nauk Medycznych, 2008).

Malwist, Miriam, "Assimilationists and Neophytes at the Time of War Orations and in the Closed Jewish Quarter," in Kermish, *To Live with Honor and Die with Honor! Selected Documents from the Warsaw Ghetto Underground Archives "O.S." (Oneg Shabbath)* (Jerusalem: Yad Vashem, 1986), pp. 620–621.

Marcus, Joseph, *Social and Political History of the Jews in Poland, 1919–1939* (Berlin: Mouton, 1983).

Markusfeld, Miriam, "Toldot Beit Hasefer Le'ahayot Tzhista BeVarsha," *Ahot BeYisrael* (Hebrew), 3 (1957), pp. 3–7.

Martin, Sean, "Zofia Szymańska and Child Welfare in Twentieth Century Poland," *NASHIM: A Journal of Jewish Women's Studies & Gender Issues*, 36 (forthcoming, Spring 2020).

Mayer, Susan, "The School That Would Not Die: The Story of the Jewish Hospital School of Nursing," (paper presented at the First International Conference on Nursing and Midwifery in the Third

Reich, "Complicity and Compassion," Limerick, Republic of Ireland, June 10–11, 2004).

McCallum, Jack Edward, *Military Medicine: From Ancient Times to the 21st Century* (Santa Barbara: ABC-CLIO, 2008), pp. 326–327.

McGregor, Katharine, Jess Melvin, and Annie Pohlman, eds., *The Indonesian Genocide of 1956: Causes, Dynamics, and Legacies* (Cham: Springer International Publishing/Palgrave Macmillan, 2018).

Meiches, Ben, and Jeff Benvenuto, eds., "Revisiting the Life and Work of Raphaël Lemkin," *Genocide Studies and Prevention*, 13:1 (2019).

Meierhenrich, Jens, "The Trauma of Genocide," *Journal of Genocide Research*, 9:4 (2007), pp. 549–573.

Melamed, Michael, "Hevrot Legmilut Hasadim," in Itzhak Gruenbaum et al., *Entziklopediya Shel Galuyot: Varsha* (Hebrew), vol. 1, (Jerusalem and Tel Aviv: Encyclopedia of the Jewish Diaspora Co., 1953), pp. 597–601.

Menczal, Jacob, and Esther Lee Marcus,"Osteoporosis among Holocaust Survivors (Abs)," *The Journal of Nutrition, Health & Aging*, 7 (2003), p. 320.

Mendelsohn, Ezra, *The Jews of East Central Europe between the World Wars* (Indiana: Indiana University Press, 1983).

______, *Zionism in Poland: The Formative Years, 1915–1926* (New Haven: Yale University Press, 1981), pp. 1–36.

Mendelsohn, Shloyme, *The Polish Jews behind the Nazi Ghetto Walls* (New York: YIVO—Yiddish Scientific Institute, 1942).

Menuhin, Naomi, "Dr. Israel Milejkowski: Ha'intelektual Hayehudi BePolin Bein Shtei Milhamot Ha'olam: Doktor Izrael Milikovski Kemikreh Mivhan" (Hebrew) (PdD diss., Ben Gurion University of the Negev, 2016).

Michalczyk, John J., ed., *Medicine, Ethics and the Third Reich: Historical and Contemporary Issues* (Kansas City: Sheed and Ward, 1994).

______, ed., *Nazi Law: From Nuremberg to Nuremberg* (London and New York, Bloomsbury Academic, 2018).

Michel, Alain, "OZE," in Gutman, Israel, ed., *Encyclopedia of the Holocaust* (New York: Macmillan, 1990).

Michman, Dan, *The Emergence of Jewish Ghettos during the Holocaust* (Jerusalem: Yad Vashem, 2011).

______, "Hapitaron Hasofi Shel She'elat Hayehudim, Hitgabshuto

Veyisumo: Matzav Hamekhkar," *Bishvil Hazikaron* (Hebrew), 42 (2001), pp. 4–21.

______, *Holocaust Historiography: A Jewish Perspective: Conceptualizations, Terminology, Approaches, and Fundamental Issues* (London: Vallentine Mitchell, 2003).

______, "Oforia Shel Nitzahon Kemafte'ah Lemikumo Shel Christopher Browning Bemapat Hamehkar Al Hapitaron Hasofi Shel She'elat Hayehudim," *Yalkut Moreshet* (Hebrew) 72 (2002), pp. 9–19.

______, "Why Did Heydrich Write the *Schnellbrief*? A Remark on the Reason and on Its Significance," *Yad Vashem Studies*, 32 (2004), pp. 433–467.

Milch, Baruch, *Can Heaven Be Void* (Jerusalem: Yad Vashem, 2003).

Mirocznik, Liza, "Beit Hasefer Le'ahayot Tzhista BeVarsha, Toldotav Veshitot Halimud Bo," *Ahot BeYisrael* (Hebrew), 9 (1963), pp. 46–48.

Mitcherlich, Alexander, and Fred Mielke, *Doctors of Infamy: The Story of Nazi Medical Crimes* (New York: H. Schuman, 1949).

Müller-Hill, Benno, *Murderous Science: Elimination by Scientific Selection of Jews, Gypsies, and Others in Germany, 1933–1945* (Plainview: Cold Spring Harbor Laboratory Press, 1998).

Muszkowska-Penson, Joanna, "Prof. Dr. Jakub Penson (1899–1971) Część I. Okres Przedwojenny I Okupacji," *Annales Academiae Medicae Gedanensis*, 32 (2002), pp. 321–330, http://pbc.gda.pl/publication/4123 (accessed March 17, 2019).

Nadav, Daniel, *Medicine and Nazism* (Jerusalem: The Hebrew University Magnes Press, 2009).

______, "Was There a 'Medicalization' of the Holocaust? SS Doctors as the Executive Arm of the German 'Biocracy' and the Perpetrators of Medical Murder," *Moreshet: Journal of the Study of the Holocaust and Antisemitism*, 16 (2019): pp. 403–459.

Nadler, Allan, "Jewish Medical Resistance during the Holocaust: Selected Papers Presented at a Conference at the YIVO Institute for Jewish Research, New York, November 1996," (unpublished manuscript).

Nagel, Thomas, "Moral Luck," in Daniel Statman, ed., *Moral Luck* (Albany: State University of New York Press, 1993), pp. 57–71.

Netzer, Shlomo, "Hama'avak Haparlementari Hayehudi Beveit

Hanivharim," in Israel Bartal and Israel Gutman, *Kiyum Veshever: Yehudei Polin Ledoroteihem* (Hebrew), vol. 2, (Jerusalem: Zalman Shazar Center, 2001), pp. 550–551.

______, *Ma'avak Yehudei Polin Al Zehuyoteihem Ha'ezrahiyot Vehale'umiyot, 1918–1922* (Hebrew) (Tel Aviv: Tel Aviv University, 1980).

______, "Polish Jewry between Two World Wars," in Nahman Tamir, ed., *Polish Jewry before the Holocaust, 1914–1939* (New York: Herzl Press Publication, 1986), pp. 212–216.

Nyiszli, Miklos, *Auschwitz: A Doctor's Eyewitness Account* (Hertfordshire: Mayflower, 1973).

Oberman, Anthony S., Tal Brosh-Nissimov, and Nachman Ash, "Medicine and the Holocaust: A Visit to the Nazi Death Camps as a Means of Teaching Medical Ethics in the Israel Defense Forces Medical Corps," *Journal of Medical Ethics*, 36:12 (December 2010), pp. 821–826.

Ofer, Dalia, "Another Glance through the Historian's Lens: Testimonies in the Study of Health and Medicine in the Ghetto," *Poetics Today*, 27 (2006), pp. 331–351.

______, "The Community and the Individual: The Different Narratives of Early and Late Testimonies and their Significance for Historians," in David Bankier and Dan Michman, eds., *Holocaust Historiography in Context: Emergence, Challenges, Polemics and Achievements* (Jerusalem: Yad Vashem, 2008), pp. 519–533.

______, "Heker Hayei Yomyom Tahat Hakibush Hanazi," *Dapim Leheker Tkufat Hashoah* (Hebrew), 10 (1993), pp. 7–39.

Offer, Miriam, "Coping with the Impossible: The Developmental Roots of the Jewish Medical System in the Ghettos," in Marcin Moskalewicz, Ute Caumanns, and Fritz Dross, eds., *Jewish Medicine Health Care in Central Eastern Europe: Shared Identities, Entangled Histories*, vol. 3, (Cham: Springer International Publishing, 2019), pp. 261–277.

______, "Ethical Dilemmas in the Work of Doctors and Nurses in the Warsaw Ghetto," *Polin: Studies in Polish Jewry*, 25 (2012), pp. 467–449.

______, *Haluk Lavan Bageto: Mabat Al Korot Harefu'a Hayehudit Bepolin Bitkufat Hashoah* (Hebrew) (Jerusalem: Yad Vashem, 2015).

______, "Jewish Medical Ethics during the Holocaust: The Unwritten Ethical Code," *Wiener klinische Wochenschrift: The Central European Journal of Medicine*, 130 (2018), pp. 172–176.

______, "Ma'arach Harefu'a Begeto Varsha Bitkufat Hashoah: Irguno Ve'etgarav Hamiktzo'iyim Bithumei Harefu'a Veha'etika Beheksher Histori" (Hebrew) (PhD diss., Bar-Ilan University, 2010).

______, "Medicine in the Shavli Ghetto in Light of the Newly Discovered Diary of Dr. Aaron Pik," in M. Grodin, ed., *Jewish Medical Resistance in the Holocaust* (NewYork, Oxford: Berghahn 2014), pp. 164–172.

______, "Refu'a Verof'im Begeto Shavli Be'ikvot Hasifat Yomano Shel Harofe Aaron Pik, Reshimot Migai Hahariga: Zihronot Ktuvim Bageto Hashavlai Lita, 1942, 1943, 1944" (Hebrew) (Master's thesis, University of Haifa, 1993).

______, "Review of *Der Arzt Hermann Strauß*, 1868–1944: *Autobiographische Notizen und Aufzeichnungen aus dem Ghetto Theresienstadt*, by H. Jenss and P. Reinicke," *Social History of Medicine*, 29:4 (2016), pp. 853–855.

______, "The Study of Jewish Medicine during the Holocaust: Its Creation and Preliminary Steps," *Korot*, 22 (2013–2014), pp. 129–154.

______, "The Study of Jewish Medicine during the Holocaust: Trends and Characteristics of Development," *Korot*, 23 (2015–2016), pp. 111–147.

Ohry, Avraham, and Amihai Levi, "Leon Pinsker, Bimlot Me'a Shana Leveidat Katovitz," in Samuel Kottek, ed., *Korot: Shnaton Letoldot Harefu'a Umada'ei Hateva* (Hebrew), vol. 8, (Jerusalem: The Hebrew University Magnes Press, 1984), pp. 326–329.

______, and Karin Ohry-Kossoy, "Dedicated Physicians in the Face of Adversity: The Association of Jewish Physicians (ZLRP) and the Jewish Health Organization (TOZ) in Poland 1921–1942," *Polin: Studies in Polish Jewry*, 25 (2013), pp. 455–462.

Ostrovsky, Mania, "Zihronoteha Shel Ahot Be'irgun Oze, 1916–1917," *Korot* (Hebrew), 11 (1995), pp. 65–72.

Parnas, Zvi, "Hevrat CENTOS," in Itzhak Gruenbaum, *Entziklopediya Shel Galuyot: Varsha* (Hebrew), vol. 1, (Jerusalem and Tel Aviv: Encyclopedia of the Jewish Diaspora Co., 1953), pp. 577–581.

Penson, Jakub,"Cechy kliniczne epidemii duru plamistego w latach

1940–1941/42 w Warszawie. Badania własne nad przemianą azotową ze szczególnym uwzględnieniem nerek. Metoda wczesnego rozpoznawania," *Polski Tygodnik Lekarski*, 46–52 (1946), pp. 1,399–1,404, 1,478–1,487, 1,538–1,542, 1,553–1,569.

Perl, Gisella, *I Was a Doctor in Auschwitz* (New York: International Universities Press, 1948).

Perzikovitz, Aaron, "Begeto Kovna," in Mark Meir Dworzecki, ed., *Hama'avak Lakiyum Velabriyut Biymei Hashoah* (Hebrew) (Jerusalem: World Jewish Congress and Physicians Association and Holocaust Survivors, 1958), pp. 34–37.

Perzyńska, Zofia, "Juliusz Zweibaum": Building Memory–Building Resilience" (lecture delivered at the Third European Conference on Nazi Medicine Warsaw and Lublin, Poland, October 3–5, 2018).

Peukert, Detlev, *Inside Nazi Germany: Conformity, Opposition and Racism in Everyday Life* (New Haven: Yale University Press, 1987).

Polish Ministry of Information, *The German New Order in Poland* (London: Polish Ministry of Information and Hutchinson, 1942), pp. 227, 558–560.

Prais, Lea, *Refugees in the Fabric of Jewish Life in Warsaw, September 1939–July 1942* (Jerusalem: Yad Vashem, 2015).

______, "Sugiyot Shel Refu'a, Etika Vemusar Begeta'ot Vilna, Kovna, VeShavli," *Yalkut Moreshet* (Hebrew), 71 (2001), pp. 23–38.

Priel, Yisrael, and Eran Dolev, "Shikulim Etiyim Be'et Eru'a Rav-Nifga'im," *Harefu'a* (Hebrew), 140 (2001), pp. 574–576.

Proctor, Robert, *Racial, Hygiene, Medicine under the Nazis* (London: Harvard University Press, 1988).

Rafes, Yulian, *Doctors and Patients Doomed to Destruction: Ethical, Human, and Professional Dimensions of Jewish Doctors in the Vilna Ghetto* (Danbury: Begell House, 2001).

______, "The Ethical and Human Dimension of Jewish Medical Resistance during the Holocaust," in Michael A. Grodin, ed., *Jewish Medical Resistance in the Holocaust* (New York, Oxford: Berghahn, 2014), p. 273.

Reis, Shmuel P., and Hedy S. Wald, "Contemplating Medicine during the Third Reich: Scaffolding Professional Identity Formation for Medical Students," *Academic Medicine: Journal of the Association of American Medical Colleges*, 90:6 (June 2015), doi: 10.1097/ACM.0000000000000716.

______, Hedy S. Wald, and Paul J. Weindling, "The Holocaust, Medicine and Becoming a Physician: The Crucial Role of Education," *Israel Journal of Health Policy Research*, 8:1 (June 2019), https://doi.org/10.1186/s13584-019-0327-3.

Ringelblum, Emanuel, "Baitrogen tsu der geshikhte fun di yidishe doktoyrim in Poylen," *Sotsiale Meditsin* (Yiddish), 9–10 (1931), pp. 127–131.

______, "Di rekhtlikhe lage fun yidishe doktoyrim in Poylen," *Sotsiale Meditsin* (Yiddish), 7–8 (1936), pp. 11–12.

______, "Tsveite reshime fun yidishe doktoyrim in Poylen," *Sotsiale Meditsin* (Yiddish), 3–4 (1933), pp. 43–47.

______, "Yidishe feldsher in Amoliker Poylen," *Sotsiale Meditsin* (Yiddish), 9–10 (1932), pp. 128–130.

______, *Żydzi w Warszawie* (Warsaw: T-wo miłośników historji, 1932).

Ritvo, Roger, and Diane Plotkin, *Sisters in Sorrow: Voices of Care in the Holocaust* (Texas: A&M University Press, 1998).

Robinson, Geoffrey B., *The Killing Season: A History of the Indonesian Massacres, 1965–1966* (Princeton: Princeton University Press, 2018).

Roelcke, Volker, "Between Professional Honor and Self-Reflection: The German Medical Associations' Reluctance to Address Medical Malpractice during the National Socialist Era," in Volker Roelcke, Sascha Topp, and Etienne Lepicard, eds., *Silence, Scapegoats, Self-Reflection: The Shadow of Medical Crimes on Medicine and Bioethics* (V&R Unipress: Göttingen, 2015), pp. 243–281.

Roland, Charles Gordon, "An Underground Medical School in the Warsaw Ghetto, 1941–1942," *Medical History*, 33 (1989), pp. 399–419.

______, *Courage under Siege: Starvation, Disease and Death in the Warsaw Ghetto* (New York: Oxford University Press, 1992).

Rom (Rotbalsam), Israel, "Mahalot Hayeladim Begeto Varsha," in Mark Meir Dworzecki, ed., *Hama'avak Lakiyum Velabriyut Biymei Hashoah* (Hebrew) (Jerusalem: World Jewish Congress and Physicians Association and Holocaust Survivors, 1958), p. 14.

Rosenbaum, Irving J., *The Holocaust and Halakhah* (New York: Ktav Publishing House, 1976).

Ross (Rosenberg), Jerzy, "Tahanat Ezra Rishona Begeto Varsha," *Yalkut Moreshet* (Hebrew), 14 (1972), pp. 67–69.

Ruderman, David, *Jewish Thought and Scientific Discoveries in Early Modern Europe* (Detroit: Wayne State University, 2001).

Rudowski, Witold Janusz, "Clandestine Medical Education in Poland, 1939–1945," *American College of Surgeons Bulletin*, 78 (1993), pp. 7–13.

Rutkowski, Boleslaw, "Jakub Penson and His Studies in Acute Renal Failure during Typhus Epidemics in Warsaw Ghetto," *Journal of Nephrology*, 17 (2004), pp. 175–179.

Rybus-Potepa, Elzbieta, and Krzysztof Marczewski, "The Nephrological Issues Raised during the Clinical Sessions in the Old Order (Jewish) Hospital of Warsaw," *Nephrology Dialysis Transplantation*, 17 (2002), pp. 2,084–2,086.

Saar, Yitzhak, "Begeto Łódź," *Dapim Refu'iyim: Hama'vak Al Hakiyum Vehabriyut Bageta'ot Biymei Hakibush Hanazi* (Hebrew), edited by Mark Meir Dworzecki, 6 (1946), pp. 38–44.

Sakowska, Ruta, "Opieka nad uchodźcami I przesiedleńcami żydowskimi w Warszawie w latach okupacji hitlerowskiej," *BŻIH*, 65–66 (1968), pp. 73–74.

Sapir, Boris, "Joint," in Itzhak Gruenbaum, *Entziklopediya Shel Galuyot: Varsha* (Hebrew), vol. 1, (Jerusalem and Tel Aviv: Encyclopedia of the Jewish Diaspora Co., 1953), p. 570.

Schaller, Dominik J., and Jürgen Zimmerer, eds., *The Origins of Genocide: Raphael Lemkin as a Historian of Mass Violence* (London and New York: Routledge, 2013).

Schwoch, Rebecca, ed., Berliner Jüdische Kassenärzte und ihr Schicksal im Nationalsozialismus (Berlin: Hentrich & Hentrich Teetz, 2009).

Segev, Tom, *The Seventh Million: The Israelis and the Holocaust* (New York: Farrar, Straus, and Giroux, 1993).

Seidelman, William E., "'Requiescat sine Pace:' Recollections and Reflections on the World Medical Association, the Case of Prof. Dr. Hans Joachim Sewering and the Murder of Babette Fröwis in Volker Roelcke, Sascha Topp, and Etienne Lepicard, eds., *Silence, Scapegoats, Self-Reflection: The Shadow of Nazi Medical Crimes on Medicine and Bioethics* (Göttingen: V & R Unipress, 1996), pp. 281–301.

Shapira, Chanina Lipa, *Lo Lishkoah Velo Lisloah: Reshimot Rofe Aliya Bishnat 1949* (Hebrew) (Jerusalem: Kiryat Sefer, 1966).

Shasha, Shaul Menashe, and Saul G. Massri, "Hafakulta Lerefu'a BePadova Uvogreha Hayehudim," *Harefu'a* (Hebrew), 141:4 (2002), pp. 388–394.

Shechter, Moshe, "Simfoniya Bilti Gmura Shel Rofim Yehudim Mishnat 1942," *Harefu'a* (Hebrew), 44:9 (1953), pp. 202–205.

Shvarts, Shifra, Penina Rotem, Yitzhak Romem, and Mordechai Shani, "Masa Hagazezet Hanishkah Shel Oze–Toz, Polin," *Harefu'a* (Hebrew), 148 (2009), pp. 265–270.

Siegel, Sari, "Between Coercion and Resistance: Jewish Prisoner–Physicians in Nazi Camps, 1940–1945" (PhD diss., University of Southern California, 2018).

______, "Treating Dr. Maximilian Samuel: A Case Study of an Auschwitz Prisoner Doctor," *Holocaust and Genocide Studies* (2014).

Šimůnek, Michal V., and Antonin Kostlán, eds., *Disappeared Science: Biographical Dictionary of Jewish Scholars from Bohemia and Moravia—Victims of Nazism, 1939–1945* (Červený Kostelec: Pavel Mervart, 2013).

Spector, Shmuel, and Geoffrey Wigoder, eds., *Encyclopedia of Jewish Life before and during the Holocaust*, vol. 3, (New York: New York University Press, 2001).

Spenser, Julian Thomas, ed., *Harefu'a Vehashoah: Ma'amarim Mitoh* Harefu'a *Ve* Mihtav Lehaver, *1946–2005* (Hebrew) (Ramat Gan: Israel Medical Association, 2007).

Stabholz, Ludwik, "Hora'at Anatomiya Bamahteret" (Hebrew) (paper presented at a conference on "The Medical Faculty in the Warsaw Ghetto and Polish–Jewish Medical Collaboration in the Holocaust," Sackler Faculty of Medicine, Tel Aviv University, May 5, 2005).

Stabholz, Thaddeus, *Seven Hells* (New York: Holocust Library, 1990).

Stark, Valeria, *Ahat Mini Elef: Yomana Shel Rof'a BeBergen-Belsen* (Hebrew) (Tel Aviv: Neografica, 1951).

Statman, Daniel, *Moral Dilemmas* (Amsterdam: Rodopi, 1995).

______, ed., *Moral Luck* (Albany: State University of New York Press, 1993).

Steier, Shmuel (Tommy), "Al Matzavam Habriyuti Shel Nitzolei Hashoah: Ha'im Kayemet Tahlua Organit Meuheret?" *Israeli Journal of Family*

Practice (Hebrew), 150 (October 2009), http://www.medicalmedia.co.il/publications/ArticleDetails.aspx?artid=2503&sheetid=158 (accessed April 5, 2020).

______, "Madua Hem Shatku Shuv? Al Matzavam Hanafshi Shel Nitzolei Hashoah Vehityahasut Hahevra Vehametaplim Eleihem," *Harefu'a* (Hebrew), 149:4 (April 2009), pp. 219–223.

Steinberg, Avraham, ed., *Entziklopediya Hilhatit Refu'it* (Hebrew) (Jerusalem: Machon Shlezinger Leheker Harefu'a Al Pi Hatorah, 1988–2009).

______, ed., *Sefer Asiya: Ma'amarim, Tamtziyot Veskirot Be'inyanei Refu'a Vehalakha* (Hebrew) (Jerusalem: Reuven Mas, 1970–2009).

Sternberg, Avraham, *Behikalet Am* (Hebrew) (Tel Aviv: Hakibbutz Hameuchad, 1973).

Strous, R., "Extermination of the Jewish Mentally-Ill during the Nazi Era—The 'Doubly Cursed,' *The Israel Journal of Psychiatry and Related Sciences*, 45:4 (February 2008), pp. 247–256.

Szereszewska, Helena, *The Last Chapter: Memoirs from Occupied Warsaw, 1940–1945* (London: Vallentine Mitchell, 1997).

Tarsi, Anita, ed., *Omanut Verefu'a Begeto Terezienstat (Terezin): Rishumim Mehashanim 1942–1944* (Haifa and Givat Hayim Ihud: The Technion, The Ruth and Bruce Rappaport Faculty of Medicine, and Beit Terezín, 2001).

Thomson, David, *Europe Since Napoleon* (Middlesex: Penguin, 1970).

Trunk, Isaiah, "Epidemics and Mortality in the Warsaw Ghetto, 1939–1942," *YIVO Annual of Jewish Social Sciences*, 8 (1953), pp. 82–122.

______, *Judenrat: The Jewish Councils in Eastern Europe under Nazi Occupation* (New York: Macmillan, 1972).

Tushnet, Leonard, "Health Conditions in the Ghetto of Lodz," *Journal of the History of Medicine and Allied Sciences*, 18 (1963), pp. 64–73.

______, *The Uses of Adversity* (New York and London: Thomas Yoseloof, 1966).

Tych, Feliks, "The Legacy of Emanuel Ringelblum and the Awareness of the Holocaust," in Israel Gutman, ed., *Emanuel Ringelblum: The Man and the Historian* (Jerusalem: Yad Vashem, 2006), pp. 7–15.

Tzeder, Shulamit, *Hamar'e Hara Sheli* (Hebrew) (Megiddo: Heshvan Publishing, 2004).

Ulrich, Herbert, ed., *National Socialist Extermination Policies, 1939–1945: Contemporary German Perspectives and Controversies* (New York and Oxford: Berghahn Books, 2000).

Uzarczyk, Kamila, "'Schluss mit der Rassenschande!' From Separation to Extermination: The Fate of Jewish Mentally Ill Patients in Germany and Occupied Poland, 1939–1942," in Sabine Hildebrandt, Miriam Offer, and Michael Grodin, eds., *Recognizing the Past in the Present: New Studies on Medicine before, during, and after the Holocaust* (New York and Oxford: Berghahn Books, 2020 forthcoming).

Van den Ende, Hannah, *Vergeet niet dat je arts bent, Joodse artsen in Nederland, 1940–1945* (Amsterdam: Boom, 2015).

Von Villiez, Anna, *Mit aller Kraft verdrängt: Entrechtung und Verfolgung "nicht arischer" Ärzte in Hamburg 1933 bis 1945* (Dölling und Galitz Verlag: Hamburg, 2009).

Wein, Abraham, ed., *Pinkas Hakehillot: Entziklopediya Shel Hayishuvim Hayehudiyim Lemin Hivasdam Ve'ad Le'ahar Shoat Milhemet Ha'olam Hashniya, Polin: Varsha Vehagalil* (Hebrew), vol. 4, (Jerusalem: Yad Vashem, 1989).

Weindling, Paul Julian, "Delousing and Resistance during the Holocaust," in Michael A. Grodin, ed., *Jewish Medical Resistance in the Holocaust* (New York, Oxford: Berghahn, 2014), pp. 49–58.

______, *Epidemics and Genocide in Eastern Europe, 1890–1945* (New York: Oxford University Press, 2000).

______, *Health, Race, and German Politics between National Unification and Nazism, 1870–1945* (Cambridge: Cambridge University Press, 1989).

Weiskopf, "Beit Haholim Hayehudi BeBudapesht Tahat Hakibush Hanatzi (1944–1945)," *Harefu'a* (Hebrew), 148:1, pp. 81–84.

Weisz, George, Andrzeh Grzybowski, and William Randall Albury, "The Fate of the Warsaw Ghetto Medical Faculty," *IMAJ*, 14 (April 2012), pp. 209–213.

______, "Henryk, Thaddeus, and Ludwik Stabholz: Three Outstanding Physicians from a Jewish Medical Family in Mid-20th Century Poland," *Korot*, 21 (2011–2012), pp. 363–372.

Wenzel, Richard P., "Control of Communicable Diseases," in Robert B. Wallace, Neal Kohatsu, and John M. Last, eds., *Wallace/Maxcy-Rosenau-Last Public Health & Preventive Medicine*, 15th ed. (New York: McGraw Hill, 2008), pp. 77–79, eBook: http://alraziuni.edu.ye/book1/nursing/Public%20Health%20and%20Preventive%20Medicine,%2015th%20ed%20(2008).pdf.

Williams, Cicely D., "A Nutritional Disease of Childhood Associated with a Maize Diet," *Archives of Disease in Childhood*, 8 (1933), pp. 423–433.

______, "Kwashiorkor: A Nutritional Disease of Children Associated with A Maize Diet," *Lancet*, 2 (1935), pp. 1,151–1,152.

Winick, Miron, *Final Stamp: The Jewish Doctors in the Warsaw Ghetto* (Bloomington: Author House, 2007).

______, ed., *Hunger Disease: Studies by the Jewish Physicians in the Warsaw Ghetto* (New York: Wiley, 1979).

______, "Hunger Disease: Studies by Jewish Physicians in the Warsaw Ghetto, Their Historical Importance and their Reference Today," http://columbia.edu/cu/epic/pdf/winick_lecture.2005

______, "Jewish Medical Resistance in the Warsaw Ghetto," in Michael A. Grodin, ed., *Jewish Medical Resistance in the Holocaust* (New York, Oxford: Berghahn, 2014), pp. 93–105.

Wistrich, Robert, "Heinrich Himmler," in Israel Gutman, ed., *Encyclopedia of the Holocaust* (New York: Macmillan, 1990).

Witkowska, Agnieszka, "Anna Braude-Heller Seen from a Distance," *NASHIM: A Journal of Jewish Women's Studies & Gender Issues*, 36 (Spring 2020, forthcoming).

Wittmann, Rebecca, *Beyond Justice: The Auschwitz Trial* (Cambridge: Harvard University Press, 2005).

Wolfgang, U. Ecrart, *Medizin in der NS-Dictatur: Ideologie, Praxis, Folgen* (Köln: Böhlan, 2012).

World Health Organization, *Controlling the Spread of Infectious Diseases*, https://www.who.int/healthsystems/topics/ health-law/chapter10.pdf (accessed April 14, 2019).

Wulf, Josef, *Das Dritte Reich und seine Vollstrecker: Die Liquidation von 500,000 Juden im Ghetto Warschau* (Berlin: Arani Verlag GmbH, 1961).

Wulman, Leon, "Hevrat Toz," in Itzhak Gruenbaum, *Entziklopediya*

Shel Galuyot: Varsha (Hebrew), vol. 1, (Jerusalem and Tel Aviv: Encyclopedia of the Jewish Diaspora Co., 1953), pp. 581–587.

______, ed., *In Fight for the Health of the Jewish People: 50 Years of OSE* (New York: World Union, OSE, and the American Committee of OSE, 1968).

______, "OZE–Hesegeha Be'avar Vetohniyoteha Latkufa Shele'ahar Hamilhama" *Harofe Ha'ivri* (Hebrew), 2 (1944), pp. 85–94.

______, Józef Tenenbaum, Leopold Lazarowitz, and Szymon Małowist, *The Martyrdom of Jewish Physicians in Poland*, ed. by Louis Falstein (New York: Medical Alliance–Association of Jewish Physicians from Poland, by Exposition Express, 1963).

Yablonka, Hanna, *Survivors of the Holocaust: Israel after the War* (London: Macmillan, 1999).

Yahil, Leni, *The Holocaust: The Fate of European Jewry, 1932–1945* (New York: Oxford University Press, 1991), p. 297.

Zabłotniak, Ryszard, "Epidemia duru plamistego wśród ludności żydowskiej w Warszawie w latach II wojny światowej," *BŻIH*, 4 (1971), pp. 3–21.

______, "Wydział lekarski w getcie warszawskim," *BŻIH*, 74 (1970), pp. 81–85.

Zborowski, Mark, and Elizabeth Herzog, *Life is with People: The Jewish Little-Town in Eastern Europe* (New York: International University Press, 1953).

Zillan, M., "Hastudentim Hayehudim Bashanim, 1915–1939," in Itzhak Gruenbaum, *Entziklopediya Shel Galuyot: Varsha* (Hebrew), vol. 6, part 2, (Jerusalem and Tel Aviv: Encyclopedia of the Jewish Diaspora Co., 1959), pp. 302–303.

Zweibaum, Juliusz, "Kurs przysposobienia Sanitarnego do walki z epidemiami w getcie warszawskim w latach, 1940–1942," *Archiwum Historii I Medycyny*, 21 (1958), pp. 355–356.

Index

Page numbers in italics refer to illustrations and page numbers ending with t refer to tables.